AF616098

MPP

33

MICHAEL J. KORNSTEIN, M.D.
Associate Professor of Pathology
Medical College of Virginia
Virginia Commonwealth University
Richmond, Virginia

with a contribution from

GEORGEAN G. deBLOIS, M.D.
Pathologist, Johnston-Willis Hospital
Assistant Clinical Professor of Pathology
Medical College of Virginia
Richmond, Virginia

Pathology of the Thymus and Mediastinum

Volume 33 in the Series

MAJOR PROBLEMS IN PATHOLOGY

W.B. SAUNDERS COMPANY
A Division of Harcourt Brace & Company
PHILADELPHIA LONDON TORONTO MONTREAL SYDNEY TOKYO

W.B. SAUNDERS COMPANY
A Division of Harcourt Brace & Company

The Curtis Center
Independence Square West
Philadelphia, Pennsylvania 19106

Library of Congress Cataloging-in-Publication Data

Kornstein, Michael J.
Pathology of the thymus and mediastinum / Michael J. Kornstein; contribution from Georgean G. deBlois.—1st ed.

p. cm.

ISBN 0–7216–4337–X

1. Thymus—Diseases. 2. Mediastinum—Diseases. 3. Thymus—Cancer. I. DeBlois, Georgean G. II. Title.

[DNLM: 1. Thymus Neoplasms—pathology. 2. Thymus Gland—pathology. 3. Mediastinum—pathology. WK 400 K84p 1995]

RC663.K67 1995 616.4′3—dc20

DNLM/DLC 94-19417

PATHOLOGY OF THE THYMUS AND MEDIASTINUM ISBN 0–7216–4337–X

Printed in the United States of America.

Last digit is the print number: 9 8 7 6 5 4 3 2 1

OTHER MONOGRAPHS IN THE SERIES MAJOR PROBLEMS IN PATHOLOGY

VIRGINIA A. LIVOLSI, M.D.
Series Editor

Published

Azzopardi: *Problems in Breast Pathology*

Katzenstein and Askin: *Surgical Pathology of Non-Neoplastic Lung Disease, 2nd ed.*

Frable: *Thin-Needle Aspiration Biopsy*

Wigglesworth: *Perinatal Pathology*

Jaffe: *Surgical Pathology of the Lymph Nodes and Related Organs, 2nd ed.*

Wittels: *Surgical Pathology of Bone Marrow*

Finegold: *Pathology of Neoplasia in Children and Adolescents*

Wolf and Neiman: *Disorders of the Spleen*

Fu and Reagan: *Pathology of the Uterine Cervix, Vagina and Vulva*

LiVolsi: *Surgical Pathology of the Thyroid*

Striker, Olson, and Striker: *Interpretation of Renal Biopsy, 2nd ed.*

Virmani, Atkinson, and Fenoglio: *Cardiovascular Pathology*

Whitehead: *Mucosal Biopsy of the Gastrointestinal Tract, 4th ed.*

Mackay, Lukeman, and Ordonez: *Tumors of the Lung*

Ellis, Auclair, and Gnepp: *Surgical Pathology of the Salivary Glands*

Nash and Said: *Pathology of AIDS and HIV Infection*

Lloyd: *Surgical Pathology of the Pituitary Gland*

Henson and Albores-Saavedra: *Pathology of Incipient Neoplasia, 2nd ed.*

Taylor and Cote: *Immunomicroscopy, 2nd ed.*

Lack: *Pathology of Adrenal and Extra-Adrenal Paraganglia*

Hammond: *Solid Organ Transplantation Pathology*

Scheuer and Lefkowitch: *Liver Biopsy Interpretation, 5th ed.*

Richardson and DeGirolami: *Pathology of the Peripheral Nerve*

Forthcoming

Frable: *Fine Needle Aspiration Biopsy, 2nd ed.*

Fox, Young, and Buckley: *Pathology of the Ovary and Fallopian Tube*

Fox: *Pathology of the Placenta, 2nd ed.*

Wigglesworth: *Perinatal Pathology, 2nd ed.*

Tomazewski: *Surgical Pathology of the Urinary Bladder, Kidney and Prostate*

Laposata: *Forensic Pathology*

Albores-Saavedra, Manivel, and Henson: *Surgical Pathology of the Gallbladder, Extrahepatic Bile Ducts and Pancreas*

To my wife and best friend, Ann Kaplan,

To my daughters, Sara Ellen and Joanna Leda,

and

To my parents

Preface

The purpose of this monograph is to provide the pathologist with updated information on mediastinal disorders. Surgeons, immunologists, pulmonologists, oncologists, radiologists, and other physicians concerned with disease of the mediastinum may also find this volume useful. The Armed Forces Institute of Pathology Fascicle on Tumors of the Thymus, by Juan Rosai and Gerald D. Levine (published in 1976), did much to organize the subject of mediastinal pathology and is still widely referenced. However, basic science has advanced considerably since that time, especially with regard to immunology and the thymus gland. Consequently, we have a better understanding of many disease processes. New techniques such as immunocytochemistry and flow cytometry have also become available.

More than ever, advances in therapy necessitate accurate diagnoses. New morphologic entities have been recognized, and new histopathologic aspects of "old" diseases have been described. This monograph presents both the "new" and the "old." Where applicable, the basic science background and the use of special techniques are also discussed. Overall, the practical, clinically useful information is emphasized.

Acknowledgments

This book is an outgrowth of a course I developed with my colleague, Dr. Georgean G. deBlois, for the United States–Canadian Academy of Pathology. The material is collected from many sources but primarily from the Hospital of the University of Pennsylvania and the Medical College of Virginia. Many cases were kindly contributed by pathologists, particularly those in the Richmond area. Drs. Carolyn Thomas, Fabio Gutierrez, Willard Milby, John Summerville, Danna Johnson, George Thomas, Mark Brownell, Jane Chatten, Ron Distefano, Ralph Beck,

Harold Dunn, William Kramer, Gary Zientek, William Todd, Tita Cua-Ng, R. Condon Hughes, Steven Zimmerman, Harry Hoke, Michael Wray, Brad Siegmund, Manuel Gonzales, David Wiecking, John Herrington, and Robert Sprague have all provided cases.

My own interest in the mediastinum, and, in particular, the thymus, derives from a preoccupation with immunology. My interest was stimulated by several people, including Dr. Virginia Utermohlen of Cornell University, Dr. Russell Tomar, then of Upstate Medical Center at Syracuse, and Dr. Steven Douglas of Children's Hospital of Philadelphia. At the University of Pennsylvania, I was fortunate to work with Drs. Burton Zweiman, Robert Lisak, and Arnold Levinson, who got me "hooked" on exploring the thymus and its relationship to myasthenia gravis. I owe much to my mentors in pathology at the University of Pennsylvania, in particular Drs. John Brooks, James Wheeler, David Elder, and Virginia LiVolsi, for getting me started as a surgical pathologist.

From Drs. William Frable, Thomas Kardos, and Paul Wakely, I have been enlightened as to the potential and the challenges of cytopathology. They and others at the Medical College of Virginia, including Drs. Saul Kay, Jonathan Ben-Ezra, Alan Harris, Margaret Grimes, Janet Stastny, Melissa Contos, and Scott Mills, as well as numerous medical students, residents, and fellows, have contributed to my continuing education by sharing their opinions and cases with me. Drs. Wakely, Ben-Ezra, and Grimes also provided me with slides and photographs. Drs. Shigeo Nakamura, Bruce Burns, and Saul Suster have given me glass slides of unusual cases. For my clinical education, particularly on lymphomas, I thank Dr. Saul Yanovich and other members of the Hematology/Oncology division at Medical College of Virginia. I thank Dr. James W. Brooks not only for sending the surgical specimens but also for providing me with the clinical information so critical to clinicopathologic studies.

I acknowledge Judith Luck, Renee Workman, Tracey Mines, Amy Perkins, and Frances Freund for their expert work in microtomy and immunohistochemistry. Virgil Mumaw and Michelle Allen provided photographic assistance. Rhonda Jackson helped with word processing. I thank Phillip Mattes for artwork and the staff of the Tompkins-McCaw Library for their assistance. The editors and staff of W.B. Saunders have been courteous and professional. Most of all, I am grateful to my wife, Ann, and daughters, Sara and Joanna, for their loving support and encouragement.

MICHAEL J. KORNSTEIN, M.D.

Contents

Chapter 1
INTRODUCTION 1
Chapter 2
THE THYMUS: HISTORICAL OVERVIEW 8
Chapter 3
THE NORMAL THYMUS 14
Chapter 4
NON-NEOPLASTIC PATHOLOGY OF THE THYMUS 34
Chapter 5
TUMORS OF THE THYMIC EPITHELIAL CELL 67
Chapter 6
LYMPHOMAS (INCLUDING HODGKIN'S DISEASE)
AND OTHER HEMATOLOGIC LESIONS 114
Chapter 7
METASTASES 158
Chapter 8
INFECTIOUS AND INFLAMMATORY CONDITIONS 164
Chapter 9
GERM CELL TUMORS 172
Chapter 10
NEUROENDOCRINE TUMORS: CARCINOID
AND PARAGANGLIOMA 191
Chapter 11
TUMORS OF NEURAL ORIGIN 201
Chapter 12
MEDIASTINAL CYSTS 210
Chapter 13
PLEURAL TUMORS 217
Chapter 14
MISCELLANEOUS LESIONS 223

APPENDIX: NOMENCLATURE FOR LEUKOCYTE
SURFACE ANTIGENS 231

INDEX 235

Chapter

1

INTRODUCTION

OVERVIEW
ANATOMY OF THE MEDIASTINUM
IMAGING
ACCESS TO THE MEDIASTINUM
Fine-needle Aspiration
Mediastinoscopy
Thoracotomy

OVERVIEW

The mediastinum is a confined space between the pleurae and contains diverse structures that give rise to a wide variety of lesions. The thymus is the organ of the anterior-superior mediastinum. Now recognized as a lymphoepithelial structure critical for the development of cell-mediated immunity, the thymus can be affected by, and contribute to, immunologic disorders. It can also be involved by neoplastic processes, usually of a lymphoid or epithelial nature. The thymus is the subject of an extensive medical literature with considerable controversy. Lymph nodes are present throughout the mediastinum. Lesions of lymph nodes account for a major portion of mediastinal pathology. The posterior mediastinum contains the vagus nerves and sympathetic chains. Neurogenic tumors are the most common neoplasm of this area. The heart occupies the middle mediastinum. Cardiovascular pathology is clearly a major subject unto itself and is therefore not included in this volume.

The mediastinal lesions most commonly encountered by the surgical pathologist are neoplasms and cysts. In a literature review encompassing 2399 patients, Davis and colleagues tabulated the frequencies of the various primary mediastinal tumors and cysts[1] (Table 1–1). Neurogenic tumors (usually ganglioneuroma, neurilemoma, or neurofibroma), cysts, and thymomas each account for approximately 20% of cases. Lymphomas and germ cell tumors each account for about 10%. Mesenchymal tumors, endocrine lesions, and primary carcinomas account for the remainder.

Among children, about 40% of cases are neurogenic tumors (usually neuroblastoma or ganglioneuroma).[2–4] Lymphomas, cysts, and germ cell tumors make up most of the remainder. Some variation occurs among the different series. Nevertheless, the major causes of a mediastinal mass are invariable and consist of neurogenic tumors, cysts, thymomas, lymphomas, and germ cell tumors. Mesenchymal tumors, primary carcinomas, and endocrine lesions are less common. Davis and colleagues also tabulated their data by location within the mediastinum[1] (Table 1–2). Thus, thymomas

Table 1–1. Primary Mediastinal Masses

Lesion	Reference and Patient Population Studied	
	Davis[1]: Adults and Children (Literature Review)	*Bower[3]: Children (< 16 yr)*
Neurogenic tumor	21%	42%
Thymoma	19%	0
Cysts	18%	24% (including duplications)
Lymphoma	13%	14%
Germ cell tumors	10%	5%
Endocrine tumors	6%	0
Mesenchymal tumors	6%	4%
Primary carcinoma	5%	0
Miscellaneous	2%	11%

Table 1–2. Distribution of Mediastinal Neoplasms[1]

	Anterior-Superior (215 Cases, or 54% of Total)	**Middle (82 Cases, or 20% of Total)**	**Posterior (103 Cases, or 24% of Total)**
Thymic neoplasms	30%	0	0
Lymphomas	20%	21%	20%
Germ cell tumors	18%	0	0
Carcinoma	13%	7%	0
Cysts	7%	60%	34%
Mesenchymal tumors	5%	9%	9%
Endocrine tumors	5%	0	2%
Neurogenic tumors	0	0	53%
Miscellaneous	2%	3%	2%
Total	100%	100%	100%

were most common in the anterior-superior mediastinum, cysts most common in the middle mediastinum, and neurogenic tumors most common in the posterior mediastinum.

Asymptomatic patients account for approximately 40% of cases and are more likely to have benign lesions than are symptomatic patients.[2, 4] In one series, 83% of patients who were asymptomatic had a benign lesion, versus 43% of symptomatic individuals.[1] Symptoms most often relate to the location of the mass and include chest pain, cough, dyspnea, recurrent respiratory infections, and dysphagia. Superior vena cava syndrome, vocal cord paralysis, Horner's syndrome, and spinal cord compression may occur. A lesion adjacent to the heart may impair cardiac performance and simulate primary heart disease. Systemic symptoms may relate to excess hormone production from endocrine tumors, leading to hypercalcemia, hypertension, Cushing's disease, or hyperthyroidism. Lymphomas, including Hodgkin's disease, are often associated with fevers. Opsomyoclonus may be associated with neuroblastoma.

ANATOMY OF THE MEDIASTINUM

The mediastinum is defined as the region in the thorax between the two pleural cavities (Fig. 1–1). It is bounded laterally by the parietal pleurae of the two lungs, anteriorly by the sternum, and posteriorly by the vertebral column. The mediastinum extends from the thoracic inlet to the diaphragm. It is divided into several compartments for descriptive purposes (Fig. 1–2). According to one scheme, the me-

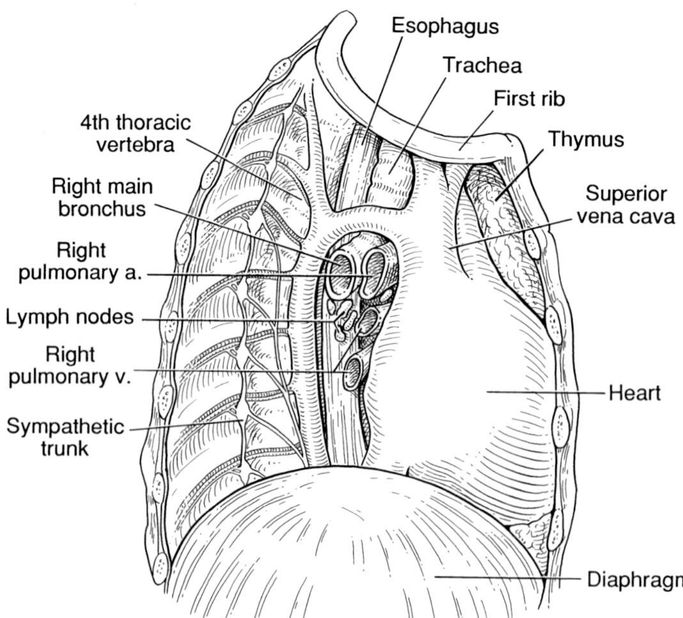

Figure 1–1. Line drawing of mediastinum from the right side demonstrates relationships of major structures (vertebrae, trachea, esophagus, heart, thymus).

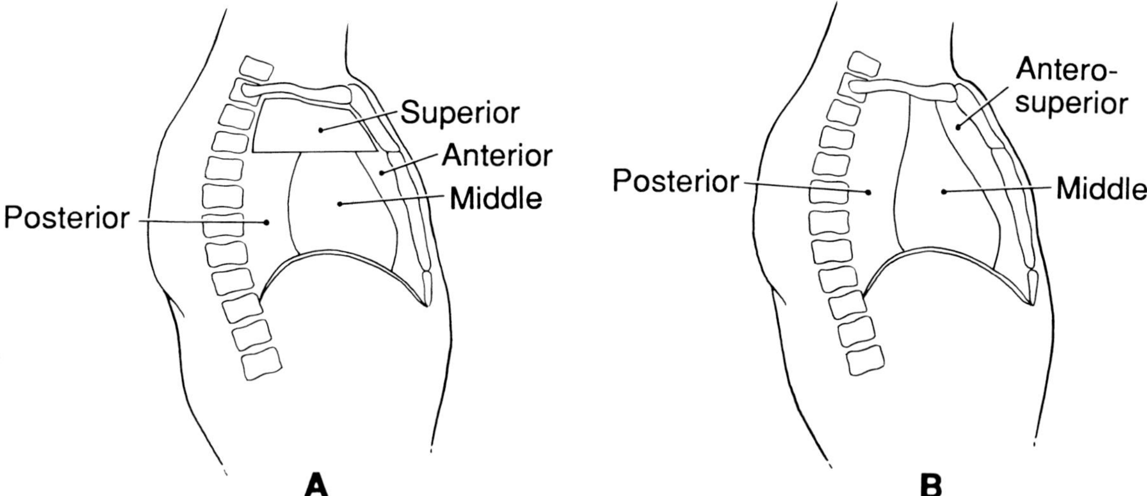

Figure 1–2. Line drawing illustrates division of mediastinum into four compartments *(A)* and three compartments *(B)*.

diastinum is divided into superior, anterior, middle, and posterior compartments. The superior mediastinum is that portion cranial to the horizontal plane extending from the lower aspect of the manubrium of the sternum to the lower border of the T4 vertebral body.[5–7] This dividing line is important anatomically because of the many structures that begin, end, or curve at this location. For example, the tracheal bifurcation and aortic arch are at this level. The superior mediastinum contains the retrosternal structures (thymus, great veins), the aortic arch with its main branches, the vagus and phrenic nerves, and the prevertebral structures (trachea, esophagus, left recurrent laryngeal nerve, thoracic duct).

The middle mediastinum contains the pericardium, heart, roots of the great vessels, phrenic nerves, tracheal bifurcation, bronchi, and hila of the lungs.[7] The mediastinum is divided into anterior and posterior portions by the pericardium.[7] According to this system, the anterior mediastinum is a small area in front of the pericardium between the pleurae. Only fat and lymph nodes are in this location. The posterior mediastinum contains the descending aorta, thoracic duct, azygos and hemiazygos veins, esophagus, vagus nerves, intercostal arteries and veins, thoracic duct, and paraspinal region.[5, 6, 8]

In a simpler scheme, the mediastinum is divided into only three parts: the anterior (or anterosuperior), middle, and posterior compartments.[9] For most purposes, this is adequate. The anterior compartment includes the thymus. The middle mediastinum includes the heart and trachea. The posterior mediastinum includes the esophagus and paravertebral area. Various other modifications to these divisions have been introduced particularly to aid in the interpretation of radiographs.[6, 9]

Lymph nodes are located throughout the mediastinum. A systematic anatomic study of the mediastinum at autopsy reported an average of 64 mediastinal nodes, of which 50 were associated with the mainstem bronchi and trachea.[10] Eleven were associated with the aorta or esophagus. The remaining three were in the anterior mediastinum. "Normal" nodes rarely exceed 2 cm in any dimension.[6]

Mediastinal nodes can be grouped in various ways based on location and drainage patterns.[6, 11] The simplest scheme includes three groups: anterior mediastinal, posterior mediastinal, and tracheobronchial (Table 1–3). There is no agreement as to exactly which nodes are hilar. According to some, this term should be applied only to nodes at the major bronchial bifurcations. Other authors include nodes more peripheral in the lung.[6] In the TNM International Staging System for lung cancer, peribronchial and ipsilateral hilar nodes are termed N_1 nodes. N_2 nodes are superior mediastinal (paratracheal), para-aortic and subaortic, and inferior mediastinal (subcarinal, paraesophageal, pulmonary ligament).[12]

IMAGING

Most mediastinal tumors can be detected on routine chest radiographs.[6, 13, 14] Additional im-

Table 1–3. Intrathoracic Lymph Nodes[6, 11]

Location	Drain From	Drain To
Anterior mediastinal Internal mammary Cardiophrenic angle Brachiocephalic	Thymus, pericardium	Tracheobronchial nodes, bronchomediastinal trunks to internal jugular/subclavian veins
Posterior mediastinal	Esophagus, pericardium, diaphragm, liver	Thoracic duct, tracheobronchial nodes
Tracheobronchial* Tracheal Bronchial Bronchopulmonary Pulmonary	Thymus, lungs, bronchi, trachea, heart, posterior mediastinum	Bronchomediastinal trunks

*Tracheobronchial nodes include four main groups: *tracheal*—on either side of the trachea; *bronchial*—in angles between trachea and bronchi and in angle between bronchi; *bronchopulmonary*—in the hilum of each lung; *pulmonary*—in the lung parenchyma.

aging techniques, including computed tomography (CT), ultrasonography, angiography, and magnetic resonance imaging (MRI), can add information regarding the precise location of the lesion within the mediastinum and its vascularity. With CT, small tumors that are not apparent on chest radiographs can be identified. Thus, patients with myasthenia gravis (who are at increased risk of having a thymoma) may benefit from CT, even if the chest radiograph is unremarkable.[14–17] Intravenous contrast aids in distinguishing mediastinal vessels from adenopathy by CT. With oral contrast, the esophagus can be well demarcated.[13] Another advantage of CT over chest radiography is its ability to detect multiple densities in the mediastinum and lungs.[18] This finding would make the diagnosis of thymoma less likely. Also, CT may detect unsuspected axillary lymphadenopathy that would raise the possibility of lymphoma in a patient with a mediastinal mass.[18]

Ultrasonography has had more limited application to the mediastinum.[13] Its advantages include (1) the ability to distinguish solid from cystic structures, (2) the ability to define masses close to the diaphragm, (3) low cost, and (4) low risk. Ultrasound waves do not transmit well through bone or lung; thus, mediastinal applications are restricted. Nevertheless, easy visualization of the biopsy needle and "real time" imaging have led some groups to prefer ultrasonography over CT and fluoroscopy for biopsy of ultrasonically detectable masses.[19, 20]

MRI is based on the magnetic properties of nuclei and is the newest imaging modality.[13, 21–24] Vascular anatomy is particularly well visualized because of the lack of any signal from circulating blood.[21] Prominent vessels are thus differentiated from lymphadenopathy without the use of contrast agents. Another advantage of MRI over CT is its ability to produce images in the coronal and sagittal planes. This permits better visualization of structures such as the trachea, vena cava, and descending aorta.[21] The thymus is better defined by MRI than by CT.[21, 24] Yet, according to a 1988 study, MRI was no better than CT in detecting thymic tumors not apparent on chest radiographs.[25]

ACCESS TO THE MEDIASTINUM

Access to the mediastinum may be required to obtain tissue for diagnosis and/or to resect or debulk a lesion.

Fine-Needle Aspiration

Fine-needle aspiration (FNA) biopsy of the mediastinum is becoming increasingly popular.[26–30] Percutaneously, a spinal needle (gauges from 18 to 25 have been used; 20 gauge or smaller is preferred[31]) is guided into the area of interest under fluoroscopy, CT, or ultrasonography. Once the needle is properly positioned, the stylet is partially withdrawn. The needle is rotated and moved up and down in short jerky motions. The stylet is then removed while the patient holds his breath. Suction is applied using a 50-ml syringe attached to the needle while the jerky motions are continued. The needle is withdrawn and its contents are smeared on slides. Air-dried slides are stained with a modified Wright's preparation, whereas alcohol-fixed smears are used for the Papanicolaou stain. Any tissue fragments are processed using standard histologic techniques. If a "cutting'' needle is used, a core of tissue can be obtained, which is processed as a surgical biopsy. Transbronchial FNA biopsy has been advocated particularly for sampling mediastinal lymph nodes in staging bronchogenic carcinoma.[32]

FNA of the mediastinum can be performed as an outpatient procedure. It is simple, quick, and safe. Diagnostic accuracy of mediastinal aspirates is not as well established as for pulmonary aspirates. Nevertheless, several small studies have reported that the correct diagnosis of a mediastinal lesion can be made by FNA in 60 to 80% of cases.[21, 26, 29, 30] One should be particularly cautious when confronted with an aspirate containing bland-appearing epithelial cells admixed with small lymphocytes. This appearance is found not only with lymphocytic thymoma but also with normal thymus, true thymic hyperplasia, and inflammation of the thymus. FitzGerald and colleagues report a case of tuberculosis of the thymus that simulated a thymoma on FNA.[33] An aspirate of normal or hyperplastic thymus is easily misinterpreted as a thymoma. Careful clinical and radiographic correlation should minimize such errors. Aspiration cytology may also be useful in the diagnosis of metastatic thymoma.[34]

FNA is indicated for diagnosis when surgical procedures are contraindicated, whether for medical reasons, because of unresectability, or because of widespread metastatic disease.[29] Another indication is to ''streamline'' the work-up. Results can be available within hours. The surgeon can better plan the surgical procedure and discuss the results with the patient. FNA can also be used to diagnose small cell carcinoma and lymphoblastic lymphoma,[35] which may not need surgical treatment. In selected cases, a benign diagnosis such as a mediastinal cyst can be established by FNA. The patient can then be followed rather than subjected to a surgical procedure.[36]

There are few contraindications to FNA.[29] The only absolute contraindications would be a patient who could not stop moving or coughing and a suspected hydatid cyst. The latter generally should not be aspirated for fear of spreading the disease. Other contraindications are relative ones. These include pulmonary arterial hypertension, advanced emphysema, suspected vascular lesions, and bleeding disorders.

Potential complications include pneumothorax, transient hemoptysis, air embolism, pneumomediastinum, and hemopericardium. However, most of these problems occur after FNA of intrapulmonary, rather than mediastinal, lesions and are either preventable or easily managed with proper techniques. Pneumothorax is the most common complication and occurs in approximately 20% of cases. Only about 25% of pneumothoraces are severe enough to require chest tube insertion for drainage.[29, 30]

The risk of local tumor spread is considered negligible when a fine needle (rather than large-bore needle) is used. Distant dissemination of tumor cells by lymphatics or small veins is a theoretical possibility; however, studies have shown no evidence of decreased survival in cancer patients who have undergone an FNA biopsy.[29]

Mediastinoscopy

Mediastinoscopy is most often used for staging bronchogenic carcinoma but is also useful in evaluating primary mediastinal disease.[37] Developed in the 1950s by Carlens, transcervical mediastinoscopy allows the surgeon to explore the superior mediastinum.[38, 39] A small transverse incision is made 1 cm above the suprasternal notch and carried down to the pretracheal muscles. These muscles are separated vertically in the midline to reach the pretracheal fascia. The fascia is incised transversely. It is then dissected off the trachea to create a ''tunnel'' into the mediastinum. The ''tunnel'' is enlarged by finger dissection, and a mediastinoscope is inserted. Paratracheal, subcarinal, and tracheobronchial lymph nodes can then be biopsied. ''Formal'' mediastinoscopy follows the plane of dissection of the trachea and therefore provides poor access to the anterior mediastinum.[40] However, modifications have been made for a more anterior approach, and some surgeons have reported good results in obtaining tissue for the diagnosis of anterior mediastinal tumors.[38]

In experienced hands, mediastinoscopy is a safe procedure. Among 2259 patients in two published series, the complication rate was 2%.[39] Fifteen percent of the complications (six patients) were considered life-threatening (hemorrhage, tracheal injury, and esophageal injury). Other complications included nerve palsy and pneumothorax. Rare cases of tumor seeding of the mediastinoscopy tract have been described.[41]

Mediastinoscopy is indicated in the evaluation of a primary mediastinal tumor in order to obtain a diagnosis. If a diagnosis of lymphoma (including Hodgkin's disease) is established, a thoracotomy may be unnecessary.[9, 38] In most cases, lymphomas are treated with chemotherapy and/or radiation; surgical excision is usually not indicated.

A transcervical approach can also be used in performing a thymectomy.[40, 42] This procedure has been used for thymectomy in myasthenia gravis patients. In some series, even thymomas have been removed transcervically. Compared with a median sternotomy, transcervical thymectomy has the advantage of a painless postoperative course and a small scar. The problems include risk of hemorrhage and pneumothorax and the possibility of leaving portions of thymus in the patient.

Advances in endoscopic surgical instruments have expanded the role of *thoracoscopy*. Landreneau and colleagues performed a complete, thoracoscopic resection of an encapsulated thymoma that was 5 cm in diameter.[43] Mediastinal cysts and a neurogenic tumor have also been resected in this manner.[44–46]

Thoracotomy

Thoracotomy allows for wider exposure of the mediastinum and is the procedure of choice for excising any mediastinal tumor. Two approaches are used. The lateral thoracotomy involves a skin excision from the posterior axillary line to the nipple line. This approach is optimal for laterally growing tumors. The median sternotomy provides bilateral access to the mediastinum. The exact procedure is variable. In one approach, the skin incision is T-shaped with the horizontal portion overlying the second costal cartilage. The vertical incision extends from the lower manubrium to the lower third of the sternum. The sternum is partially sectioned vertically to obtain access to the mediastinum.[42]

Complication rates for thoracotomy up to 15% are reported, with operative mortality rates of 3 to 10%.[47] As expected, bleeding and infections are the most common complications. In particular, mediastinitis is a major infectious complication of median sternotomy.[48]

Summary

The mediastinum may be affected by a wide variety of pathologic processes. The most common mass lesions are neurogenic tumors, cysts, thymomas, lymphomas, and germ cell tumors. Nearly half of patients are asymptomatic at the time of diagnosis. When present, symptoms usually relate to the location of the mass. Anatomically, the mediastinum can be divided into compartments. Thymoma is the most common neoplasm of the anterior mediastinum. Lymphomas are the most common tumor of the middle mediastinum. In the posterior mediastinum, neurogenic tumors are most common. Tumors can be detected by various imaging techniques, including routine chest radiographs, CT, ultrasonography, and MRI. FNA and mediastinoscopy are useful diagnostic techniques. Thoracoscopy and thoracotomy can be used to biopsy or excise mass lesions.

REFERENCES

1. Davis RD Jr, Oldham HN Jr, Sabiston DC Jr. Primary cysts and neoplasms of the mediastinum: recent changes in clinical presentation, methods of diagnosis, management, and results. Ann Thorac Surg 1987; 44:229–237.
2. Silverman NA, Sabiston DC Jr. Mediastinal masses. Surg Clin North Am 1980; 60:757–777.
3. Bower RJ, Liesewetter WB. Mediastinal masses in infants and children. Arch Surg 1977; 112:1003–1009.
4. Blegvad S, Lippert H, Simper LB, Dybdahl H. Mediastinal tumours. A report of 129 cases. Scand J Thorac Cardiovasc Surg 1990; 24:39–42.
5. Belfast School of Radiography. The anatomy of the mediastinum. Radiography 1971; 37:39–42.
6. Heitzman ER. The Mediastinum: Radiologic Correlations with Anatomy and Pathology. Saint Louis: CV Mosby, 1977:1–42.
7. Williams PL, Warwick R. Gray's Anatomy, 36th edition. Philadelphia: WB Saunders, 1980:1251–1252.
8. Shields TW, Reynolds M. Neurogenic tumors of the thorax. Surg Clin North Am 1988; 68:645–668.
9. Rosenberg JC. Neoplasms of the mediastinum. *In* DeVita VT Jr, Hellman S, Rosenberg SA, eds. Cancer: Principles and Practice of Oncology. Philadelphia: JB Lippincott, 1989:706–724.
10. Beck E, Beattie EJ Jr. The lymph nodes in the mediastinum. J Int Coll Surg 1958; 29:247–251.
11. Williams PL, Warwick R. Gray's Anatomy, 36th edition. Philadelphia: WB Saunders, 1980:799–800.
12. Mackay B, Lukeman JM, Ordonez NG. Structure and function of the respiratory tissues. *In* Tumors of the Lung. Philadelphia: WB Saunders, 1991:1–20.
13. Aronberg DJ, Evens RG. Radiologic evaluation of the mediastinum. Curr Probl Diagn Radiol 1985; 14:1–35.
14. Batra P, Brown K, Steckel R. Diagnostic imaging techniques in mediastinal malignancies. Am J Surg 1988; 156:4–10.
15. Rivner MH, Swift TR. Thymoma: diagnosis and management. Semin Neurol 1990; 10:83–88.
16. Hale DA, Cohen AJ, Schaefer P, Jordan D, Thompson LD, Bellamy RF, Edwards FH, Barry MJ. Computerized tomography in the evaluation of myasthenia gravis. South Med J 1990; 83:414–416.

17. Moore AV, Korobkin M, Powers B, Olanow W, Ravin CE, Putman CE, Breiman RS, Ram PC. Thymoma detection by mediastinal CT: patients with myasthenia gravis. AJR 1992; 138:217–222.
18. Rebner M, Gross BH, Robertson JM, Pennes DR, Spizarny DL, Glazer GM. CT evaluation of mediastinal masses. Comput Radiol 1987; 11:103–110.
19. Yang P-C, Lee YC, Yu C-J, Chang D-B, Wu H-D, Lee L-N, Kuo S-H, Luh K-T. Ultrasonographically guided biopsy of thoracic tumors: a comparison of large-bore cutting biopsy with fine-needle aspiration. Cancer 1992; 69:2553–2560.
20. Saito T, Kobayashi H, Sugama Y, Tamaki S, Kawai T, Kitamura S. Ultrasonically guided needle biopsy in the diagnosis of mediastinal masses. Am Rev Respir Dis 1988; 138:679–684.
21. Jereb M, Us-Krasovec M. Transthoracic needle biopsy of mediastinal and hilar lesions. Cancer 1977; 40:1354–1357.
22. Swensen SJ, Ehman RL, Brown LR. Magnetic resonance imaging of the thorax. J Thorac Imag 1990; 4:19–33.
23. Bisset GS. Pediatric thoracic applications of magnetic resonance imaging. J Thorac Imag 1989; 4:51–57.
24. Molina PL, Siegel MJ, Glazer HS. Thymic masses on MR imaging. AJR 1990; 155:495–500.
25. Emskotter T, Trampe H, Lachenmayer L. Magnetic resonance imaging in myasthenia gravis. An alternative to mediastinal computerized tomography. Dtsch Med Wochenschr 1988; 113:1508–1510.
26. Adler OB, Rosenberger A, Peleg H. Fine-needle aspiration biopsy of mediastinal masses: evaluation of 136 experiences. AJR 1983; 140:893–896.
27. Tao L-C. Introduction. *In* Guides to Clinical Aspiration Biopsy: Lung, Pleura, and Mediastinum. New York: Igaku-Shoin, 1988:2–10.
28. Tao L-C. Primary mass lesions of the mediastinum. *In* Guides to Clinical Aspiration Biopsy: Lung, Pleura, and Mediastinum. New York: Igaku-Shoin, 1988:273–328.
29. Weisbrod GL. Percutaneous fine-needle aspiration biopsy of the mediastinum. Clin Chest Med 1987; 8:27–41.
30. Linder J, Olsen GA, Johnston WW. Fine-needle aspiration biopsy of the mediastinum. Am J Med 1986; 81:1005–1008.
31. Westcott JL. Needle aspiration biopsy of pulmonary, hilar, and mediastinal masses. Clin Chest Med 1984; 5:365–377.
32. Baker JJ, Solanki PH, Schenk DA, Van Pelt C, Ramzy I. Transbronchial fine needle aspiration of the mediastinum. Importance of lymphocytes as an indicator of specimen adequacy. Acta Cytol 1990; 34:517–523.
33. FitzGerald JM, Mayo JR, Miller RR, Jamieson WRE, Baumgartner F. Tuberculosis of the thymus. Chest 1992; 102:1604–1605.
34. Hoda SA, Warren GP, Zaman MB. Extrathoracic metastatic malignant thymoma. Diagnosis by aspiration cytology. Arch Pathol Lab Med 1991; 115:399–401.
35. Kardos TF, Maygarden SM, Blumberg AK, Wakely PE Jr, Frable WJ. Fine needle aspiration biopsy in the management of children and young adults with peripheral lymphadenopathy. Cancer 1989; 63:703–707.
36. Nath PH, Sanders C, Holley HC, McElvein RB. Percutaneous fine needle aspiration in the diagnosis and management of mediastinal cysts in adults. South Med J 1988; 81:1225–1228.
37. Puhakka HJ, Lippo K, Tala E. Mediastinoscopy in relation to clinical evaluation. Scand J Thorac Cardiovasc Surg 1990; 24:43–45.
38. Sarrazin R. Surgical approach of thymic tumors. *In* Sarrazin R, Vrousos C, Vincent F, eds. Thymic Tumors. Basel: Karger, 1989:25–33.
39. Ginsberg RJ. Evaluation of the mediastinum by invasive techniques. Surg Clin North Am 1987; 67:1025–1035.
40. Clarke DB. Technical aspects of thymectomy. *In* Givel J-C, ed. Surgery of the Thymus. Berlin: Springer-Verlag, 1990:255–263.
41. Hoyer ER, Leonard CE, Hazuka MB, Wechsler-Jentzsch K. Mediastinoscopy incisional metastasis: a radiotherapeutic approach. Cancer 1992; 70:1612–1615.
42. Merlini M, Clarke DB. Surgical approaches. *In* Givel J-C, ed. Surgery of the Thymus. Berlin: Springer-Verlag, 1990:247–253.
43. Landreneau RJ, Dowling RD, Castillo WM, Ferson PF. Thoracoscopic resection of an anterior mediastinal tumor. Ann Thorac Surg 1992; 54:142–144.
44. Landreneau RJ, Dowling RD, Ferson PF. Thoracoscopic resection of a posterior mediastinal neurogenic tumor. Chest 1992; 102:1288–1290.
45. Lewis RJ, Caccavale RJ, Sissler GE. Imaged thoracoscopic surgery: a new thoracic technique for resection of mediastinal cysts. Ann Thorac Surg 1992; 53:318–320.
46. Naunheim KS, Andrus CH. Thoracoscopic drainage and resection of giant mediastinal cyst. Ann Thorac Surg 1993; 55:156–158.
47. Neef H. The role of surgery in diagnosis and treatment of mediastinal malignancies. Lung 1990; 168(Suppl):1153–1161.
48. Grossi EA, Culliford AT, Kreiger KH, Kloth D, Press R, Baumann FG, Spencer FC. A survey of 77 major infectious complications of median sternotomy: a review of 7949 consecutive operative procedures. Ann Thorac Surg 1985; 40:214–222.

Chapter

2

THE THYMUS: HISTORICAL OVERVIEW

ETYMOLOGY
FUNCTION
ANATOMY AND HISTOLOGY
STATUS THYMICOLYMPHATICUS
MYASTHENIA GRAVIS

The thymus has puzzled investigators for thousands of years. Many controversies have been generated; some of them remain unsolved to this day. The history of man's investigation of the thymus is not readily available in the medical literature; yet the numerous "wrong alleys" that were taken illustrate how medical knowledge advances.

ETYMOLOGY

The etymology of the word "thymus" is uncertain. One theory is that the thymus was so named because of its resemblance to the thyme plant[1–3] (Fig. 2–1). Similarly, venereal warts were named "thymia" because of their resemblance to thyme.[1] A member of the mint family, thyme was well known to the early Greeks, who burned it as incense in religious ceremonies. Therefore, the word "thyme" derives from the Greek *thymos,* meaning "soul, spirit, incense, or sacrifice."[1–3]

Another etymologic theory concerns the early anatomists' belief that the thymus was the location of the soul. Thus, "thymus" may derive directly from the Greek word for soul.[1] According to Crotti, Galen regarded the thymus as the "center of courage and affection."[3] Therefore, the word thymus may derive from the Greek word for "courage," which is also the word for "heart." Another possibility is that early anatomists recognized the close physical relationship between the thymus and the heart, and thereby devised the word "thymus."[4] The first theory (related to the thyme plant) is generally favored.[1, 2]

The first description of the thymus gland ("a soft mass with a white secretion") may be the one found in one of the earliest written medical documents, the Ebers papyrus (1550

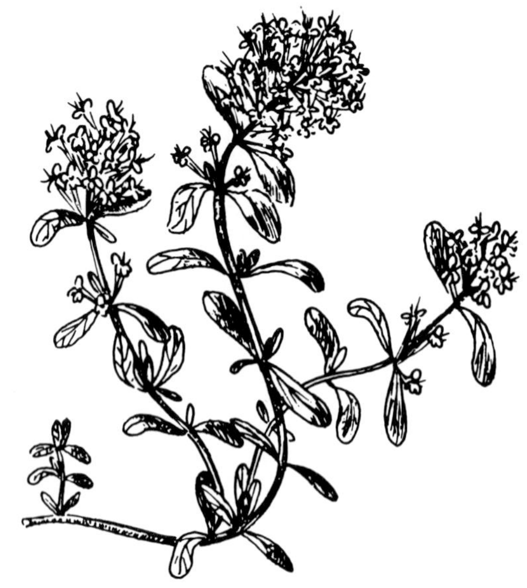

Figure 2–1. *Thymus serpyllum* (wild, or creeping, thyme). (From Gabriel I. Herb Identifier and Handbook, New York: Sterling; 1974:221; adapted from the German version, Wiesbaden: Falken-Verlag, 1970, reprinted with permission of Falken-Verlag.)

B.C.E.),[5] The reference, however, is obscure, and it is not clear exactly what is being alluded to.

The first known written use of the word thymus was by the Greek physician Rufus of Ephesus.[1,6] Rufus was the "great link" between Hippocrates (460–375 B.C.E.), whose extant writings never mention the thymus, and Galen (130–200 C.E.), the noted Greek physician of Rome. Although Galen is frequently credited with naming the thymus,[3,7] Rufus uses the word before Galen was born.[6] Rufus' anatomic knowledge derived from the dissection of monkeys. Interestingly, in other works, Rufus describes the medicinal uses of herbs. Thyme is recommended as part of concoctions for treating diverse ailments, including arthritis, melancholy, and jaundice.[8] Besides his contributions to nomenclature, Rufus is credited with describing bubonic plague.

FUNCTION

The function of the thymus has been debated since the time of Galen. Galen believed the thymus functioned as a cushion:

> For nature has spread this very large and also very soft gland [the thymus] beneath the . . . sternum, so that the bone itself may not come in contact with the vena cava . . .[9]

He claimed that the thymus supported the vena cava and its "many ramifications" in this region. Indeed, wherever a suspended vessel branches, "[Nature] places a gland to fill up the space at the junction."[9] Galen also recognized that the thymus is large in newborn animals and becomes smaller with age.[2,10]

Apparently, little was written about the thymus for the next 1400 years or so. Vesalius is credited with the first printed sketch of the thymus in 1543,[2] and Platter described death from an enlarged thymus in 1614 (see "Status Thymicolymphaticus"). Later in the seventeenth century, investigators again began to speculate on the function of the thymus. Its prominent location next to the heart and its large size in the neonatal period suggested that the thymus had an important purpose. In 1650, Glisson wrote that the thymus served as a source of nutrition for the fetus. He related an abnormal thymus to the development of rickets.[2] In 1706, Bidloo believed that the thymus prevented expansion of the lungs before birth.[2] Others considered the thymus to be a receptacle for chyme or a producer of milk as a supplement to breast milk.[3] These beliefs stemmed from the finding that cutting the thymus produces a white fluid.

In the late 1700s, Hewson described the human lymphatic system and suggested that the thymus is an accessory to the lymph glands. He thought that the thymus acted as "an auxiliary to the lymphatic system for the purpose of forming more of the central particles [i.e., lymphocytes] of the blood" for which there are a greater need in the fetus and newborn.[11] This would account for the larger size of the thymus in early life. If the thymus was important, then removing it should have serious consequences. A debate on the "essentiality" of the thymus stirred considerable interest.[2,3] In 1845, Restelli surgically removed the thymus gland from 72 sheep, 23 dogs, and 3 calves. None survived more than a few weeks. Therefore, Restelli claimed, the gland was essential to life. Friedleben performed thymectomies on goats and dogs without any loss of life for months after surgery. He did find slowed growth and loss of stamina when very young puppies were thymectomized.

In the following years, many sheep, dogs, rabbits, frogs, chicks, guinea pigs, rats, mice, and other animals were subjected to thymectomy to determine whether the thymus was essential for life. The net result depended on what species was studied and when the thymectomy was performed. Some animals developed a fatal wasting syndrome if thymectomized in the neonatal period. In other species, neonatal thymectomy had no apparent effect. Some animals developed rickets. Undoubtedly, the high perioperative mortality rate, as in the Restelli study, was related to causes (such as infection) other than the loss of the thymus. Similarly, rickets most likely resulted from nutritional deprivations unrelated to the thymectomy.[12]

Another method of investigating thymic function was to feed the organ to various animals and observe its effects.[2,3] Conflicting results were obtained. Some reported that the thymus stimulated the rate of growth in frogs and rats but delayed their sexual maturation. Others found no effect. In an article in the *Journal of the American Medical Association* in 1900, Solis-Cohen described the therapeutic value of ingesting the thymus gland.[13] Several commercial oral preparations of desiccated lamb or calf thymus were available for "affectations of metabolism," such as Graves' disease. The reasons for these therapeutic effects were unclear, but the effects were ascribed by some to the nutritional value of the thymus rather than to any association with its function.

For many years, investigators debated whether the thymus is an endocrine organ.[14] In 1776, Haller wrote that the thymus, thyroid, and spleen are ductless glands that secrete special substances into the veins. Other investigators described excretory ducts from the thymus to various structures such as veins, esophagus, trachea, pericardium, and pleura.[3] Citing clinical observations, researchers postulated that the thymus secretes substances that have a variety of effects, including the prevention of cancer, regulation of normal growth, lowering of calcium, and development of myasthenia gravis.[15] In 1966, Goldstein and others identified thymic hormones with biologic activity on lymphocytes.[16]

The current appreciation of the thymus as a central organ of the immune system developed during the 1960s.[17, 18] Cooper, Good, Miller, and others described two distinct compartments of the lymphoid system, one thymus-dependent and the other related to the production of immunoglobulins.[19, 20] In 1967, DiGeorge and others described impaired cell-mediated immunity in patients with congenital absence of the thymus.[21] In the 1970s, two major advances occurred. One was the discovery that T-cell responses were restricted by the major histocompatibility complex. The second was the discovery that T cells possess surface antigens related to their function and stage of differentiation.[18] In the 1980s, the nature of the T-cell antigen receptor was elucidated. Also, the process of intrathymic maturation of T cells became better understood.[18]

ANATOMY AND HISTOLOGY

The basic histology of the thymus (including the lobular configuration, cortex and medulla, lymphoid cells, and reticulum cells) was understood by the mid-nineteenth century.[22] Beginning in the late seventeenth century, anatomists described a "central cavity" in the thymus[3, 14] (Fig. 2–2). For two centuries, a debate ensued as to the existence of such a cavity. Eventually, it became apparent that the central cavity was an artifact of dissection.

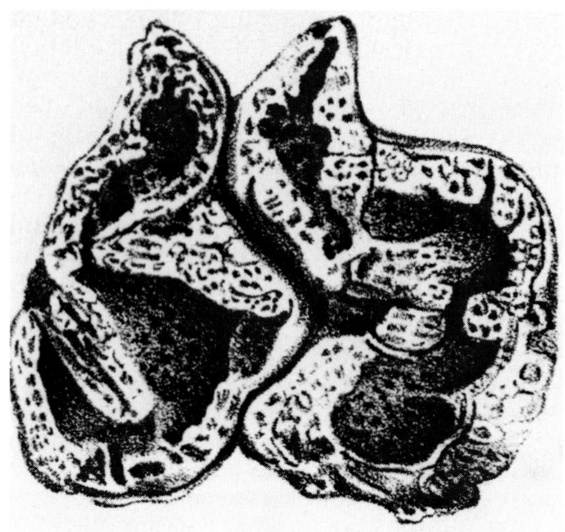

Figure 2–2. A fetal thymus gland illustrating the "central cavity," now known to be an artifact of dissection. (From Cooper A. The Anatomy of the Thymus Gland. Philadelphia: Lea & Blanchard, 1845.)

In 1846, an English physician and anatomist, Arthur Hill Hassall, wrote one of the first histology books.[23] He illustrated the concentric structures termed compound cells of the thymus, which were later called Hassall's corpuscles.[24] In the text,[25] Hassall quoted an earlier description of these structures from an 1845 essay by Sir John Simon. A debate followed as to the genesis of Hassall's corpuscles. One theory proposed a vascular origin. Another suggested that Hassall's corpuscles developed from persistent thymopharyngeal ducts.[26]

Beginning in the middle of the nineteenth century, a debate developed between those who believed the thymus to be lymphoid and those who believed it to be an epithelial organ.[3] Numerous theories were proposed. Some investigators believed in the "transformation theory" (i.e., that thymic epithelial cells directly transformed into lymphocytes). Some considered the lymphoid cells to be in fact epithelial, with only a *resemblance* to actual lymphocytes. Others believed in the "migration theory," which held that the lymphocytes "invade" the thymus from elsewhere.[3]

STATUS THYMICOLYMPHATICUS

In 1614, Felix Platter reported on a 5-month-old healthy infant who died suddenly.[1, 27] At autopsy, Platter found a prominent thymus and attributed the death to "mors thymica" (i.e., death caused by suffocation from pressure on the trachea by the thymus). The idea that thymic hyperplasia could compromise the trachea was debated for the next three centuries.

In 1889, Paltauf described status thymicolymphaticus, a condition characterized by thymic hyperplasia, along with hyperplasia of the entire lymphatic system.[3] These patients were also described as frequently having a reduced caliber of the aorta and arterial system, and affected males often had a female distribution of pubic hair. Patients with this disorder are "pale, yellowish in color . . . . The skin is thick, pasty looking; the hair is poorly developed . . . . Some patients have a diminished resistance; they are more vulnerable to bacterial and toxic influences."[3]

In subsequent years, the concept that an enlarged thymus could cause sudden death led to tragic results. Support for the idea was obtained from autopsies wherein no cause for a child's sudden death was apparent.[2, 28, 29] In these cases, the death was often attributed to a large thymus. Clinically, the syndrome of status thymicolymphaticus became widely accepted. It could be congenital or acquired and was characterized by increased susceptibility to a variety of physical and chemical agents. Diagnostic criteria were vague and included enlarged tonsils, pale skin, and, of course, a large thymus.[30] A French surgeon, Victor Veau, advocated thymectomy for "thymic asthma," a condition characterized by "recurrent difficulty in breathing associated with stridor and cyanosis."[4, 31] An animal model appeared to support the existence of status thymicolymphaticus. Removal of adrenal glands and gonads in rabbits induced hyperplasia of the thymus and lymphoid tissues.[32] This finding supported the belief that status lymphaticus develops because of "insufficient functional activity" of the adrenal and sex glands.

With the development of radiation therapy in the early 1900s, the accepted practice was to irradiate children whose chest radiographs showed prominent thymic shadows. The problem, however, was that normal ranges for thymic size were not established. Also, the subtleties of chest radiography (such as the effect of inspiration versus expiration on the size of the thymic shadow) were not appreciated. Consequently, up to half of all children were reported to have an enlarged thymus. Those admitted for tonsillectomy with an enlarged thymus were irradiated. In an upstate New York county, for example, 1% of all children born between 1939 and 1945 received radiation therapy to the thymus.[28]

In 1926, the Status Lymphaticus Investigation Committee was organized by the Medical Research Council of Great Britain and the Pathological Society of Great Britain and Ireland. Seven hundred and ten autopsy records were studied. In a 1931 report, this committee reached several conclusions, including the following: (1) a large thymus in itself cannot be considered a cause of death, (2) there is no association between lymphoid hyperplasia and weight of the thymus, and (3) there is no association between arterial hypoplasia or feminism in males and a large thymus.[33]

Despite this report, along with the reports of Hammar and many others, the practice of irradiating an "enlarged" thymus continued into the 1950s. Because of their experience performing autopsies, many pathologists remained convinced even into the 1960s that an enlarged thymus could cause sudden death.[34] In contrast, among 12,000 autopsies on infants under 1 year of age at the Chicago Lying-In Hospital, death was never attributed to thymic enlargement, according to Potter and Craig.[35] In later years, persons irradiated as children have shown an increased risk of cancer, particularly carcinoma of the thyroid and breast.[29, 36]

MYASTHENIA GRAVIS

The first reports (from autopsies) of an association between thymic tumors and myasthenia gravis were in 1901 by Oppenheim and by Weigert.[4, 37, 38] An enlarged thymus or thymoma was associated with myasthenia gravis by numerous subsequent investigators.[4, 12] Aware of these reports, the German surgeon Ernst Sauerbruch performed a thymectomy on a patient with exophthalmic goiter, enlarged thymus, and myasthenia gravis. Sauerbruch apparently believed that he was treating the hyperthyroidism as well as the myasthenia. After surgery, the patient experienced improvement of her myasthenia gravis, but the hyperthyroidism was not affected. This case was reported by Schumacher and Roth in 1912.[4, 39] Five years later, Haberer reported a partial transcervical thymectomy in a 27-year-old man with myasthenia gravis. Improvement was noted after surgery despite an absence of evident thymic enlargement.[4, 40]

In 1936, the American surgeon Alfred Blalock removed a cystic thymic tumor from a patient with myasthenia gravis at Vanderbilt University.[4, 12] The patient's myasthenia improved postoperatively, and she was entirely well for 4 years. In 1939, Blalock performed the first total thymectomy for the sole purpose of treating myasthenia gravis. In 1941, Blalock moved to Johns Hopkins, where he continued to treat myasthenia gravis patients by removal of all thymic tissue, even in the absence of a thymic tumor. In his first report, five of six patients improved after surgery.[41] In his later review of 20 patients treated by thymectomy, 13 were "cured" or improved.[42] However, Blalock became disappointed by the unpredictability of a response to thymectomy. Gradually, he lost interest in surgery of the thymus and devoted his time to cardiac surgery, where he pioneered surgical correction of the tetralogy of Fallot.[4] Over the next 40 years, a debate ensued as to the value of thymectomy for myasthenia gravis. Despite a lack of knowledge as to its mechanism of action, most would now agree that thymectomy is an accepted treatment modality for this disorder.[4] Radiation to the thymus has also been tried as a therapeutic modality for myasthenia gravis but without much success.[42]

The histopathology of the thymectomy specimens from Blalock's myasthenia gravis patients was reported by Sloan in 1943.[43] This appears to be the first thorough description of non-neoplastic changes in the myasthenic thymus. In contrast to previous reports describing an enlarged or "persistent" thymus in myasthenia gravis, the 10 thymus glands in this study were no larger than normal glands and had weights within the normal range. However, Sloan also notes that patients with myasthenia gravis tend to have thymus glands with less involution than do patients with other chronic illnesses of similar duration. Sloan describes germinal centers in the thymic medulla of 7 of the 10 myasthenia gravis cases and increased medullary lymphocytes in all cases. He contradicts previous reports of epithelial hyperplasia in the myasthenic thymus.

SUMMARY

The thymus has had a controversial history (Table 2–1). The word "thymus" probably derives from the resemblance of the organ to the thyme plant. The function of the thymus was a subject of debate for nearly 2000 years. Only since the 1960s has its role in cell-mediated immunity become accepted. Misunderstanding of the normal size and function of the thymus had tragic consequences.

Much of the misleading data generated in the investigations of the thymus arose from failure to consider a "control" sample. Lack of controls for neonatal thymectomy led Restelli to conclude erroneously that the adult thymus was essential for life. The absence of controls for sudden-death investigations led to the irradiation of children for status thymicolymphaticus. What are the errors in our present understanding of the thymus? Only "thyme" will tell . . . .

Table 2–1. History of the Thymus

~100 C.E.	First known written use of the word thymus by Rufus
1614	Mors thymica: death due to enlarged thymus described by Platter
1889	Status thymicolymphaticus described by Paltauf
1901	First association of myasthenia gravis with thymic tumor by Oppenheim and Weigert
1939	First thymectomy to treat myasthenia gravis by Blalock
1960s	Demonstration of the thymus as a central organ for cell-mediated immunity by Miller, Good, Cooper, and others
1966	Identification of thymic hormone by Goldstein
1967	Congenital absence of the thymus: association with immunodeficiency by DiGeorge and others
1970s to 1990s	Description of thymic microenvironment, role of thymus in T-cell development (see Chapter 3), classification of thymic tumors (see Chapter 5)

REFERENCES

1. Spees EK. Thymos primer. JAMA 1969; 207:1436–1439.
2. Cardarelli NF. Historical antecedents. *In* Cardarelli NF, ed. The Thymus in Health and Senescence, volume I: Thymus and Immunity. Boca Raton, FL: CRC Press, 1989:5–20.
3. Crotti A. The thymus gland. *In* Thyroid and Thymus. Philadelphia: Lea & Febiger, 1922:607–693.
4. Givel J-C. Historical review. *In* Givel J-C, ed. Surgery of the Thymus. Berlin: Springer-Verlag, 1990:1–10.
5. Ebbell B. The Papyrus Ebers. Copenhagen: Levin & Munksgaard, 1937:121.
6. Daremberg C. Oeuvres de Rufus d'Ephese. Paris: Imprimerie Nationale, 1879:156.
7. Thomson WAR. Black's Medical Dictionary. London: A. and C. Black, 1981:876–877.
8. Daremberg C, ed. Oeuvres de Rufus d'Ephese. Paris: Imprimerie Nationale, 1879:270, 386–387, 649.
9. Galen. On the Usefulness of the Parts of the Body. May MT, trans. Ithaca: Cornell University Press, 1968:286.
10. Galen. On the Usefulness of the Parts of the Body. May MT, trans. Ithaca: Cornell University Press, 1968:283 (footnote).
11. Hewson W. The works of William Hewson, F.R.S. Ed. Gulliver G, ed. London: Sydenham Society, 1846:255.
12. Blalock A, Mason MF, Morgan HJ, Riven SS. Myasthenia gravis and tumors of the thymic region. Ann Surg 1939; 110:544–561.
13. Solis-Cohen S. The therapeutic uses of the thymus gland. JAMA 1900; 35:421–424.

14. Cooper A. The Anatomy of the Thymus Gland. Philadelphia: Lea & Blanchard, 1845.
15. Cardarelli NF. Thymic hormones: an introduction. *In* Cardarelli NF, ed. The Thymus in Health and Senescence. Boca Raton, FL: CRC Press, 1989:161–178.
16. Goldstein AL, Slater FD, White A. Preparation, assay and partial purification of a thymic lymphocytopoietic factor (thymosin). Proc Natl Acad Sci U S A 1966; 56:1010–1017.
17. Cardarelli NF. The thymus and immunology. *In* Cardarelli NF, ed. The Thymus in Health and Senescence. Boca Raton, FL: CRC Press, 1989:81–132.
18. Miller JFAP. Three decades of T-ology. Thymus 1990; 16:131–142.
19. Cooper MD, Peterson RDA, Good RA. A new concept of the cellular basis of immunity. J Pediatr 1965; 67:907 (abstract).
20. Miller JF. Immunological function of the thymus. Lancet 1961; 2:748–749.
21. DiGeorge AM, Lischner HW, Dacou C, Arey JB. Absence of the thymus. Lancet 1967; 1:1387.
22. Cardarelli NF. Developmental anatomy and morphology of the thymus. *In* Cardarelli NF, ed. The Thymus in Health and Senescence, volume I: Thymus and Immunity. Boca Raton, FL: CRC Press, 1989:21–42.
23. Blau JN. Hassall—physician and microscopist. Br Med J 1968; 2:617–619.
24. Hassall AH. The Microscopic Anatomy of the Human Body in Health and Disease, volume 2. London: S. Highley, 1849:131.
25. Hassall AH. The Microscopic Anatomy of the Human Body in Health and Disease, volume 1. London: S. Highley, 1849:478.
26. Jaboslow BN. Genesis of Hassall's corpuscles. Nature 1967; 215:408–409.
27. Ruhrah J. Pediatrics of the Past. New York: Paul B. Hoeber, 1925:239.
28. Pifer JW, Toyooka ET, Murray RW, Ames WR, Hempelmann LH. Neoplasms in children treated with X rays for thymic enlargement. I. Neoplasms and mortality. J Natl Cancer Inst 1963; 31:1333–1356.
29. Saenger EL, Silverman FN, Sterling TD, Turner ME. Neoplasia following therapeutic irradiation for benign conditions in childhood. Radiology 1960; 74:889–904.
30. Jaffe HL. Thymus gland. *In* Piersol GM, Bortz EL, eds. The Cyclopedia of Medicine. Philadelphia: FA Davis, 1935:97–110.
31. Veau V. Rapport sur la chirurgie du thymus. C R Assoc Fr Pediatr 1910; 1:77–126.
32. Marine D, Manley OT, Baumann EJ. The influence of thyroidectomy, gonadectomy, suprarenalectomy, and splenectomy on the thymus gland of rabbits. J Exp Med 1924; 40:429–443.
33. Young M, Turnbull HM. An analysis of the data collected by the Status Lymphaticus Investigation Committee. J Pathol Bacteriol 1931; 34:213–258.
34. Symmers WStC. The thymus gland. *In* Wright GP, Symmers WStC, eds. Systemic Pathology. New York: American Elsevier, 1967:275–284.
35. Potter EL, Craig JM. Thymus and glands of internal secretion. *In* Pathology of the Fetus and Infant. Chicago: Year Book Medical, 1975:317–343.
36. Hildreth NG, Shore RE, Dvoretsky PM. The risk of breast cancer after irradiation of the thymus in infancy. N Engl J Med 1989; 321:1281–1284.
37. Weigert C. Pathogisch-Anatomischer Beirtrag Zur Erbschen Krankheit (myasthenia gravis). Neurol Zentralbl 1901; 20:397–601.
38. Oppenheim H. Die myasthenische Paralyse (Bulbarparalyse ohne anatomischen Befund). Berlin: Karger, 1901:119–123.
39. Schumacher ED, Roth J. Thymektomie bei einem Fall von Morbus Basedowi mit Myasthenie. Mitt Grenzgeb Med Chir (Jena) 1912; 25:746–765.
40. von Haberer H. Zur klinischen Bedeutung der Thymusdruse. Arch Klin Chir 1917; 109:193–248.
41. Blalock A, Harvey AM, Ford FR, Lillianthal JL. The treatment of myasthenia gravis by removal of the thymus gland. JAMA 1941; 117:1529–1533.
42. Blalock A. Thymectomy in the treatment of myasthenia gravis, report of 20 cases. J Thorac Surg 1944; 13:316–339.
43. Sloan HE. The thymus in myasthenia gravis: with observations on the normal anatomy and histology of the thymus. Surgery 1943; 13:154–174.

Chapter

3

THE NORMAL THYMUS

ANATOMY
HISTOLOGY
Lymphocytes
Epithelial Cells
Hassall's Corpuscles
Nurse Cells
Mononuclear Phagocytes
Myoid Cells
Other Cells
NEUROENDOCRINE FEATURES
AGE-RELATED CHANGES
EMBRYOLOGY
PHYLOGENY
FUNCTION

ANATOMY

The thymus is located in the anterior and superior mediastinum (Fig. 3–1). It overlies the pericardium, the aortic arch and its branches, the left brachiocephalic vein, and the trachea.[1] Superiorly, it extends to the lower aspect of the thyroid gland. Anterior to the thymus are the sternum, adjacent portions of the upper four costal cartilages, and the sternothyroid and sternohyoid muscles. In a young adult, the thymus is typically V-shaped with two lobes extending down from the neck[2] (Fig. 3–2). The upper poles of the thymus are joined to the lower poles of the thyroid by the thyrothymic ligament.[3] The two thymic lobes join at various levels in the superior mediastinum and extend over the pericardium, usually to about the level of the fourth costal cartilage. Variations in gross morphology are common. For example, the thymus may be shaped like an X or an inverted V. Unilobed and trilobed thymuses have been described.[2] The infant's thymus is pink. In older individuals, the thymus becomes yellow because of fat deposition.

The arterial supply of the thymus varies[4] but derives principally from the internal thoracic, superior thyroid, and inferior thyroid arteries.[1,5] Lateral thymic arteries arise from the internal thoracic artery at the lateral border of the thymus. Superior thymic arteries arise from inferior thyroid arteries as collaterals or terminal branches. Posterior thymic arteries are less common and arise from either the brachiocephalic trunk or the left common carotid. Accessory thymic arteries arise from superior thyroid, subclavian, and thyrocervical arteries. Direct branches from the aorta or brachiocephalic artery may also occur.[2] The arterial blood supply of the thymus has many variations and often differs even from one side of the organ to the other.

Arterioles penetrate into the thymic capsule and course through the interlobular trabecula. At the corticomedullary junction, the arterioles give rise to capillaries that extend into the cortex and medulla. The venous system drains into the left brachiocephalic, internal thoracic, and inferior thyroid veins. Small veins from the cortex form a venous plexus on the posterior capsule. A single vein often leaves the medial side of each lobe. These veins fuse to form a larger vein ("the great vein of Keynes"), which drains into the left brachiocephalic vein. A lateral vein from each side drains into the superior vena cava (right) and left brachiocephalic vein (left).[4]

Afferent lymphatics are not described in the thymus.[4] In the mouse, perivascular spaces around the postcapillary venules open into terminal lymphatic vessels at the corticomedullary junction and in the medulla.[4,6] This seems to be one route for mature T cells to exit the

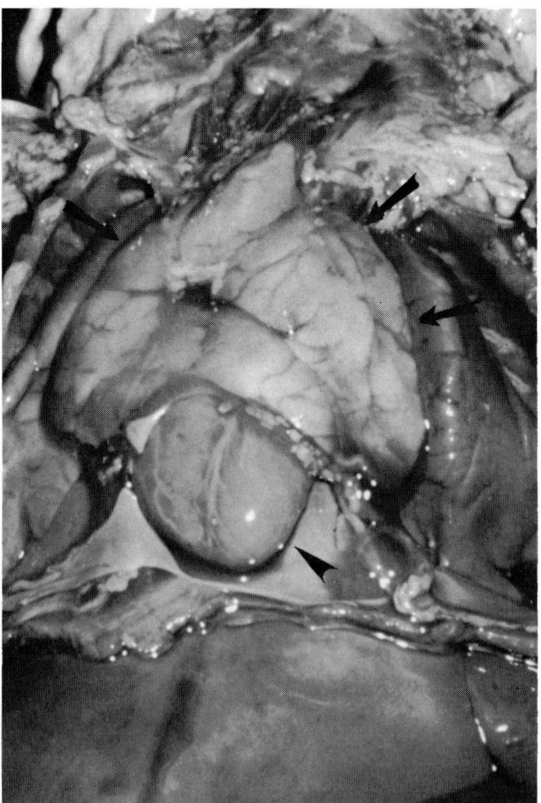

Figure 3–1. This photograph of the mediastinum in a neonate at autopsy demonstrates the location of the thymus (*arrows*) between the lungs and overlying the heart (*arrowhead*).

thymus. The lymphatic vessels within the thymus join to form larger lymphatic vessels that run with blood vessels to the capsule. From there, the efferent lymphatic vessels drain into the brachiocephalic, tracheobronchial, and parasternal lymph nodes.

The innervation of the thymus is now an active area of investigation. Most of the studies have been done in laboratory animals.[7–11] The thymus is innervated by sympathetic nerves arising from thoracic ganglia of the sympathetic chain and by parasympathetic nerves from the vagus, recurrent laryngeal, and phrenic nerves. The thymus receives afferent innervation from the nodose ganglia of the vagus nerve and from the dorsal root ganglia.[9] In an immunohistochemical study, Al-Shawaf and colleagues describe sympathetic nerves that enter the rat thymus with the vessels and then are distributed in the subcapsular area and corticomedullary junction. Parasympathetic nerves also enter the gland with the vessels and are distributed to both cortex and medulla.[12]

In the human thymus, noradrenergic nerve-like fibers (immunoreactive for tyrosine hydroxylase and neurofilament) are present within the medulla.[13] Peptidergic nerve-like fibers (immunoreactive for pituitary hormones) have been identified in the thymic cortex and medulla.[13] Although the innervation of the thymus is incompletely understood, the potential for communication between the nervous system and the immune system in the thymus is intriguing. Innervation of the thymus gland during embryogenesis may be critical to its development.[11]

The size of the thymus varies widely. This subject was studied extensively during the investigations of status thymolymphaticus[14–17] (see Chapter 2). These studies found that, on average, the thymus increases in absolute weight until adolescence and then gradually diminishes. However, weight varied widely at any given age. In a more recent study, Steinmann studied 136 thymuses from apparently healthy individuals who died suddenly.[18] No statistically significant difference was found among the different age groups (newborn to 107 years) (Table 3–1). In this study, there was no evidence that the thymus grows until puberty; the entire range of thymic sizes was reached during the first months of life. In 1980, Kendall et al. studied 574 thymuses from individuals who died suddenly.[4, 19] They also reported marked variation in thymic weight at any given age. The mean thymic weights increased slightly during the first decade and decreased thereafter.

Reasons for the discrepancies among the

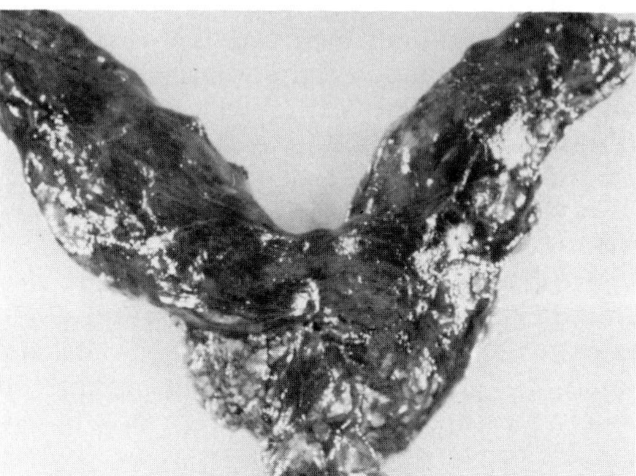

Figure 3–2. Thymectomy specimen from a 22-year-old woman with myasthenia gravis demonstrates normal gross configuration of the thymus in a young adult. The upper poles extend into the neck, while the lower portion of the organ is within the anterior-superior mediastinum.

Table 3–1. Wet Weight and Volume of Thymus in Apparently Healthy Persons Who Died Suddenly

		Weight (g)		Volume (ml)	
Age (years)	Number Studied	*Mean*	*Standard Deviation*	*Mean*	*Standard Deviation*
0–1	6	27.3	16.4	26.8	16.1
2–4	4	28.0	19.3	27.9	10.4
5–9	7	22.1	9.2	21.5	8.8
10–14	5	21.5	6.1	21.1	6.4
15–19	9	20.2	10.3	19.3	10.1
20–24	18	21.6	9.5	23.0	10.6
25–29	9	23.1	11.8	23.7	11.9
30–34	5	25.5	9.9	27.6	11.2
35–44	17	21.9	9.2	22.2	10.5
45–54	14	24.8	12.8	26.5	12.4
55–64	15	21.3	9.5	23.5	10.4
65–84	17	23.8	16.1	25.6	17.0
85–90	5	18.2	5.4	20.4	6.8
91–107	5	12.4	6.9	13.4	7.2
	136 total	22.8 average	12.5 average	23.4 average	11.9 average

various studies are not apparent. Nevertheless, the conclusion is clear: the weight of the "normal" thymus is extremely variable at any age. However, a range of 5 to 50 g will encompass virtually all normal thymuses from birth through adulthood. The weight of the thymus as a percentage of total body mass is greatest at or near the time of birth.[5, 20]

HISTOLOGY

Microscopically, the infant thymus has a lobular configuration with each lobule surrounded by fibrous tissue[21] (Fig. 3–3). The lobules are separated into darkly staining cortex and lightly staining medulla. The cortex and medulla are composed predominantly of lymphocytes ("thymocytes") and epithelial cells (Fig. 3–4). The lymphocytes are more closely packed in the cortex than in the medulla. Also, the cortical lymphocytes are less mature than those in the medulla.

Within the cortex, the blood vessels are separated from the thymic parenchyma by a single layer of epithelial cells joined by desmosomes.[20, 22] This arrangement is unique; it seems consistent with the concept of a blood-thymus barrier and the thymus as an "immunologically privileged" site. However, this concept has been challenged in studies showing antigens entering the thymus by a transcapsular route or via the medulla.[20, 23, 24] Nevertheless, the blood-thymus barrier may exist to some extent and may account for the finding that the thymus is an immunologically privileged site relatively removed from immune surveillance. For example, investigators have used the thymus as a site for islet cell allograft transplantation in an animal model for diabetes.[25]

Between the vessels and the epithelial cells is the perivascular space.[22] The perivascular spaces are continuous with the connective tissue surrounding the thymic lobules. During fetal development, the perivascular spaces form when the thymic anlage is invaginated by blood vessels and surrounding mesenchyme. The epithelial cells that line the perivascular space in the cortex merge with the medullary epithelial cells at the corticomedullary junction. Hence, the well-defined perivascular space in the cortex is absent or incomplete in the medulla. Vessels within the perivascular space include arterioles, capillaries, venules, and lymphatics. Other contents of the perivascular space include collagen, fibroblasts, small nerves, macrophages, mast cells, eosinophils, plasma cells, and lymphocytes.[22]

Lymphocytes

Prothymocytes enter the thymus from the bone marrow and migrate to the outer cortex and possibly the corticomedullary junction.[26] With maturation, the thymic lymphocytes are thought to move from the outer cortex toward the medulla. Medullary lymphocytes then mi-

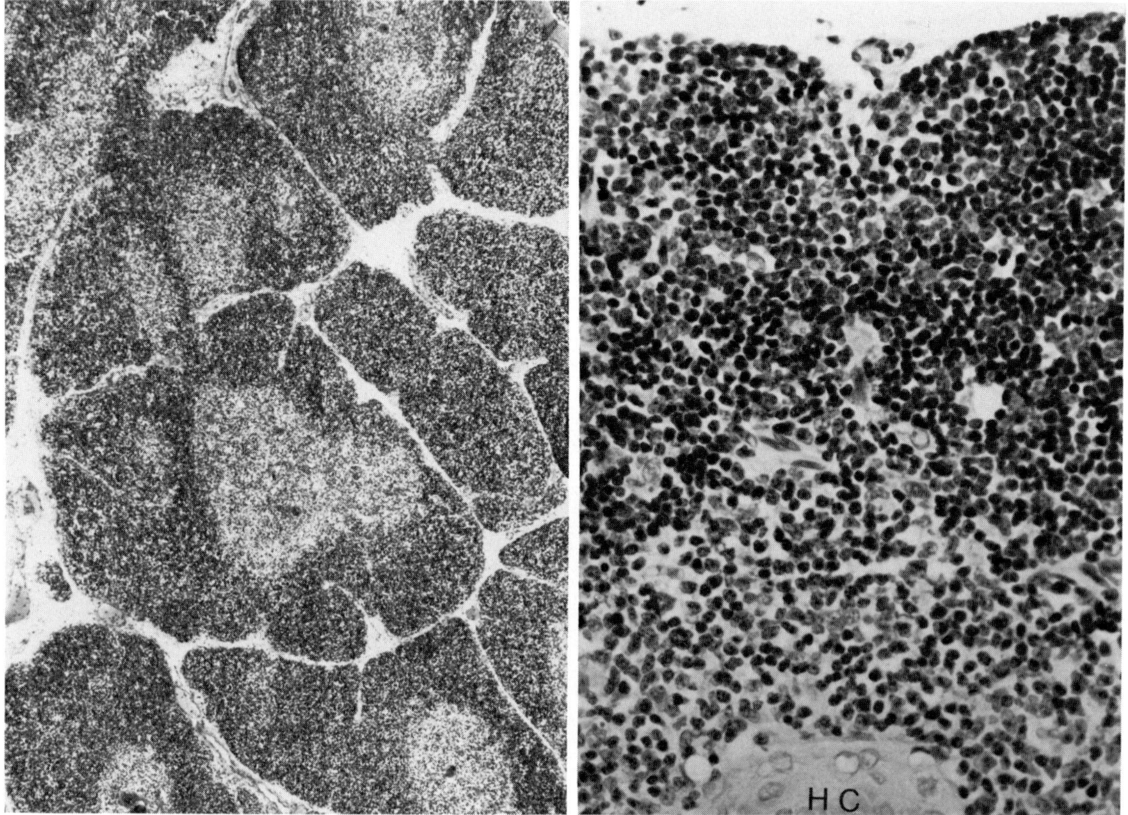

Figure 3–3. *Left,* Microscopic appearance of the thymus in an infant. Note the lobular architecture, corticomedullary differentiation, and thin fibrous septa between lobules. The lighter-staining area within the central portion of the lobule is the medulla. *Right,* Photograph at a higher magnification illustrates the cortex in the upper half and the medulla in the lower portion. A Hassall's corpuscle (*HC*) is present within the medulla (H&E: left, ×40; right, ×400).

grate from the thymus into the peripheral circulation, where they function as mature T cells. The cortical lymphocytes are larger, because they are less mature. Monoclonal antibodies to cell surface markers (defined by cluster of differentiation, or "CD" numbers) delineate stages of thymic lymphocyte maturation[27, 28] (Fig. 3–5).

Approximately 80% of thymic lymphocytes are positive for CD1 (including virtually all of those in the cortex) and co-express CD4 and CD8 molecules[29] (Fig. 3–6). These cortical lymphocytes are described as "double-positive" (CD4+CD8+). Double-negative cells are few in number (1 to 2% of thymic lymphocytes) and are concentrated in the subcapsular area of the outer cortex. The remaining thymic lymphocytes express either CD4 or CD8 and are located predominantly in the medulla. As in the peripheral blood, the CD4/CD8 ratio is approximately 2:1.

The single-positive thymic lymphocytes are immunocompetent and presumably circulate to the peripheral lymphoid tissue. The medullary lymphocytes appear to exit the thymus via veins and lymphatics at the corticomedullary junction. CD3 is a molecule associated with the T-cell antigen receptor. Double-positive cells express low levels of surface CD3, whereas most single-positive cells express high levels.[29] CD3 is present initially within the cytoplasm. With maturation, the CD3 is expressed on the surface.[30] Cortical lymphocytes bind to the lectin peanut agglutinin (PNA) and contain heat-stable antigen (HSA), whereas mature T cells do not.[24]

A critical event in T-cell development is expression of the T-cell antigen receptor (TCR).[29] Rearrangement and expression of the TCR are needed for the T cell to recognize antigen in association with self–major histocompatibility complex antigens (see later).

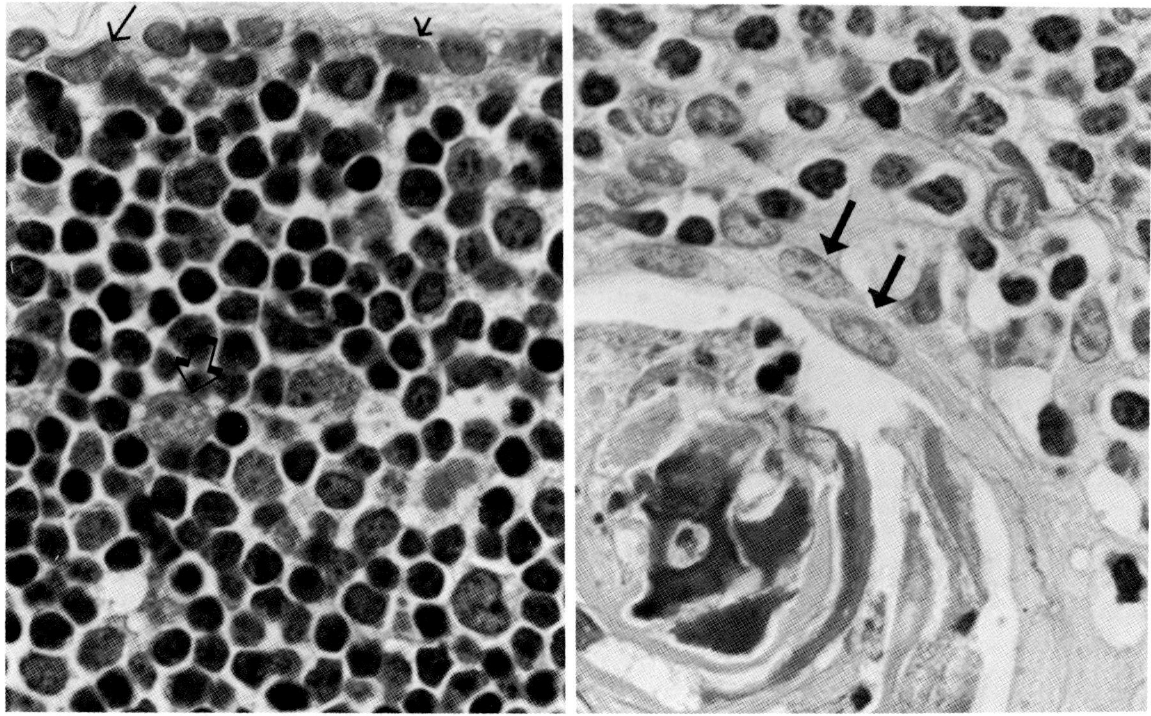

Figure 3–4. Light-microscopic appearance of epithelial cell subpopulations. *Left,* The subcapsular epithelial cells (*thin arrows*) are spindled in shape and have inconspicuous nucleoli. The cortical epithelial cells (*thick arrow*) have round nuclei with prominent nucleoli. *Right,* The medullary epithelial cells (*arrows*) surrounding the Hassall's corpuscle are spindled with inconspicuous nucleoli (H & E, ×1000).

The TCR is a disulfide-linked polypeptide heterodimer composed of two chains closely associated with the CD3 complex. Two major types of TCR have been identified. One type contains alpha and beta polypeptide chains. The alpha-beta TCR is expressed in nearly all T cells. The other TCR type contains gamma and delta polypeptide chains. The gamma-delta TCR is expressed on about 2% of T cells in lymphoid tissue. The gamma-delta T cells lack CD4 and CD8; their function is not understood.

Most immature thymic lymphocytes that are negative for both CD4 and CD8 (double negatives) have mRNA for the beta chain of the TCR.[26, 31] Cells that have mRNA for both beta and alpha chains are more mature (weakly positive for CD4 and CD8). In these cells, the

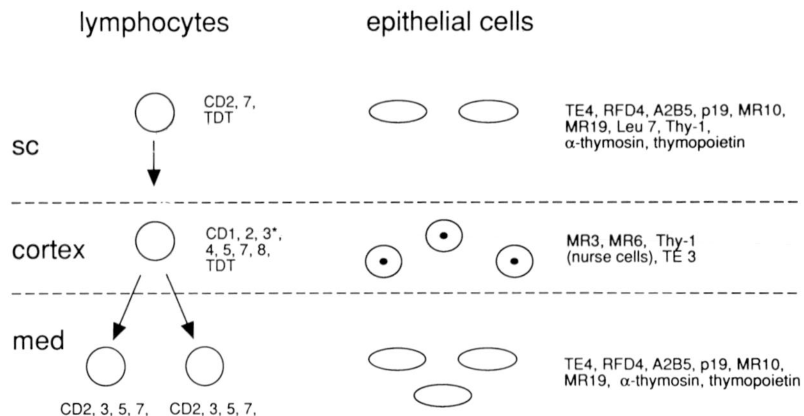

Figure 3–5. Cell markers in the thymus. On the left, stages of thymic lymphocyte maturation are illustrated with the corresponding phenotype. On the right, epithelial cell subsets are illustrated along with their corresponding immunoreactivity to various antibodies. *sc,* subcapsular cortex; *med,* medulla; *CD,* clusters of differentiation; *TDT,* terminal deoxynucleotidyl transferase. *CD3 is expressed in the perinuclear region of early thymic lymphocytes in the cortex. Then, with maturation of the cell, CD3 emerges on the surface.[30] (See text.)

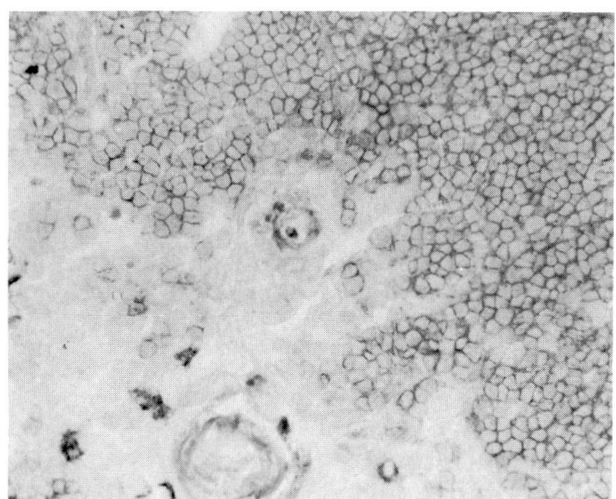

Figure 3–6. Immunoperoxidase stain on frozen section demonstrates localization of CD1-positive lymphocytes predominantly in the cortex (top and right). Fewer positive cells are present in the medulla (lower left) (×200).

TCR is assembled in the cytoplasm and expressed on the cell surface at low levels. With further maturation comes an increased density of TCRs. Gamma-delta TCRs are limited to a subset of double-negative cells.[29]

Most thymic lymphocytes die in situ by a process of programmed cell death ("apoptosis").[32] In particular, the vast majority of double-positive thymic lymphocytes appear to die within the thymic cortex. Relatively few cortical lymphocytes give rise to single-positive, immunocompetent T cells.[29] Investigators have speculated that the large percentage of dying cells may reflect the elimination of autoreactive lymphocytes.[32]

Adhesion molecules may be important in intrathymic T-cell differentiation. The integrins are one group of such molecules that mediate cell adhesion.[33, 34] In the normal human thymus, different subpopulations of lymphocytes express different integrins.[35] For example, the integrin VLA-4 (very late activation antigen-4) is a fibronectin receptor, and is expressed by cortical lymphocytes. Interaction between VLA-4 on the lymphocytes and fibronectin on the epithelial cells may be important in T-cell maturation.

Another integrin, VLA-6, is a ligand for laminin, a basement membrane component, and is expressed by medullary lymphocytes.[35] VLA-6 expression may relate to the ability of the medullary lymphocytes to emigrate from the thymus into the peripheral blood. H-CAM (CD44) and LECAM-1 (Leu 8, peripheral lymph node homing receptor) are other adhesion molecules that function as homing receptors. Both are expressed predominantly by medullary lymphocytes.[36, 37] In addition, these antigens are present on a small subset of immature lymphocytes that co-express the progenitor cell antigen, CD34. These data suggest that adhesion molecules may be involved in homing of prothymocytes to the thymus as well as homing of medullary T cells to peripheral blood and tissues.[37, 38]

B lymphocytes can also be identified in the thymus.[39, 40] They are present in the medulla and within the perivascular space. They express the pan B-cell antigens CD19, CD20, and CD22, as well as surface immunoglobulin M (IgM). Unlike B cells of germinal centers and surrounding mantle zones, the medullary B cells are negative for CD21. Another cell population in the medulla expresses B-cell markers and has a dendritic morphology. These cells have been called asteroid cells, and their origin is unclear.[39] Asteroid cells have a dendritic morphology (Fig. 3–7). Perhaps they are a subset of interdigitating dendritic cells.

In the perivascular space, B cells may form germinal centers. Although germinal centers are associated with autoimmune disorders (e.g., myasthenia gravis), they may be present in apparently healthy individuals.[41]

Epithelial Cells

The thymic epithelial cells provide the framework within which T lymphocytes mature. Thymic epithelial cells are morphologically heterogeneous. Descriptions of various subsets of thymic epithelial cells have been based on light-microscopic appearance, anti-

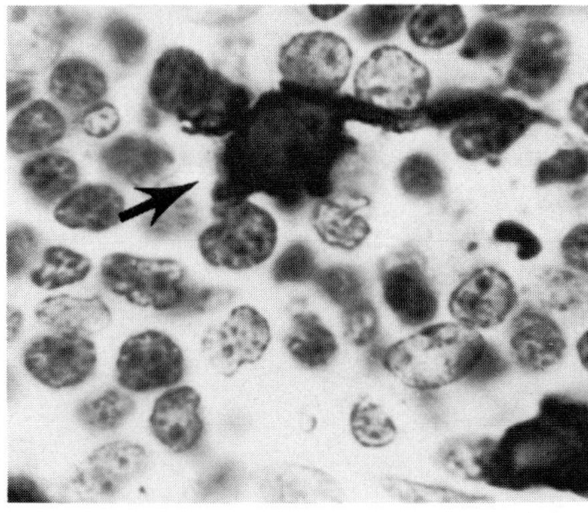

Figure 3–7. Immunoperoxidase stain for CD20 in paraffin-embedded tissue demonstrates "asteroid" cell (*arrow*) within the thymic medulla (×400).

gen expression, and ultrastructure[3, 42–44] (Fig. 3–8; see Figs. 3–4, 3–5). A flattened, or "spindled," epithelial cell is present along the inner surface of the thymic capsule ("subcapsular"), interlobular septa, and perivascular spaces. In the cortex, the epithelial cell nuclei tend to be round and have conspicuous, central nucleoli. These cells have long, cytoplasmic processes. Medullary epithelial cells vary in appearance, with either spindled or round nuclei.

Ultrastructurally, subcapsular and perivascular spindled epithelial cells form a basal lamina.[20, 44] Together with vascular endothelium, the surrounding epithelial cells are believed to form the structural basis for the "blood-thymus" barrier. Kendall and others[43, 44] have divided thymic epithelial cells into six types based on electron-microscopic appearance. The subcapsular, spindled cells are type 1. Cortical epithelial cells have been divided into "pale" cells with electron-lucent cytoplasm (type 2), "intermediate" cells with variable electron density (type 3), and "dark" cells with electron-dense cytoplasm (type 4). All have abundant desmosomes. The pale cells are predominantly in the outer cortex. They have prominent nucleoli, well-developed Golgi cells, and occasional electron-dense granules. The intermediate cells are in the mid-to-deep cortex and have a more irregular nucleus, more vacuoles, and lysosome-like inclusions. The dark cells (Fig. 3–8) have cytoplasmic processes with numerous tonofilaments and polyribosomes. Secretory granules are frequently present. These cells are in the deep cortex, where they are often associated with pyknotic lymphocytes. All of these types of cortical epithelial cells are also present in the medulla. In addition, the medulla contains "undifferentiated" epithelial cells with sparse cytoplasm (type 5). Also in the medulla are large epithelial cells with abundant tonofilaments, well-developed rough endoplasmic reticulum, and numerous cytoplasmic vesicles (type 6). These cells are located adjacent to Hassall's corpuscles.

Like other epithelial cells, those in the thymus express cytokeratin[45] (Fig. 3–9). Cytokeratins are a complex family of intermediate filaments that have been divided into at least 19 types based on molecular weights. Different types of cytokeratin have been detected in epithelial cells located in the different areas of the thymus.[45, 46] For example, an antibody to cytokeratin 18 labels a subset of medullary epithelial cells. Cytokeratins 8 and 19 are expressed by most epithelial cells throughout the thymus.

Subpopulations of thymic epithelial cells have been identified on the basis of antigen expression[42, 47–50] (see Fig. 3–5). One group of antigenically defined thymic epithelial cells is located in the subcapsular cortex and medulla. These cells contain thymic hormones (thymopoietin and thymosin-α-1). The subcapsular and medullary epithelial cells are labeled with certain monoclonal antibodies (e.g., TE-4, A2B5, anti-p19). Cortical epithelium is labeled by other antibodies (e.g., TE-3, MR3, MR6).

The subcapsular and medullary epithelia

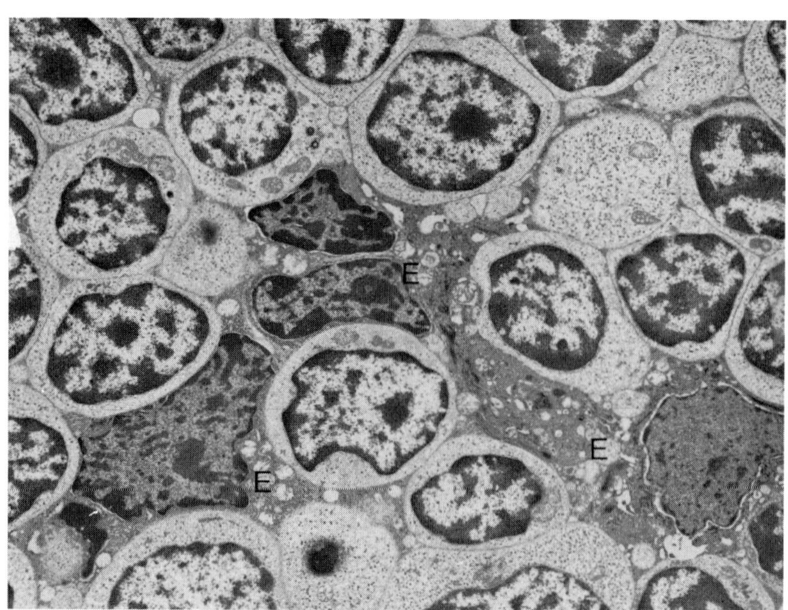

Figure 3–8. Electron micrograph illustrates epithelial cells (*E*) and lymphocytes in thymic cortex. The cytoplasmic processes of the epithelial cells intertwine among the lymphocytes. The epithelial cell cytoplasm appears darker (more electron-dense) than that of the lymphocytes. These epithelial cells correspond to the type 4 subset as described in the text (×2800).

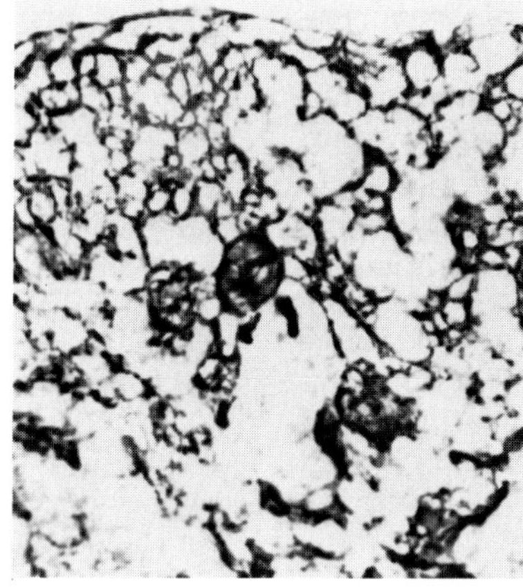
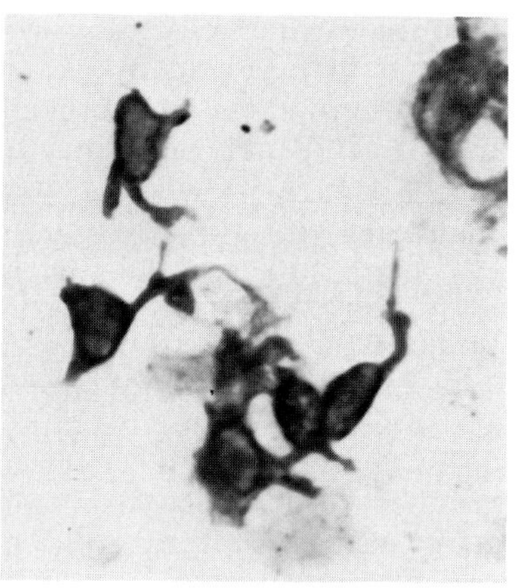

Figure 3–9. Immunoperoxidase staining of thymic epithelial cells for cytokeratin. *Left,* A frozen section of normal thymus shows the dendritic pattern of staining in the cortex (top) and medulla (bottom) (immunoperoxidase stain on frozen section using cocktail of different anticytokeratin antibodies, ×400). *Right,* The morphology of the epithelial cells in a cytospin preparation (note the dendritic cytoplasmic processes). (Immunoperoxidase stain on cytospin preparation using same antibody cocktail, ×1000).

differ in some respects. The antigen Thy-1 is expressed by subcapsular epithelial cells and by nurse cells in the cortex. Leu 7 is expressed by subcapsular epithelium. Neither Thy-1 nor Leu 7 is present on medullary epithelium. Interestingly, none of the monoclonal antibodies developed against thymic epithelium is thymus-specific. For example, A2B5 labels neuroendocrine tissues, including pancreatic islet cells, adrenal medulla, anterior pituitary, medullary carcinomas of the thyroid, and neuroblastomas. TE-4 and anti-p19 label the basal layer of squamous epithelium.

Expression of major histocompatibility complex (MHC) antigens by thymic epithelial cells is believed to be important in the immunologic development of T cells.[51, 52] Class I (HLA-A, B, C) and class II (HLA-DR) MHC antigens are expressed by thymic epithelial cells.[53] Some authors have reported that the cortical epithelial cells express primarily the class II determinants, whereas medullary cells express both.[51] Others find that the medullary epithelial cells lack HLA-DR.[54] The HLA-DR–positive interdigitating dendritic cells in the thymic medulla may obscure the epithelial cells and make the interpretation of staining patterns difficult. This problem may explain the discrepancies among the different studies.

Hassall's Corpuscles

Epithelial cells in the thymic medulla form concentric "swirls" of keratinizing cells, called Hassall's corpuscles (HCs). These structures may undergo cystic degeneration and calcification (Fig. 3–10). Mucin (sulfated acid mucopolysaccharide) may be present within the epithelial cells of HCs and in individual med-

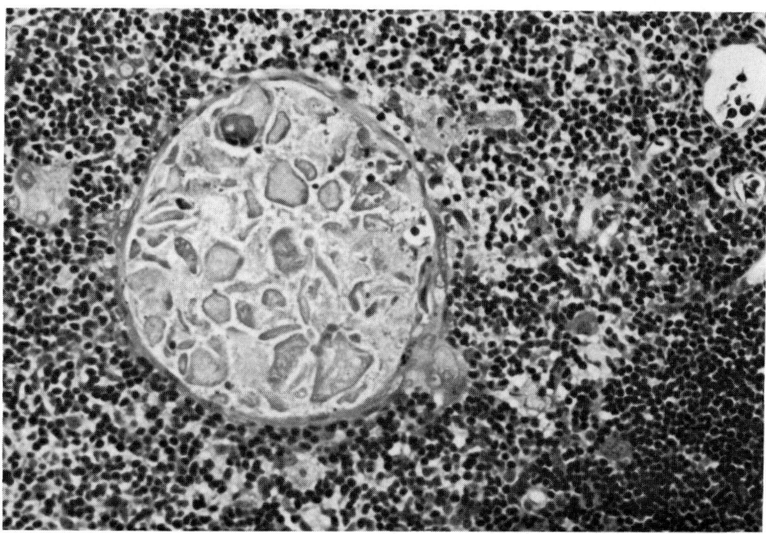

Figure 3–10. Dilated Hassall's corpuscle containing keratinous debris (H & E, ×200).

ullary epithelial cells.[55] Rarely, columnar epithelium may be identified. Other cell types (e.g., lymphocytes, macrophages, eosinophils, plasma cells, mast cells) may be found within the HCs. Embryologically, HCs first appear at 12 to 14 weeks of gestation.[56, 57] Large, cystic HCs predominate in the elderly.[56]

HCs are sites of antigen and antibody localization.[56, 58] They increase in number after antigen is injected into the thymus of hamsters and following parenteral antigen administration in guinea pigs.[56, 59] In humans, increased numbers of HCs have been noted during the acute stages of infectious diseases.[56] Investigators have postulated that HCs participate in phagocytosing and removing dead cells from the thymus.[56] Thymic hormones have also been localized to HCs.[60] HCs express high-molecular-weight cytokeratin and share other antigens with epidermal keratinocytes.[45, 61–63] A theory that HCs are a vestigial remnant of the thymopharyngeal duct is unlikely to be correct, because HCs are formed in vitro by cultured thymic epithelial cells.[64]

Nurse Cells

Nurse cells are a subset of thymic epithelial cells located predominantly in the cortex (types 2 and 3; see "Epithelial Cells").[20, 65] A single nurse cell contains up to 200 thymic lymphocytes within its cytoplasm. The cells within the cytoplasm are intact, maturing T cells. When isolated in vitro, the intracytoplasmic cells are surrounded by vacuolar membranes.[66] There is a debate about whether nurse cells are present in vivo or occur only as an artifact of isolation. One study did identify nurse cells with intravacuolar lymphocytes in sections of murine thymus after depletion of cortisone-sensitive lymphocytes.[67] Another study identified a ring-like staining pattern by immunoperoxidase with anti–epithelial cell antibodies on sections of human thymus.[65] The ring-like structures were interpreted as nurse cells. Investigators have reached different conclusions about whether the lymphocytes within the nurse cells proliferate.[65, 68] The thymic nurse cell may provide a specialized microenvironment for T-cell differentiation, maturation, deletion, and selection.[65, 69]

Mononuclear Phagocytes

Different types of mononuclear phagocytes can be identified in the thymus[70–73] (Table 3–2). Interdigitating dendritic cells are located in the medulla and corticomedullary junction. Macrophages are readily identifiable in the cortex and are also present in the medulla. Interdigitating cells and macrophages are closely related. They express common antigens[74] and may derive from the same bone marrow precursor.[75] According to one hypothesis, blood monocytes enter the thymus at the corticomedullary region, where they transform into macrophages. Some of these cells migrate to the cortex, where they become cortical macrophages. Others migrate to the medulla, where they form interdigitating cells.[24, 71]

In the rat, HLA-DR–positive bone marrow cells migrate to the thymus, where they develop the morphologic (elongated, invaginated nucleus and pale cytoplasm) and cytochemical (acid phosphatase positivity) features of interdigitating cells.[75] Some have Birbeck granules, typical of epidermal Langerhans cells. In culture, human thymic dendritic cells express the CD1 (T6) antigen, as do Langerhans cells.[49, 76] Thus, Langerhans cells in the thymus are a subset of dendritic cells.

Functionally, the cortical macrophages may be involved in the removal and phagocytosis of thymic lymphocytes.[24] Some of the macrophages and the interdigitating dendritic cells may function in antigen presentation to lymphocytes. These cells also produce soluble factors.[77] In particular, thymic dendritic cells are

Table 3–2. Interdigitating Cells and Macrophages[49, 70–74, 76]

Characteristic	Interdigitating Cells	Macrophages
Location	Medulla, corticomedullary region	Cortex, medulla, connective tissue septa
Phenotype	ATPase, HLA-DR, S100, MAC-1, MAC-2, CD1,* LN2, RFD-1	Esterase, lysozyme, weak ATPase, acid phosphatase, weak HLA-DR, MAC-1, MAC-2, RFD-7
Ultrastructure	Complex cytoplasmic processes, tubulovesicular structures, occasional Birbeck granules	Lysosomes, phagolysosomes

*Thymic interdigitating dendritic cells express CD1 (T6) in culture[76]; a minority appear to express CD1 in situ by immunocytochemistry.[49]

immunoreactive for interleukin-1, which can potentiate thymocyte proliferation. Interleukin-1 production may also be linked to HLA-DR expression.

Myoid Cells

Thymic cells with characteristics of striated muscle were first recognized in frogs and salamanders in 1888. In 1905, they were first observed in the human thymus by Hammar, who called them "myoid cells."[78] Ultrastructurally, myoid cells have myofilaments and dense patches typical of striated muscle. The cross-striations are not apparent by light microscopy. (In contrast, the striations are readily identifiable in birds and reptiles.) Human myoid cells can be demonstrated within the thymic medulla using immunoperoxidase techniques (Fig. 3–11). These cells react with antibodies to muscle markers, including myoglobin, actin, desmin, the M-component of creatine kinase, and beta-enolase.[78, 79] Morphologically, myoid cells are round to spindle-shaped cells. Embryologically, they first appear at the 8th week of gestation in humans.[80]

There is conflicting evidence concerning the derivation of thymic myoid cells. Using the quail-chick hybrid, Nakamura and Ayer–Le Lievre found the myoid cells to have a neural crest origin.[81] However, their finding is contradicted by Seifert and Christ. Also using the quail-chick hybrid, these authors found myoid cells to be derived from the axially located prechordal head mesoderm, similar to branchiomeric muscle.[82] Zoltowska found myoid cell positivity for both cytokeratin and desmin and postulated a common origin for both epithelial cells and myoid cells.[83] By electron microscopy, myoid cells may have desmosomal connections to epithelial cells.[84] Furthermore, cells have been identified with both tonofilaments and myofilaments. This close relationship between myoid and epithelial cells has been cited as evidence that both derive from a common precursor.[84]

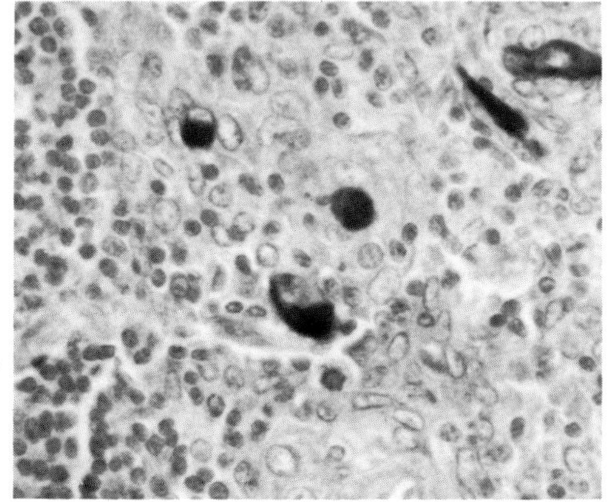

Figure 3–11. Immunoperoxidase stain using an antibody to desmin, an intermediate filament of muscle, demonstrates myoid cells (darkly staining) within the thymic medulla (×400).

Some investigators report that myoid cells tend to increase in number as the thymic parenchyma atrophies.[78] No consistent relationship with myasthenia gravis (MG) is evident (personal observations), although a pathogenic role for myoid cells in MG has been proposed. The function of myoid cells is unknown. One theory is that myoid cells present antigens of skeletal muscle within the thymus to induce self-tolerance.[82]

Other Cells

Mast cells, eosinophils, and plasma cells can be identified in the thymus. These cells are located in connective tissue areas such as the fibrous septa and perivascular spaces.[22] Eosinophils are more numerous in the thymus of infants and children than in the thymus of adults.[85, 86] In human fetal thymus, granulocytic and erythroid precursors have been described within the connective tissue and around small vessels in the cortex.[87]

Parathyroid tissue is occasionally located within the thymus[88] (Fig. 3–12). This is not surprising given the close association between parathyroid and thymus glands during embryogenesis (see later). Sebaceous glands have been reported to be closely associated with thymic epithelium.[89] Because sebaceous glands are ectodermal in origin, this finding was interpreted as supporting an ectodermal contribution to thymic development (see later). Salivary gland tissue has been noted in the thymus, also presumably on a developmental basis.[21]

NEUROENDOCRINE FEATURES

Thymic hormones are capable of inducing differentiation antigens on early precursor cells. They are thought to represent a physiologic signal in vivo that leads to differentiation of pre–T cells in the thymus. Thymic hormones also may enhance various helper and

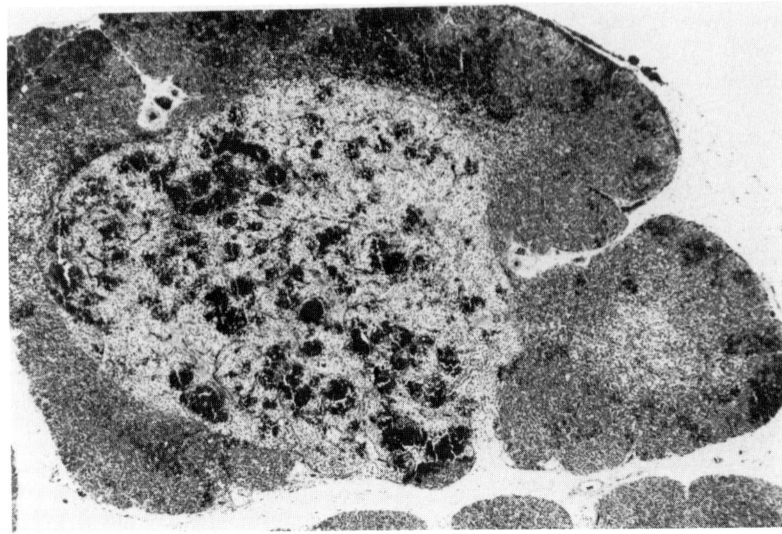

Figure 3–12. A parathyroid gland is present within the thymus (H & E, ×40).

suppressor functions of mature T cells. Four distinct thymic hormones have been described: thymopoietin, thymosin-α-1, thymulin (formerly facteur thymique serologique), and thymic humoral factor (Table 3–3).

All are polypeptides with molecular weights from 800 to 5500 daltons. Thymopoietin and thymulin are produced only by the thymic epithelium. Thymosins are a series of peptides that are synthesized in many organs. Besides the thymic hormones, thymic epithelial cells contain oxytocin and vasopressin, as demonstrated by immunoperoxidase and confirmed by dot blot studies of messenger RNA.[90] Another neuropeptide, beta-endorphin, has also been found in fetal and neonatal thymus as measured by radioimmunoassay.[91] The oxytocin- and vasopressin-positive cells are distributed in the subcapsular cortex and medulla. A similar distribution has been reported for cells that immunoreact with antibodies to thymulin, thymopoietin, and thymosin-α-1.[42, 43]

Batanero and colleagues reported epithelial cells in the human thymus that contain somatostatin and the anterior pituitary hormones (follicle-stimulating hormone, luteinizing hormone, thyroid-stimulating hormone, adrenocorticotropic hormone, growth hormone, and prolactin).[92] Most of the hormones localized to scattered epithelial cells in the medulla. Follicle-stimulating hormone immunoreactivity occurred predominantly in the cortical epithelial cells. An antibody to human chorionic gonadotropin (HCG) labeled most medullary lymphocytes and scattered lymphocytes in the cortex. By two-color immunofluorescence, HCG immunoreactivity was restricted to CD3-positive cells.

The thymus, in particular, and the immune system, in general, have complex interactions with the endocrine system.[93–97] These interactions have been demonstrated in animal models (Table 3–4).

Hypophysectomy causes atrophy of the thymus in rodents, and thymectomy causes degranulation of anterior pituitary cells. In 1924, Marine and colleagues reported that adrenalectomized rabbits had thymic hyperplasia.[98] Thyroidectomy induced thymic involution, whereas gonadectomy delayed involution. In more recent studies using laboratory animals, some hormones (e.g., prolactin, growth hormone, thyroxin) have increased thymic size,

Table 3–3. Thymic Hormones

Thymopoietin
Thymosin-α-1
Thymulin
Thymic humoral factor

Table 3–4. Endocrine Interactions with the Thymus

Endocrine Substance/Maneuver	Effect on Thymic Size
ACTH/adrenal steroids/catecholamines	Decrease
Adrenalectomy	Increase
Sex hormones	Decrease
Castration	Increase
Thyroid hormones	Increase
Thyroidectomy	Decrease

whereas others (glucocorticoids, sex hormones) have caused thymic involution.[93, 96] Some authors have postulated an effect of the thymus on reproductive function.[99]

Besides hormones, the thymus produces various cytokines and growth factors, including interleukin-1 interleukin-6, and granulocyte-monocyte colony–stimulating factor.[100–102] Transforming growth factor beta is synthesized in the developing murine and bovine thymus and has regulatory effects on T lymphocytes.[103–105] Epidermal growth factor receptors are present on thymic epithelial cells.[106]

Synthesis of thymic hormones is affected by hormones from other sites.[107] For example, injection of triiodothyronine in mice increases the numbers of thymulin-containing cells.[96] Adrenalectomy and castration of mice result in an initial decrease in thymulin-containing cells followed by an increase to three times the number of cells in "sham-operated" control animals.[96]

In vitro, glucocorticoids and sex steroids (progesterone, estradiol, and testosterone) are potent stimulators of thymulin production and release. However, corticosteroids and sex hormones are also cytolytic to cortical lymphocytes and cause thymic involution in vivo.[107, 108]

Haynes and others have developed monoclonal antibodies that identify the cells containing thymopoietin and thymosin-α-1 in the subcapsular cortex and medulla.[42, 109] One of these antibodies (A2B5) also reacts with neurons and other endocrine cells (see earlier). The markers of thymic hormone-containing thymic epithelium (TE-4, p19, A2B5) are also expressed on the basal layer of squamous epithelium. Such similarities between the thymus and skin suggest some common functions. For example, the skin may be a site for extrathymic T-cell maturation.[42, 110]

HCG has also been identified in scattered epithelial cells of the thymic medulla.[111] By immunoelectron microscopy, HCG was shown in the perinuclear space and rough endoplasmic reticulum. In contrast, HCG of endocrine cells in the stomach is present within various types of granules. Thymic epithelial cells lack the dense core granules (by electron microscopy and immunoperoxidase for chromogranin, a neuroendocrine granule–associated protein) typical of endocrine cells.

Another neuroendocrine feature of the thymus is the presence of Kultschitzky's cells within the medulla.[112, 113] These cells are readily demonstrable in the thymus of birds and reptiles using chromaffin or argyrophil stains. Ultrastructurally, these cells have dense core granules similar to those of polypeptide hormone–producing cells elsewhere. As in other foregut-derived organs, Kultschitzky's cells in the thymus are non-argentaffin. Argyrophil-positive cells are infrequent in the human thymus but have been described.

AGE-RELATED CHANGES

With aging, the thymus becomes replaced by fat (Fig. 3–13). According to Steinmann, the lipomatous atrophy represents a "final state" of involution.[18] Earlier changes (in children and young adults) include an increase in the thymic perivascular space. Connective tissue septa become replaced by fat tissue. The fat does not actually infiltrate the thymic parenchyma. The outer cortex becomes free of lymphocytes, and the medulla becomes smaller. Hassall's corpuscles may become cystic. Beyond the age of 50, the thymus is mostly fat surrounded by a fibrous capsule. Scattered islands of thymic parenchyma allow the tissue to be identified. The corticomedullary organization becomes less clear. An "inverse" appearance results from the cellular perivascular space surrounding remaining cortex. The epithelial cells may become spindled or form rosette-like structures.[21]

From 1 to 25 years of age, the perivascular space grows while the thymic lymphoid tissue decreases.[18] From age 25 to 40 years, both the lymphoid tissue and the perivascular space decrease, and fatty atrophy develops. After age 40, the lymphoid tissue of the thymus continues to decrease. The involution continues beyond the age of 90. Thymosin-containing cells decrease in number progressively beginning around 13 years of age.[50] However, terminal deoxynucleotidyl transferase (TDT)–positive lymphocytes can be identified in the thymus of elderly individuals, and the medullary epithelium continues to secrete the thymic hormone thymulin.[24] These findings suggest that the thymus contains differentiating T cells and continues to function in some capacity throughout life.

EMBRYOLOGY

The embryology of the thymus has been studied since the early 1900s, although estab-

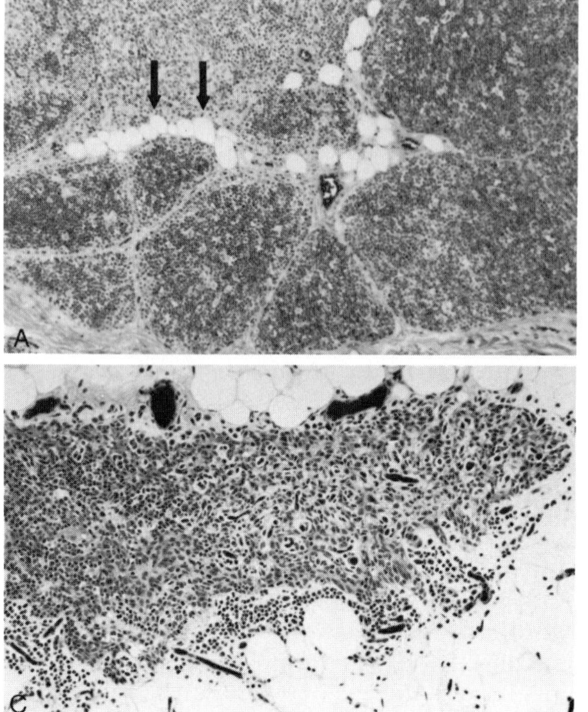

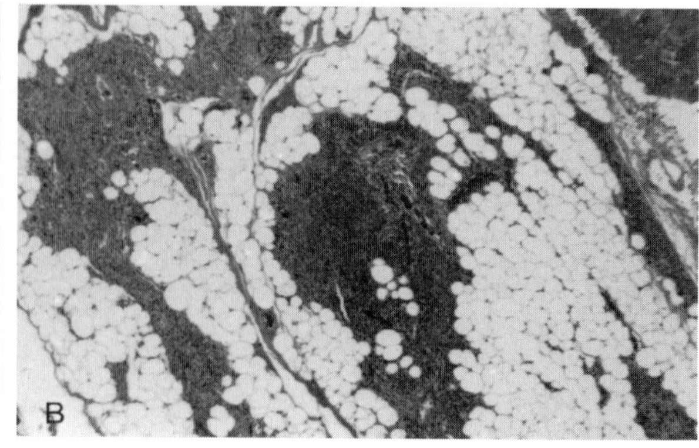

Figure 3–13. Age-related changes in the thymus. *A*, The thymus of a young adult shows early infiltration of adipose tissue along the septa (*arrows*) (H & E, ×40). *B*, The thymus of an older adult has more extensive fatty replacement (H & E, ×40). *C*, Higher magnification demonstrating depletion of lymphocytes with loss of corticomedullary differentiation in the thymus of an older adult (H & E, ×100).

lished ideas have been challenged in recent years. At the 4th week of human development, five pairs of outpouchings form along the lateral walls of the pharyngeal gut[114] (Fig. 3–14). At the same time, pharyngeal grooves ("clefts") become visible on the surface of the embryo. Beginning in the 5th week of development, the ventral portion of the third pharyngeal pouch differentiates into the thymic primordium, while the dorsal portion becomes parathyroid tissue. The thymus may also have a minor contribution from the fourth pouch. The second, third, and fourth pharyngeal clefts merge into the cervical sinus, which also may contribute to thymic embryogenesis.[115] With further development, the thymus separates from the pharynx. The bud-like thymic primordium elongates and becomes a cylindrical structure, its long axis oriented medially and caudally. With proliferation of the lining cells, the hollow cylindrical structure (termed thymopharyngeal duct, or thymic cord) becomes a solid stalk.[116–119]

The bilateral stalks descend into the superior mediastinum, where the pair is joined together by connective tissue.[80, 119, 120] The inferior portions enlarge and form the bulk of the gland. The proximal portion of each epithelial cord atrophies. Remnants may persist and develop into cysts (see Chapter 4).

During its descent, the thymic tissue passes behind the thyroid gland and sternocleidomastoid muscles. Thus, not surprisingly, thymic tissue can persist in the neck. In an autopsy study, Wenglowski found cervical thymic tissue in 20% of adults and 33% of infants.[121] Damiani and colleagues found thymic tissue in or adjacent to about 1% of surgically removed thyroid glands.[122] Gilmour described thymus within the neck and within the thyroid gland.[88] Ectopic thymic tissue has been identified in the retrocarinal fat,[123] neck,[124, 125] tympanic cavity,[126] and extrathymic anterior mediastinal fat.[127] These tissues can give rise to ectopic thymic cysts and thymic tumors.

Gilmour also described epithelial structures in fetuses in the area of the parathyroids and thymus.[118] Vesicular, canalicular, and gland-like formations were present on the surface of the parathyroid glands and close to the upper pole of the thymus. Some of the formations were traced to the thymic cord and thymus. Gilmore named these epithelial rudiments "canals of Kursteiner" after the author who is credited with initially describing them. These structures may persist into adult life (Fig. 3–15).

Since the earliest studies, there has been controversy about a possible dual origin of

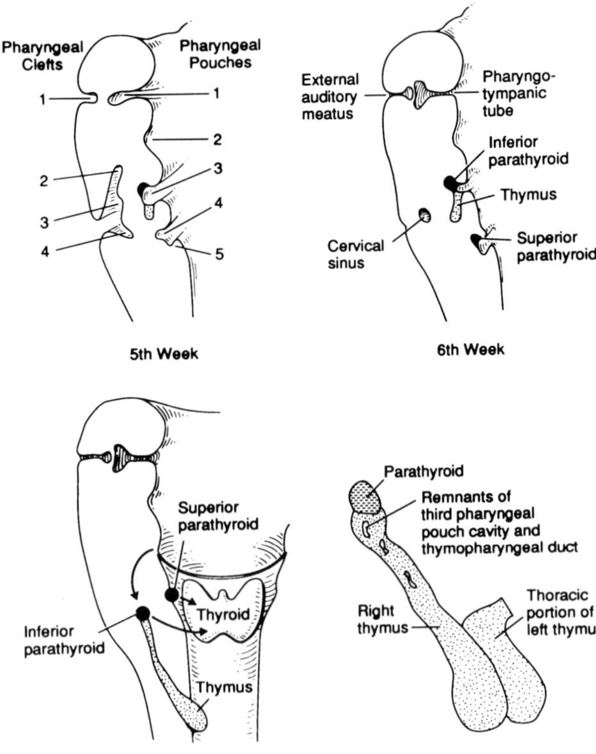

Figure 3–14. Embryology: drawings demonstrate the origin of the thymus from the third branchial pouch.

thymic epithelial cells. Some investigators have believed that the pharyngeal pouch endoderm develops into the thymic medulla, while the branchial cleft ectoderm gives rise to the cortex.[24, 128] Different investigators interpret the accumulated data to either support or refute the dual origin of thymic epithelial cells.[24, 47, 129] Indeed, Norris and Weller each studied the same collection of embryos and reached opposite conclusions in this regard.[115, 130]

More recently, immunohistochemical studies have shown that at an early stage of development (7 weeks), the human thymic epithelial cells all express common antigens. Moreover, antibodies that label different subsets of thymic epithelium in the adult mark all of the epithelial cells in the early fetal thymus.[47, 109] Although the evidence is incomplete, it is possible that thymic epithelial cells derive from a common stem cell.

Mesenchymal cells form the surrounding connective tissue and septa of the thymus. In mice, the mesenchymal cells have an inductive influence on the thymic epithelium, thereby allowing the epithelial cells to proliferate. In a quail-chick hybrid, the mesenchymal cells of the thymic capsule and septa were found to originate from the neural crest.[131] Mesenchyme derived from the neural crest (''ectomesenchyme'') rather than from mesoderm was also identified in many other structures in the head and neck, including the dermis of the face and neck, walls of major vessels near the heart, and connective tissue of the lower jaw and tongue.

Haynes and colleagues have questioned the neural crest origin of mesenchyme in the human thymus. They developed a monoclonal antibody, A2B5, which labels neural and neural crest–derived cells. In the thymus, this antibody labels subcapsular and medullary epithelial cells. Another antibody, TE-7, labels the connective tissue in the thymic capsule and septa as well as the fibrous stroma in every tissue tested.[109] Thus, these data suggest that if there is a neural crest–derived element in the thymus, it would be the subcapsular and medullary epithelial cells rather than connective tissue.

In laboratory animals, the thymus depends on the neural crest for development. Ablation of regions of the neural crest in chick embryos results in a markedly small or absent thymus.[128] Neural crest ablation leads to abnormal development of the heart, great vessels, thyroid, and parathyroid glands. A similar range of defects

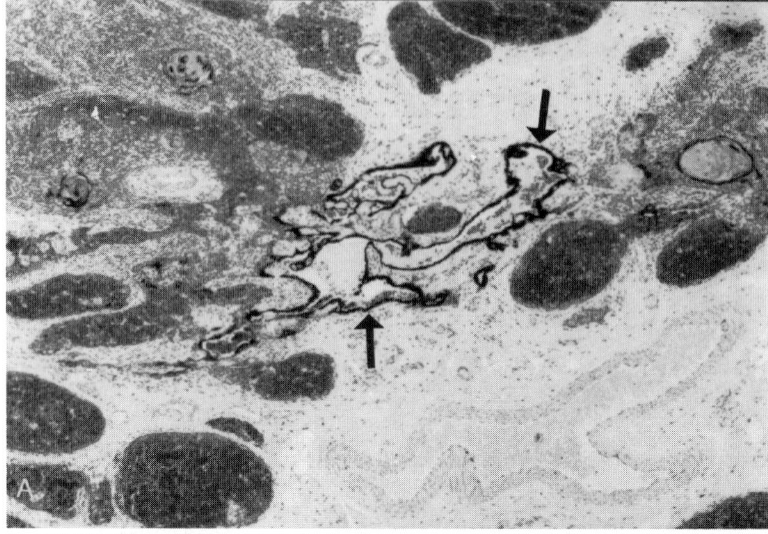

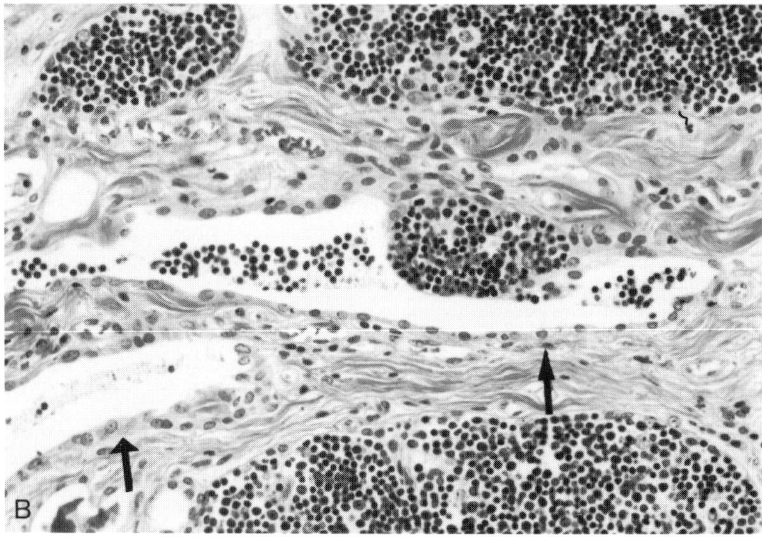

Figure 3–15. Canalicular structures within thymus gland from a 22-year-old patient with myasthenia gravis. *A*, An immunoperoxidase stain for cytokeratin highlights these structures (*arrows*) (×40). *B*, Their histologic appearance on a routine H & E stain (*arrows*) (×200).

is observed in humans with the DiGeorge syndrome (see Chapter 4). One hypothesis is that impaired thymic development from neural crest ablation results from loss of the inductive functions of the ectomesenchyme. Thus, the neural crest is important for thymic development. Whether the neural crest is the origin for any thymic cells or has an inductive influence only is unclear.

At 9 weeks of development, the primordial thymus becomes indented by mesenchymal septa, which by 17 weeks reach the corticomedullary junction.[20] Cells from the septa appear to enter the medulla. These cells may be precursors of the thymic interdigitating cells.[80] Also, Norris believed that during this process of lobulation, ectodermal epithelial cells from the thymic surface "break off" and get displaced into the medulla. He thought Hassall's corpuscles derived from these displaced cells.[115] This idea of displaced ectodermal cells has been used to explain a common ectodermal origin for outer cortical and medullary epithelial cells.[24]

The thymus also begins to attract circulating lymphoid cells during the 9th week.[80] These thymic lymphoid stem cells presumably arise in either the yolk sac or the liver.[29] Chemotactic factors, including beta-$_2$-microglobulin, attract the stem cells to the thymus.[38] In the mouse, the early thymic lymphocytes are double-negative (CD4−CD8−). Several days later, double-positive and then single-positive cells develop. In the human, corticomedullary differentiation becomes evident at 14 weeks.[80] By 17 weeks, the differentiation is complete. In the cortex, large, immature-appearing cells with mitotic activity are found primarily in the outer cortex. Smaller, more mature lymphoid cells populate the inner cortex and medulla. The thymus continues to increase in size until birth.

The embryology of the thymus is complex and incompletely understood. All cell layers, including the neural crest, appear to be involved in normal thymic development. Which thymic cells derive from the various embryonic structures is not clear. Differences in development between laboratory animals and humans may account for some of the conflicting data. The embryology of the thymus has implications for the study of thymic tumors (see Chapter 5).

PHYLOGENY

From an evolutionary standpoint, the thymus is an ancient organ.[47, 132, 133] Its development from the pharyngeal pouch may be related to the feeding habits of ancestral vertebrates. In fish, antigens can enter the body through the gills. The presence of antigens in this area may have influenced the development of lymphoid tissue at this location. The thymus is present in all jawed vertebrates (gnathostomata), including those whose ancestors first appeared 400 million years ago. The thymus may have evolved from lymphocytic accumulations in the pharynx of more primitive animals.

Throughout evolution, the thymus maintained its origin from the pharyngeal tissue, although the exact contributions from each pharyngeal pouch differ in different vertebrates. The morphology of the thymus has also remained constant. The histologic appearance with cortex and medulla populated by epithelial cells and lymphocytes characterizes the thymus in all vertebrates. Only the size of Hassall's corpuscles varies in different species. (In the mouse, for example, Hassall's corpuscles are inconspicuous.) Lampert and Ritter believe that this uniformity among species supports epithelial cell derivation from a common stem cell. Otherwise, diverse origins should have produced different appearances.[47]

FUNCTION

The thymus functions as the central organ of the cell-mediated (T cell) immune system. Cellular immunity includes cytotoxic T cells (most of which express CD8), such as those that kill virally infected cells. Delayed type hypersensitivity (e.g., the tuberculin reaction) and transplant rejection are other manifestations of cellular immunity. T cells also regulate the immune system. Some T cells (CD4+) "help" B cells and other lymphocytes; other T cells (CD8+) suppress the immune response. T lymphocytes become "educated" as they pass through the thymus. During this process, T cells learn to distinguish "self" from "nonself." The cellular mechanisms for this process are gradually becoming better understood.

T cells do not respond to free antigen.[29] They only recognize antigens bound to cell surface molecules encoded by the MHC. Moreover, they recognize antigens bound only to self-MHC (i.e., MHC molecules encountered by the T cells in the thymus during their development). CD4-positive cells recognize antigen together with class II MHC antigens, whereas CD8-positive cells recognize class I antigens. By positive selection, those cells with self-MHC specificity are allowed to differentiate into mature T cells. This process occurs in the thymus.[134] Using transgenic mice, Berg and colleagues found that expression of class II MHC antigens by cortical epithelial cells was sufficient for positive selection to occur.[135]

Another feature of cell-mediated immunity is self-tolerance. This refers to the inability of T cells to respond against self-antigens. There seems to be more than one explanation for this finding. Some antigens are "sequestered." For example, T cells reactive to antigens in the brain are present in normal individuals. However, these antigens are sequestered under normal circumstances.

Many self-antigens are constantly exposed to the immune system, without evident reaction. One theory is that autoreactive T cells are "deleted" in the thymus.[29] Some data suggest that tolerance may be induced in the medulla by contact with macrophages and/or dendritic cells. Another theory is that autoreactivity is actively suppressed. Multiple mechanisms of tolerance probably exist. The process by which certain T cells are selected and others are deleted remains an area of active research.

SUMMARY

The thymus is the central organ for cell-mediated immunity and is located in the anterosuperior mediastinum. Its size and weight vary widely. As a percentage of total body mass, the weight of the thymus is greatest in the newborn period. Histologically, the thymus has a cortex and medulla composed primarily of epithelial cells, maturing T lymphocytes, and interdigitating dendritic cells. Subpopulations of the different cell types can be identified by studying antigen expression. Myoid cells are a numerically minor cellular element of unknown function that have ultrastructural and immunohistochemical features of muscle. Thymic epithelial cells secrete hormones capable of inducing T-cell differentiation. Complex interactions between the thymus and the endocrine system have been described.

Embryologically, the thymus derives principally from the third pharyngeal pouch. The thymus develops as paired organs that descend into the superior mediastinum and join together. By processes of positive and negative selection in the thymus, T cells become able to respond to certain antigens and not to respond to others.

REFERENCES

1. Williams PL, Warwick R. Gray's Anatomy, 36th edition. Philadelphia: WB Saunders, 1980:780–784.
2. Sarrazin R, Gabell P, Dyon J-F. Anatomical background of the thymus. *In* Sarrazin R, Vrousos C, Vincent F, eds. Thymic Tumors. Basel: Karger, 1989:1–8.
3. Rosai J, Levine GD. Tumors of the Thymus. Washington, DC: Armed Forces Institute of Pathology, 1976:1–21.
4. Kendall MD. Anatomy. *In* Givel J-C, ed. Surgery of the Thymus. Berlin: Springer-Verlag, 1990:19–26.
5. Di Marino V, Argeme M, Brunet C, Coppens R, Bonnoit J. Macroscopic study of the adult thymus. Surg Radiol Anat 1987; 9:51–62.
6. Kato S. Intralobular lymphatic vessels and their relationship to blood vessels in the mouse thymus. Light- and electron-microscopic study. Cell Tissue Res 1988; 253:181–187.
7. Felten DL, Felten SY. Innervation of the thymus. *In* Kendall MD, Ritter MA, eds. Thymus Update 2: T Lymphocyte Differentiation in the Human Thymus. Chur, Switzerland: Harwood Academic Publishers, 1989:73–88.
8. Bulloch K. A comparative study of the autonomic nervous system innervation of the thymus in the mouse and chicken. Intern J Neurosci 1988; 40:129–140.
9. Magni F, Bruschi F, Kasti M. The afferent innervation of the thymus gland in the rat. Brain Res 1987; 424:379–385.
10. Novotny GEK, Sommerfeld H, Zirbes T. Thymic innervation in the rat: a light and electron microscopical study. J Comp Neurol 1990; 302:552–561.
11. Bulloch K, Cullen MR, Schwartz RH, Longo DL. Development of innervation within syngeneic thymus tissue transplanted under the kidney capsule of the nude mouse: a light and ultrastructural microscope study. J Neurosci Res 1987; 18:16–27.
12. Al-Shawaf AA, Kendall MD, Cowen T. Identification of neural profiles containing vasoactive intestinal polypeptide, acetylcholinesterase and catecholamines in the rat thymus. J Anat 1991; 174:131–143.
13. de Leeuw F-E, Jansen GH, Batanero E, van Wichen DF, Huber J, Schuurman H-J. The neural and neuroendocrine component of the human thymus I. Nerve-like structures. Brain Behav Immun 1992; 6:234–248.
14. Boyd E. Growth of the thymus: its relation to status thymicolymphaticus and thymic symptoms. Am J Dis Child 1927; 33:867–879.
15. Young M, Turnbull HM. An analysis of the data collected by the Status Lymphaticus Investigation Committee. J Pathol Bacteriol 1931; 34:213–258.
16. Hammar JA. Die menschen thymus in gesundheit undkrankheit. Z Mikrosk Anat Forsch 1926; 6(Suppl):107–208.
17. Hammar JA. Die menschen thymus in gesundheit undkrankheit. Z Mikrosk Anat Forsch 1928; 16(Suppl):733–771.
18. Steinmann GG. Changes in the human thymus during aging. Curr Top Pathol 1986; 75:43–88.
19. Kendall MD, Johnson HRM, Singh J. The weight of the human thymus gland at necropsy. J Anat 1980; 131:485–499.
20. von Gaudecker B. Functional histology of the human thymus. Anat Embryol 1991; 183:1–15.
21. Suster S, Rosai J. Histology of the normal thymus. Am J Surg Pathol 1990; 14:284–303.
22. Kendall MD. The morphology of perivascular spaces in the thymus. Thymus 1989; 13:157–164.
23. Stet RJM, Wagenaar-Hilbers JP, Nieuwenhuis P. Thymus localization of monoclonal antibodies circumventing the blood-thymus barrier. Scand J Immunol 1987; 25:441–446.
24. Kendall MD. Functional anatomy of the thymic microenvironment. J Anat 1991; 177:1–29.
25. Posselt AM, Naji A, Roark JH, Markmann JF, Barker CF. Intrathymic islet transplantation in the spontaneously diabetic BB rat. Ann Surg 1991; 214:363–373.
26. Boyd RL, Hugo P. Towards an integrated view of thymopoiesis. Immunol Today 1991; 12:71–79.
27. Knapp W, Dorken B, Gilks WR, Rieber EP, Schmidt RE, Stein H, von dem Borne AEGKr, eds. Leucocyte Typing IV: White Cell Differentiation Antigens. Oxford: Oxford University Press, 1989.
28. Reinherz EL, Kung PC, Goldstein G, Levey RH, Schlossman SF. Discrete stages of human intrathymic differentiation: analysis of normal thymocytes and leukemic lymphoblasts of T-cell lineage. Proc Natl Acad Sci U S A 1980; 77:1588–1592.
29. Sprent J. T lymphocytes and the thymus. *In* Paul WE, ed. Fundamental Immunology. New York: Raven Press, 1989:69–93.
30. Swerdlow SH, Angermeier PA, Hartman AL. Intrathymic ontogeny of the T cell receptor associated CD3 (T3) antigen. Lab Invest 1988; 58:421–427.
31. Nikolic-Zugic J. Phenotypic and functional stages in the intrathymic development of alpha beta T cells. Immunol Today 1991; 12:65–70.
32. Kendall MD. The cell biology of cell death in the thymus. *In* Kendall MD, Ritter MA, eds. Thymus Update 3: The Role of the Thymus in Tolerance Induction. Chur, Switzerland: Harwood Academic Publishers, 1990:53–76.
33. Shimizu Y, Newman W, Tanaka Y, Shaw S. Lymphocyte interactions with endothelial cells. Immunol Today 1992; 13:106–112.

34. Albelda SM. Role of integrins and other cell adhesion molecules in tumor progression and metastasis. Lab Invest 1993; 68:4–17.
35. Ruco LP, Paradiso P, Pittiglio M, Diodoro MG, Gearing AJH, Mainiero F, Gismondi A, Sanatoni A, Baroni CD. Tissue distribution of very late activation antigens-1/6 and very late activation antigen ligands in the normal thymus and in thymoma. Am J Pathol 1993; 142:765–772.
36. Picker LJ, Terstappen LW, Rott LS, Streeter PR, Stein H, Butcher EC. Differential expression of homing-associated adhesion molecules by T cell subsets in man. J Immunol 1990; 145:3247–3255.
37. Shortman K, Wilson A, van Ewijk W, Scollay R. Phenotype and localization of thymocytes expressing the homing receptor-associated antigen MEL-14: arguments for the view that most mature thymocytes are located in the medulla. J Immunol 1987; 138:342–351.
38. Dunon D, Imhof BA. Mechanisms of thymus homing. Blood 1993; 81:1–8.
39. Hofmann WJ, Momburg F, Moller P, Otto HF. Intra- and extrathymic B cells in physiologic and pathologic conditions: immunohistochemical study on normal thymus and lymphofollicular hyperplasia of the thymus. Virchows Arch [A] 1988; 412:431–442.
40. Isaacson PG, Norton AJ, Addis BJ. The human thymus contains a novel population of B lymphocytes. Lancet 1987; 2:1488–1491.
41. Middleton G. The incidence of follicular structures in the human thymus at autopsy. Aust J Exp Biol Med Sci 1967; 45:189–199.
42. Haynes BF. The human thymic microenvironment. Adv Immunol 1984; 36:87–142.
43. Kendall MD. Histology. *In* Givel J-C, ed. Surgery of the Thymus. Berlin: Springer-Verlag, 1990:27–43.
44. van de Wijngaert FP, Kendall MD, Schuurman H-J, Rademakers LHPM, Kater L. Heterogeneity of epithelial cells in the human thymus: an ultrastructural study. Cell Tissue Res 1984; 237:227–237.
45. Laster AJ, Itoh T, Palker TJ, Haynes BF. The human thymic microenvironment: thymic epithelium contains specific keratins associated with early and late stages of epidermal keratinocyte maturation. Differentiation 1986; 31:67–77.
46. Fukai I, Masaoka A, Hashimoto T, Yamakawa Y, Mizuno T, Tanamura O. Cytokeratins in normal thymus and thymic epithelial tumors. Cancer 1993; 71:99–105.
47. Lampert IA, Ritter MA. The origin of the diverse epithelial cells of the thymus: is there a common stem cell? *In* Kendall MD, Ritter MA, eds. Thymus Update 1: The Microenvironment of the Human Thymus. Chur, Switzerland: Harwood Academic Publishers, 1989:5–25.
48. Kampinga J, Berges S, Boyd RL, Brekelmans P, Colic M, van Ewijk W, Kendall MD, Ladyman H, Nieuwenhuis P, Ritter MA, Schuurman H-J, Tournefier A. Thymic epithelial antibodies: immunohistological analysis and introduction of nomenclature. Summary of the Epithelium Workshop held at the 2nd Workshop "The Thymus. Histophysiology and Dynamics in the Immune System." Thymus 1989; 13:165–173.
49. Janossy G, Bofill M, Trejdosiewicz LK, Willcox HNA, Chilosi M. Cellular differentiation of lymphoid subpopulations and their microenvironments in the human thymus. Curr Top Pathol 1986; 75:89–125.
50. Hirokawa K, McClure JE, Goldstein AL. Age-related changes in localization of thymosin in the human thymus. Thymus 1982; 4:19–29.
51. Weissman IL. Nursing the thymus [editorial]. Lab Invest 1986; 55:1–4.
52. Carbone FR, Bevan MJ. Major histocompatibility complex control of T cell recognition. *In* Paul WE, ed. Fundamental Immunology. New York: Raven Press, 1989:541–567.
53. Rouse RV, Weissman IL. Microanatomy of the thymus: its relationship to T cell differentiation. Ciba Found Symp 1981; 84:161–177.
54. Henry K. The thymus—what's new. Histopathology 1989; 14:537–548.
55. Henry K, Farrer-Brown G. Color Atlas of Thymus and Lymph Node Histopathology. Chicago: Year Book, 1982:9–44.
56. Gilhus NE, Matre R, Tonder O. Hassall's corpuscles in the thymus of fetuses, infants, and children: immunological and histochemical aspects. Thymus 1985; 7:123–135.
57. Kater L. A note on Hassall's corpuscles. Contemp Top Immunobiol 1973; 2:101–109.
58. Blau JN. Antigen and antibody localization in Hassall's corpuscles. Nature 1967; 215:1073–1075.
59. Sherman JD, Adner MM, Dameshek W. Experimental production of germinal follicles in the thymus. Relationship of Hassall's corpuscles to germinal follicle formation. Ann N Y Acad Sci 1965; 124:105–117.
60. Savino W, Huang PC, Corrigan A, Berrih S, Dardenne M. Thymic hormone-containing cells. V. Immunohistological detection of metallo-thionein within the cells bearing thymulin (a zinc-containing hormone) in human and mouse thymuses. J Histochem Cytochem 1984; 32:942–946.
61. Lobach DF, Scearce RM, Haynes BF. The human thymic microenvironment. Phenotypic characterization of Hassall's bodies with the use of monoclonal antibodies. J Immunol 1985; 134:250–257.
62. Bonnefoy JY, Reano A, Schmitt D, Thivolet J. Thymic Hassall's corpuscles—epidermis antigenic relations defined by a common glycoprotein in man (GP 37). Thymus 1984; 6:387–394.
63. Laster AJ, Haynes BF. Characterization of a monoclonal antibody, RTE-21, that binds to keratohyalin granule-associated proteins in epithelial cells of human skin and thymus. Clin Immunol Immunopathol 1986; 41:130–144.
64. Itoh T, Kasahara S, Aizu S, Kato K, Takeuchi M, Mori T. Formation of Hassall's corpuscles in vitro by the thymic epithelial cell line IT-26R21 of the rat. Cell Tissue Res 1982; 226:469–476.
65. Dipasquale B, Tridente G. Immunohistochemical characterization of nurse cells in normal human thymus. Histochemistry 1991; 96:499–503.
66. De Waal Malefijt R, Leene W, Roholl PJM, Wormmeester J, Hoeben KA. T cell differentiation within thymic nurse cells. Lab Invest 1986; 55:25–34.
67. Leene W, De Waal Malefijt R, Roholl PJM, Hoeben KA. Lymphocyte depletion in thymic nurse cells: a tool to identify in situ lympho-epithelial complexes having thymic nurse cell characteristics. Cell Tissue Res 1988; 253:61–68.
68. Brelinska R. Thymic nurse cells: division of thymocytes within complexes. Cell Tissue Res 1989; 258:637–643.
69. Hiramine C, Hojo K, Koseto M, Nakagawa T, Mukasa A. Establishment of a murine thymic epithelial cell line capable of inducing both thymic nurse cell for-

mation and thymocyte apoptosis. Lab Invest 1990; 62:41–54.
70. Timens W, Boes A, Rozeboom-Uiterwijk T, Poppema S. Immuno-architecture of human fetal lymphoid tissues. Virchows Arch [A] 1988; 413:563–571.
71. Sminia T, van Asselt AA, van de Ende MB, Dijkstra CD. Rat thymus macrophages: an immunohistochemical study on fetal, neonatal and adult thymus. Thymus 1986; 8:141–150.
72. Pelletier M, Tautu C, Landry D, Montplaisir S, Chartrand C, Perreault C. Characterization of human thymic dendritic cells in culture. Immunology 1986; 58:263–270.
73. Nakahama M, Mohri N, Mori S, Shindo G, Yokoi Y, Machinami R. Immunohistochemical and histometrical studies of the human thymus with special emphasis on age-related changes in medullary epithelial and dendritic cells. Virchows Arch [B] 1990; 58:245–251.
74. Nabarra B, Papiernik M. Phenotype of thymic stromal cells: an immunoelectron microscopic study with anti-IA, anti-MAC-1, and anti-MAC-2 antibodies. Lab Invest 1988; 58:524–531.
75. Duijfestijn AM, Barclay AN. Identification of the bone marrow-derived Ia positive cells in the rat thymus: a morphological and cytochemical study. J Leukoc Biol 1984; 36:561–568.
76. Barthelemy H, Pelletier M, Landry D, Lafontaine M, Perreault C, Tautu C, Montplaisir S. Demonstration of OKT6 antigen on human thymic dendritic cells in culture. Lab Invest 1986; 55:540–545.
77. Ruco LP, Pisacane A, Pomponi D, Stoppacciaro A, Pescarmona E, Rendina EA, Santoni A, Boraschi D, Tagliabue A, Uccini S, Baroni CD. Marcophages and interdigitating reticulum cells in normal human thymus and thymomas: immunoreactivity for interleukin-1 alpha, interleukin-1 beta and tumour necrosis factor alpha. Histopathology 1990; 17:291–299.
78. Sato T, Tamaoki N. Myoid cells in the human thymus and thymoma revealed by three different immunohistochemical markers for striated muscle. Acta Pathol Jpn 1989; 39:509–519.
79. Drenckhahn D, von Gaudecker B, Muller-Hermelink HK, Unsicker K, Groschel-Stewart U. Myosin and actin containing cells in the human postnatal thymus: ultrastructural and immunohistochemical findings in normal thymus and in myasthenia gravis. Virchows Arch [B] 1979; 32:33–45.
80. von Gaudecker B. The development of the human thymus microenvironment. Curr Top Pathol 1986; 75:1–41.
81. Nakamura H, Ayer–Le Lievre C. Neural crest and thymic myoid cells. Curr Top Dev Biol 1986; 20:111–115.
82. Seifert R, Christ B. On the differentiation and origin of myoid cells in the avian thymus. Anat Embryol 1990; 181:287–298.
83. Zoltowska A. Myoid and epithelial cell differentiation in myasthenic thymuses. Thymus 1991; 17:237–248.
84. Henry K. The human thymus in disease with particular emphasis on thymitis and thymoma. *In* Kendall MD, ed. The Thymus Gland. London: Academic Press, 1981:85–111.
85. Bhathal PS. Eosinophil leucocytes in the child's thymus. Australas Ann Med 1965; 14:210–213.
86. Dourov N. L'examen microscopique du thymus au cours de la periode perinatale. Ann Pathol 1982; 2:255–261.
87. Taylor CR, Skinner JM. Evidence for significant hematopoiesis in the human thymus. Blood 1976; 47:305–313.
88. Gilmour JR. Some developmental abnormalities of the thymus and parathyroids. J Pathol Bacteriol 1941; 52:213–218.
89. Wolff M, Rosai J, Wright DH. Sebaceous glands within the thymus: report of three cases. Hum Pathol 1984; 15:341–343.
90. Geenen V, Robert F, Defresne M-P, Boniver J, Legros J-J, Franchimont P. Neuroendocrinology of the thymus. Horm Res 1989; 31:81–84.
91. Jevremovic M, Terzic M, Kartaljevic G, Popovic V, Rosic B, Filipovic S. The determination of immunoreactive beta-endorphin concentration in the human fetal and neonatal thymus. Horm Metab Res 1991; 23:623–624.
92. Batanero E, de Leeuw F-E, Jansen GH, van Wichen DF, Huber J, Schuurman H-J. The neural and neuroendocrine component of the human thymus. II. Hormone immunoreactivity. Brain Behav Immun 1992; 6:249–264.
93. Kendall MD. Anatomical and physiological factors influencing the thymic microenvironment. *In* Kendall MD, Ritter MA, eds. Thymus Update 1: The Microenvironment of the Human Thymus. Chur, Switzerland: Harwood Academic Publishers, 1989:27–65.
94. Khansari DN, Murgo AJ, Faith RE. Effects of stress on the immune system. Immunol Today 1990; 11:170–175.
95. Fabris N, Mocchegiani E, Mariotti S, Paccini F, Pinchera A. Thyroid-thymus interactions during development and aging. Horm Res 1989; 31:85–89.
96. Dardenne M, Savino W, Bach J-F. Modulation of thymic endocrine function by thyroid and steroid hormones. Intern J Neurosci 1988; 39:325–334.
97. Mocchegiani E, Paolucci P, Balsamo A, Cacciari E, Fabris N. Influence of growth hormone on thymic endocrine activity in humans. Horm Res 1990; 33:248–255.
98. Marine D, Manley OT, Baumann EJ. The influence of thyroidectomy, gonadectomy, suprarenalectomy, and splenectomy on the thymus gland of rabbits. J Exp Med 1924; 40:429–443.
99. Bloom DF, Bloch GJ, Gorski RA. Effects of thymectomy on reproductive function and behavior. Physiol Behav 1992; 52:291–298.
100. Wainberg MA, Numazaki K, Destephano L, Wong I, Goldman H. Infection of human thymic epithelial cells by human cytomegalovirus and other viruses: effect on secretion of interleukin-1-like activity. Clin Exp Immunol 1988; 72:415–421.
101. Le PT, Kurtzberg J, Brandt SJ, Niedel JE, Haynes BF, Singer KH. Human thymic epithelial cells produce granulocyte and macrophage colony-stimulating factors. J Immunol 1988; 141:1211–1217.
102. Le PT, Lazorick S, Whichard LP, Yang Y-C, Clark SC, Haynes BF, Singer KH. Human thymic epithelial cells produce IL-6, granulocyte-monocyte-csf, and leukemia inhibitory factor. J Immunol 1990; 145:3310–3315.
103. Millan FA, Denhez F, Kondaiah P, Akhurst RJ. Embryonic gene expression patterns of TGF beta-1, beta-2, and beta-three suggest different developmental functions in vivo. Development 1991; 111:131–143.
104. Ellingsworth LR, Brennan JE, Fok K, Rosen DM, Bentz H, Piez KA, Seyedin SM. Antibodies to the N-terminal portion of cartilage-inducing factor A and transforming growth factor beta. J Biol Chem 1986; 261:12362–12367.

105. Inge TH, McCoy KM, Susskind BM, Barrett SK, Zhao G, Bear HD. Immunomodulatory effects of transforming growth factor-beta on T lymphocytes: induction of CD8 expression in the CTLL-2 cell line and in normal thymocytes. J Immunol 1992; 148:3847–3856.
106. Fava RA, Piltch AS. Histological distribution of the 35 kd protein substrate of the epidermal growth factor receptor/kinase in thymus. J Histochem Cytochem 1987; 35:1309–1315.
107. Kendall MD. Anatomical and physiological factors influencing the thymic environment. *In* Kendall MD, Ritter MA, eds. Thymus Update 1: The Microenvironment of the Human Thymus. Chur, Switzerland: Harwood Academic Publishers, 1988:27–65.
108. Willcox N. The thymus in myasthenia gravis patients, and the in vivo effects of corticosteroids on its cellularity, histology, and functions. *In* Kendall MD, Ritter MA, eds. Thymus Update 2: T Lymphocyte Differentiation in the Human Thymus. Chur, Switzerland: Harwood Academic Publishers, 1989:105–124.
109. Haynes BF, Scearce RM, Lobach DF, Hensley LL. Phenotypic characterization and ontogeny of mesodermal-derived and endocrine epithelial components of the human thymic microenvironment. J Exp Med 1984; 159:1149–1168.
110. Elbe A, Kilgus O, Strohal R, Payer E, Schreiber S, Stingl G. Fetal skin: a site of dendritic epidermal T cell development. J Immunol 1992; 149:1694–1701.
111. Fukayama M, Hayashi Y, Shiozawa Y, Maeda Y, Koike M. Human chorionic gonadotropin in the thymus: an immunocytochemical study on discordant expression of subunits. Am J Pathol 1990; 136:123–129.
112. Rosai J, Levine G, Weber WR, Higa E. Carcinoid tumors and oat cell carcinomas of the thymus. Pathol Annu 1976; 11:201–226.
113. Rosai J, Higa E. Mediastinal endocrine neoplasm, of probable thymic origin, related to carcinoid tumor. Clinicopathologic study of 8 cases. Cancer 1972; 29:1061–1074.
114. Langman J. Medical Embryology. Baltimore: Williams & Wilkins, 1981:273–276.
115. Norris EH. The morphogenesis and histogenesis of the thymus gland in man: in which the origin of the Hassall's corposcles of the human thymus is discovered. Contrib Embryol 1938; 166:191–221.
116. Shier KJ. The thymus according to Schambacher: medullary ducts and reticular epithelium of thymus and thymomas. Cancer 1981; 48:1183–1199.
117. Shier KJ. The morphology of the epithelial thymus: observations on lymphocyte-depleted and fetal thymus. Lab Invest 1963; 12:316–326.
118. Gilmour JR. The embryology of the parathyroid glands, the thymus, and certain associated rudiments. J Pathol Bacteriol 1937; 45:507–522.
119. Leong ASY. Thymic cysts. *In* Givel J-C, ed. Surgery of the Thymus. Berlin: Springer-Verlag, 1990:71–77.
120. Wick MR. Mediastinal cysts and intrathoracic thyroid tumors. Semin Diagn Pathol 1990; 7:285–294.
121. Wenglowski R. Ueber die halsfistein und cysten. Arch Klin Chir 1912; 100:789–892.
122. Damiani S, Filotico M, Eusebi V. Carcinoma of the thyroid showing thymoma-like features. Virchows Arch [A] 1991; 418:463–466.
123. Fukai I, Funato Y, Mizuno T, Hashimoto T, Masaoka A. Distribution of thymic tissue in the mediastinal adipose tissue. J Thorac Cardiovasc Surg 1991; 101:1099–1102.
124. Spigland N, Bensoussan AL, Blanchard H, Russo P. Aberrant cervical thymus in children: three case reports and review of the literature. J Pediatr Surg 1990; 25:1196–1199.
125. Bale PM, Sotelo-Avila C. Maldescent of the thymus: 34 necropsy and 10 surgical cases, including 7 thymuses medial to the mandible. Pediatr Pathol 1993; 13:181–190.
126. Hagens EW. Malformation of the auditory apparatus in the newborn. Arch Otolaryngol 1932; 15:671–680.
127. Masaoka A, Nagaoka Y, Kotake Y. Distribution of thymic tissue at the anterior mediastinum: current procedures in thymectomy. J Thorac Cardiovasc Surg 1975; 70:747–754.
128. Bockman DE, Kirby ML. Neural crest function in thymus development. Immunol Ser 1989; 45:451–467.
129. Muller-Hermelink HK, Marino M, Palestro G. Pathology of thymic epithelial tumors. Curr Top Pathol 1986; 75:208–268.
130. Weller GL. Development of the thyroid, parathyroid, and thymus glands in man. Contrib Embryol 1933; 141:95–138.
131. Le Lievre CS, Le Douarin NM. Mesenchymal derivatives of the neural crest: analysis of chimaeric quail and chick embryos. J Embryol Exp Morph 1975; 34:125–154.
132. Manning MJ. A comparative view of the thymus in vertebrates (abstract). J Anat 1981; 132:439–440.
133. Manning MJ. A comparative view of the thymus in vertebrates. *In* Kendall MD, ed. The Thymus Gland. London: Academic Press, 1981:7–20.
134. Benoist C, Mathis D. Positive selection of the T cell repertoire: where and when does it occur? Cell 1989; 58:1027–1033.
135. Berg LJ, Pullen AM, Fazekas de St Groth B, Mathis D, Benoist C, Davis MM. Antigen/MHC-specific T cells are preferentially exported from the thymus in the presence of their MHC ligand. Cell 1989; 58:1035–1046.

Chapter

4

NON-NEOPLASTIC PATHOLOGY OF THE THYMUS

GERMINAL CENTER HYPERPLASIA (LYMPHOFOLLICULAR HYPERPLASIA)

STRESS-RELATED CHANGES

TRUE THYMIC HYPERPLASIA (THYMIC HYPERPLASIA WITH MASSIVE ENLARGEMENT, MASSIVE THYMIC HYPERPLASIA)

CONGENITAL THYMIC DISORDERS
- DiGeorge Syndrome
- Primary Immunodeficiency Disorders and Thymic Dysplasia

ACQUIRED IMMUNODEFICIENCY SYNDROME (AIDS)

BONE MARROW TRANSPLANTATION

CYCLOSPORIN A

INFECTIONS

ANOXIA

MALNUTRITION

VASCULITIS

RADIATION

DOWN'S SYNDROME

CYSTS

TOXIC AGENTS

GERMINAL CENTER HYPERPLASIA (LYMPHOFOLLICULAR HYPERPLASIA)

Germinal center hyerplasia refers to the presence of germinal centers within the thymus (Fig. 4–1). The germinal centers appear to be within the medulla, and the expanded medulla seems to produce a thinning of the cortex. Actually, the germinal centers are within the perivascular (or paraseptal) space.[1, 2] Some authors advocate use of the term thymitis to describe these changes in the thymic microenvironment.[3, 4] The borders of the perivascular space can be demonstrated around the germinal centers with a reticulin stain (Fig. 4–2) or by immunoperoxidase staining with an antibody to laminin, a component of the basement membrane.[1, 5] The germinal centers vary in number and size.[6] They are not uniformly distributed, and thus, several sections from different areas of the thymus may need to be examined.[7] Follicular hyperplasia of the thymus has been associated with myasthenia gravis, but is not specific to this disorder.

Myasthenia gravis (MG) is an autoimmune disease characterized clinically by muscle weakness accentuated by fatigue.[8] Eighty to ninety percent of patients have serum antibody to the nicotinic acetylcholine receptor of skeletal muscle. The antibody binds to the receptor and interferes with neuromuscular transmission at the motor endplate. Although this aspect of the disease is well understood, the reason that these patients develop the autoantibody is not known.

Histologically, thymic abnormalities occur in approximately 80% of MG patients.[9] In the United States, about 10% of patients have a thymoma (see Chapter 5), and approximately two thirds of patients with MG have germinal centers in the thymus.[10] Because of these histologic changes, the thymus is thought to have a role in the pathogenesis of this disorder.

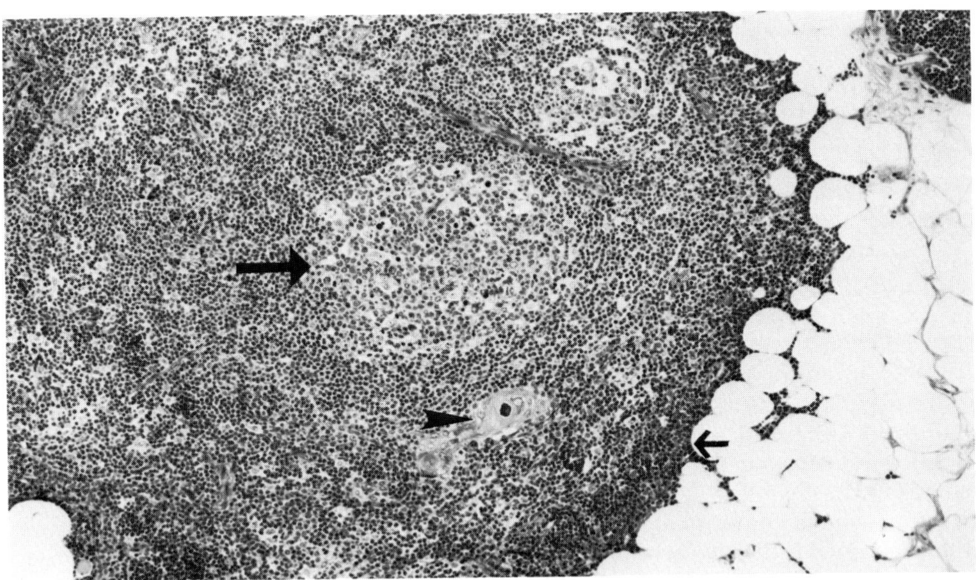

Figure 4–1. Thymus from a 22-year-old with myasthenia gravis illustrates germinal center *(large arrow)*, Hassall's corpuscle *(arrowhead)*, and thinned cortex *(small arrow)* (H & E, ×100).

One hypothesis is that autosensitization against the acetylcholine receptor (AchR) occurs in the thymus. A possible source of AchR in the thymus is the myoid cell. The myoid cell is an actin- and desmin-containing cell with Z bands characteristic of skeletal muscle[8] (see Chapter 3.) It is a minor cell population numerically but has been demonstrated to express AchR.[11, 12] With the polymerase chain reaction, messenger RNA for the alpha chain of the AchR has been identified in nonlymphoid cells of the mouse thymus and in human thymic epithelial cell lines.[13] Similar findings have been reported for human thymus and thymoma from MG patients.[14]

The evidence is conflicting as to whether myoid cells are more or less numerous in the MG-affected thymus. Some investigators report increased myoid cells in MG,[15] others find myoid cells decreased,[16] and yet others find no difference between MG-affected and normal thymus.[17, 18]

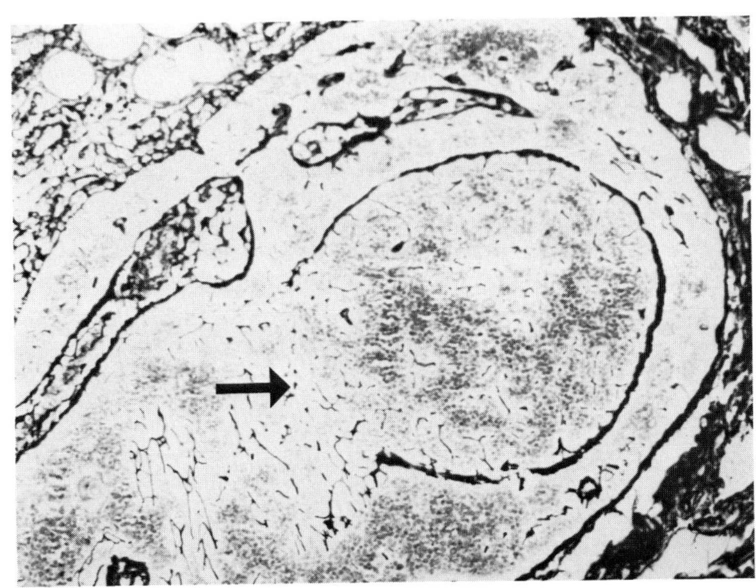

Figure 4–2. Silver stain demonstrates reticulin surrounding germinal center. In one area, the reticulin appears fenestrated *(arrow)* (H & E, ×100).

Other cell types in the thymus, including subsets of epithelial cells[11, 12] and lymphocytes,[19] also contain antigens cross-reactive with antibodies to AchR. Perhaps some immunologic breakdown leads to antibody production against the AchR. The antibody would then also react with AchR at motor endplates throughout the body. The thymic germinal centers would be a manifestation of the immune response at the site of sensitization. Interleukin production has been demonstrated in the MG-affected thymus and may be involved in this immune response.[20] Interestingly, in the experimental model for MG, animals immunized with AchR develop symptoms similar to those of MG but do not have histologic changes in the thymus.[21]

In vitro studies have demonstrated anti–acetylcholine receptor antibody production by thymic B cells.[22] Furthermore, the level of antibody production generally correlates with the numbers of germinal centers. Those patients with more numerous thymic germinal centers tend to have higher autoantibody titers.[23, 24] Seronegative patients have fewer and smaller germinal centers.[25] Immunoperoxidase studies on frozen sections of MG-affected thymus have demonstrated no abnormality in distribution of T-cell subsets.[26] B cells localize primarily to the germinal centers in the pattern typical for lymphoid follicles elsewhere, with immunoglobulin D (IgD)-positive cells in the mantle zone and IgM-positive cells in both the mantle and germinal center.[26] Using immunofluorescence on cell suspensions, Ferrio and colleagues found a decreased percentage of cortical lymphocytes (CD1+) and increased B cells (CD20+) in the MG-affected thymus.[27] These findings are in accord with the immunohistologic data.

The perivascular space of the MG-affected thymus may be expanded not only by germinal centers but also by T cells and scattered B cells. These areas have been described as "lymph-node-like" because they contain T-cell zones (resembling paracortex of lymph nodes) as well as germinal centers. Unlike the thymic parenchyma, these lymphocytic areas contain no epithelial cells.[3, 25, 28] (Fig. 4–3). As in the lymph node, the T-cell zones contain fibronectin.[5]

The lymph-node-like T-cell areas are present in the thymus of MG patients in whom the germinal centers are less prominent or absent.[25, 29] Some investigators have found the T-cell zones to be a more constant feature of the MG-affected thymus than germinal centers.[25, 28] Like the germinal centers, the T-cell areas may represent a response to intrathymic antigens. Wirt and colleagues have questioned whether the changes described in the MG-affected thymus are unique to this disorder. They find similar changes in patients without MG or other immune-mediated disease.[30] They suggest that thymic B-cell activation is a "final common pathway" resulting from various antigenic stimuli.

The histologic changes associated with MG have been interpreted as representing lymph-node-like tissue pushing into the thymic medulla from the perivascular space. The fenestrated basement membrane near the germinal centers (see Fig. 4–2) suggests breakdown of the barrier separating the perivascular space from the thymic parenchyma.[5] This breakdown may allow for communication among the various epithelial and lymphoreticular cells. Perhaps this breakdown allows for autosensitization against AchR.

Another reported finding associated with

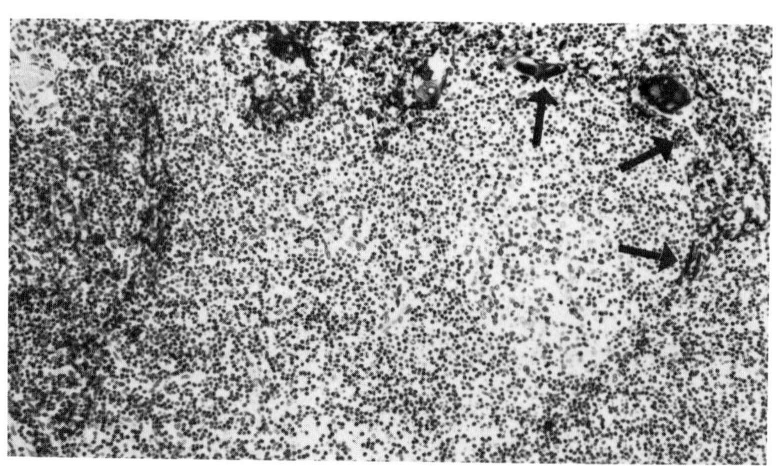

Figure 4–3. Thymus from a myasthenia gravis patient. Immunoperoxidase stain for cytokeratin shows lymphoid tissue that appears to "push" the medullary epithelium aside *(arrows)* (H & E, ×100).

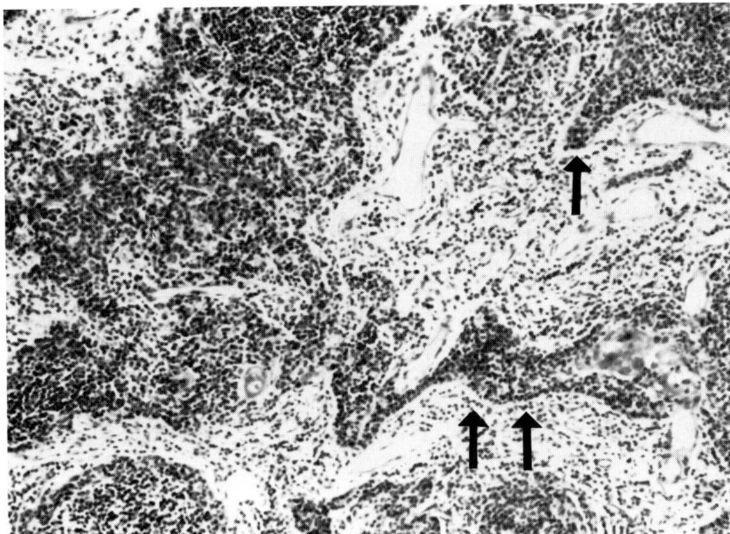

Figure 4–4. Thymus from a myasthenia gravis patient demonstrates prominent bands of medullary epithelium *(arrows)* and intervening lymphoid tissue (H & E, ×100).

the MG-affected thymus is hyperplasia of medullary epithelium.[4, 28, 31] In normal thymus, the medulla contains a loose network of epithelial cells. In the MG-affected thymus, the medulla may contain bands of epithelial cells (Fig. 4–4). These bands are separated from the lymph-node-like areas (T-cell zones and germinal centers) by a layer of laminin. It is not clear to this author whether the bands of medullary epithelium result from epithelial hyperplasia or from compression of normal medulla by the lymph-node-like areas. Increased mucus secretion by the epithelial cells, particularly in Hassall's corpuscles, has also been described in MG.[31]

Occasional patients with MG have thymic involution with strands of thymic parenchyma scattered within adipose tissue[3] (Fig. 4–5). The atrophic MG-affected thymus has only minor changes in the perivascular space. Thymic involution is more common in male patients over the age of 40 years, whereas follicular hyperplasia tends to occur in females under the age of 40 years.[32] MG patients with thymic follicular hyperplasia have an increased incidence of other autoimmune disorders, includ-

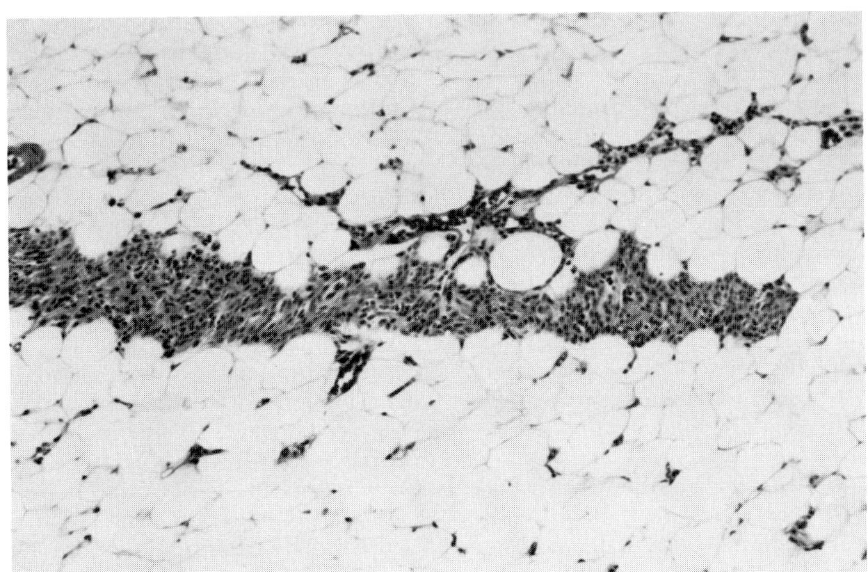

Figure 4–5. Thymus from an older myasthenia gravis patient illustrates atrophic changes. Strands of thymic tissue within fat have few lymphocytes and lack corticomedullary differentiation (H & E, ×100).

ing rheumatoid arthritis, systemic lupus erythematosus, and thyroiditis.[33] Investigators have reported differences in human leukocyte antigen (HLA) associations between these two groups.[32, 34] The younger group is associated with HLA-A1, -B8, and -DRw3, whereas the older group is associated with HLA-A3, -B7, and -DRw2.

MG patients have been reported to develop "histioeosinophilic granulomas" in the thymus.[35] These lesions occurred only in patients who had had a diagnostic pneumomediastinum prior to thymectomy. The lesions resemble histiocytosis X (eosinophilic granuloma) except that they are located only within the capsule and septa of the thymus. They do not have the immunohistochemical and ultrastructural characteristics of histiocytosis X (i.e., they have no S100 and lack Birbeck granules).

Halicek and Rosai believe the histioeosinophilic granulomas are the thymic counterpart to reactive eosinophilic pleuritis, a nonspecific reaction to pleural injury associated in many cases with spontaneous pneumothorax.[35] Of interest, those MG patients who developed these thymic granulomas had a significantly increased probability of remission compared with those who did not have granulomas. At the current time, diagnostic pneumomediastinum has been replaced by newer imaging techniques. Thus, thymic histioeosinophilic granuloma may be of historic interest only.

Because of histologic changes in the thymus, thymectomy has long been advocated as a therapeutic option. Most patients (60 to 80%) will improve after thymectomy,[36–39] although no controlled study has ever evaluated this treatment modality. Some investigators advocate an extended mediastinal dissection. The extended procedure includes splitting the sternum and removing all mediastinal fat that might contain thymic tissue.[40] Others claim that an extended thymic resection is unnecessary.[37] The reason for improvement after thymectomy is not clear. No changes in lymphocyte subsets have been found in patients after thymectomy.[41] Autoantibody titers do decrease, but the titer does not always correlate with disease activity.[42] There is no consistent relationship between extent of thymic germinal center hyperplasia and course of disease.[6, 43]

It is important to realize that individuals without MG also have germinal centers in the thymus. Thymic germinal centers occur in patients with other autoimmune disorders, including systemic lupus erythematosus, rheumatoid arthritis, rheumatic heart disease, Graves' disease, Hashimoto's thyroiditis, and Addison's disease.[1, 4, 44] Michie and Gunn biopsied the thymus in patients with thyroid disease at the time of thyroidectomy.[44] These authors found thymic germinal centers in 38% of patients (29 of 77) with thyrotoxicosis and in 2 of 4 patients with Hashimoto's disease. Thymic germinal centers have also been reported in patients with the acquired immunodeficiency syndrome (AIDS)[45, 46] and multiple sclerosis.[47]

Even healthy individuals may have thymic germinal centers. Indeed, in one autopsy study, healthy young adults who died suddenly were as likely to have germinal centers in the thymus as were patients with MG.[48] Follicles were not present in neonatal thymus. Thymic germinal centers were less common in patients with illness and advancing age.[48, 49] The MG patients do have larger and more numerous thymic germinal centers, especially when compared with hospitalized patients in autopsy studies. Also, as discussed above, the MG-affected thymus has other changes in addition to germinal centers. However, the specificity of these changes for MG requires further study.

One common misconception is that the thymus in MG patients is enlarged. This does not seem to be the case.[1, 10] Thymic hyperplasia in MG patients refers to the presence of germinal centers and should more precisely be termed "germinal center hyperplasia" or "lymphofollicular hyperplasia" of the thymus. A study comparing actual size or weight of the thymus in untreated MG patients with that of age- and sex-matched controls has not been done to this authors's knowledge. In an early report by Castleman and Norris, the weight of non-neoplastic MG-affected thymuses was within normal limits.[10] In a study of patients with thyroid disease, Michie and colleagues found that the size of the thymus was unrelated to the presence of germinal centers.[50]

The New Zealand mouse (strain NZB), an animal model for autoimmune disease, develops thymic germinal centers.[51] The germinal centers develop between 3 and 9 months of age. They tend to occur earlier and, on average, are more extensive in females. The germinal centers in the NZB mice are thought to be evidence of generalized autoimmune disease rather than a primary thymic disease process. The nonobese diabetic mouse, an animal model for human type I (autoimmune) diabetes, also develops thymic germinal centers.[52] Mice of other strains without immune disorders do not have germinal centers in the thymus. Thus, laboratory animals appear to develop thymic germinal centers as a manifestation of systemic autoimmune disorders.

Perhaps the germinal centers in the human MG-affected thymus are a manifestation of systemic autoimmune disease rather than a primary thymic disease process. One wonders whether thymectomy would have the same effect in other autoimmune disorders that it has in myasthenia. Indeed, thymectomy has been performed in small numbers of patients with other autoimmune disorders but with limited success.[53]

STRESS-RELATED CHANGES

As discussed earlier, the thymus undergoes progressive involution with age (see Chapter 3). The thymus may also involute much more quickly as a reaction to various stimuli, including malnutrition, trauma, and illness.[54–57] In laboratory animals, physiologic events such as pregnancy and lactation also induce thymic involution.[58] The involution is reversible, and its extent correlates with the duration of the stimulus.

The degree of involution can be appreciated both by measuring thymic weight and by assessing the histologic changes. Thymic weight as a measure of involution is complicated by age-related differences and marked variability among normal individuals. Thus, microscopic examination is a better method to study involution.

Van Baarlen and colleagues correlated changes in thymic histology with duration of illness at autopsy in 234 fetuses and children.[54] No changes in thymic histology occurred in those who died within 12 hours. Histiocytes containing debris of phagocytosed lymphocytes appeared in the cortex in most cases after 12 to 24 hours. The lymphophagocytosis became more prominent and produced a "starry sky" appearance in the cortex after 24 to 48 hours (Fig. 4–6). Also, the cortex began to thin.

With increasing duration of illness, the distinction between the cortex and medulla was less evident as the thymus became depleted of cortical lymphocytes (Fig. 4–7). An "inverted" histologic pattern resulted from the lymphocytes being depleted in the cortex but preserved in the medulla. Increasing separation of the lobules was also noted. By 72 hours of illness, the thymus appeared severely involuted. No further histologic changes were evident beyond 72 hours. An additional feature noted by Dourov is the presence of numerous lipid-laden cells within the atrophic thymic lobules and connective tissue of infants treated with large doses of adrenocorticotropic hormone (ACTH) and in those dying after long illnesses.[55] The digestion of cellular material

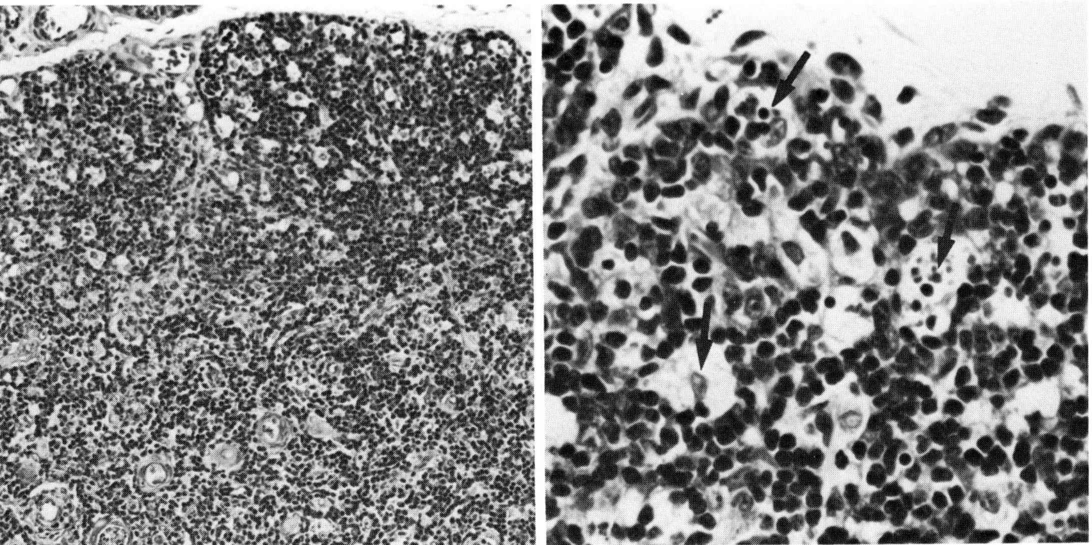

Figure 4–6. Early stress-related histologic changes in the thymus. *Left,* The earliest change is the "starry sky" appearance of the cortex (H & E, ×100). *Right,* With higher magnification, the white spaces in the cortex can be identified as the tingible-body macrophages *(arrows)* (H & E, ×400).

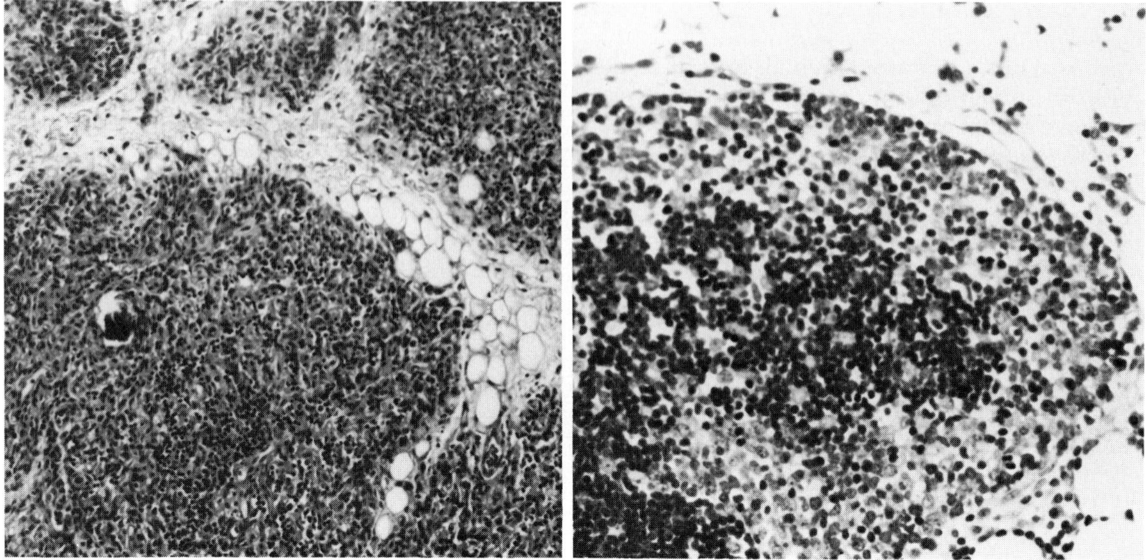

Figure 4–7. With prolonged stress of several days, the cortical lymphocytes become progressively depleted. *Left,* Corticomedullary differentiation becomes inapparent as illustrated on the left. Also note the calcified Hassall's corpuscle in the left central portion of the photograph. The medullary lymphocytes are relatively unaffected (H & E, ×100). *Right,* Progressive depletion of cortical lymphocytes may result in the inverted appearance in which the medulla is more cellular than the cortex (H & E, ×200).

results in accumulation of lipid. Dourov also noted that Hassall's corpuscles usually persist and may become cystic.

Van Baarlen and colleagues studied phenotypic changes in acute thymic involution.[57] In severe involution, they found a depletion of CD1-positive, cortical lymphocytes, whereas the phenotypically mature lymphocytes in the medulla were unchanged. Similarly, the expression of Ki-67, a marker of proliferating cells, decreased in the subcapsular and cortical areas with higher grades of involution. The epithelial cells were generally unaffected as to reactivity with cytokeratin and antiepithelial cell antibodies, although decreased immunoreactivity for thymosin alpha-1 and beta-4 was noted. HLA-DR expression by medullary interdigitating dendritic cells decreased with increasing involution.

The acute involutional changes have been attributed to endogenous steroid production as a response to stress.[56] Similar histologic findings have been reported in laboratory animals following glucocorticoid injection.[55, 59, 60] After in vitro glucocorticoid exposure, cortical lymphocytes undergo "apoptosis" (i.e., changes characteristic of cell death). Twelve to sixteen hours after the first injection, the cortex has the starry sky appearance. Maximum involution is reached 3 to 6 days after the last dose. At this time, the cortex is reduced to one fourth its normal thickness. The organ lacks lobulation. An inverted microscopic appearance results because medullary lymphocytes are relatively steroid resistant.[56] Mast cells are increased in the capsule and interlobular septa.[60]

Histologically, epithelial cells appear relatively unaffected by steroids. However, epithelial cells do express glucocorticoid receptors. In mice, hydrocortisone injection modulates the expression of high-molecular-weight cytokeratin and decreases thymulin secretion.[61]

With cessation of steroids, the thymus regenerates. By 10 to 12 days after the last dose of hydrocortisone, the mouse thymus appears histologically normal.[59]

TRUE THYMIC HYPERPLASIA (THYMIC HYPERPLASIA WITH MASSIVE ENLARGEMENT, MASSIVE THYMIC HYPERPLASIA)

True thymic hyperplasia (TTH) refers to an actual increase in thymic size. Normal thymic size was studied extensively in the early 1900s (see Chapter 2). However, some of the data have been criticized for excluding "exceptionally heavy thymuses."[62] More recently, Steinmann studied the weight and volume of the thymus in individuals who died suddenly[62] (see

Chapter 3, Table 3–1). According to his data, the thymus grows only during the first year of life. Almost the entire range of sizes is reached during the first months of life.

Kendall and colleagues studied 574 coroners' autopsies and found a slight decrease in mean weight with age. However, marked variation occurred at all ages.[63] Nevertheless, all thymus glands in their study weighed less than 55 g. If TTH is considered to involve a thymus weighing more than two standard deviations above the mean,[64] then the definition according to Steinmann's data (using the maximum normal age-specific range) would be a condition in which the thymus weighs more than 67 g. Arliss and colleagues define massive thymic hyperplasia as a condition in which a normal-appearing thymus weighs more than 100 g.[65]

Clinically, TTH occurs in three settings: in individuals without pre-existing disease, those recovering from stress, and those with other disorders, usually hyperthyroidism (Table 4–1). Grossly, the normal thymic configuration is usually retained, although some reports describe an encapsulated tumor-like mass[64, 66, 67] (Fig. 4–8).

Histologically, TTH has the appearance of normal thymus. Adipose tissue may be present.[64, 65] Unlike thymolipoma, true thymic hyperplasia should have only a minor component of adipose tissue.

Of more importance is the separation of TTH from lymphocytic thymoma. The former should retain normal lobular architecture with well-defined cortex and medulla. Hassall's corpuscles are readily identifiable. In contrast, a lymphocytic thymoma should have a fibrous capsule and broad fibrous bands. Corticomedullary differentiation is absent or relatively indistinct. Hassall's corpuscles are infrequent.

Table 4–1. True Thymic Hyperplasia

Idiopathic
"Rebound"
Hyperthyroidism (and, less commonly, other disorders)

Lymphoblastic lymphoma must also be considered. On fine-needle aspiration of TTH or on small biopsy specimens, the finding of terminal deoxynucleotidyl transferase in lymphoblasts might lead to the erroneous diagnosis of lymphoblastic lymphoma or lymphocytic thymoma.[68] Immunoperoxidase stains for cytokeratin help to identify the epithelial cells of a thymoma or thymic hyperplasia but would not distinguish between these two entities. Knowledge of the clinical setting is also important.

Histologically confirmed TTH is uncommon, and the literature on the subject is limited to case reports and small series.[64–80] The idiopathic form occurs usually in asymptomatic patients; a routine chest radiograph leads to the diagnosis. The ages of the patients range from 7 months to 21 years (Table 4–2). An occasional patient has respiratory difficulty.[66, 81] Some have a lymphocytosis in the peripheral blood. For example, a 1-year-old pa-

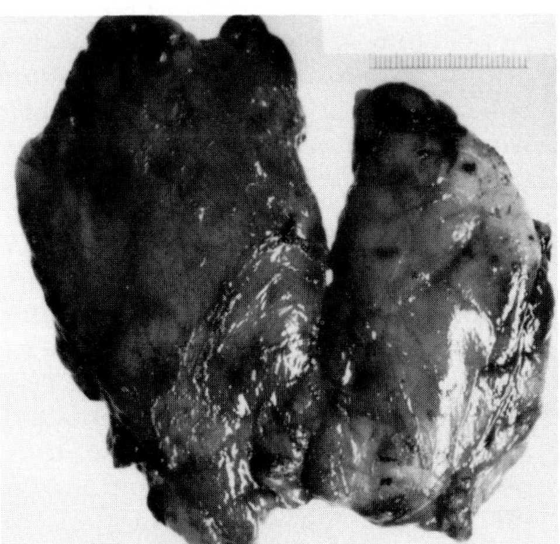

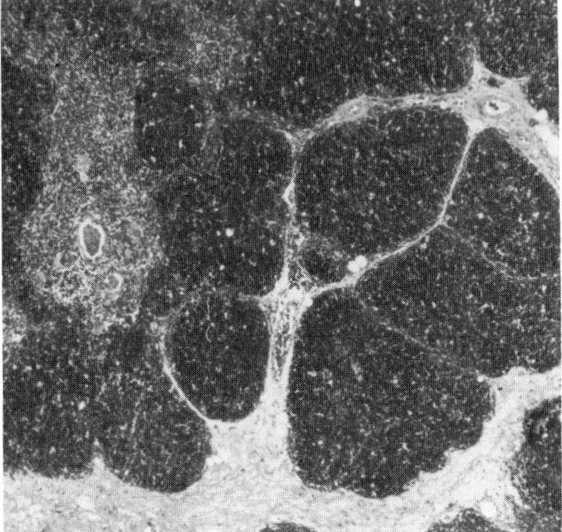

Figure 4–8. *Left*, Gross appearance of true thymic hyperplasia. The enlarged thymus (77 g) was excised from a 16-year-old with a testicular mixed germ cell tumor. The patient was thought to have a mediastinal mass after completing chemotherapy. Note the thymus has maintained its normal bilobed configuration. *Right*, Microscopic appearance showing lobules with corticomedullary differentiation (H & E, ×40).

Table 4–2. Idiopathic True Thymic Hyperplasia: Review of Literature

Age	Sex	Thymus Weight (g)	Peripheral Blood	Symptoms	Reference
10 years	f	93	Normal	Cough	71
5 years	f	(bx)	Leukocytosis	None	71
11 years	f	(bx)		None	71
7 months	m	224	Lymphocytosis		70
1 year	m	420	Lymphocytosis	Dyspnea	66
4 years	f	800	Lymphocytosis	Enteritis	79
22 months	f	550		None	67
11 years	m	324	Normal	Dyspnea	64
14 years	m	490	Normal	None	64
15 years	m	680	Lymphocytosis	Hepatitis	65
16 years	m	230	Normal	None	72
12 years	m	120	Normal	Dyspnea	72
14 years	m	840		Dyspnea	72
5 years	m	950	Lymphocytosis	Dyspnea	72
12 years	m	245		Dyspnea	73
21 years	m	105		Sepsis	74
15 years	f	102		Diabetes mellitus	80

tient is reported who presented with respiratory distress and had an absolute lymphocytosis of 15,200/mm^3 with 92% T cells (E-rosette positive lymphocytes).[66] The lymphocytosis resolved after surgical excision of a 420-g thymus.

An early report suggested an abnormality in T-cell maturation.[71] More recent studies have demonstrated the normal distribution of T cells, epithelial cells, and myoid cells.[73, 76, 82] Most asymptomatic patients are infants or young children. However, a 21-year-old who died of fulminant meningococcal sepsis was reported to have a 105-g histologically normal thymus.[74]

An enlarged thymus gland may regress transiently after steroid therapy.[83] Thus, a course of steroids has been advocated to obtain a better cardiac image on chest radiographs in selected patients[83] and to support a diagnosis of TTH.[84] However, most reports of oral steroid administration to reduce TTH show unsuccessful results.[66, 67, 81, 84] Moreover, response to steroids does not distinguish TTH from a thymic malignancy. Not only lymphoma, but also thymoma may reduce in size in response to steroids.

The second group of patients have "rebound" TTH. In these cases, a preceding stress is identified. For example, Lee et al. report a 22-month-old infant with a large mediastinal mass noted 1 month after hospitalization for second-degree burns on both lower extremities.[67] When excised, the 550-g specimen had the histologic appearance of normal thymus. Gelfand and colleagues reported 5 children (ages 5 to 12 years) with thymic hyperplasia after burn injuries.[85] The enlargement occurred 5 to 9 months after the injury. In three patients who did not have surgery, the thymus decreased in size over 3 to 10 months. Rebound thymic enlargement has also been reported after surgery for congenital heart disease.[86]

Rebound TTH may also occur after chemotherapy. Patients with Hodgkin's disease, germ cell tumors, and childhood neoplasms have been reported to develop thymic hyperplasia.[77, 82, 87–91] Radiographically, these mediastinal lesions arouse suspicion of recurrent or residual malignancy. When excised, the mass appears to be normal thymus (Fig. 4–8). Thus, TTH may occur as a rebound reaction to stress, including aggressive chemotherapy. The reported cases are in children or young adults.

TTH may also occur in association with lymphoma at the time of diagnosis. Nomori and colleagues reported a case of non-Hodgkin's lymphoma in a 14-year-old.[75] At presentation, the child underwent excision of a 125-g mediastinal mass that turned out to be TTH. A diffuse mixed small- and large-cell lymphoma was diagnosed in mediastinal lymph nodes, which also had features of angiofollicular hyperplasia (Castleman's disease) (see Chapter 6). The authors suggest that the TTH and Castleman's disease–like changes both represent an unusual immune response to the lymphoma. Alternatively, this case may represent the coincidental occurrence of idiopathic TTH and lymphoma.

TTH may be a frequent occurrence; however, only the unusually large cases get biopsied or excised. For example, radiographic studies document frequent thymic enlargement after chemotherapy. Kissin and colleagues studied 200 patients (ages 16 to 50) with malignant teratoma of the testis by serial computed tomography (CT) scans.[92] The size of the thymus was assessed on initial and follow-up scans. The authors found an enlarging thymus in 14 of 120 patients (12%) who had received chemotherapy. Thymic enlargement occurred from 3 to 14 months (mean = 7.5 months) after beginning chemotherapy. The thymic volume increased up to 64 times. One patient underwent surgical excision, which confirmed the diagnosis of TTH (thymic weight 160 g). One of 80 patients who did not receive chemotherapy (orchiectomy only) developed minimal thymic enlargement.

Interestingly, among the patients who received chemotherapy, those with thymic enlargement had a significantly better disease-free survival rate (93% vs. 78% with mean follow-up of 45 months, chi-squared test with $P < 0.02$). Thus, thymic enlargement is a common phenomenon after chemotherapy. It must be considered in patients suspected of having residual or recurrent disease in the anterior mediastinum. As Kissin and colleagues suggest, perhaps the thymic enlargement is a good prognostic factor because it relates to restoration of immunity.

The third group of patients with TTH have an associated (usually endocrinologic) disorder, such as Graves' disease.[77, 78, 93] Pardo-Mindan and colleagues report an association of sarcoidosis with TTH.[94] A single case was reported with Beckwith-Weidemann syndrome.[95] Potter and Craig describe increased size of the thymus relative to total body weight in anencephaly.[96] They attribute it to lack of ACTH. An enlarged thymus has also been reported in Addison's disease and following castration.[94a]

Thymic enlargement is a common feature of hyperthyroidism and, in particular, Graves' disease.[77, 78, 93, 97–101] The first report of an association between Graves' (Basedow's) disease and an enlarged thymus is attributed to Cooper in 1845.[102] Eighty-three to ninety-one percent of patients with Graves' disease have been reported to have a hyperplastic thymus.[103] Suspecting a role for the thymus in the pathogenesis of the disease, early investigators advocated thymectomy as treatment.[104] Graves' disease has been associated with both lymphofollicular hyperplasia and TTH.[50, 97] Thymic enlargement has also been reported in a child receiving L-thyroxine for primary hypothyroidism.[105]

In a 1967 report, Michie and colleagues studied the radiographic size of the thymus (using pneumomediastinography) and the histologic appearance of thymic biopsies in patients with thyroid disease.[50] They found the size of the thymus (measured as maximum sagittal cross-sectional area) to be significantly greater in patients with thyrotoxicosis and chronic thyroiditis compared with those having nontoxic nodular goiter. Patients with thyrotoxicosis had a significantly higher ratio of thymic parenchyma to adipose tissue than did those with nontoxic goiter. Treatment of the hyperthyroidism often results in regression of the thymic hyperplasia.[93, 98]

Laboratory studies have confirmed a relationship between the thymus and the thyroid. In a 1924 study, Marine and colleagues found that thyroidectomy in rabbits hastened thymic involution.[106] In a more recent report, mice treated with tri-iodothyronine developed significant hyperplasia of the thymus.[107] Both epithelial cells and thymic lymphocytes proliferate after thyroid hormone administration. Thyroid hormones also induce thymic epithelial cells to synthesize and secrete thymic hormones.[108] Immunoglobulins isolated from the serum of two of six patients with Graves' disease induced proliferation of thymic lymphocytes in vitro.[109] In 1992, Villa-Verde and colleagues demonstrated thyroid hormone receptors on thymic epithelium.[110]

CONGENITAL THYMIC DISORDERS

Congenital deficiencies of cell-mediated immunity may be associated with maldevelopment (''dysplasia''), aplasia, or hypoplasia of the thymus. The term dysplasia is used to describe apparent abnormal thymic development (as defined by histopathology) and does not imply any preneoplastic condition.

DiGeorge Syndrome

The first report of congenital absence of the thymus is credited to Harington, who in 1829 reported an infant dying with convulsions. The infant was found at autopsy to have no thymus.[111] He reported the case with the intent that ''we may hereafter succeed in discovering the physiology of an apparatus apparently of great importance to foetal and infantile organization.''[111] One hundred and thirty-eight years later, DiGeorge was credited with recognizing the significance of thymic aplasia in cellular immune deficiency.[112, 113] His description of the disorder provided evidence for the role of the thymus in cell-mediated immunity. DiGeorge suggested the name "Harington syndrome" after the author of the original report.[113] However, Good and colleagues began referring to the "DiGeorge syndrome"[114]; "Harington syndrome" never caught on.

The DiGeorge syndrome (or the DiGeorge anomaly) results from malformations of the third and fourth pharyngeal pouch derivatives. The disorder has also been referred to as the III-IV pharyngeal pouch syndrome.[115] In addition to an absent thymus, associated conditions include absence of parathyroid glands, defects in the great vessels, malformation of the ears, abnormal facies (hypoplastic nose, micrognathia, hypertelorism), esophageal atresia, thyroid aplasia/hypoplasia, absence of calcitonin-containing cells in the thyroid, and endocardial cushion defects.[115–118] Lack of ossification of the hyoid bone during the first month of life is more common in the complete DiGeorge syndrome than in the partial syndrome or normal individuals.

In the complete DiGeorge syndrome, the thymus is absent.[115, 119, 120] In the partial, or incomplete, DiGeorge syndrome, the thymus is hypoplastic but histologically normal (i.e., normal lobulation and corticomedullary differentiation with Hassall's corpuscles). It is often "undescended" (i.e., in the cervical region). The region medial to the submandibular salivary gland is a common site for ectopic thymus.[121] At autopsy examination, a thorough search should be made for thymus tissue. The posterior tongue, pharynx, anterior neck structures, anterior and superior mediastinum, and pericardium are removed en bloc, fixed, and serially sectioned. After looking along the carotid artery from the aorta to the base of the skull, one should examine the submandibular salivary gland area before diagnosing thymic agenesis.[115, 121, 122]

Although small, the thymus is histologically normal or may have stress-related changes.[115] The thymus in partial DiGeorge syndrome must be distinguished from thymic dysplasia, in which a vestigial thymic remnant has few lymphoid cells and rare, if any, Hassall's corpuscles. In patients with complete or partial DiGeorge syndrome, defective cellular immunity can be attributed to the deficiency in thymic tissue. Thymic function can be assessed by in vitro tests such as numbers of CD4-positive lymphocytes in the peripheral blood and in vitro phytohemagglutinin proliferation responses.

Several series of DiGeorge syndrome patients have been published.[115, 117, 119, 120, 123–125] Most patients come to medical attention in the first days of life because of congenital heart disease or hypocalcemic seizures. Virtually all patients with DiGeorge syndrome (partial or complete) have congenital heart disease or aortic arch abnormalities. (Interrupted aortic arch and persistent truncus arteriosus are the two most common anomalies.[125]) In these seven series, only 3 of 131 patients with partial or complete DiGeorge syndrome did not have congenital heart disease.

Patients who survive beyond the neonatal period may develop recurrent infections. Lymphocytopenia and low numbers of T cells are common in the complete DiGeorge syndrome but infrequent in the incomplete syndrome. Cell-mediated immunity may be absent or depressed.[119] Conley and colleagues noted a high incidence of mental retardation in patients who survived infancy.[120] The occurrence of central nervous system (CNS) anomalies (hypoplasia of corpus callosum, microcephaly, arhinencephalia) suggests that retardation is sometimes a part of the syndrome.

Animal studies provide clues to the pathogenesis of DiGeorge syndrome. Ablation of the neural crest in chick embryos leads to a thymus that is markedly reduced in size but that has normal corticomedullary differentiation.[126, 127] In addition, abnormalities of the heart, great vessels, thyroid, and parathyroids occur simultaneously with aberrant thymic development. These abnormalities are similar to those which occur in the DiGeorge syndrome. Thus, the laboratory data suggest that the DiGeorge syndrome may result from defective development of the neural crest.

The cause of maldevelopment of the neural crest appears to be heterogeneous.[118] DiGeorge syndrome has been associated with teratogens (e.g., alcohol, retinoids) and maternal diabetes. Work with experimental animals suggests similarities between the fetal alcohol syndrome and DiGeorge syndrome.[128] In addition, chromosomal abnormalities and associations with other syndromes (e.g., Zellweger, Kallmann syndromes) have been described. A partial deletion of chromosome 22 has been reported, particularly in the familial cases.[123, 124] Other cytogenetic abnormalities have also been found. Twenty percent of abnormalities involve chromosome 22. Most cases are sporadic, although familial cases (some with autosomal dominant and autosomal recessive modes of inheritance) have been described.[118, 125]

Many patients have a minimal defect in cell-mediated immunity, which often improves with time.[118] Severe, persistent immunologic deficiency can be corrected by transplanted cultured thymic tissue or by bone marrow transplantation.[118, 119, 129, 130] A recent review suggests that the immune deficiency can be successfully treated in most patients.[118] However, most patients die in early infancy from congenital heart disease.[125]

Primary Immunodeficiency Disorders and Thymic Dysplasia

Primary immunodeficiency disorders can be divided into those that affect predominantly humoral, or B-cell, immunity, and those that affect predominantly cell-mediated, or T-cell, immunity.[130, 131] The latter are referred to as "combined" immunodeficiencies. Because T cells regulate B cells, cell-mediated immunodeficiencies are commonly associated with abnormalities of both the B- and T-cell systems. The thymus is frequently abnormal ("dysplastic") histologically in those disorders that have prominent defects in T-cell function.[129, 132]

Severe combined immunodeficiency (SCID) diseases are a spectrum of disorders characterized by marked T- and B-cell dysfunction.[131, 133–135] About 20% of patients with SCID have a deficiency of adenosine deaminase (ADA), an enzyme necessary for T-cell maturation.[135, 136] About 4% of SCID patients have a deficiency of purine nucleoside phosphorylase.[137] Another uncommon type of SCID, the "bare lymphocyte" syndrome, is associated with defective expression of histocompatibility antigens. Reticular dysgenesis is associated with impaired development of T and B lymphocytes as well as defective myeloid cell differentiation. SCID may be inherited in an autosomal or X-linked recessive form. Other congenital immunodeficiencies (e.g., ataxia-telangiectasia, Wiskott-Aldrich syndrome) are associated with less severe immunologic defects.

Thymic biopsy may be performed to evaluate a patient with a suspected congenital immunodeficiency.[138] The procedure is performed under general anesthesia by an extrapleural transcervical route. The upper pole of the thymus is sampled. Approximately 1 cm^3 of tissue is obtained. In a series of 19 biopsies reported by Borzy et al., the only complication was a wound infection (in two patients). Specimens should be divided, with one portion fixed in formalin or B5 for routine microscopic examination and another portion snap-frozen in liquid nitrogen for surface marker studies.

The heterogeneity of the congenital immunodeficiencies is illustrated by the range of thymic histopathology in these disorders.[132, 138] The thymic morphology in congenital immunodeficiencies ranges from normal (lobular configuration, corticomedullary differentiation, Hassall's corpuscles) to total dysplasia (loss of architectural organization, small lobules containing undifferentiated-appearing, "embryonal" epithelial cells and devoid of lymphocytes; no corticomedullary differentiation or Hassall's corpuscles). Occasional lymphocytes may be seen in less severe cases. Several investigators have classified the histologic appearance into various categories.[138–140] However, the histopathology does not always correlate with the clinical and laboratory immunologic assessment.

Gosseye and colleagues proposed that the histologic appearance of the thymus in SCID is a dynamic process with different patterns dependent on the duration or severity of the disease process.[139] The earliest changes resemble severe atrophy. In these cases, lymphocytes range from absent to numerous. When numerous, they are concentrated in the central part of the lobules, producing an "inverted" thymic appearance. The gland appears lobulated, and Hassall's corpuscles are present. These authors found this pattern in five patients with SCID. They note that in these atrophic-appearing glands, some lobules were histologically identical to dysplasia.

In addition to the severe atrophy, three other patterns were recognized in patients with SCID.[138] In simple dysplasia, lobules were irregular, small, and separated by fibrous or fibroadipose tissue (Fig. 4–9). No corticomedullary differentiation or Hassall's corpuscles were present, and lymphoid cells were sparse. In some cases, the peripheral cells of the lobules formed a denser layer, one or two cells thick. Occasionally, a multinucleated giant cell may be identified within the lobules. Dysplasia with stromal corticomedullary differentiation was another pattern. In these patients, the thymic lobules were larger, and the outer portion of the lobule appeared denser than the central part. Again, lymphoid cells were sparse, and Hassall's corpuscles absent. The final pattern was dysplasia with pseudoglandular ap-

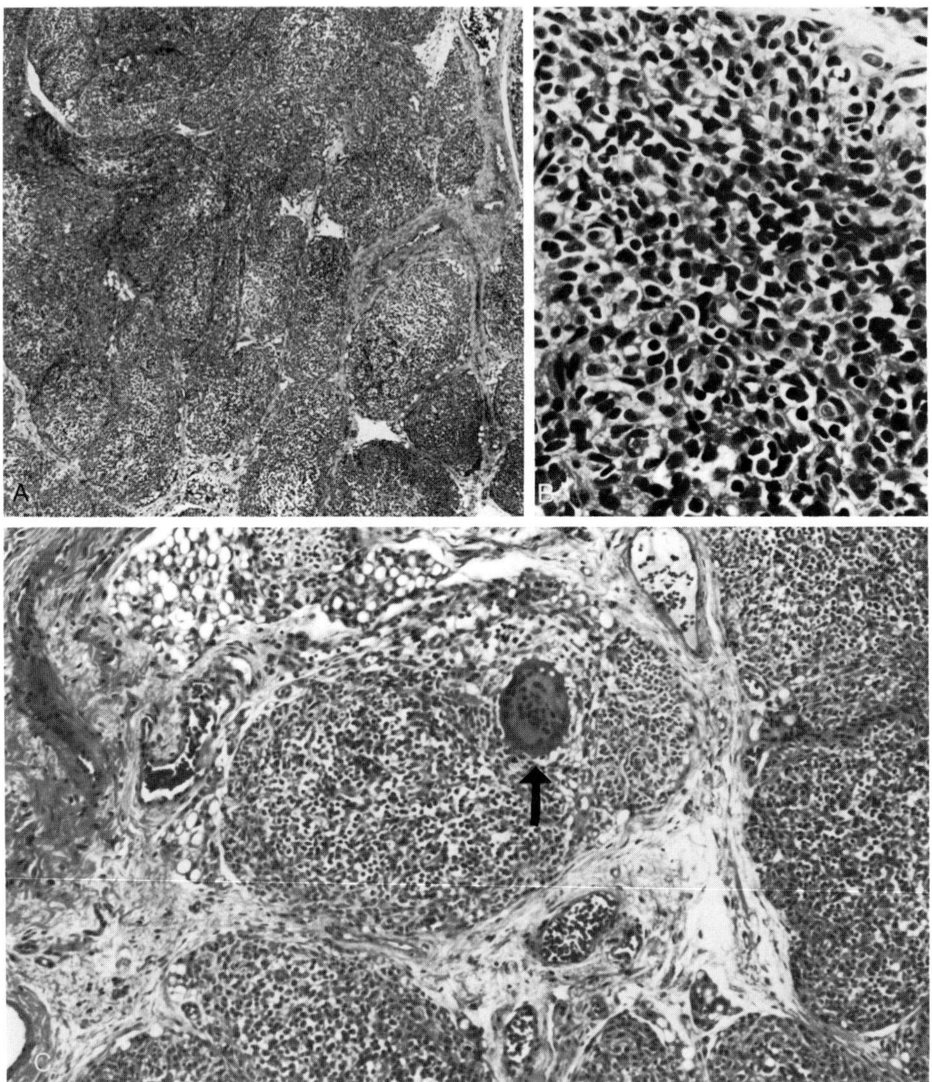

Figure 4–9. *A* and *B*, Histologic appearance of "simple" dysplasia of the thymus in an infant with severe combined immunodeficiency (SCID). Note abnormal lobular pattern, lack of corticomedullary differentiation, absence of Hassall's corpuscles, and decreased thymic lymphocytes (*A*, H & E, ×100; *B*, H & E, ×400). *C*, Thymus from another infant with SCID. Note the multinucleated giant cell (H & E, ×200).

pearance. In this group, the lobules were small and numerous, and they resembled the acini of a glandular organ with nuclei arranged at the periphery. Lymphoid cells were sparse, and Hassall's corpuscles were absent.

Haynes and colleagues have demonstrated abnormalities of epithelial surface markers in the dysplastic thymus of two patients with SCID and one with Nezelof syndrome (cellular immunodeficiency with normal serum immunoglobulins).[133] In addition, scattered, phenotypically immature T cells (positive for CD2, negative for CD4 and CD8) were present in the SCID-affected thymus, whereas the Nezelof syndrome–affected thymus contained many mature T cells (80% CD4+: 20% CD8+). By radioimmunoassay, thymosin-alpha-1 levels per gram of tissue were markedly lower in the SCID patient's thymus compared with the Nezelof syndrome thymus. Stallmach studied the thymus in four cases of SCID and found a small population of phenotypic cortical lymphocytes.[141]

The pathogenesis of SCID and other immunodeficiencies remains unclear. Is the thymic abnormality primary or secondary? In other words, does thymic dysplasia cause the T-cell abnormalities, or are the thymic changes a result of defective T cells? The cell marker studies suggest that immature T cells are present in the SCID-affected thymus but are unable to differentiate.[133, 142] Many cases appear to result from an intrinsic defect in the lymphoid cells rather than from an inherent thymic defect.

Some of the debate as to the location of the abnormality has come from studying patients with ADA-deficient SCID.[143] Initial reports indicated that the thymus in ADA-deficient (ADA−) SCID patients appeared involuted and had Hassall's corpuscles. In contrast, the thymus of SCID patients with normal ADA (ADA+) had the classic findings of dysplasia.[143] Blood vessels were reported to be larger in the ADA− than in the ADA+ SCID-affected thymus. Authors speculated that the ADA− thymus involuted after its population by lymphoid cells. In utero, maternal ADA would allow normal thymic development. With birth, deficiency of ADA would then lead to arrested thymic development. The larger blood vessels in the ADA− thymus were interpreted as histologic evidence of a previously functioning gland. However, subsequent investigators have found the ADA+ and ADA− SCID-affected thymus indistinguishable in most cases.[144, 145]

Thus, the more recent evidence from the ADA− patients suggests that the changes of thymic dysplasia may result from an enzyme deficiency affecting lymphocyte differentiation rather than from an inherent defect in the thymus. Using an animal model, Shores and colleagues provided additional evidence that lymphocyte-epithelial interactions are necessary for normal thymic development.[146] In SCID-affected mice, normal organization and maturation of thymic medullary epithelial cells did not occur in the absence of T cells bearing the T-cell antigen receptor. However, in the presence of receptor-bearing T cells, the thymus developed normally.

The fundamental problem in the SCID-affected mice seems to be abnormal recombinase activity that impairs the rearrangement of T-cell receptor and immunoglobulin genes.[134] Therefore, the basic problem in SCID may be with the lymphocytes and not the thymus. Maturing T cells appear to be necessary for normal thymic development.

Further support for this concept is the finding that in patients with SCID, the thymus may become functional after bone marrow transplantation. In these patients, normal T-cell precursors are provided by the bone marrow transplant.[135] Finally, histologic changes similar to those in SCID have been described in adults with AIDS and in children with graft-versus-host disease.[147–149] Thus, the "dysplastic" features of the thymus in SCID may be acquired and, therefore, may not necessarily reflect abnormal thymic development.

Omenn's syndrome ("familial reticuloendotheliosis with eosinophilia") is a type of SCID characterized by phenotypically normal T cells, elevated IgE, and eosinophilia.[150] A proliferative defect in T cells has been described. Patients have gradual onset of dermatitis, lymphadenopathy, and hepatosplenomegaly during the first and second months of life. Investigators have suggested antigenic stimulation as the pathogenesis for the associated manifestations of this disorder. Others have suggested that the disorder results from intrauterine graft-versus-host disease in a fetus with SCID. The thymus in these patients is similar to the thymus of patients with SCID. The thymus is small with abnormal lobulation, marked lymphoid depletion, and absence of Hassall's corpuscles.

The "bare lymphocyte" syndrome (major histocompatibility complex, or MHC, deficiency syndrome) is a form of SCID characterized by defective expression of histocompatibility (HLA) antigens (class I and/or class II) on peripheral blood mononuclear cells.[151, 152] Patients have impaired T-cell immunity and frequently have hypogammaglobulinemia. Schuurman and colleagues studied the thymus in two patients with this disorder.[153] They found the thymus to have a normal histologic appearance (lobulation, corticomedullary differentiation, Hassall's corpuscles). Immunohistologic studies revealed the normal distribution of T-cell phenotypes. However, unlike normal thymus, cortical epithelial cells did not express HLA class I (HLA-A, -B, -C) antigens. Class II (HLA-DR) antigens were present only on nonepithelial stromal cells in the thymic medulla. Interestingly, these authors found class I antigens on medullary lymphocytes, despite their absence on peripheral blood cells. These data indicate that normal phenotypic maturation of T cells occurs despite abnormalities in HLA expression.

X-linked lymphoproliferative syndrome is an immunodeficiency characterized by an unusual susceptibility to Epstein-Barr virus (EBV). When infected with EBV, patients with X-linked lymphoproliferative syndrome may develop fatal infectious mononucleosis.[154–157] They also may develop hypogammaglobulinemia, aplastic anemia, and/or malignant lymphoma. Purtilo described the histopathology of the thymus gland in fatal cases of X-linked lymphoproliferative syndrome.[157] During the first 2 weeks of EBV infection, the thymus increases in size because of an immunoblastic infiltrate. The corticomedullary differentiation is absent. Lymphocytes and immunoblasts infiltrate the connective tissue. Degenerating Hassall's corpuscles and multinucleated giant cells can be seen in the medulla. Patients who die during the third or fourth weeks of EBV infection show lymphocyte depletion. Hassall's corpuscles may be absent or calcified. Plasma cells and plasmacytoid lymphocytes infiltrate the residual lobules and connective tissue. In patients who die beyond 4 weeks after onset of EBV infection, the thymus may be infiltrated by a monomorphic large cell characteristic of malignant lymphoma.

Information on the morphology of the thymus in other primary immunodeficiencies is scant. Borzy et al. described the thymus in two patients with ataxia-telangiectasia.[138] The thymus was small but with normal lobulation. Neither corticomedullary demarcation nor Hassall's corpuscles were present. The epithelial cells were "plump," with many showing nuclear atypia and hyperchromatism. Small lymphocytes were admixed with the epithelial cells. Nuclear atypia has also been observed in other organs of patients with ataxia-telangiectasia.[158]

Wiskott-Aldrich syndrome is an X-linked disorder characterized by thrombocytopenia, eczema, and varying degrees of immunodeficiency (both humoral and cell-mediated).[131, 159] Impaired expression of a surface glycoprotein sialophorin (CD43) has been described on lymphocytes from patients with this disorder.[160] The thymus in patients with Wiskott-Aldrich syndrome is usually reported as normal in structure.[161, 162] In one case, a dysplastic thymus was found. It was described as having a rudimentary lobular architecture with absent corticomedullary differentiation. Scattered lymphocytes, plasma cells, and partly calcified Hassall's corpuscle–like structures were also present.[161]

Another immunodeficiency results from absence of CD18 expression on peripheral blood cells.[163] CD18 is the beta chain component of three cell surface glycoproteins, LFA-1, CR3 receptor, and p150,95. Each has a distinctive alpha chain (CD11a, -11b, and -11c, respectively). If the beta chain is abnormal, the alpha chains are not expressed.[131] These glycoproteins are involved in adherence of phagocytes and lymphocytes to endothelium. CD11-CD18 deficiency is an autosomal recessive disorder characterized by granulocytosis, recurrent infections, and impaired adhesion functions of phagocytes. Severe hypoplasia of lymphoid tissues along with lymphopenia has been reported.[164] In one case, the thymus was described as hypoplastic with indistinct medulla and cortex. Scattered lymphocytes were present. Hassall's corpuscle–like structures were difficult to find. Nunoi and colleagues suggest that defective lymphocyte homing processes result from absent adherence proteins and result in lymphoid hypoplasia.[164]

The most effective therapy for primary, severe T-cell immunodeficiencies is bone marrow transplantation. Excellent results (97% cure rate) have been reported with SCID patients treated by HLA-identical bone marrow transplantation.[165] Similar treatment has also been successful in Wiskott-Aldrich syndrome.[159] Gene therapy may be effective in patients with ADA− SCID. Using this procedure, the gene for ADA can be inserted into the patient's chromosome to replace the defective gene.[166] Preliminary results of gene therapy in patients with ADA− SCID are encouraging.[167] When chromosomal defects for these disorders become better defined, curative gene therapy may be available in the future for many patients with primary immunodeficiencies.

ACQUIRED IMMUNODEFICIENCY SYNDROME (AIDS)

Biopsy of the thymus has been used to help distinguish AIDS from the congenital immunodeficiency syndromes.[46, 168] Joshi and colleagues described the histopathology of thymic biopsies in 11 AIDS patients ranging from 6 to 36 months of age[46] (Fig. 4–10). They found three patterns (Table 4–3).

Table 4–3. The Thymus in AIDS

Change	Description
Severe stress-related changes ("precocious involution")	Small size/weight, lymphocyte depletion, obscured corticomedullary distinction, microcystic changes in Hassall's corpuscles
Changes similar to those of thymic dysplasia ("dysinvolution")	As above, but lacking Hassall's corpuscles
"Thymitis"	Normal size/weight, medullary germinal centers, plasma cells

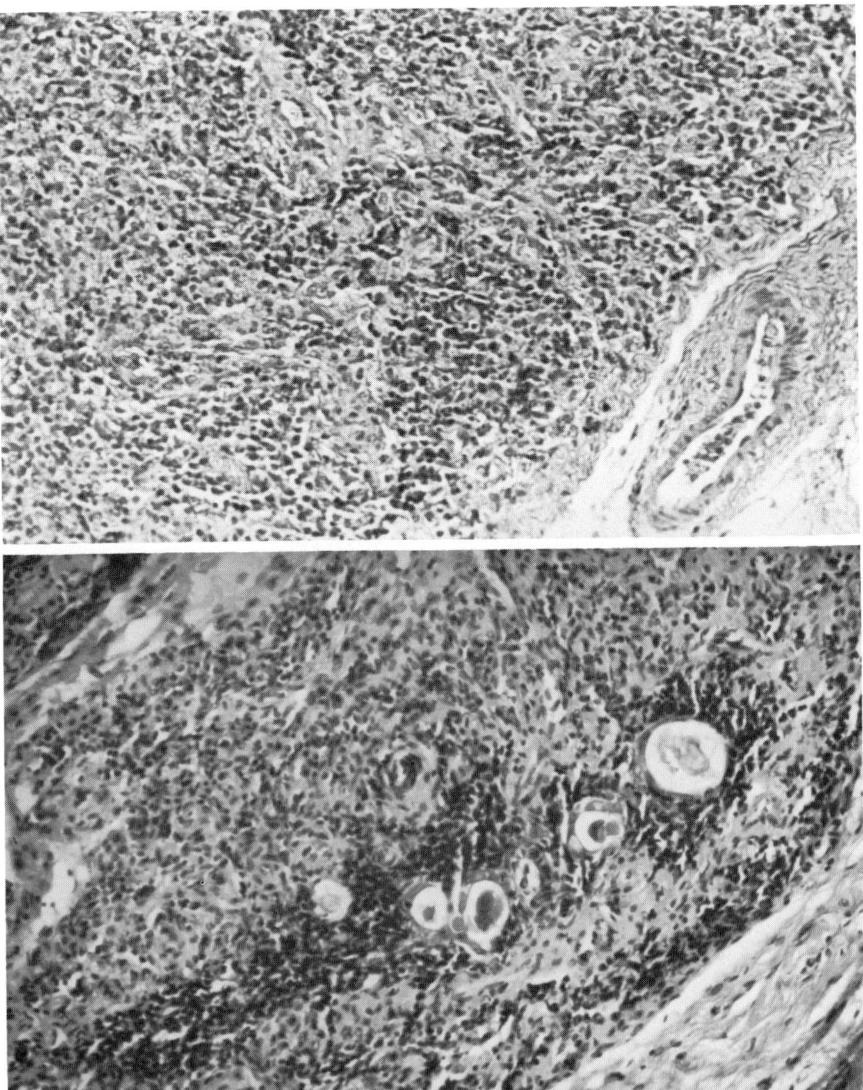

Figure 4–10. Thymic biopsies from children with acquired immunodeficiency syndrome. *Top*, The thymus shows "dysinvolution," characterized by normal blood vessels, loss of corticomedullary differentiation, profound lymphocytic depletion, and absence of Hassall's corpuscles (H & E, ×100). (From Joshi VV, et al. Thymic biopsy in children with acquired immunodeficiency syndrome. Arch Pathol Lab Med 1986; 110:837–842.) *Bottom*, The thymus shows precocious involution, or severe atrophy, with loss of corticomedullary differentiation, lymphocyte depletion, and microcystic Hassall's corpuscles (H & E, ×100). (From Joshi VV, et al. Pathology of suspected acquired immune deficiency syndrome in children: a study of eight cases. Pediatr Pathol 1984; 2:71–87.)

Two of the 11 patients had precocious involution of the thymus. This is described as involution beyond that expected for the patient's age and out of proportion to the patient's stress. The features are (1) normal anatomic location, configuration, and blood vessels, (2) reduction in size and weight, and (3) severe lymphocyte depletion, obscured corticomedullary differentiation, and microcystic changes in most of the Hassall's corpuscles.

The second pattern was seen in two patients and is described as thymic involution mimicking thymic dysplasia, or "dysinvolution." In these cases, the thymus was similar to that of precocious involution but lacking in Hassall's corpuscles.

The third pattern was "thymitis" and occurred in seven of the patients. The features of this pattern include normal anatomic location, weight, and blood vessels, with the presence of germinal centers in the medulla. In addition, lymphocytes and plasma cells were prominent in some cases and obscured the corticomedullary differentiation. Multinucleated giant cells were present in the medulla of one patient.

Thus, in contrast to severe combined immunodeficiency syndromes, thymic biopsy in children with AIDS reveals a gland of normal anatomic location, normal configuration, and normal blood vessels, and, in most cases, with less severe reductions in lymphoid cells and Hassall's corpuscles. The changes of thymitis are not described in congenital immunodeficiency disorders. Joshi and colleagues speculate that the changes of thymitis, precocious involution, and dysinvolution represent different stages of thymic epithelial cell injury in children with AIDS.[46]

Several autopsy series have reported the histopathology of the thymus in AIDS.[169–175] Marked involution is a constant finding and is more extensive than in other chronically ill patients of similar age. Depletion of both lymphocytes and epithelial cells has been described. Corticomedullary differentiation is rarely apparent. Another variable feature is infiltration by mature plasma cells. The plasma cells are most prominent in the fat adjacent to the cords of involuted thymus. Intrathymic blood vessels often show adventitial hyalinization with "onion-skin" patterns. Occasional multinucleated giant cells, patchy areas of fibrosis, and epithelial rosettes have also been reported.[170] The nuclear inclusions of cytomegalovirus (CMV) have been identified within the thymus in AIDS patients with disseminated CMV infection.[172, 174]

A striking finding has been the frequent absence of Hassall's corpuscles at autopsy.[169, 170, 175] In the series of Grody et al., Hassall's corpuscles were absent in 5 of 14 AIDS patients. In the other patients, all of the Hassall's corpuscles were calcified. Microcystic dilatation of Hassall's corpuscles has been described in pediatric autopsy cases.[171, 176] Total absence or complete calcification of Hassall's corpuscles was not seen in control groups composed of patients without AIDS. Chronically ill patients without AIDS had marked thymic involution, but Hassall's corpuscles were present with little or no calcification. The thymus of infants with "stress atrophy" had severe lymphocyte depletion, but Hassall's corpuscles were present. However, absence or complete calcification of Hassall's corpuscles is not a specific finding for AIDS, because it has been reported in primary immunodeficiencies and graft-versus-host disease (see Table 4–4).

Indeed, Schuurman and colleagues found no major differences between the thymus of AIDS patients and the thymus of control subjects.[147] They studied the thymus from autopsies of eight AIDS patients (seven adults and one child). The controls included thymic tissue from autopsies of four patients with primary immune deficiency (one with ataxia-telangiectasia and three with congenital agammaglobulinemia) and seven patients who received allogeneic bone marrow transplants. They reported that all of the thymus specimens were severely involuted with diminished or absent lymphocytes and Hassall's corpuscles. Some specimens had a lobule-like appearance, whereas others appeared as "guirlandes" (i.e., stalks of epithelium connected to each other). These authors found no histologic features to distinguish patients with AIDS from the control subjects.

Furthermore, Schuurman and colleagues performed in-situ hybridization using a probe for HIV-1 messenger RNA and found low numbers of positive cells in the AIDS-affected thymus. They conclude that the thymus of AIDS

Table 4–4. The Thymus in Selected Immunodeficiencies and Stress

Disorder	Size	Location	Lobulations	Lymphocytes	Cortico-Medullary Differentiation	Hassall's Corpuscles
DiGeorge	Absent					
Partial DiGeorge	Small	Often undescended	Normal	Normal	Normal	Normal
SCID	Small	Normal	Normal to absent	Numerous to sparse	"Inverted" or absent	Normal to absent
AIDS	Normal to small	Normal	Normal	Normal to sparse	Normal to absent	Normal to absent
Stress	Small	Normal	Normal	Decreased	Normal, absent, or "inverted"	Normal

patients does not show evidence of specific destruction. Unlike the study of thymic biopsies by Joshi and colleagues,[46] the report by Schuurman et al. includes only autopsied patients and includes almost only adults. Thus, the latter authors are studying "end-stage" disease, which may not reflect the early changes observed by Joshi et al. Also, the thymic lesions in children with AIDS show a wider spectrum than do the lesions of adults.[168]

Immunohistologic analyses of the thymus in AIDS report absence of cells expressing the phenotype of thymic cortical lymphocytes.[177] Depletion of CD4-positive cells and resulting predominance of CD8 cells has been noted. The epithelial cells express the antigens present in the normal thymus. However, the normal compartmentalization of cortical and medullary epithelial cells is lost in some cases. In contrast to normal thymus, the thymus in AIDS patients shows no thymosin-positive cells as studied by immunohistochemistry. Reduction in thymulin-containing cells has also been found.[178] Thymosin alpha-1 and beta-4 are elevated in some patients, whereas thymulin is decreased.[179, 180]

Both thymic lymphocytes and epithelial cells can be infected with HIV-1 using in vitro techniques.[181–183] HIV-1 has been demonstrated by viral isolation and polymerase chain reaction in the thymus of fetuses born to infected mothers.[184, 185] According to one hypothesis advocated by Joshi and Oleske, early intrauterine infection could lead to abnormal thymic development and the histologic changes similar to thymic dysplasia.[168]

Baskin and colleagues studied the thymus in an animal model for AIDS: simian immunodeficiency virus (SIV)-infected rhesus monkeys.[186] They report thymic involution from loss of lymphocytes within 8 weeks of inoculation. Virus was identified in thymic lymphocytes and macrophages within 2 weeks. The involution occurred in animals that were not clinically ill. Therefore, the involution may not be entirely stress-related. There was no evidence of thymic epithelial cell destruction. Hassall's corpuscles were present even in the most severely involuted glands. Virus could not be identified within the epithelial cells of the thymus.

The destruction of the immune system by HIV-1 infection and the associated changes in the thymus have led investigators to attempt immunologic reconstitution in these patients. Immunotherapy with thymus transplantation and thymic hormones has been reported but with limited success.[177, 187–193]

BONE MARROW TRANSPLANTATION

The thymus in bone marrow transplant patients is affected by multiple factors, including the patient's underlying disease, preparative regimens such as radiation therapy and/or chemotherapy, immunosuppressive drugs such as cyclosporin A, endogenous corticosteroids (the "stress response"), and possible graft-versus-host disease. In general, the changes are similar to those of stress-induced involution.

Thomas and colleagues studied the thymus at autopsy from 12 patients who had received allogeneic bone marrow transplants for acute leukemia.[194] Most of the patients had died of infection or hemorrhage, with or without graft-versus-host disease. In all cases, the thymus showed marked involution with depletion of lymphocytes, absence of corticomedullary differentiation, and extensive fatty replacement. Hassall's corpuscles varied in size and number. Some were cystic or calcified. Tingible-body macrophages were often present around the Hassall's corpuscles. Plasma cells were frequent within the residual thymic epithelium and connective tissue. These authors also studied the thymus at autopsy from three acute leukemia patients who received chemotherapy but no bone marrow transplant. The histologic appearance of the thymus in the nontransplanted patients was similar.

Immunohistologic studies of the thymus were similar in bone marrow transplant recipients and nongrafted leukemia patients. The few lymphocytes were mature T cells; no immature lymphocytes (positive for terminal deoxynucleotidyl transferase) were present. In two cases, the authors demonstrated that the lymphocytes had the HLA type of the host, not of the donor. Thus, there was no evidence of engraftment. Most of the epithelial cells expressed the phenotype of subcapsular and medullary epithelium. Small foci of cortical epithelium were present, which lacked the normal expression of HLA-DR.

In patients who survive for over 2 months, increasing numbers of mature, small lymphocytes in the perivascular space have been described.[195] Most reports of long-term survivors describe thymic involution. However, most of the patients have died after long illnesses. Rare cases of thymic reconstitution after bone marrow transplantation have been reported. Muller-Hermelink and colleagues described reconstitution of the thymus in a child who died in an automobile accident 5 years after bone marrow transplantation for acute leukemia.[196] The thymus appeared smaller than average with fewer Hassall's corpuscles. However, the cortical and medullary areas were well-delineated and had normal numbers of lymphocytes.

Studies of the thymus in laboratory animals permit the investigation of graft-versus-host disease (GVH) in the absence of underlying disease and drugs.[197] GVH refers to the clinical syndrome caused by the attack of immunocompetent donor lymphoid cells against host organs. In mice, mild GVH is associated with infiltration of Hassall's corpuscles by lymphocytes. Moderate and severe GVH results in a marked reduction in thymic size with decrease in lymphocytes, loss of corticomedullary differentiation, and absence of Hassall's corpuscles. Ultrastructural examination reveals epithelial cell damage characterized by prominent cytoplasmic vacuolization. In some animals with severe GVH, the thymus becomes so atrophic that, in one study, it could not be located despite *en bloc* dissection and serial sectioning.[197]

Seemayer and colleagues noted the similarity between the histologic appearance of the thymus in murine GVH and in children with congenital immunodeficiency.[197] In addition, Seemayer and Bolande reported an infant with transfusion-induced GVH whose involuted thymus lacked lymphocytes, corticomedullary differentiation, and Hassall's corpuscles.[149] A similar case but in an older child was reported by Gartner.[148] The thymus in these cases resembled that in patients with congenital immunodeficiency. The authors speculated that some of the congenital immunodeficiencies may result from maternal lymphocytes engrafting in the developing fetus and causing a GVH reaction. An alternative explanation would be that the changes in the thymus are nonspecific (i.e., they may result from a variety of causes).

In a follow-up article, Seemayer and colleagues used the same animal model of GVH but adrenalectomized one group of mice.[168] The adrenalectomized animals had GVH in the absence of the corticosteroid-mediated stress response. The marked reduction in thymic size and the depletion of cortical lymphocytes did not occur in the adrenalectomized animals. However, both groups had changes in the medulla, including increased numbers of medullary lymphocytes with epithelial cell disorganization and disappearance of Hassall's corpuscles. Thus, these authors concluded that the thymic medullary epithelial cell injury results from GVH disease and not from corticosteroids.

Other investigations in laboratory animals provide further evidence that the thymus is a direct target of the GVH reaction.[198] The attack on the thymus in GVH may lead to loss of self-tolerance and subsequent development of autoimmune disorders. Indeed, bone marrow transplant patients with chronic GVH frequently develop disorders resembling autoimmune diseases such as Sjögren's syndrome and systemic lupus erythematosus.[199] In animals with chronic GVH, the thymus remains markedly atrophic.[200]

CYCLOSPORIN A

Cyclosporin A is an immunosuppressive drug that has improved survival of solid organ allografts and helps to prevent GVH in bone marrow transplant patients.[201] In vitro studies indicated that cyclosporin A inhibits production of interleukin-2 (IL2) and IL2 receptors. At pharmacologic doses in laboratory animals, the drug caused thymic involution.[202] The mean thymic weight decreased to 68% of control weight after 1 week of therapy. Histologically, the predominant effect is a decrease in the size of the medulla from approximately 50% of the thymic lobule to less than 10%. The medullary epithelial cells and Hassall's corpuscles are virtually eliminated. The transition from cortical ("double positive") to medullary ("single positive") lymphocyte is blocked both in vitro and in vivo.[201] The changes appear reversible with a return to normal histologic appearance 4 weeks after cessation of therapy. This maturational arrest may explain some of the immunosuppressive effects of cyclosporin. FK-506 is another immunosuppressive drug with effects comparable to those of cyclosporin.[203] It induces similar changes in the thymus.

INFECTIONS

Most of the changes in thymic histology associated with acute infection are stress-related. In general, no specific histologic changes are identified in patients dying of infectious diseases.[204] Exceptions would be the rare examples of viral inclusions within thymic cells. CMV and adenovirus inclusions have been described in the thymus of patients dying of disseminated disease.[172, 174, 195]

In laboratory animals, the mouse thymic virus causes severe thymic necrosis due to lysis of CD4-positive lymphocytes.[205] Thymic necrosis in newborn mice is the basis for the standard infectivity assay. Newborn mice infected with CMV develop thymic involution histologically resembling that seen with the glucocorticoid-mediated stress reaction.[206] Other viruses have similar effects.[206] Studies have shown that thymic epithelial cells can be infected in vitro with various organisms, including trypanosomes, measles, HIV-1, and CMV.[207] Infection of the thymic epithelial cell may be important in the pathophysiology of various infectious disorders.

Congenital viral infections frequently result in an atrophic thymus. However, the patients are studied at autopsy, and multiple factors probably contribute to the thymic atrophy. For example, autopsied patients with congenital rubella are described with an atrophic thymus depleted of lymphocytes and with few Hassall's corpuscles.[208] Laboratory studies suggest that intrauterine viral infection of the thymus may result in tolerance. The virus is seen as a "self" antigen, and the animal is unable to eliminate it.[209]

In 1850, Paul Dubois, a French obstetrician, published a study of cysts in the thymus of the newborn.[210] They had been first described 21 years earlier by Cruveilhier, according to Oliver.[211] Dubois considered the cysts to be abscesses because they had purulent contents. All of his cases were in patients with congenital syphilis, and he therefore thought the cysts were of syphilitic origin.[210] Subsequent studies (reviewed by Oliver[211]) confirmed the association and demonstrated spirochetes within the cysts. However, later reports indicated that cystic Hassall's corpuscles containing inflammatory cells are a nonspecific finding.[96, 212]

In congenital syphilis, the thymus is atrophic.[96, 211] The lobules are small and depleted of lymphocytes; corticomedullary differentiation is absent. The interlobular connective tissue is increased and dense. This marked increase in connective tissue was emphasized in an early review by Jacobi.[213] Hassall's corpuscles are present. Rarely, cystic Hassall's corpuscles become infiltrated with neutrophils and granular debris. These structures have been called Dubois' abscesses. These necrotic areas may be apparent on gross inspection. They must be distinguished from areas of liquefaction in an otherwise normal thymus as a result of postmortem degeneration.

Granulomas in the thymus may be associated with generalized or localized tuberculosis, histoplasmosis, or other fungal infection; the histopathology is the same as that seen in other organs.[214] Rare examples of tuberculosis apparently confined to the thymus have been described.[215] A case of tuberculosis simulating a thymic tumor has been reported.[215] Granulomas may also occur with ruptured thymic cysts.

ANOXIA

Petechial hemorrhages in the thymic cortex are associated with anoxia.[96] The hemorrhages in a newborn are commonly associated with abruptio placentae. The lesions are grossly visible on the surface and within the parenchyma of the thymus. Similar hemorrhages are usually present under the pleura and epicardium.

MALNUTRITION

Atrophy of the thymus and other lymphoid organs has been noted in malnourished children.[55, 216–219] The thymus has been described as an "early barometer of nutrition" by Simon (in 1845).[220] In the malnourished child, the thymus is atrophic but retains its lobulated appearance. One Ugandan autopsy series of 10 patients with kwashiorkor (a syndrome affecting young children and resulting from protein deficiency) reported an average thymic weight of 4.4 g compared with an age-matched control average weight of 37 g.[220] Patients had died of acute infections. Corticomedullary differentiation is lost because of depletion of cortical lymphocytes. Hassall's corpuscles have cystic dilation. These changes are indistinguishable from the stress-related involution described earlier. The thymic changes may have clinical significance, because malnutrition has been associated with impairment of T-cell function and increased susceptibility to fatal infections. Indeed, infections are a confounding factor in the autopsy series and may explain the thymic involution. However, according to Smythe and colleagues, the impaired T-cell function precedes the onset of serious infections.[219]

VASCULITIS

Allergic angiitis and granulomatosis (Churg-Strauss syndrome) has been reported to involve the thymus. Jessurun and colleagues reported a 14-year-old male who presented with multiple skin lesions and an anterior mediastinal mass.[221] Histologic examination of the excised mass revealed confluent granulomas with central necrosis. Arteries and small veins were infiltrated by histiocytes, eosinophils, and giant cells. Destruction of vessels was demonstrated by focal fibrinoid necrosis and fragmentation of the elastica. The thymus adjacent to these lesions was infiltrated by eosinophils and occasional multinucleated giant cells. Special stains for acid-fast bacilli and fungi yielded negative results. Multiple skin biopsies showed eosinophilia along with vasculitis. Subsequently, the patient developed pulmonary nodules. Steroid therapy resulted in near disappearance of skin and lung lesions.

Histologically, the necrotizing vasculitis (involving small arteries, veins, and capillaries), granulomas, and eosinophilia are characteristic of allergic angiitis and granulomatosis. Unlike this case, most patients with the disorder have histories of asthma. Presentation with a thymic mass is unusual. Microscopically, the differential diagnosis of the thymic tumor includes Hodgkin's disease, Langerhans cell granulomatosis, and infections such as tuberculosis. The lack of atypical cells, presence of vasculitis, and absence of acid-fast bacilli would favor the diagnosis of allergic angiitis and granulomatosis. Histioeosinophilic granuloma would also be a diagnostic consideration, as discussed earlier. However, histioeosinophilic granuloma is limited to the thymic capsule and septa. Moreover, it has been described only in MG patients who have had a diagnostic pneumomediastinum.

RADIATION

Radiation to the thymus of laboratory animals produces marked depletion of lymphocytes.[200] The changes are indistinguishable from acute GVH. Six weeks after total body irradiation followed by autologous bone marrow transplantation, the dog thymus repopulates with lymphocytes. By 10 months following radiation, the thymus appears histologically normal.

DOWN'S SYNDROME

Patients with Down's syndrome have an increased susceptibility to infection and are at higher than average risk for developing leukemia and lymphoma. Investigators have studied the thymus in these patients for clues as to the nature of their immunosuppression. Indeed, most patients with Down's syndrome have histologic changes in the thymus. Larocca and colleagues studied the thymus from 35 Down's syndrome patients either at autopsy or at surgery for congenital heart disease.[222] Age-matched control organs obtained at autopsy or heart surgery were also studied.

Compared with controls, the thymus of Down's syndrome patients had cortical thinning with poor corticomedullary differentiation. In addition, most cases showed septal fibrosis and enlarged, cystic Hassall's corpuscles. In the control patients, the thymus had cortical lymphocyte depletion without other abnormalities. Alterations in thymic lymphocyte subpopulations have been reported in Down's syndrome, with decreased numbers of phenotypic cortical cells, compared with findings in age-matched control subjects.[223] Other reports found overexpression of cytokines (tumor necrosis factor alpha and interferon gamma) and adhesion molecules in the thymus of patients with Down's syndrome.[224, 225] Thus, abnormalities in the thymus may reflect the altered immune system associated with Down's syndrome.

CYSTS

Thymic cysts are uncommon.[226–228] In a series of 230 patients with primary cysts and tumors of the mediastinum, 11 (5%) had thymic cysts.[229] Thymic cysts may be located in the neck, particularly in the anterior cervical triangle near the thyroid, but occur most often in the anterior-superior mediastinum.[1, 230–233] The cervical thymic cysts frequently have a pedicle extending into the mediastinum.[230] The mediastinal thymic cysts usually occur in asymptomatic patients between the ages of 20 and 50 years. If infected, the cyst may rapidly enlarge.[234]

Radiographically, the cysts are circumscribed mass lesions of uniform density. They may be "rimmed" by calcification. Size varies from 1 to 18 cm. Grossly, the cysts have a smooth fibrous capsule and may be unilocular or multilocular (Figs. 4–11, 4–12, 4–13). The fluid may be clear, turbid, or hemorrhagic. The epithelial lining may be flattened, cuboidal, columnar with or without cilia, transitional, or squamous. The epithelial lining may show pseudoepitheliomatous hyperplasia (Fig. 4–14) and simulate a squamous cell carcinoma.[226, 235] Carcinoma may be excluded

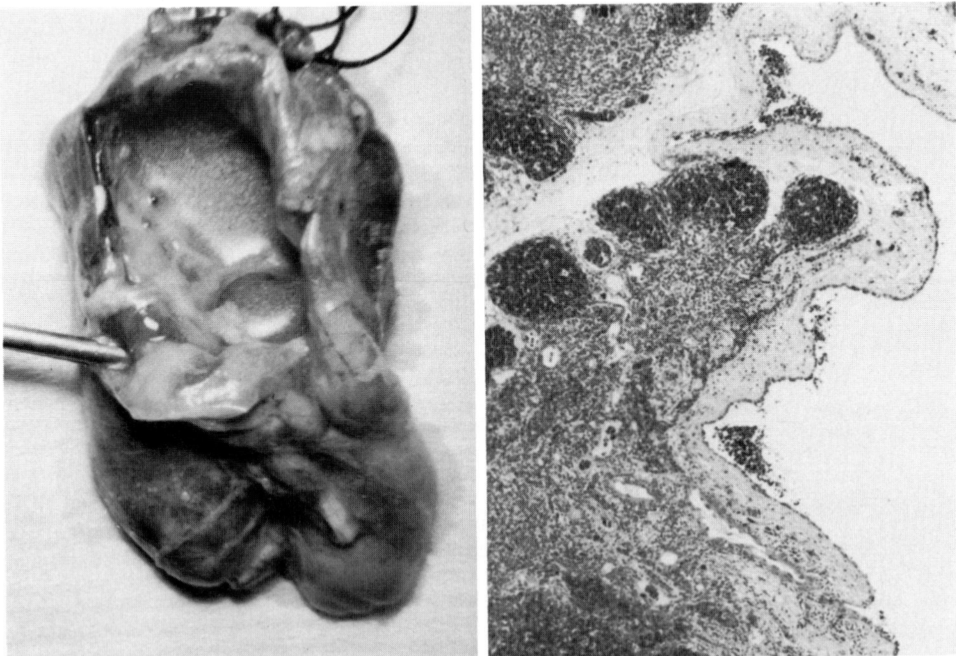

Figure 4–11. *Left,* A unilocular thymic cyst excised from the neck of a 9-year-old child. A smooth-walled cavity is apparent. (Courtesy of Dr. Jane Chatten, Children's Hospital of Philadelphia.) *Right,* Microscopically, the epithelial lining is identified. Thymic tissue is present within the cyst wall (left half of photograph). The lining epithelium varies from cuboidal or columnar to squamous (H & E, × 40).

by the finding of cytologically bland epithelial cells lacking mitotic figures. Cholesterol clefts and granulomas with foreign body giant cells and hemosiderin-laden macrophages are commonly found within the cyst wall (Fig. 4–15).

Thymic tissue within the cyst wall is necessary for the diagnosis of a thymic cyst. The thymic tissue may be abundant or fragmentary. It typically shows corticomedullary differentiation and Hassall's corpuscles, both solid and cystic. The thymic epithelium may appear as elongated, branching strands of cells within the fibrous tissue of the cyst wall (see Fig. 4–13). In the absence of thymic tissue, no specific diagnosis other than benign cyst can be made. Differentiation from other benign mediastinal cysts would be impossible.

Suster and Rosai reported a series of 18 patients with mediastinal, multilocular thymic cysts.[236] Patients ranged in age from 15 to 76 years; males outnumbered females five to one. Most patients were asymptomatic, and the lesions were identified on routine chest radiographs. Some had symptoms such as chest pain and dyspnea.

Grossly, multilocular thymic cysts are described as soft, rubbery masses ranging from 3 to 17 cm in greatest dimension. On cut section, there are multiloculated cavities filled with dark blood or gray-brown fluid. These lesions may be well-circumscribed and easily excised, or they may adhere to surrounding structures. The cysts are lined by squamous, columnar (sometimes ciliated), or cuboidal epithelium. Some have pseudoepitheliomatous hyperplasia. The cysts are filled with desquamated epithelium and debris. The cyst walls are fibrous and may have marked acute and chronic inflammation. Well-formed germinal centers are common (see Fig. 4–14). Thymic tissue is present within the cyst walls.

Most thymic cysts appear to be congenital and may originate from cystic dilatation of branchial pouch remnants.[227, 237] Cervical cysts may occur in an undescended thymus.[121] A congenital origin is favored by the finding that cervical thymic cysts are frequently associated with other endocrine gland tissue (parathyroid and thyroid).[230] A case report of a mediastinal thymic cyst containing parathyroid and salivary gland tissue ("choristoma of the thymus") suggests that some of these cysts result from abnormal development.[238] Thymic tissue in the skin adjacent to an apparent branchial sinus

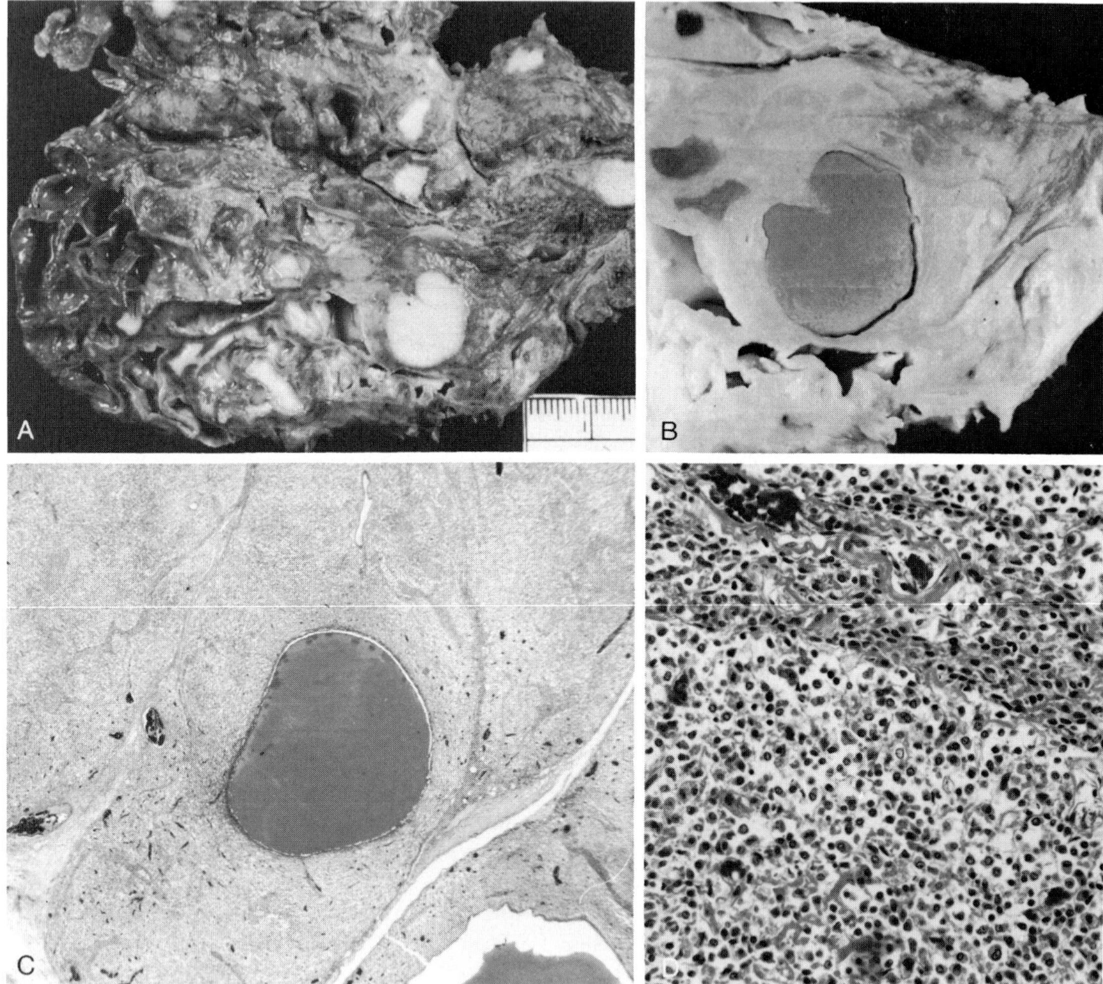

Figure 4–12. *A,* A cross-sectioned, formalin-fixed, multilocular thymic cyst. The lesion was found at autopsy in the anterior mediastinum of a 26-year-old patient with AIDS and widespread infection. Some cystic areas contain proteinaceous material, whereas others appear empty. *B,* A closer view shows more detail of the cyst wall. *C,* Microscopically, the protein-filled cysts are surrounded by a cellular infiltrate (H & E, ×40). *D,* Higher magnification of the solid areas reveals numerous chronic inflammatory cells admixed with epithelium (H & E, ×200).

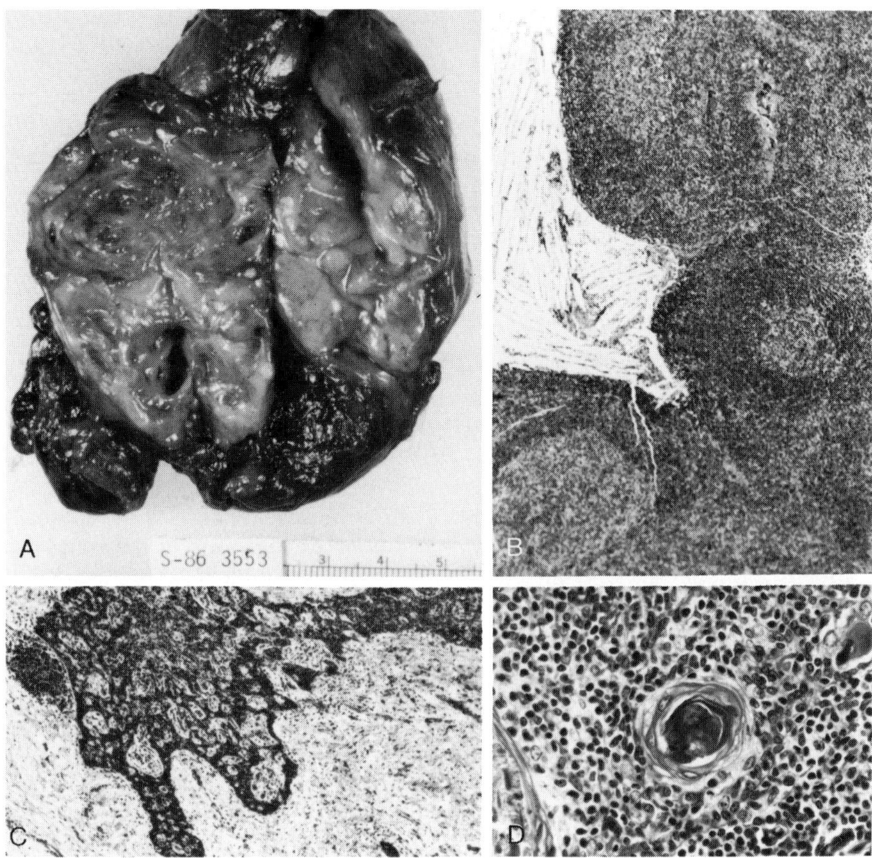

Figure 4–13. *A*, Gross photograph of a multilocular thymic cyst excised from the anterior mediastinum of a 27-year-old. *B*, Prominent reactive germinal centers around a cystic space (H & E, ×40). *C*, Thymic epithelium within the fibrous wall of a cyst forms interlacing, elongated strands of cells (H & E, ×100). *D*, Hassall's corpuscles are present among the lymphocytes and plasma cells (H & E, ×200).

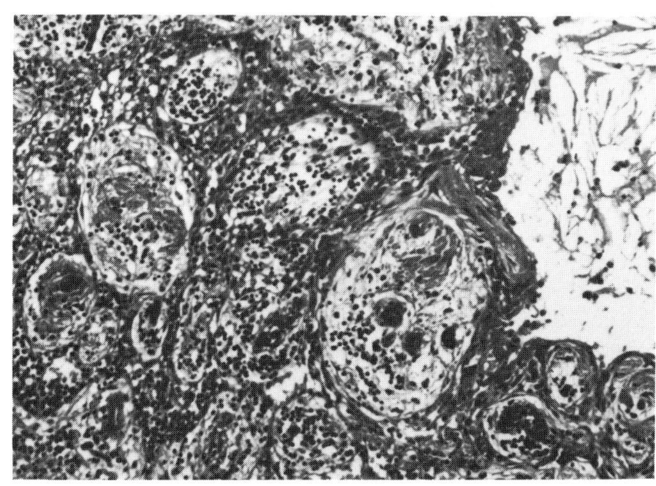

Figure 4–14. Proliferation of the epithelium lining a thymic cyst ("pseudoepitheliomatous hyperplasia") (H & E, ×200).

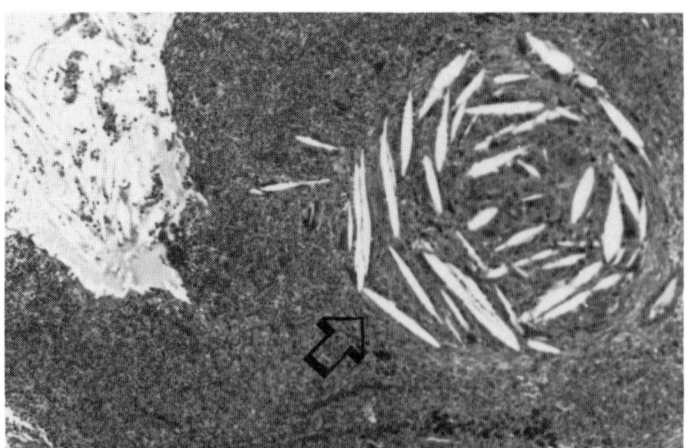

Figure 4–15. Cholesterol granuloma within the wall of a thymic cyst *(arrow)* (H & E, ×40).

has been reported in association with bilateral cleft lip and palate.[121]

Some investigators have suggested that the multilocular thymic cyst is an acquired lesion distinct from the congenital unilocular thymic cyst. Suster and Rosai speculate that cystic changes occur in branchial pouch derivatives as a result of an inflammatory cell infiltrate.[236] Other examples include branchial cleft cysts in the neck, branchial cleft-like cysts of the thyroid in association with thyroiditis,[239] and benign lymphoepithelial cysts in the parotid gland of patients with AIDS.[240]

Multilocular thymic cysts have been associated with other disorders, including Sjögren's syndrome and aplastic anemia, suggesting the possibility of an immune-mediated pathogenesis.[236] This author has seen one multilocular thymic cyst removed at autopsy from an AIDS patient with widespread infection (see Fig. 4–12). Suster and Rosai cite another case occurring in an HIV-positive individual.[236] Thymic cysts have been described in MG patients.[241] Thymic cysts have been reported in patients who had previous thoracic surgery, suggesting a pathogenic role for surgical trauma.[242]

Most thymic cysts can be completely excised.[236] Multilocular cysts may adhere to or infiltrate adjacent structures. In such cases, radiation therapy has been used postoperatively. Rarely, the cyst may recur. Thoracoscopy rather than thoracotomy has been advocated for resection of mediastinal cysts.[243, 244]

Other cystic thymic lesions must be considered whenever the diagnosis of thymic cyst is entertained. Thorough sampling of the lesion is critical to the correct diagnosis. Some cases of multilocular thymic cysts are associated with thymoma or thymic carcinoma. In the series by Suster and Rosai, 2 of 18 patients had a lymphocytic thymoma within the cyst wall, and another 2 had thymic carcinoma.[236] Cystic thymomas have been reported in which most of the lesion appears similar to a multilocular thymic cyst.[245] Focally within the wall of the apparent cyst, solid sheets of epithelial cells typical of a thymoma are present.

Hodgkin's disease and non-Hodgkin's lymphoma (see Chapter 6) may be associated with thymic cysts.[246–248] Cystic seminomas occur where only scattered tumor cells are present among the lymphoid tissue in the cyst wall.[249] Finally, a rare case of squamous cell carcinoma has been described within a thymic cyst.[250]

TOXIC AGENTS

Many chemicals and drugs are known to have a suppressive or carcinogenic effect on the immune system. For example, increased risk of developing lymphoma may be associated with exposure to herbicides.[251, 252] Perhaps some of these effects relate to the toxicity of these substances on the thymus. Most of the research concerning the thymus in immunotoxicology has necessarily involved laboratory animals. For example, halogenated aromatic hydrocarbons are environmental pollutants.[253] Dioxins are the protoype of this class of compounds. At low doses in mice, dioxins cause thymic atrophy, with their predominant effect on the cortex. The thymic cortical epithelial cell is especially susceptible to the toxic effect, although high doses also affect thymic lymphocytes by inducing apoptosis.

Human studies have involved immunologic assessment in populations exposed to relatively high levels of these chemicals. These substances reach the environment as a by-product of man-made chemicals. Municipal incinerators and electrical fires are among the sources. The compounds then contaminate the soil in surrounding areas. Studies of highly exposed populations have shown short-term alterations in T-cell subsets (e.g., decreased CD4/CD8 ratio). One study of low-level exposure to dioxin revealed significantly lower serum levels of thymosin alpha-1.[253]

Organotins are another class of chemicals that induce thymic atrophy.[254] These substances are used in a variety of circumstances, including plastic stabilizers and agricultural fungicides. These compounds appear to affect the immature lymphocytes of the thymic cortex in laboratory animals.

Thymic hypoplasia has been reported in a newborn with intrauterine exposure to isotretinoin (Accutane).[255] The drug, a form of retinoic acid used for facial acne, was begun 2 weeks before conception and was discontinued at 12 weeks of gestation. A nodule of 3 mm was all the thymus that could be identified in the infant. The nodule had normal lobulations and marked depletion of lymphocytes. Corticomedullary differentiation and Hassall's corpuscles were present. The infant had virtually no peripheral T cells and died of pneumonia at 9 weeks of age. The hypoplastic thymus is only one component of retinoic acid embryopathy. Other features include malformations of the central nervous system, congenital heart disease, and craniofacial abnormalities. Laboratory animals exposed in utero to retinoic acid have severe hypoplasia of the thymus along with incomplete descent.[256]

SUMMARY

The thymus is affected by many systemic illnesses. Thymic follicular hyperplasia is associated with myasthenia gravis but is not specific to this disorder. Stress induces a reversible thymic involution. The effects of stress are often difficult to separate from the effects of systemic illness (such as infections, malnutrition) or therapy (such as bone marrow transplantation). An increase in the size of the thymus (true thymic hyperplasia) may occur as a "rebound" phenomenon following stress, with hyperthyroidism, or with no apparent cause. Congenital and acquired immunodeficiencies are often associated with histologic changes in the thymus. Thymic cysts may appear as mass lesions in the neck or mediastinum. Although benign, they must be carefully evaluated to exclude a neoplastic process. Thymic epithelial tumors, Hodgkin's disease, non-Hodgkin's lymphomas, and germ cell tumors may all have a cystic component.

REFERENCES

1. Rosai J, Levine GD. Tumors of the thymus. Washington, DC: Armed Forces Institute of Pathology, 1976:34–98.
2. Hofmann WJ, Moller P, Otto HF. Thymic hyperplasia II. Lymphofollicular hyperplasia of the thymus. An immunohistologic study. Klin Wochenschr 1992; 65:53–60.
3. Kirchner T, Schalke B, Melms A, von Kugelgen T, Muller-Hermelink HK. Immunohistological patterns of non-neoplastic changes in the thymus in myasthenia gravis. Virchows Arch [B] 1986; 52:237–257.
4. Henry K. The human thymus in disease with particular emphasis on thymitis and thymoma. *In* Kendall MD, ed. The Thymus Gland. London: Academic Press, 1981: 85–111.
5. Bofill M, Janossy G, Willcox N, Chilosi M, Trejdosiewicz LK, Newsom-Davis J. Microenvironments in the normal thymus and thymus in myasthenia gravis. Am J Pathol 1985; 119:463–473.
6. Moran CA, Suster S, Gil J, Jagirdar J. Morphometric analysis of germinal centers in nonthymomatous patients with myasthenia gravis. Arch Pathol Lab Med 1990; 114:689–691.
7. Grody WW, Jobst S, Keesey J, Herrmann C Jr, Naeim F. Pathologic evaluation of thymic hyperplasia in myasthenia gravis and Lambert-Eaton myasthenic syndrome. Arch Pathol Lab Med 1986; 110:843–846.
8. Drachman, DB. Myasthenia gravis. N Engl J Med 1994; 330:1797–1810.
9. Castleman B. The pathology of the thymus gland in myasthenia gravis. Ann N Y Acad Sci 1966; 135:496–503.
10. Castleman B, Norris EH. The pathology of the thymus in myasthenia gravis. Medicine 1949; 28:27–58.
11. Schluep M, Willcox N, Vincent A, Dhoot GK, Newsom-Davis J. Acetylcholine receptors in human thymic myoid cells in situ: an immunohistological study. Ann Neurol 1987; 22:212–222.
12. Kirchner T, Tzartos S, Hoppe F, Schalke B, Wekerle H, Muller-Hermelink HK. Pathogenesis of myasthenia gravis. Acetylcholine receptor-related antigenic determinants in tumor-free thymuses and thymic epithelial tumors. Am J Pathol 1988; 130:268–280.
13. Wheatley LM, Urso D, Tumas K, Maltzman J, Loh E, Levinson AI. Molecular evidence for the expression of nicotinic acetylcholine receptor alpha-chain in mouse thymus. J Immunol 1992; 148:3105–3109.
14. Hara Y, Ueno S, Uemichi T, Takahashi N, Yorifuji S, Fujii Y, Tarui S. Neoplastic epithelial cells express alpha-subunit of muscle nicotinic acetylcholine receptor in thymomas from patients with myasthenia gravis. FEBS Lett 1991; 279:137–140.
15. van de Velde RL, Friedman NB. Thymic myoid cells and myasthenia gravis. Am J Pathol 1970; 59:347–368.
16. Sato T, Tamaoki N. Myoid cells in the human thymus and thymoma revealed by three different immunohistochemical markers for striated muscle. Acta Pathol Jpn 1989; 39:509–519.
17. Furuya A, Kobayashi T, Kameda N, Tsukagoshi H. Human myasthenia gravis thymic myoid cells: de novo immunohistochemical and intracellular electrophysiological studies. J Neurol Sci 1991; 101:208–220.
18. Drenckhahn D, von Gaudecker B, Muller-Hermelink HK, Unsicker K, Groschel-Stewart U. Myosin and actin containing cells in the human postnatal thymus: ultrastructural and immunohistochemical findings in normal thymus and in myasthenia gravis. Virchows Arch [B] 1979; 32:33–45.
19. Fuchs S, Schmidt-Hopfeld I, Tridente G, Tarrab-Hazdai R. Thymic lymphocytes bear a surface antigen which cross-reacts with acetylcholine receptor. Nature 1980; 287:162–164.
20. Emlie D, Crevon MC, Cohen-Kaminsky S, Peuchmaur M, Devergne O, Berrih-Aknin S, Galanaud P. In situ production of interleukins in hyperplastic thymus from myasthenia gravis patients. Hum Pathol 1991; 22:461–468.
21. Meinl E, Klinkert WEF, Wekerle H. The thymus in myasthenia gravis: changes typical for the human disease are absent in experimental autoimmune myasthenia gravis of the Lewis rat. Am J Pathol 1991; 139:995–1008.

22. Levinson AI, Lisak RP, Zweiman B, Kornstein M. Phenotypic and functional analysis of lymphocytes in myasthenia gravis. Springer Semin Immunopathol 1985; 8:209–233.
23. Lisak RP, Levinson AI, Zweiman B, Kornstein MJ. Antibodies to acetylcholine receptor and tetanus toxoid: in vitro synthesis by thymic lymphocytes. J Immunol 1986; 137:1221–1225.
24. Scadding GK, Vincent A, Newsom-Davis J, Henry K. Acetylcholine receptor antibody synthesis by thymic lymphocytes: correlation with thymic histology. Neurology 1981; 31:935–943.
25. Willcox N, Schluep M, Ritter MA, Newsom-Davis J. The thymus in seronegative myasthenia gravis patients. J Neurol 1991; 238:256–261.
26. Kornstein MJ, Brooks JJ, Anderson AO, Levinson AI, Lisak RP, Zweiman B. The immunohistology of the thymus in myasthenia gravis. Am J Pathol 1984; 117:184–194.
27. Ferrio MF, Durelli L, Massazza U, Cavallo R, Poccardi G, Maggi G, Casadio C, Di Summa M, Bergamini L. Intrathymic lymphoid cell differentiation in myasthenia gravis: an immunophenotypic study. Ital J Neurol Sci 1991; 12:569–573.
28. Schluep M, Willcox N, Ritter MA, Newsom-Davis J, Larche M, Brown AN. Myasthenia gravis thymus: clinical, histological and culture correlations. J Autoimmun 1988; 1:445–467.
29. Eimoto T, Kusano T, Ando K, Kikuchi M, Shirakusa T, Kawanami S. Nonneoplastic and nonhyperplastic thymus in myasthenia gravis: an immunohistochemical study with double immunoenzymatic labeling of basement membrane and cellular components. Am J Clin Pathol 1990; 94:36–43.
30. Wirt DP, Grogan TM, Nagle RB, Copeland JG, Richter LC, Rangel CS, Sjchuchardt M, Fosse J, Layton JM. A comprehensive immunotopographic map of human thymus. J Histochem Cytochem 1988; 36:1–12.
31. Henry K, Farrer-Brown G. Color Atlas of Thymus and Lymph Node Histopathology. Chicago: Year Book, 1982:9–44.
32. Compston AS, Vincent A, Newsom-Davis J, Batchelor JR. Clinical, pathological, HLA antigen and immunological evidence for disease heterogeneity in myasthenia gravis. Brain 1980; 103:579–601.
33. Aarli JA, Gilhus NE, Matre R. Myasthenia gravis with thymoma is not associated with an increased incidence of non-muscle autoimmune disorders. Autoimmunity 1992; 11:159–162.
34. Spurkland A, Gilhus NE, Renningen KS, Aarli JA, Vartdal F. Myasthenia gravis patients with thymus hyperplasia and myasthenia gravis patients with thymoma display different HLA associations. Tissue Antigens 1991; 37:90–93.
35. Halicek F, Rosai J. Histioeosinophilic granulomas in the thymuses of 29 myasthenic patients: a complication of pneumomediastinum. Hum Pathol 1984; 15:1137–1144.
36. Fischer JE, Grinvalski HT, Nussbaum MS, Sayers HJ, Cole RE, Samaha FJ. Aggressive surgical approach for drug-free remission from myasthenia gravis. Ann Surg 1987; 205:496–503.
37. Papatestas AE, Genkins G, Kornfield P, Eisenkraft JB, Fagerstrom RP, Pozner J, Aufses AH Jr. Effects of thymectomy in myasthenia gravis. Ann Surg 1987; 206:79–88.
38. Mulder DG, Graves M, Herrmann C. Thymectomy for myasthenia gravis: recent observations and comparisons with past experience. Ann Thorac Surg 1989; 48:551–555.
39. Scadding GK, Havard CW, Lange MJ, Domb I. The long term experience of thymectomy for myasthenia gravis. J Neurol Neurosurg Psychiatry 1985; 48:401–406.
40. Nussbaum MS, Rosenthal GJ, Samaha FJ, Grinvalsky HT, Quinlan JG, Schmerler M, Fischer JE. Management of myasthenia gravis by extended thymectomy with anterior mediastinal dissection. Surgery 1992; 112:681–688.
41. Cox A, Lisak RP, Skolnik P, Zweiman B. Effect of thymectomy on blood T-cell subsets in myasthenia gravis. Ann Neurol 1986; 19:297–298.
42. Vincent A, Newsom-Davis J, Newton P, Beck N. Acetylcholine receptor antibody and clinical response to thymectomy in myasthenia gravis. Neurology 1983; 33:1276–1282.
43. Reinglass JL, Brickel ACJ. The prognostic significance of thymic germinal center proliferation in myasthenia gravis. Neurology 1973; 23:69–72.
44. Michie W, Gunn A. The thyroid, the thymus and autoimmunity. Br J Clin Pract 1966; 20:9–13.
45. Prevot S, Audouin J, Andre-Bougaran J, Griffais R, le Tourneau A, Fournier JG, Diebold J. Thymic pseudotumorous enlargement due to follicular hyperplasia in a human immunodeficiency virus sero-positive patient: immunohistochemical and molecular biological study of viral infected cells. Am J Clin Pathol 1992; 97:420–425.
46. Joshi VV, Oleske JM, Saad S, Gadol C, Connor E, Bobila R, Minnefor AB. Thymus biopsy in children with acquired immunodeficiency syndrome. Arch Pathol Lab Med 1986; 110:837–842.
47. Trotter JL, Ferguson TF, Garvey WF. Studies on the thymus from patients with multiple sclerosis and myasthenia gravis. J Neuroimmunol 1982; 3:99–111.
48. Middleton G. The incidence of follicular structures in the human thymus at autopsy. Aust J Exp Biol Med Sci 1967; 45:189–199.
49. Vetters JM, Barclay RS. The incidence of germinal centres in thymus glands of patients with congenital heart disease. J Clin Pathol 1973; 26:583–591.
50. Michie W, Beck JS, Mahaffy RG, Honein EF, Fowler G. Quantitative radiological and histological studies of the thymus in thyroid disease. Lancet 1967; 1:691–695.
51. Burnet FM, Holmes MC. Thymic changes in the mouse strain NZB in relation to the auto-immune state. J Pathol 1964; 88:229–241.
52. Savino W, Boitard C, Bach J-F, Dardenne M. Studies on the thymus in nonobese diabetic mouse. I. Changes in the microenvironmental compartments. Lab Invest 1991; 64:405–417.
53. D'Andrea V, Malinovsky L, Ambrogi V, Artico M, Capuano LG, Buccolini F, de Antoni E. Thymectomy as treatment of autoimmune diseases other than myasthenia gravis. Thymus 1993; 21:1–10.
54. van Baarlen J, Schuurman H-J, Huber J. Acute thymus involution in infancy and childhood: a reliable marker for duration of acute illness. Hum Pathol 1988; 19:1155–1160.
55. Dourov N. Thymic atrophy and immune deficiency in malnutrition. Curr Top Pathol 1986; 75:127–150.
56. Colic M, Lilic D. The effect of trauma on the thymus. *In* Kendall MD, Ritter MA, eds. Thymus Update 4: The Thymus in Immunotoxicology. Chur, Switzerland: Harwood Academic Publishers, 1991:3–34.
57. van Baarlen J, Schuurman H-J, Reitsma R, Huber J.

Acute thymus involution during infancy and childhood: immunohistology of the thymus and peripheral lymphoid tissues after acute illness. Pediatr Pathol 1989; 9:261–275.
58. Ito T, Hoshino T. Studies of the influences of pregnancy and lactation on the thymus in the mouse. Z Zellforsch 1962; 57:667–678.
59. Ito T, Hoshino T. Histological changes of the mouse thymus during involution and regeneration following administration of hydrocortisone. Z Zellforsch 1962; 56:445–464.
60. van Haelst U. Light and electron microscopic study of the normal and pathological thymus of the rat. II. The acute thymic involution. Z Zellforsch 1967; 80:153–182.
61. Savino W, Cirne-Lima E, Soares JFT, Leite-De-Moraes MDC, Ono IPC, Dardenne M. Hydrocortisone increases the numbers of KL1 + cells, a discrete thymic epithelial cell subset characterized by high molecular weight cytokeratin expression. Endocrinology 1988; 123:2557–2564.
62. Steinmann GG. Changes in the human thymus during aging. *In* Muller-Hermelink HK, ed. The Human Thymus: Histophysiology and Pathology. Berlin: Springer-Verlag, 1986:43–88.
63. Kendall MD, Johnson HRM, Singh J. The weight of the human thymus gland at necropsy. J Anat 1980; 131:485–499.
64. Lack EE. Thymic hyperplasia with massive enlargement: report of two cases with review of diagnostic criteria. J Thorac Cardiovasc Surg 1981; 81:741–746.
65. Arliss J, Scholes J, Dickson PR, Messina JJ. Massive thymic hyperplasia in an adolescent. Ann Thorac Surg 1988; 45:220–222.
66. O'Shea PA, Pansatiankul B, Farnes P. Giant thymic hyperplasia in infancy: immunologic, histologic, and ultrastructural observations [abstract]. Lab Invest 1978; 38:391.
67. Lee Y, Moallem S, Clauss RH. Massive hyperplastic thymus in a 22 month old infant. Ann Thorac Surg 1979; 27:356–358.
68. Riazmontazer N, Bedayat G. Aspiration cytology of an enlarged thymus presenting as a mediastinal mass: a case report. Acta Cytol 1993; 37:427–430.
69. Judd RL. Massive thymic hyperplasia with myoid cell differentiation. Hum Pathol 1987; 18:1180–1183.
70. Katz SM, Chatten J, Bishop HC, Rosenblum H. Massive thymic enlargement: report of a case of gross thymic hyperplasia in a child. Am J Clin Pathol 1977; 68:786–790.
71. Nezelof C, Normand C. Tumor-like massive thymic hyperplasia in childhood: a possible defect of T-cell maturation, histological and cytoenzymatic studies of three cases. Thymus 1986; 8:177–186.
72. Ricci C, Pescarmona E, Rendina EA, Venuta F, Ruco LP, Baroni CD. True thymic hyperplasia: a clinicopathologic study. Ann Thorac Surg 1989; 47:741–745.
73. Judd RL, Welch SL. Myoid cell differentiation in true thymic hyperplasia and lymphoid hyperplasia. Arch Pathol Lab Med 1988; 112:1140–1144.
74. Williams DJ. True thymic hyperplasia: an unrecognized cause of cardiac murmur? Thymus 1988; 12:135–137.
75. Nomori H, Ishihara T, Torikata C, Harigaya K, Mikata A. A case of massive true thymic hyperplasia with non-Hodgkin's lymphoma. Chest 1990; 98:1304–1305.
76. Ruco LP, Rosati S, Palmieri B, Pescarmona E, Rendina EA, Baroni CD. True thymic hyperplasia: a histological and immunohistochemical study. Histopathology 1989; 15:640–643.
77. Pendlebury SC, Boyages S, Koutts J, Boyages J. Thymic hyperplasia associated with Hodgkin's disease and thyrotoxicosis. Cancer 1992; 70:1985–1987.
78. Ichiki S, Komatsu C, Ogata H, Mitsudome A. A case of myasthenia gravis complicated with hyperthyroidism and thymic hyperplasia in childhood. Brain Dev 1992; 14:164–166.
79. Rasore-Quartino A, Rebizzo F, Romagnoli G. Iperplasia gigante del timo nell'infanzia. Pathologica 1992; 71:711–715.
80. Oh KS, Weber AL, Borden S IV. Normal mediastinal mass in late childhood. Pediatr Radiol 1971; 101:625–628.
81. Lamesch AJ. Massive thymic hyperplasia in infants. Z Kinderchir 1983; 38:16–18.
82. Due W, Dieckmann K-P, Stein H. Thymic hyperplasia following chemotherapy of a testicular germ cell tumor. Cancer 1989; 63:446–449.
83. Caffey J, Silbey R. Regrowth and overgrowth of the thymus after atrophy induced by the oral administration of adrenocorticosteroids to human infants. Pediatrics 1960; 26:762–770.
84. Barcia PJ, Nelson TG. Hyperplasia of the thymus and thymic neoplasms in children. Milit Med 1979; 144:799–801.
85. Gelfand DW, Goldman AS, Law EJ, MacMillan BG, Larson D, Abston S, Schreiber JT. Thymic hyperplasia in children recovering from thermal burns. J Trauma 1972; 12:813–817.
86. Rizk G, Cueto L, Amplatz K. Rebound enlargement of the thymus after successful corrective surgery for transposition of the great vessels. Am J Roentgenol 1972; 116:528–530.
87. Carmosino L, DeBenedetto A, Feffer S. Thymic hyperplasia following successful chemotherapy: a report of two cases and review of the literature. Cancer 1985; 56:1526–1528.
88. Cohen M, Hill CA, Cangir A, Sullivan MP. Thymic rebound after treatment of childhood tumors. AJR 1980; 135:151–156.
89. Shin MY, Ho K-J. Diffuse thymic hyperplasia following chemotherapy for nodular sclerosing Hodgkin's disease: an immunologic rebound phenomenon. Cancer 1983; 51:30–33.
90. Durkin W, Durant J. Benign mass lesions after therapy for Hodgkin's disease. Arch Intern Med 1979; 139:333–336.
91. Langer CJ, Keller SM, Erner SM. Thymic hyperplasia with hemorrhage simulating recurrent Hodgkin's disease after chemotherapy-induced complete remission. Cancer 1992; 70:2082–2086.
92. Kissin CM, Husband JE, Nicholas D, Eversman W. Benign thymic enlargement in adults after chemotherapy: CT demonstration. Radiology 1987; 163:67–70.
93. White S, Hall JB, Little A. An approach to mediastinal masses associated with hyperthyroidism. Chest 1986; 90:691–693.
94. Pardo-Mindan FJ. Immunological aspects of sarcoidosis associated with true thymic hyperplasia. Allerg Immunopathol (Paris) 1980; 8:91–96.
94a. Goldstein G, Mackay IR. The Human Thymus. London: William Heinemann Medical Books, 1969.
95. Balcom RJ, Hakanson DO, Werner A, Gordon LP. Massive thymic hyperplasia in an infant with Beckwith-Wiedemann syndrome. Arch Pathol Lab Med 1985; 109:153–155.

96. Potter EL, Craig JM. Thymus and glands of internal secretion. *In* Pathology of the Fetus and Infant. Chicago: Year Book Medical, 1975:317–333.
97. Judd R, Bueso-Ramos C. Combined true thymic hyperplasia and lymphoid hyperplasia in Graves' disease. Pediatr Pathol 1990; 10:829–836.
98. Rose JS, Lam C. Thymic enlargement in association with hyperthyroidism. Pediatr Radiol 1982; 12:37–38.
99. Bergman TA, Mariash CN, Oppenheimer JH. Anterior mediastinal mass in a patient with Graves' disease. J Clin Endocrinol Metab 1982; 55:587–588.
100. Fyfe B, Dominguez F, Poppiti RJ. Thymic hyperplasia: a clue to the diagnosis of hyperthyroidism. Am J Forensic Med Pathol 1990; 11:257–260.
101. Beddingfield GW, Campbell DC Jr, Hood RH Jr, Dooley BN. Simultaneous disorders of thyroid and thymus: report of two cases. Ann Thorac Surg 1967; 4:445–450.
102. Cooper A. The Anatomy of the Thymus Gland. Philadelphia: Lea & Blanchard, 1845.
103. Cardarelli NF. Thymus pathology and disease states. *In* Cardarelli NF, ed. The Thymus in Health and Senescence, volume 1: Thymus and Immunity. Boca Raton, Florida: CRC Press, 1989:133–160.
104. Halsted WS. The significance of the thymus gland in Graves' disease. Bull Johns Hopkins Hosp 1914; 25:223–234.
105. Yulish BS, Owens RP. Thymic enlargement in a child during therapy for primary hypothyroidism. AJR 1980; 135:157–158.
106. Marine D, Manley OT, Baumann EJ. The influence of thyroidectomy, gonadectomy, suprarenalectomy, and splenectomy on the thymus gland of rabbits. J Exp Med 1924; 40:429–443.
107. Scheiff JM, Cordier AC, Haumont S. Epithelial cell proliferation in thymic hyperplasia induced by triiodothyronine. Clin Exp Immunol 1977; 27:516–521.
108. Fabris N, Mocchegiani E, Mariotti S, Paccini F, Pinchera A. Thyroid-thymus interactions during development and aging. Horm Res 1989; 31:85–89.
109. Wortsman J, McConnachie P, Baker JR, Burman KD. Immunoglobulins that cause thymocyte proliferation from a patient with Graves' disease and an enlarged thymus. Am J Med 1988; 85:117–121.
110. Villa-Verde DMS, Defresne M-P, Vannier-Dos-Santos MA, Dussault JH, Boniver J, Savino W. Identification of nuclear triiodothyronine receptors in the thymic epithelium. Endocrinology 1992; 131:1313–1320.
111. Harington H. Absence of the thymus gland. London Med Gaz 1829; 3:314.
112. Lischner HW. DiGeorge syndrome(s). J Pediatr 1972; 81:1042–1044.
113. DiGeorge AM. Congenital absence of the thymus and its immunologic consequences: concurrence with congenital hypoparathyroidism. Birth Defects Original Article Series 1968; 4:116–123.
114. Good RA, Peterson RDA, Perey DY, Finstad J, Cooper MD. The immunological deficiency diseases of man: consideration of some questions asked by these patients with an attempt at classification. Birth Defects Original Article Series 1968; 4:17–39.
115. Robinson HB. DiGeorge's or the III-IV pharyngeal pouch syndrome: pathology and a theory of pathogenesis. Perspect Pediatr Pathol 1973; 2:173–206.
116. Burke BA, Johnson D, Gilbert EF, Drut RM, Ludwig J, Wick M. Thyrocalcitonin-containing cells in the DiGeorge anomaly. Hum Pathol 1987; 18:355–360.
117. Thomas RA, Landing BH, Wells TR. Embryologic and other developmental considerations of thirty-eight possible variants of the DiGeorge anomaly. Am J Med Genet Suppl 1987; 3:43–66.
118. Hong R. The DiGeorge anomaly. Immunodefic Rev 1991; 3:1–14.
119. Muller W, Peter HH, Wilken M, Juppner H, Kallfelz HC, Krohn HP, Miller K, Rieger CHL. The DiGeorge syndrome I. Clinical evaluation and course of partial and complete forms of the syndrome. Eur J Pediatr 1988; 147:496–502.
120. Conley ME, Beckwith JB, Mancer JF, Tenckhoff L. The spectrum of the DiGeorge syndrome. J Pediatr 1979; 94:883–890.
121. Bale PM, Sotelo-Avila C. Maldescent of the thymus: 34 necropsy and 10 surgical cases, including 7 thymuses medial to the mandible. Pediatr Pathol 1993; 13:181–190.
122. Huber J, Zegers BJM, Schuurman H-J. Pathology of congenital immunodeficiencies. Semin Diagn Pathol 1992; 9:31–62.
123. Kelley RI, Zackai EH, Emanuel BS, Kistenmacher M, Greenberg F, Punnett HH. The association of the DiGeorge anomalad with partial monosomy of chromosome 22. J Pediatr 1982; 101:197–200.
124. de la Chapelle A, Herva R, Koivisto M, Aula P. A deletion in chromosome 22 can cause DiGeorge syndrome. Hum Genet 1981; 57:253–256.
125. Van Mierop LHS, Kutsche LM. Cardiovascular anomalies in DiGeorge syndrome and importance of neural crest as a possible pathogenetic factor. Am J Cardiol 1986; 58:133–137.
126. Bockman DE, Kirby ML. Neural crest function in thymus development. Immunol Ser 1989; 45:451–467.
127. Bockman DE, Kirby ML. Dependence of thymus development on derivatives of the neural crest. Science 1984; 223:498–500.
128. Sulik KK, Johnston MC, Daft PA, Russell WE, Dehart DB. Fetal alcohol syndrome and DiGeorge anomaly: critical ethanol exposure periods for craniofacial malformations as illustrated in an animal model. Am J Med Genet Suppl 1986; 2:97–112.
129. Nezelof Ch. Pathology of the thymus in immunodeficiency states. *In* Muller-Hermelink HK, ed. The Human Thymus: Histophysiology and Pathology. Berlin: Springer-Verlag, 1986:151–177.
130. Buckley RH. Advances in the diagnosis and treatment of primary immunodeficiency diseases. Arch Intern Med 1986; 146:377–384.
131. Buckley RH. Immunodeficiency diseases. *In* deShazo RD, Smith DL, eds. Primer on allergic and immunologic diseases. JAMA 1992; 268:2797–2806.
132. Neuhaus TJ, Briner J. Morphology of original and transplanted thymuses in severe combined immunodeficiency. Pediatr Pathol 1986; 5:251–270.
133. Haynes BF, Warren RW, Buckley RH, McClure JE, Goldstein AL, Henderson FW, Hensley L, Eisenbarth GS. Demonstration of abnormalities in expression of thymic epithelial surface antigens in severe cellular immunodeficiency diseases. J Immunol 1983; 130:1182–1189.
134. Cooper MD, Butler JL. Primary immunodeficiency diseases. *In* Paul WE, ed. Fundamental Immunology. New York: Raven Press, 1989:1033–1057.
135. Fischer A. Severe combined immunodeficiencies. Immunodefic Rev 1992; 3:83–100.
136. Doherty PJ, Pan S, Mulloy JC, Thompson E, Thorner P, Barankiewiecz J, Roifman CM, Cohen A. Adenosine deaminase and thymocyte maturation. Scand J Immunol 1991; 33:405–410.

137. Markert ML. Purine nucleoside phosphorylase deficiency. Immunodefic Rev 1991; 3:45–81.
138. Borzy MS, Schulte-Wisserman H, Gilbert E, Horowitz SD, Pellett J, Hong R. Thymic morphology in immunodeficiency diseases: results of thymic biopsies. Clin Immunol Immunopathol 1979; 12:31–51.
139. Gosseye S, Diebold N, Griscelli C, Nezelof C. Severe combined immunodeficiency disease: a pathological analysis of 26 cases. Clin Immunol Immunopathol 1983; 29:58–77.
140. Landing BH, Yutuc IL, Swanson VL. Clinicopathologic correlations in immunologic deficiency diseases of children, with emphasis on thymic histologic patterns. *In* Kobayashi N, ed. Immunodeficiency: Its Nature and Etiological Significance in Human Diseases. Baltimore: University Park Press, 1978:3–35.
141. Stallmach Th. Thymic lymphocytes and thymic epithelial cells in four cases of congenital immunodeficiency. In Vivo 1991; 5:249–254.
142. Hitzig WH, Landolt R, Muller G, Bodmer P. Heterogeneity of phenotypic expression in a family with Swiss-type agammaglobulinemia: observations on the acquisition of agammaglobulinemia. J Pediatr 1971; 78:968–980.
143. Meuwissen HJ, Pollara B, Pickering RJ. Combined immunodeficiency disease associated with adenosine deaminase deficiency. J Pediatr 1975; 86:169–181.
144. Hirschhorn R, Vawter GF, Kirkpatrick JA, Rosen FS. Adenosine deaminase deficiency: frequency and comparative pathology in autosomally recessive severe combined immunodeficiency. Clin Immunol Immunopathol 1979; 14:107–120.
145. Ratech H, Hirschhorn R, Greco MA. Pathologic findings in adenosine deaminase deficient-severe combined immunodeficiency. Am J Pathol 1989; 135:1145–1156.
146. Shores EW, van Ewijk W, Singer A. Disorganization and restoration of thymic medullary epithelial cells in T cell receptor-negative scid mice: evidence that receptor-bearing lymphocytes influence maturation of the thymic microenvironment. Eur J Immunol 1991; 21:1657–1661.
147. Schuurman H-J, Krone WJA, Broekhuizen R, van Baarlen J, van Veen P, Goldstein AL, Huber J, Goudsmit J. The thymus in acquired immune deficiency syndrome: comparison with other types of immunodeficiency diseases and the presence of components of human immunodeficiency virus type 1. Am J Pathol 1989; 134:1329–1338.
148. Gartner JG. Thymic involution with loss of Hassall's corpuscles mimicking thymic dysplasia in a child with transfusion-associated graft-versus-host disease. Pediatr Pathol 1991; 11:449–456.
149. Seemayer TA, Bolande RP. Thymic involution mimicking thymic dysplasia: a consequence of transfusion induced graft versus host disease in a premature infant. Arch Pathol Lab Med 1980; 104:141–144.
150. Businco L, DiFazio A, Ziruolo MG, Boner AL, Valletta EA, Ruco LP, Vitolo D, Ensoli B, Paganelli R. Clinical and immunological findings in four infants with Omenn's syndrome: a form of severe combined immunodeficiency with phenotypically normal T cells, elevated IgE, and eosinophilia. Clin Immunol Immunopathol 1987; 44:123–133.
151. Touraine J-L. The bare-lymphocyte syndrome: report on the registry. Lancet 1981; 1:319–323.
152. Schuurman H-J, Zegers BJM. The thymus in MHC deficiency syndrome: implications for immune function. *In* Kendall MD, Ritter MA, eds. Thymus Update 2: T Lymphocyte Differentiation in the Human Thymus. Chur, Switzerland: Harwood Academic Publishers, 1989:89–103.
153. Schuurman H-J, van de Wijngaert FP. The thymus in "bare lymphocyte" syndrome: significance of expression of major histocompatibility complex antigens on thymic epithelial cells in intrathymic T cell maturation. Hum Immunol 1985; 13:69–82.
154. Kornstein MJ, Weber J, Luck JB, Massey GV, Strom S, McWilliams NB. Epstein-Barr virus-associated lymphoproliferative disorder: applications of immunoperoxidase and molecular biologic techniques. Arch Pathol Lab Med 1989; 113:481–484.
155. Purtilo D. X-linked lymphoproliferative syndrome: an immunodeficiency disorder with acquired agammaglobulinemia, fatal infectious mononucleosis, or malignant lymphoma. Arch Pathol Lab Med 1981; 105:119–121.
156. Harrington DS, Weisenburger DD, Purtilo DT. Epstein-Barr virus-associated lymphoproliferative lesions. Clin Lab Med 1988; 8:97–118.
157. Purtilo DT. Immunopathology of infectious mononucleosis and other complications of Epstein-Barr virus infections. *In* Sommers S, Rosen PP, eds. Pathology Annual, 1980, Part 1. New York: Appleton-Century-Crofts, 1980:253–299.
158. Aguilar MJ, Kamoshita S, Landing BH, Boder E, Sedgwick RP. Pathological observations in ataxia-telangiectasia: a report on five cases. J Neuropathol Exp Neurol 1968; 27:659–676.
159. Standen GR. Wiskott-Aldrich syndrome: a multidisciplinary disease. J Clin Pathol 1991; 44:979–982.
160. Park JP, Rosenstein YJ, Remold-O'Donnell E, Bierer BE, Rosen FS, Burakoff SJ. Enhancement of T-cell activation by the CD43 molecule whose expression is defective in Wiskott-Aldrich syndrome. Nature 1991; 350:706–709.
161. Huber J. Experience with various immunologic deficiencies in Holland. Birth Defects Original Article Series 1968; 4:53–66.
162. Cooper MD, Chase HP, Lowman JT, Krivit W, Good RA. Immunologic defects in patients with Wiskott-Aldrich syndrome. Birth Defects Original Article Series 1968; 4:378–387.
163. Gallin JI. Inflammation. *In* Paul WE, ed. Fundamental Immunology. New York: Raven Press, 1989:721–733.
164. Nunoi H, Yanabe Y, Higuchi S, Tsuchiya H, Yamamoto J, Matsuda I, Naito M, Takahashi K, Fujita K, Uchida M, Kobayashi K, Jono M, Malech H. Severe hypoplasia of lymphoid tissues in Mo1 deficiency. Hum Pathol 1988; 19:753–759.
165. Fischer A, Landais P, Friedrich W, Morgan G, Gerritsen B, Fasth A, Porta F, Griscelli C, Goldman SF, Levinsky R, Vossen J. European experience of bone-marrow transplantation for severe combined immunodeficiency. Lancet 1990; 336:850–853.
166. Ferrari G, Rossini S, Nobili N, Maggioni D, Garofalo A, Giavazzi R, Mavvilio F, Bordignon C. Transfer of the ADA gene into human ADA-deficient T lymphocytes reconstitutes specific immune functions. Blood 1992; 80:1120–1124.
167. Blaese RM, Culver KW. Gene therapy for primary immunodeficiency disease. Immunodefic Rev 1992; 3:329–349.
168. Joshi VV, Oleske JM. Morphologic findings in children with acquired immune deficiency syndrome: pathogenesis and clinical implications. Pediatr Pathol 1990; 10:155–165.

169. Grody WW, Fligiel S, Naeim F. Thymus involution in the acquired immunodeficiency syndrome. Am J Clin Pathol 1985; 84:85–95.
170. Seemayer TA, Laroche AC, Russo P, Malebranche R, Arnoux E, Guerin J-M, Pierre G, Dupuy J-M, Gartner JG, Lapp WS, Spira TJ, Elie R. Precocious thymic involution manifest by epithelial injury in the acquired immunodeficiency syndrome. Hum Pathol 1984; 15:469–474.
171. Joshi VV, Oleske JM, Minnefor AB, Singh R, Bokhari T, Rapkin RH. Pathology of suspected acquired immune deficiency syndrome in children: a study of eight cases. Pediatr Pathol 1984; 2:71–87.
172. Guarda LA, Luna MA, Smith JL Jr, Mansell PWA, Gyorkey F, Roca AN. Acquired immune deficiency syndrome: postmortem findings. Am J Clin Pathol 1984; 81:549–557.
173. Reichert CM, O'Leary TJ, Levens DL, Simrell CR, Macher AM. Autopsy pathology in the acquired immunodeficiency syndrome. Am J Pathol 1983; 112:357–382.
174. Welch K, Finkbeiner W, Alpers CE, Blumenfeld W, Davis RL, Smuckler EA, Beckstead JH. Autopsy findings in the Acquired Immune Deficiency Syndrome. JAMA 1984; 252:1152–1159.
175. Elie R, Laroche AC, Arnoux E, Guerin J-M, Pierre G, Malebranche R, Seemayer TA, Dupuy J-M, Russo P, Lapp WS. Thymic dysplasia in acquired immunodeficiency syndrome. N Engl J Med 1983; 308:841–842.
176. Joshi VV, Oleski JM. Pathologic appraisal of the thymus gland in acquired immunodeficiency syndrome in children: a study of four cases and a review of the literature. Arch Pathol Lab Med 1985; 109:142–146.
177. Schuurman H-J, van Baarlen J, Krone WJA, Huber J. The thymus in the acquired immune deficiency syndrome. *In* Kendall MD, Ritter MA, eds. Thymus Update 1: The Microenvironment of the Human Thymus. Chur, Switzerland: Harwood Academic Publishers, 1988:171–189.
178. Savino W, Dardenne M, Marche C, Trophilme D, Dupuy J-M, Pekovic D, Lapointe N, Bache J-F. Thymic epithelium in AIDS: an immunohistologic study. Am J Pathol 1986; 122:302–307.
179. Dardenne M, Bach J-F, Safai B. Low serum thymic hormone levels in patients with acquired immunodeficiency syndrome. N Engl J Med 1983; 309:48–49.
180. Naylor PH, Friedman-Klein A, Hersch E, Erdos M, Goldstein AL. Thymosin beta-1 and thymosin beta-4 in serum: comparison of normal, cord, homosexual and AIDS serum. Int J Immunopharmacol 1986; 8:667–676.
181. Schnittman SM, Denning SM, Greenhouse JJ, Justement JS, Baseler M, Kurtzberg J, Haynes BF, Fauci AS. Evidence for susceptibility of intrathymic T cell precursors and their progeny carrying T cell antigen receptor phenotypes TCR alpha beta+ and TCR gamma delta+ to human immunodeficiency virus infection: a mechanism for CD4+ (T4) lymphocyte depletion. Proc Natl Acad Sci U S A 1990; 87:7727–7731.
182. Numazaki K, Goldman H, Bai X-Q, Wong I, Wainberg MA. Effects of infection by HIV-1, cytomegalovirus, and human measles virus on cultured human thymic epithelial cells. Microbiol Immunol 1989; 33:733–745.
183. De Rossi A, Calabro ML, Panozzo M, Bernardi D, Caruso B, Tridente G, Chieco-Bianchi L. In vitro studies of HIV-1 infection in thymic lymphocytes: a putative role of the thymus in AIDS pathogenesis. AIDS Res Hum Retroviruses 1990; 6:287–298.
184. Mano H, Chermann J-C. Fetal human immunodeficiency virus type 1 infection of different organs in the second trimester. AIDS Res Hum Retroviruses 1991; 7:83–88.
185. Courgnaud V, Laure F, Brossard A, Bignozzi C, Goudeau A, Barin F, Brechot C. Frequent and early in utero HIV-1 infection. AIDS Res Hum Retroviruses 1991; 7:337–341.
186. Baskin GB, Murphey-Corb M, Martin LN, Davison-Fairburn B, Kuebler D. Thymus in simian immunodeficiency virus-infected rhesus monkeys. Lab Invest 1991; 65:400–407.
187. Dwyer JM, Wood CC, McNamara J, Kinder B. Transplantation of thymic tissue into patients with AIDS: an attempt to reconstitute the immune system. Arch Intern Med 1987; 147:513–517.
188. Hermans P, Clumeck N. Preliminary results on clinical and immunological effects of thymus hormone preparations in AIDS. Med Oncol Tumor Pharmacother 1989; 6:55–58.
189. Trainin N. Prospects of AIDS therapy by thymic humoral factor, a thymic hormone. Nat Immun Cell Growth Regul 1990; 9:155–159.
190. Chachoua A, Green MD, Valentine F, Muggia FM. Phase I/II trial of thymostimulin in opportunistic infections of the acquired immune deficiency syndrome. Cancer Invest 1989; 7:225–229.
191. Phair J. Therapy for acquired immunodeficiency syndrome: implantation of cultured thymic fragments. Arch Intern Med 1986; 146:1074–1075.
192. Dupuy J-M, Gilmore N, Goldman H, Tsoukas C, Pekovic D, Chausseau J-P, Duperval R, Joly M, Pelletier L, Thibaudeau Y. Thymic epithelial cell transplantation in patients with acquired immunodeficiency syndrome: evidence for infection by HIV-1 of newly differentiated T cells at the site of transplantation. Thymus 1991; 17:205–218.
193. Danner SA, Schuurman H-J, Lange JMA, Meyling FHJG, Schellekens PThA, Huber J, Kater L. Implantation of cultured thymic fragments in patients with acquired immunodeficiency syndrome. Arch Intern Med 1986; 146:1133–1136.
194. Thomas JA, Sloane JP, Imrie SF, Ritter MA, Schuurman H-J, Huber J. Immunohistology of the thymus in bone marrow transplant recipients. Am J Pathol 1986; 122:531–540.
195. Beschorner WE, Hutchins GM, Elfenbein GJ, Santos GW. The thymus in patients with allogeneic bone marrow transplants. Am J Pathol 1978; 92:173–181.
196. Muller-Hermelink HK, Sale GE, Borisch B, Storb R. Pathology of the thymus after allogeneic bone marrow transplantation in man. Am J Pathol 1987; 129:242–256.
197. Seemayer TA, Lapp WS, Bolande RP. Thymic involution in murine graft-versus-host reaction. Am J Pathol 1977; 88:119–133.
198. Fukushi N, Arase H, Wang B, Ogasawara K, Gotohda T, Good RA, Onoe K. Thymus: a direct target tissue in graft-versus-host reaction after allogeneic bone marrow transplantation that results in abrogation of induction of self-tolerance. Proc Natl Acad Sci U S A 1990; 87:6301–6305.
199. Weiden P, Sale GE, Shulman HM. Human marrow transplantation: an overview. *In* Sale GE, Shulman HM, eds. The Pathology of Bone Marrow Transplantation. Chicago: Year Book Medical, 1984:1–10.
200. Sale GE. Pathology of the lymphoreticular system. *In* Sale GE, Shulman HM, eds. The Pathology of Bone Marrow Transplantation. Chicago: Year Book Medical, 1984:171–191.

201. Ritter MA, Ladyman HM. The effects of cyclosporin on the thymic microenvironment and T cell development. *In* Kendall MD, Ritter MA, eds. Thymus Update 4: The Thymus in Immunotoxicology. Chur, Switzerland: Harwood Academic Publishers, 1991: 157–177.
202. Beschorner WE, Namnoum JD, Hess AD, Shinn CA, Santos GW. Cyclosporin A and the thymus: immunopathology. Am J Pathol 1987; 126:487–496.
203. Thomson AW, Pugh-Humphreys RGP. The antilymphocytic properties of FK-506 and its influence on the thymic environment. *In* Kendall MD, Ritter MA, eds. Thymus Update 4: The Thymus in Immunotoxicology. Chur, Switzerland: Harwood Academic Publishers, 1991:93–127.
204. Smith SM, Ossa-Gomez LJ. A quantitative histologic comparison of the thymus in 100 healthy and diseased adults. Am J Clin Pathol 1981; 76:657–665.
205. Morse SS. Thymic necrosis following oral inoculation of mouse thymic virus. Lab Anim Sci 1989; 39:571–574.
206. Schwartz JN, Daniels CA, Klintworth GK. Lymphoid cell necrosis, thymic atrophy, and growth retardation in newborn mice inoculated with murine cytomegalovirus. Am J Pathol 1975; 79:509–519.
207. Savino W. The thymic microenvironment in infectious diseases. Mem Inst Oswaldo Cruz 1990; 85:255–260.
208. Berry CL, Thompson EN. Clinico-pathological study of thymic dysplasia. Arch Dis Child 1968; 43:579–584.
209. King C-C, Jamieson BD, Reddy K, Bali N, Concepcion RJ, Ahmed R. Viral infection of the thymus. J Virol 1992; 66:3155–3160.
210. Dubois P. Du diagnostic de la syphilis consideree comme une des causes possibles de la mort du foetus. Gaz Med Paris 1850; 5:392.
211. Oliver J. Syphilitic disease of the thymus in infants and the mode of origin of the Dubois abscesses. Am J Dis Child 1917; 13:158–166.
212. Benjamin EL. Dubois' sequestra of the thymus gland of nonsyphilitic origin. Am J Dis Child 1930; 39:586–590.
213. Jacobi A. Contributions to the anatomy and pathology of the thymus gland. Trans Assoc Am Phys 1888; 3:297–319.
214. Roth SI. The endocrine glands. *In* Ioachim HL, ed. Pathology of Granulomas. New York: Raven Press, 1983:449–462.
215. FitzGerald JM, Mayo JR, Miller RR, Jamieson WRE, Baumgartner F. Tuberculosis of the thymus. Chest 1992; 102:1604–1605.
216. Linder J. The thymus gland in secondary immunodeficiency. Arch Pathol Lab Med 1987; 111:1118–1122.
217. Ohshima T, Nakaya T, Saito K, Maeda H, Nagano T. Child neglect followed by marked thymic involution and fatal systemic pseudomonas infection. Int J Leg Med 1991; 104:167–171.
218. Purtilo DT, Connor DH. Fatal infections in protein-calorie malnourished children with thymolymphatic atrophy. Arch Dis Child 1975; 50:149–152.
219. Smythe PM, Schonland M, Brereton-Stiles GG, Loening WEK, Mafoyane A, Parent MA, Vos GH. Thymolymphatic deficiency and depression of cell-mediated immunity in protein-calorie malnutrition. Lancet 1971; 2:939–943.
220. Mugerwa JW. The lymphoreticular system in kwashiorkor. J Pathol 1971; 105:105–109.
221. Jessurun J, Azevedo M, Saldana M. Allergic angiitis and granulomatosis (Churg-Strauss syndrome): report of a case with massive thymic involvement in a non-asthmatic patient. Hum Pathol 1986; 17:637–639.
222. Larocca LM, Lauriola L, Ranelletti FO, Piantelli M, Maggiano N, Ricci R, Capelli A. Morphological and immunohistochemical study of Down syndrome thymus. Am J Med Genet Suppl 1990; 7:225–230.
223. Larocca LM, Piantelli M, Valitutti S, Castellino F, Maggiano N, Musiani P. Alterations in thymocyte subpopulations in Down's syndrome (Trisomy 21). Clin Immunol Immunopathol 1988; 49:175–186.
224. Murphy M, Insoft RM, Pike-Nobile L, Derbin KS, Epstein LB. Overexpression of LFA-1 and ICAM-1 in Down syndrome thymus. J Immunol 1993; 150:5696–5703.
225. Murphy M, Friend DS, Pike-Nobile L, Epstein LB. Tumor necrosis factor-alpha and interferon-gamma expression in human thymus: localization and overexpression in Down syndrome. J Immunol 1992; 149:2506–2512.
226. Wick MR. Mediastinal cysts and intrathoracic thyroid tumors. Semin Diagn Pathol 1990; 7:285–294.
227. Leong ASY. Thymic cysts. *In* Givel J-C, ed. Surgery of the Thymus. Berlin: Springer-Verlag, 1990:71–77.
228. Davis RD, Oldham HN Jr, Sabiston DC Jr. Primary cysts and neoplasms of the mediastinum: recent changes in clinical presentation, methods of diagnosis, management, and results. Ann Thorac Surg 1987; 44:229–237.
229. Cohen AJ, Thompson L, Edwards FH, Bellamy RF. Primary cysts and tumors of the mediastinum. Ann Thorac Surg 1991; 51:378–386.
230. Guba AM, Adam AE, Jaques DA, Chambers RG. Cervical presentation of thymic cysts. Am J Surg 1978; 136:430–436.
231. Krech WG, Storey CF, Umiker WC. Thymic cysts: a review of the literature and report of two cases. J Thorac Surg 1954; 27:477–493.
232. Indeglia RA, Shea MA, Grage TB. Congenital cysts of the thymus gland. Arch Surg 1967; 94:149–152.
233. Bieger RC, McAdams AJ. Thymic cysts. Arch Pathol 1966; 82:535–541.
234. Wagner CW, Vinocur CD, Weintraub WH, Golladay S. Respiratory complications in cervical thymic cysts. J Pediatr Surg 1988; 23:657–660.
235. Michael M, Havlicek F. Pseudo-epitheliomatous hyperplasia in thymic cysts. Histopathology 1991; 19:281–282.
236. Suster S, Rosai J. Multilocular thymic cyst: an acquired reactive process: a study of 18 cases. Am J Surg Pathol 1991; 15:388–398.
237. Fahmy S. Cervical thymic cysts: their pathogenesis and relationship to branchial cysts. J Laryngol Otol 1974; 88:47–60.
238. Breckler IA, Johnston DG. Choristoma of the thymus. Am J Dis Child 1956; 92:175–178.
239. Louis DN, Vickery AL, Rosai J, Wang CA. Multiple branchial cleft-like cysts in Hashimoto's thyroiditis. Am J Surg Pathol 1989; 13:45–49.
240. Kornstein MJ, Parker GA, Mills AS. Immunohistology of the benign lymphoepithelial lesion in AIDS-related lymphadenopathy: a case report. Hum Pathol 1988; 19:1359–1361.
241. Peacey SR, Belchetz PE. Graves' disease: associated ocular myasthenia gravis and a thymic cyst. J R Soc Med 1993; 86:297–298.
242. Jaramillo P, Perez-Atayde A, Griscom NT. Apparent association between thymic cysts and prior thoracotomy. Radiology 1989; 172:207–209.

243. Lewis RJ, Caccavale RJ, Sissler GE. Imaged thoracoscopic surgery: a new thoracic technique for resection of mediastinal cysts. Ann Thorac Surg 1992; 53:318–320.
244. Naunheim KS, Andrus CH. Thoracoscopic drainage and resection of giant mediastinal cyst. Ann Thorac Surg 1993; 55:156–158.
245. Suster S, Rosai J. Cystic thymomas: a clinicopathologic study of ten cases. Cancer 1992; 69:92–97.
246. Murray JA, Parker AC. Mediastinal Hodgkin's disease and thymic cysts. Chest 1984; 71:282–284.
247. Kaesberg PR, Foley DB, Pellett J, Hafez GR, Ershler WB. Concurrent development of a thymic cyst and mediastinal Hodgkin's disease. Med Pediatr Oncol 1988; 16:293–294.
248. Baron RL, Sagel SS, Baglan RJ. Thymic cysts following radiation therapy for Hodgkin's disease. Radiology 1981; 141:593–597.
249. Burns BF, McCaughey WTE. Unusual thymic seminomas. Arch Pathol Lab Med 1986; 110:539–541.
250. Leong ASY, Brown JH. Malignant transformation in a thymic cyst. Am J Surg Pathol 1984; 8:471–475.
251. Blair A. Herbicides and non-Hodgkin's lymphoma: new evidence from a study of Saskatchewan farmers. J Natl Cancer Inst 1990; 82:544–545.
252. Morrison HI, Wilkins K, Semenciw R, Mao Y, Wigle D. Herbicides and cancer. J Natl Cancer Inst 1992; 84:1866–1874.
253. Schuurman H-J, de Waal EJ, van Loveren H, Vos JG. The toxicity of dioxin to the thymus. *In* Kendall MD, Ritter MA, eds. Thymus Update 4: The Thymus in Immunotoxicology. Chur, Switzerland: Harwood Academic Publishers, 1991:35–56.
254. Penninks AH, Pieters RHH, Snoeij NJ, Seinen W. Organotin-induced thymic atrophy. *In* Kendall MD, Ritter MA, eds. Thymus Update 4: The Thymus in Immunotoxicology. Chur, Switzerland: Harwood Academic Publishers, 1991:57–79.
255. Cohen M, Rubinstein A, Li JK, Nathenson G. Thymic hypoplasia associated with isotretinoin embryopathy. Am J Dis Child 1987; 141:263–266.
256. Shenefelt RE. Morphogenesis of malformations in hamsters caused by retinoic acid: relation to dose and stage at treatment. Teratology 1972; 5:103–118.

Chapter

5

TUMORS OF THE THYMIC EPITHELIAL CELL

THYMOMA
Clinical Features
Gross Pathology
Histopathology
Frozen Sections
Cytopathology
Histochemistry
Immunohistochemistry
Molecular Pathology
Electron Microscopy
Prognostic Factors
Surgical Pathology Report
Prognosis and Therapy
THYMIC CARCINOMA
Clinical Features
Gross Pathology
Histopathology
Prognostic Factors
Therapy
Comments
THYMIC EPITHELIAL CELL TUMORS IN ANIMALS
PATHOGENESIS OF THYMIC EPITHELIAL TUMORS

Tumors derived from the thymic epithelial cell include thymomas and thymic carcinomas. The term thymoma refers to a thymic epithelial cell tumor that is bland cytologically. Although frequently associated with a prominent lymphocytic infiltrate, the neoplastic cell is epithelial. Thymic carcinoma is an epithelial cell tumor that is malignant cytologically. In the past, the term thymoma referred to any tumor involving the thymus. Thus, seminoma-like thymoma (mediastinal seminoma) and granulomatous thymoma (Hodgkin's disease) are terms used in the older literature.[1, 2] Thymic carcinoid is another example of a lesion that has been included with thymomas.

Therefore, in interpreting the extensive medical literature on thymoma, one must be cautious in comparing studies that use different terminology. Another problem is the accuracy of the diagnosis. In today's pathology practice, morphologic examination alone may be insufficient. For example, immunoperoxidase studies are often helpful, especially in discriminating between large-cell lymphoma and epithelial thymoma. Many older series of thymomas undoubtedly include some large-cell lymphomas among the reported thymomas.

Some authors have used the term malignant thymoma to refer to both invasive thymoma and thymic carcinoma. In 1978, Levine and Rosai proposed subdividing malignant thymoma into two groups.[3] Type 1 are cytologically benign, but invasive or metastatic. Type 2 are cytologically malignant (thymic carcinoma).

A simpler system has been advocated.[4] Thymomas should be subdivided into the invasive and noninvasive categories only. The term malignant thymoma should be avoided, because it gets confused with thymic carcinoma. The term thymic carcinoma should be used for cytologically malignant thymic epithelial tumors (see Table 5–1).

THYMOMA

Clinical Features

Thymomas are among the most common primary neoplasms of the anterior mediastinum[5] (see Chapter 1). They occur most fre-

Table 5–1. Thymic Epithelial Tumors

Levine and Rosai, 1978	Current	Definition
Thymoma	Thymoma, noninvasive	Cytologically benign thymic epithelial tumor without invasion through capsule or evidence of metastatic disease
Malignant thymoma, type 1	Thymoma, invasive	Cytologically benign thymic epithelial tumor with invasion through capsule and/or metastatic disease
Malignant thymoma, type 2	Thymic carcinoma	Cytologically malignant thymic epithelial tumor

quently in older adults. Among six series comprising a total of 875 thymomas, patients ranged from 2 to 90 years of age, with a mean age of 50 (Table 5–2). Females outnumbered males 53% to 47%. Forty-three percent of patients had myasthenia gravis. The percentage of myasthenia gravis patients varies among different series depending on the referral pattern of the reporting institution. Occasional patients with thymoma develop myasthenia gravis after the tumor is removed. Among myasthenia gravis patients, the tumors tend to occur at a slightly earlier age.

Thymomas have been reported in children as young as 9 months of age.[6–9] However, some of the childhood cases reported as thymoma probably represent lymphoblastic lymphoma.[6, 10] Nevertheless, the diagnosis of many childhood thymomas has been well documented by immunohistochemistry and electron microscopy. Most cases come to medical attention because of local symptoms from a large mediastinal mass. Rare childhood cases associated with myasthenia gravis[11] or hypoplastic anemia[7] have been described.

About 10% of patients with thymoma have various disorders other than myasthenia gravis[12–31] (Table 5–3). The most common are hypogammaglobulinemia and pure red cell aplasia. These disorders may precede, arise concurrently with, or follow the resection of a thymoma.

The association between thymoma and hypogammaglobulinemia has been called Good's syndrome after the author of the original description.[32–34] Patients with Good's syndrome are generally older adults. However, one case of an 8-year-old child with this disorder has been reported.[32] Besides the hypogammaglobulinemia, patients often develop anemia from pure red cell aplasia. Bacterial, viral, and fungal infections may follow. The immunodeficiency is generally attributed to a decreased number of B cells as demonstrated in bone marrow and peripheral blood.[35] Although some patients have changes in cellular immunity, T cells are usually present in normal numbers. Two cases have been reported in which the patient's T cells lacked the OKT4 epitope of T-cell antigen CD4.[36, 37] Because this CD4 variant may be present in apparently healthy individuals, its significance is not clear. In one case, the lymphocytes in the thymoma were also noted to lack the OKT4 epitope.[36]

Rarely, patients with a lymphocytic thymoma have T-cell lymphocytosis in the peripheral blood.[38–40] The patient may then be misdiagnosed as having leukemia or disseminated lymphoma. Unlike a lymphoid malignancy, the thymoma-associated lymphocytosis resolves if the tumor can be successfully treated. Leukocyte counts have been as high as 30×10^9/L with as much as 80% lymphocytes. The reported patients have not had lymphadenopathy. Bone marrow aspirates have shown up to 30% mature-appearing lymphocytes, and bone

Table 5–2. Clinical Features of Thymoma Based on Selected Clinicopathologic Studies

First Author/Date	No. of Cases	Age Range/Mean	Male/Female	% MG
Verley/1985[14]	200	5–80/50	93/107	53%
Hofmann/1985*[13]	98	2–77/45	44/54	35%
Lewis/1987[12]	283	16–90/52	136/147	46%
Kornstein/1988†[68]	126	12–82/54	64/62	47%
Pescarmona/1990[75]	83	21–83/49	39/44	30%
Wilkins/1991[76]	85	13–81/?	39/46	41%
Overall	875 (total)	2–90/50 (average)	415/460 (47%/53%)	42% (average)

*The Hofmann series includes three cases of thymic carcinoma. Also, in the Hofmann series, 19% of cases could not be evaluated for invasiveness.

†The Kornstein series includes 95 thymomas in the publication plus another 31 thymomas reviewed since the manuscript was written.

Table 5–3. Thymoma-Associated Disorders*

Alopecia areata	Mucocutaneous candidiasis
Aplastic anemia	Myocarditis
Autoimmune hemolytic anemia	Myopathy
Crohn's disease	Pemphigus vulgaris
Dermatomyositis	Pernicious anemia
Essential thrombocytosis	Polymyositis
Graves' disease	Pure red cell aplasia
Hypogammaglobulinemia	Sarcoidosis
Kaposi's sarcoma	Sjögren's disease
Limbic encephalitis	Systemic lupus erythematosus
Minimal change nephropathy	Ulcerative colitis
Mixed collagen vascular disease	Various malignancies (see text)

*See text for references.

marrow biopsies may have aggregates of small lymphocytes. A case has been reported of an unresectable thymoma associated with T-cell chronic lymphocytic leukemia.[41] The latter condition involved not only the peripheral blood, but also the skin, lymph nodes, liver, kidney, adrenal gland, and lungs. Other reports describe T-cell lymphoblastic leukemia/ lymphoma in patients with thymoma.[42, 42a]

The question arises as to whether the lymphocytes in the thymoma can "spill out" into the peripheral blood and thereby account for the lymphocytosis. One case report demonstrated a thymoma-associated lymphocytosis to have a mature T-cell phenotype (positive for T-cell markers CD2, 3, 5, and 7; negative for CD1 and terminal deoxynucleotidyl transferase). Gene rearrangement studies revealed germ line configuration for the T-cell receptor beta chain gene.[40] Thus, if other cases are similar, thymoma-associated lymphocytosis can be distinguished from disseminated lymphoma, chronic lymphocytic leukemia, and acute lymphoblastic leukemia on the basis of immunologic and molecular biologic studies. The pathogenesis of the lymphocytosis is unclear. Medeiros and colleagues speculated that it results from an imbalance in immune regulation.[40] Alternatively, perhaps, the lymphocytes from the thymoma do disseminate to the peripheral blood. However, like the cortical lymphocytes in the normal thymus, they may be capable of maturation, either within the tumor or elsewhere.

In a clinicopathologic study from the Mayo Clinic, 17% of thymoma patients also had another primary tumor.[12] A series from the M.D. Anderson Cancer Center found second primary tumors in 11 of 52 thymoma patients (21%).[43] These percentages vary with the patient population. For example, another series found that only 7% of thymoma patients had second malignancies.[44] In this author's series, the percentage was 3%. Similarly, among studies of myasthenia gravis patients with thymoma, the percentage of patients with another malignancy ranged from 5% to 18%.[45]

The second primary tumors have included carcinomas of the breast, lung, stomach, kidney, cervix, endometrium, and ovary. Sarcoma, multiple myeloma, leukemia, and lymphoma (including Hodgkin's disease) have been reported as rare associations with thymoma.[45–51] One study found that extrathymic malignancies occurred significantly more often among myasthenia gravis patients with thymoma than among those myasthenic patients without thymoma.[45] Confounding variables in these studies include the effects of thymectomy, medications, and radiation therapy. Thus, thymoma patients may have an increased risk of a second malignancy, but a more thorough investigation of this subject is needed before reaching a definite conclusion.

A single case report describes a patient with both the acquired immunodeficiency syndrome (AIDS) and a spindle cell thymoma.[52] Given the apparent rarity of this association, it seems unlikely that there is any direct relationship between these two disorders.

Approximately one third of patients with thymoma come to medical attention because of a mediastinal mass detected on a routine chest radiograph.[13] In about 50% of cases, the patient presents because of an associated syndrome, usually myasthenia gravis. The remaining patients present with local symptoms such as chest pain, cough, dyspnea, or superior vena cava syndrome. Occasional thymomas (4% in this author's series) are found incidentally during heart surgery for coronary artery bypass grafts.

Although nearly all thymomas occur in the anterior mediastinum, occasional cases have been described in the posterior mediastinum, lungs, pleura, and neck.[13, 53–60] A thymoma adjacent to the right hemidiaphragm was reported by Jansen and Johnson.[61] Thymomas may occur adjacent to or within the thyroid gland.[12, 62] Such tumors may be difficult to diagnose definitively as a thymoma.[63] Moran and colleagues described eight thymomas that presented as pleural masses, some of which encased the lung and grossly simulated diffuse mesothelioma.[64] Rarely, a thymoma may present as an endobronchial lesion with the tumor extending from the mediastinum into the lung.[65–67]

Ectopic hamartomatous thymoma is an uncommon, benign tumor that presents in adults as a mass in the neck (near the sternoclavicular joint).[59] It is a biphasic neoplasm composed of spindled cells admixed with epithelial elements (squamous or glandular). Some cases have adipose tissue within the tumor. Both the spindled and epithelial elements contain immunoreactive cytokeratin. Despite its name, there is no evidence relating this tumor to the thymus. It may arise from branchial remnants.

Other tumors of the neck that may relate to the thymus include the "spindle epithelial tumor with thymus-like differentiation" (SETTLE) and the "carcinoma showing thymus-like differentiation" (CASTLE).[59] The former is a spindle cell tumor of the thyroid with sclerotic fibrous bands and mucinous glands. The latter is a malignant thyroid neoplasm resembling the lymphoepithelioma-like thymic carcinoma or squamous cell carcinoma of the thymus. The evidence linking these tumors to the thymus is mostly limited to rather subtle histologic similarities. The SETTLE has some re-

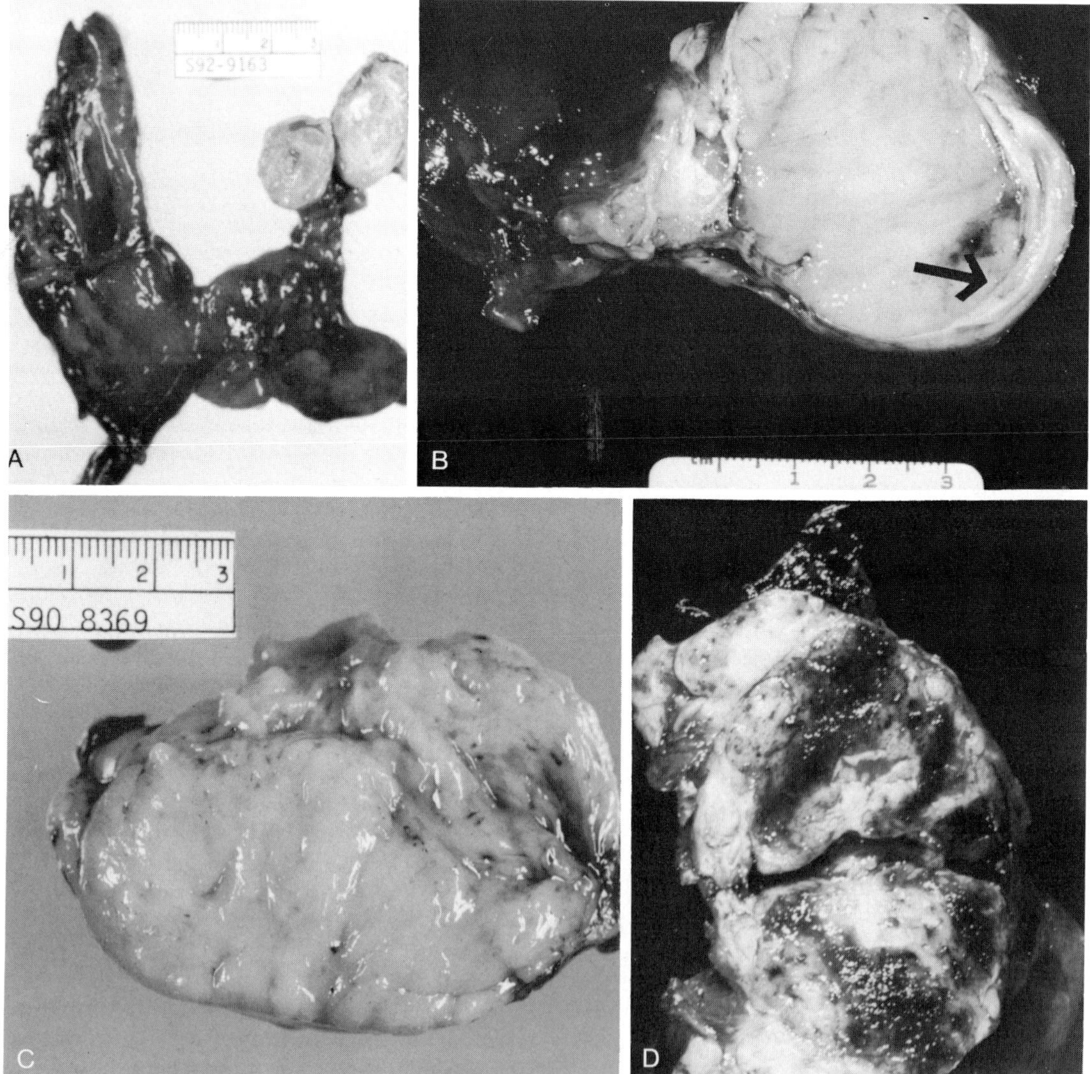

Figure 5–1. Photographs of thymomas illustrate varied gross appearances. *A*, A noninvasive, spindled epithelial thymoma (bisected) is present at an upper pole of the thymus. The lesion was resected from a 47-year-old male with myasthenia gravis. *B*, This noninvasive thymoma (mixed lymphocytic and epithelial) has a prominent capsule *(arrow)*. The tumor was resected from a 32-year-old male with myasthenia gravis. *C*, This lymphocytic thymoma with microscopic invasion through the capsule was excised from the anterior mediastinum of a 79-year-old male. Only a thin fibrous capsule was present. Grossly, the "flesh-like" appearance simulates a lymphoma. *D*, This epithelial thymoma from a 59-year-old female with myasthenia gravis is shown invading the lung. Areas of hemorrhage are prominent.

semblance to spindle cell thymoma. In one case, ectopic thymus was present in the vicinity of the tumor. The CASTLE has lobulations, occasional perivascular spaces, and Hassall's corpuscle–like structures. Both are indolent neoplasms.

Clinical-pathologic studies have identified a small percentage (about 5%) of invasive thymomas that metastasize outside the thoracic cavity.[12, 14, 68] Rarely, a perfectly ordinary-appearing lymphocytic, mixed, or epithelial thymoma will develop widespread metastases.[69] Most thymic epithelial tumors that metastasize are cytologically malignant[70] and should be diagnosed as thymic carcinoma. However, the clinicopathologic studies in the literature do not always make the distinction between thymoma and thymic carcinoma.

Sites of metastases include the chest wall, pleura, lung, bone (rib, vertebra, sternum), spleen, and lymph nodes (most commonly supraclavicular and mediastinal). Thymomas often disseminate within the thorax as pleural plaques. Unusual cases may present with a metastasis, such as a solitary mass in the lung.[71] A case of a thymoma metastatic to an inguinal hernia sac has been reported.[72]

In this author's series, a patient with an invasive thymoma had a large spleen on a follow-up examination 1 month after thymectomy. Splenectomy revealed a metastatic thymoma histologically similar to his mediastinal neoplasm. After receiving mediastinal radiation, the patient was well, without evidence of disease, for 7 years. Thus, the finding of distant metastases does not necessarily indicate the imminent demise of the patient.

Gross Pathology

Most thymomas are well circumscribed, firm, tan-to-gray masses with a fibrous capsule and vague lobulation (Fig. 5–1). Sizes up to 34 cm in greatest dimension have been reported.[70] In grossly nonneoplastic thymus, microscopic foci of epithelial cells (1 mm or less in diameter) have been interpreted as "microscopic thymomas," although they probably have no clinical significance.[70, 73] Patients with myasthenia gravis tend to have smaller tumors, presumably because they are detected earlier.[12] Cystic changes are common (Fig. 5–2). Some tumors are entirely cystic and simulate a thymic cyst.[74] Grossly invasive thymomas infiltrate surrounding structures, including pleura, lungs, pericardium, great vessels, chest wall, diaphragm, phrenic nerve, and trachea.[13] Adherence to adjacent structures is commonly noted at surgery but does not necessarily indicate true invasion.[12]

Depending on the study, 29 to 72% of thymomas are invasive. In some studies, invasion is defined microscopically,[68, 75, 76] whereas in other reports, invasion is determined by gross examination only.[12–14] Careful gross examination is needed to determine where the tumor may extend beyond its fibrous capsule.

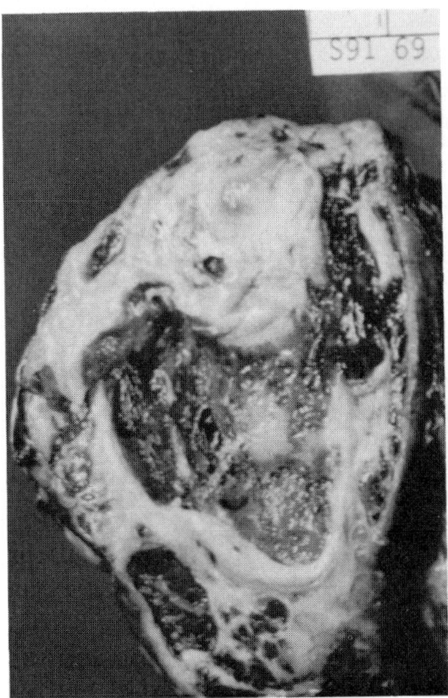

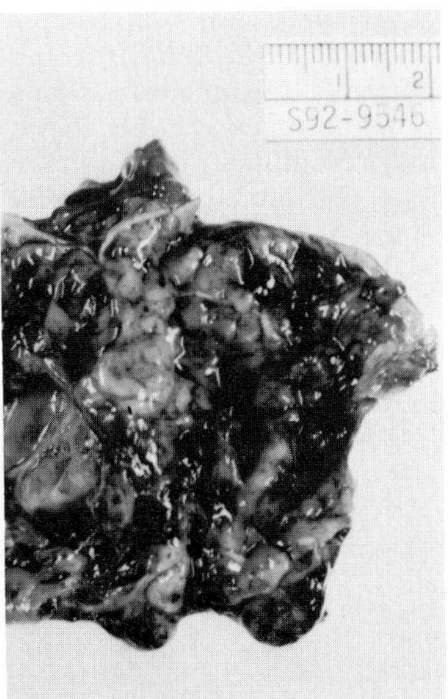

Figure 5–2. Thymomas with cystic changes. *Left,* This invasive thymoma (bisected) demonstrates a prominent cystic cavity. It was excised from a 42-year-old female with myasthenia gravis. Implants of tumor were noted on the patient's diaphragm. *Right,* This cystic mass has been opened to reveal a hemorrhagic wall with white thickened areas. It was removed from the anterior mediastinum of a 39-year-old woman. Histologically, the thickened areas represent a mixed lymphocytic and epithelial thymoma with microscopic invasion into the surrounding tissue.

Histopathology

Thymomas are characterized by the proliferation of epithelial cells with or without an associated lymphocytic infiltrate. Traditionally, thymomas are classified histologically by the number of associated lymphocytes[12, 77] (Table 5–4). Other histologic features are summarized in Table 5–5.

In lymphocytic thymoma, more than two thirds of the cells are lymphocytes (Fig. 5–3). The lymphocyte nuclei are frequently enlarged with folded membranes. Mitoses may be frequent. This appearance may resemble a lymphoblastic lymphoma. Recognition of the epithelial cell component is important to distinguish thymoma from lymphoblastic lymphoma. Epithelial cells that are larger and have more prominent nucleoli are interspersed among the lymphocytes. They may be present as individual cells or clusters. The epithelial cells are round or polygonal with vesicular nuclei. Distinct nucleoli are usually present. Lymphocytic thymomas may have "medullary differentiation" (i.e., areas of the tumor with fewer lymphocytes) (Fig. 5–4). These areas, which appear lighter on routinely stained sections, may have Hassall's corpuscles. Morphologically and immunologically, these areas resemble the thymic medulla.[78]

Another pattern occasionally present in lymphocytic thymoma is a "starry sky" appearance, created by tingible-body macrophages[70] (see Fig. 5–4). A similar pattern is associated with Burkitt's lymphoma. However, the mediastinum is an uncommon location for Burkitt's lymphoma, and the lymphocytes in a thymoma have more diffuse nuclear chromatin than they do in Burkitt's lymphoma. Most importantly, the identification of an epithelial element together with the lymphocytes permits recognition of thymoma.

In predominantly epithelial thymoma, lymphocytes are less numerous (accounting for less than one third of cells) or absent, whereas mixed thymomas have approximately equal numbers of each cell type (Figs. 5–5 and 5–6). Occasional epithelial cells may be large and multinucleated. However, cytologic evidence of malignancy (hyperchromasia, large nucleoli, frequent mitoses) would indicate a diagnosis of thymic carcinoma. The tumor cells of a predominantly epithelial or mixed thymoma may vary in size and shape. They may be large with round-to-polygonal, vesicular nuclei and abundant cytoplasm.

Table 5–4. Traditional Classification of Thymomas[12, 68]

Category	Definition
Lymphocytic	>⅔ of cells are lymphocytes
Mixed lymphocytic and epithelial	Approximately equal numbers of lymphocytes and epithelial cells
Predominantly epithelial	>⅔ of cells are epithelial
Spindled	Predominantly epithelial tumor with prominent fusiform cells

Table 5–5. Histologic Features of Thymomas

Histologic Feature	% of Thymomas (in Author's Series)
Fibrous bands	85%
Perivascular spaces	72%
Hassall's corpuscles	14%
Cysts	19%
Squamous differentiation	10%
Medullary differentiation	16%
Germinal centers within tumor	6%

Spindled thymomas are tumors in which the epithelial component is elongated, or spindled, in shape (Fig. 5–7). Nucleoli are inconspicuous. Some authors disregard the number of lymphocytes in the definition of spindle cell thymoma.[14] Others refer to spindle cell thymoma as a variant of the predominantly epithelial type.[12]

Fibrous bands and prominent perivascular spaces are present in most thymomas. The fibrous bands separate the tumor into lobules (Fig. 5–8). Typically, a broad fibrous capsule is present and may contain calcifications. Perivascular spaces surround the small blood vessels within the tumor (Fig. 5–9). The area between the vessel and the adjacent epithelial cells may contain red blood cells, lymphocytes, and macrophages. It may be filled with proteinaceous material and become hyalinized.

Thymomas can produce a wide spectrum of histologic appearances. Spindled epithelial cells may appear in parallel bundles or whorls. The epithelial cells may have a storiform pattern and simulate a fibrous histiocytoma. Epithelial thymomas may assume a reticular pattern (Fig. 5–10). Prominent, "staghorn"-shaped vessels may be present in a pattern similar to that of a hemangiopericytoma (Fig. 5–11). Thymomas may contain rosettes (cells arranged around an open space) or pseudoro-

Text continued on page 78

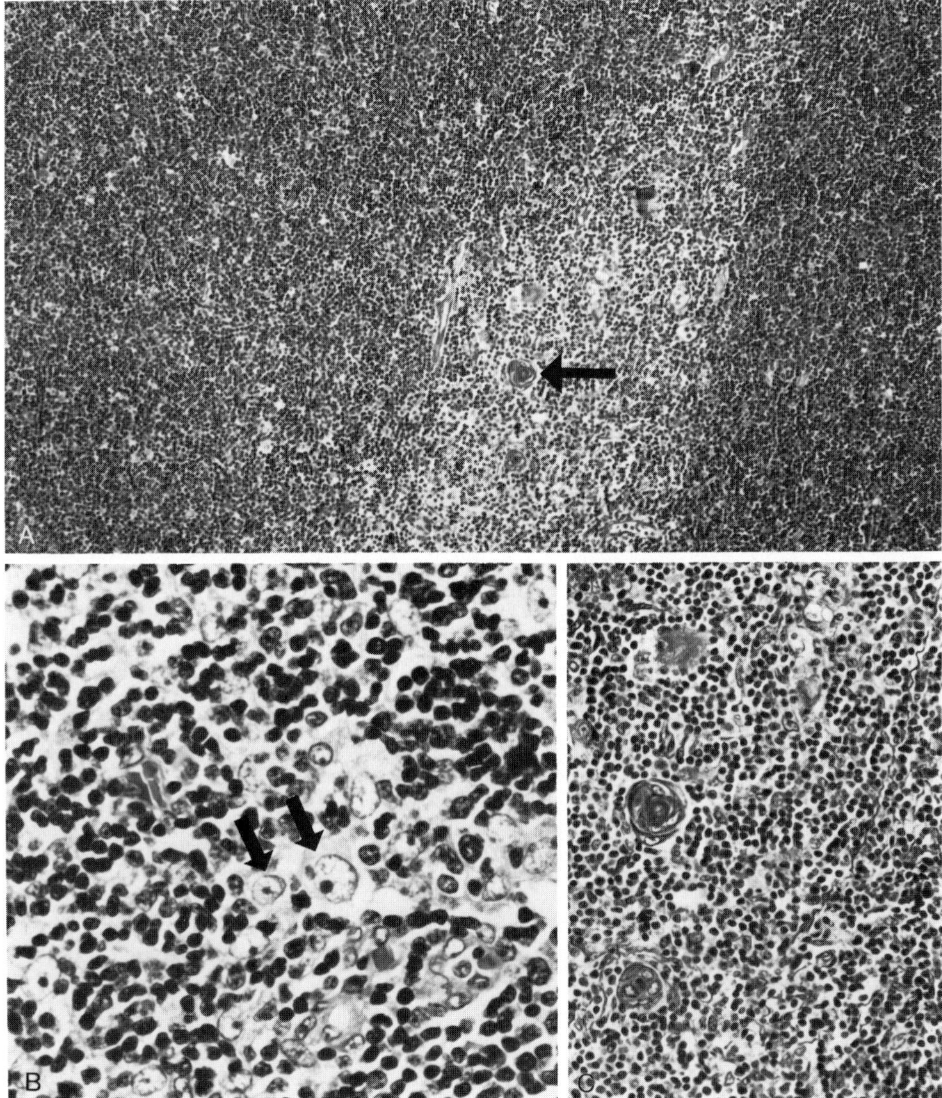

Figure 5–3. *A*, Lymphocytic thymoma with medullary differentiation. Lighter areas resemble thymic medulla in that the lymphocytes are less dense and Hassall's corpuscles *(arrow)* may be present (×100). *B*, With higher magnification, the epithelial cells *(arrows)* can be distinguished from lymphocytes. The epithelial cells have vesicular chromatin and prominent nucleoli (H & E ×400). *C*, Hassall's corpuscles are seen within the area of medullary differentiation (H & E ×200).

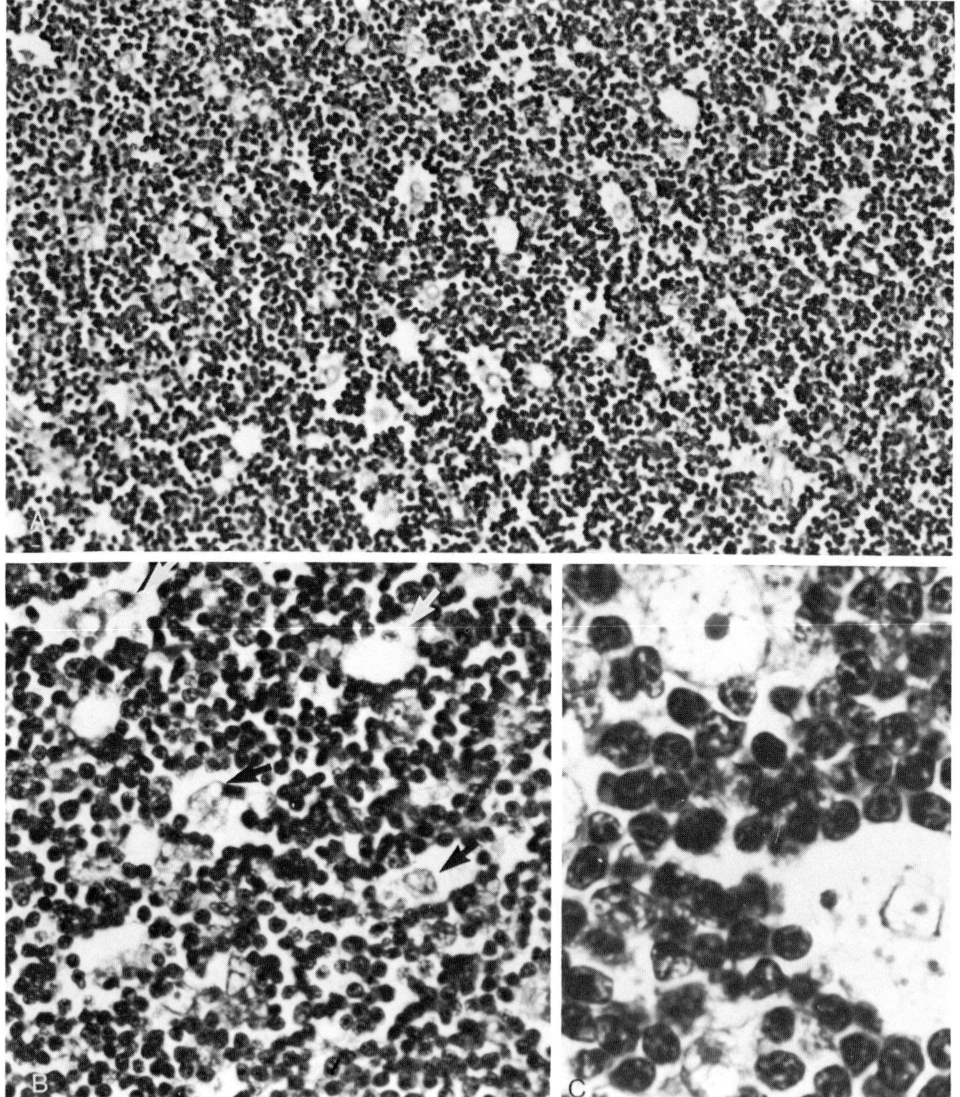

Figure 5–4. *A*, Lymphocytic thymoma with a "starry sky" appearance (H & E ×200). *B*, With higher magnification, the tingible-body macrophages *(arrows)* are seen to create the "starry sky" pattern (H & E ×400). *C*, An epithelial cell (top) and tingible-body macrophage (bottom right) within a lymphocytic thymoma (H & E ×1000).

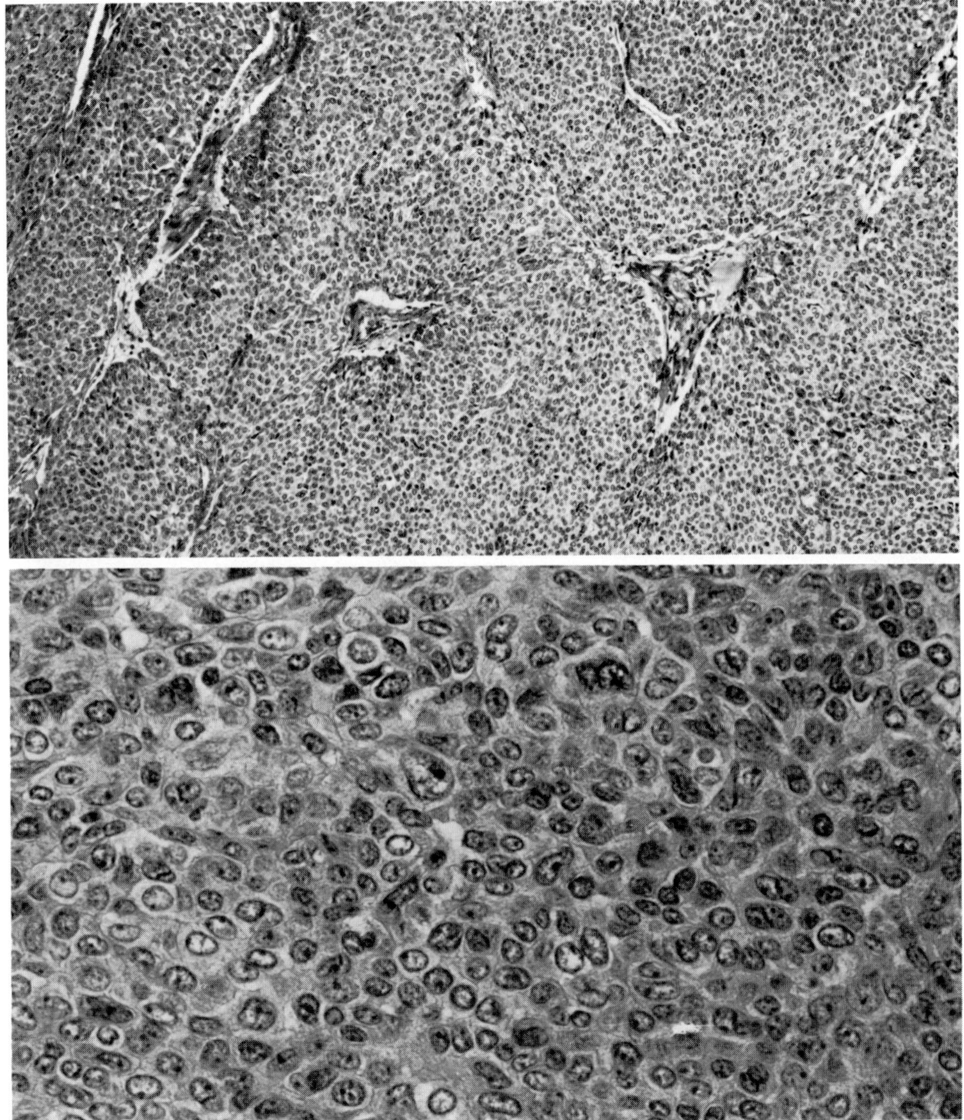

Figure 5–5. An epithelial thymoma is characterized by sheets of bland-appearing epithelial cells. Cellular atypia (cells with larger nuclei and nucleoli) is present. (*Top*, H & E ×40; *bottom*, H & E ×400.)

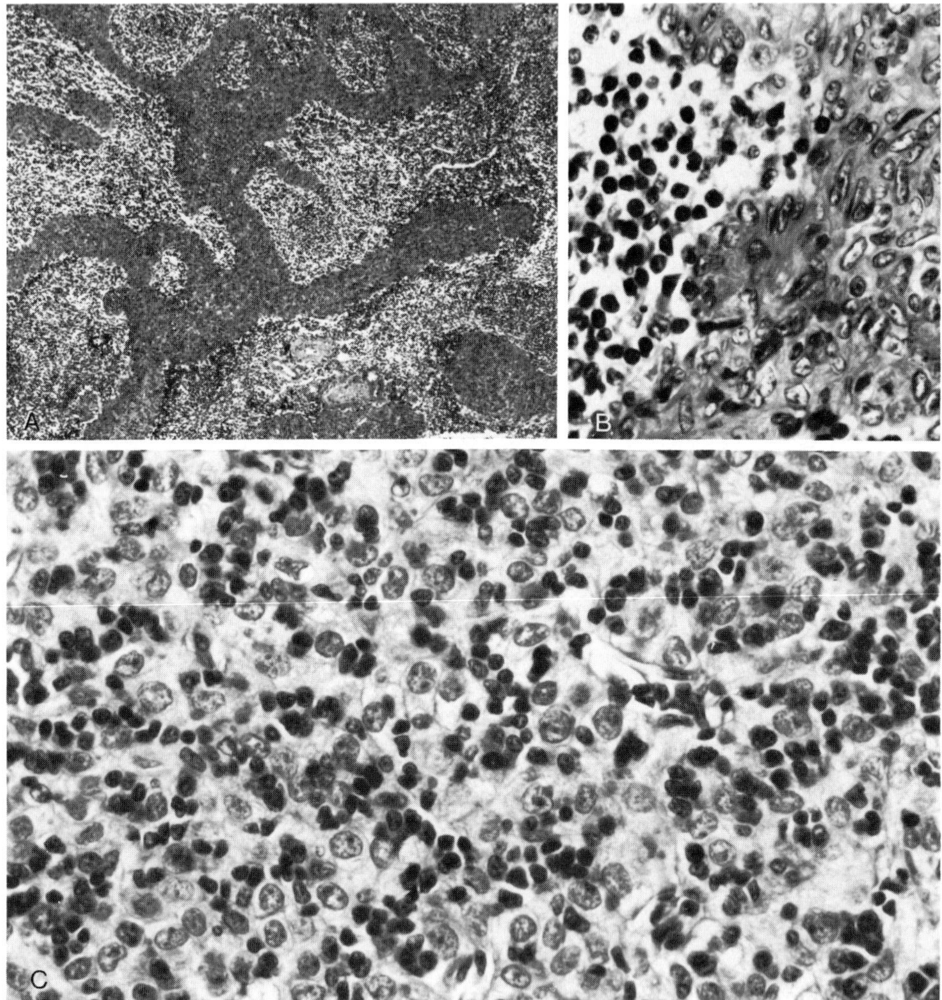

Figure 5–6. Mixed lymphocytic and epithelial thymomas are shown. Both components are present in approximately equal proportion. In the tumor illustrated in *A* and *B*, the epithelial cells are present in bands (*A*, H & E ×40; *B*, H & E ×400). *C*, Another tumor has intermixed lymphocytes and epithelial cells (H & E ×400).

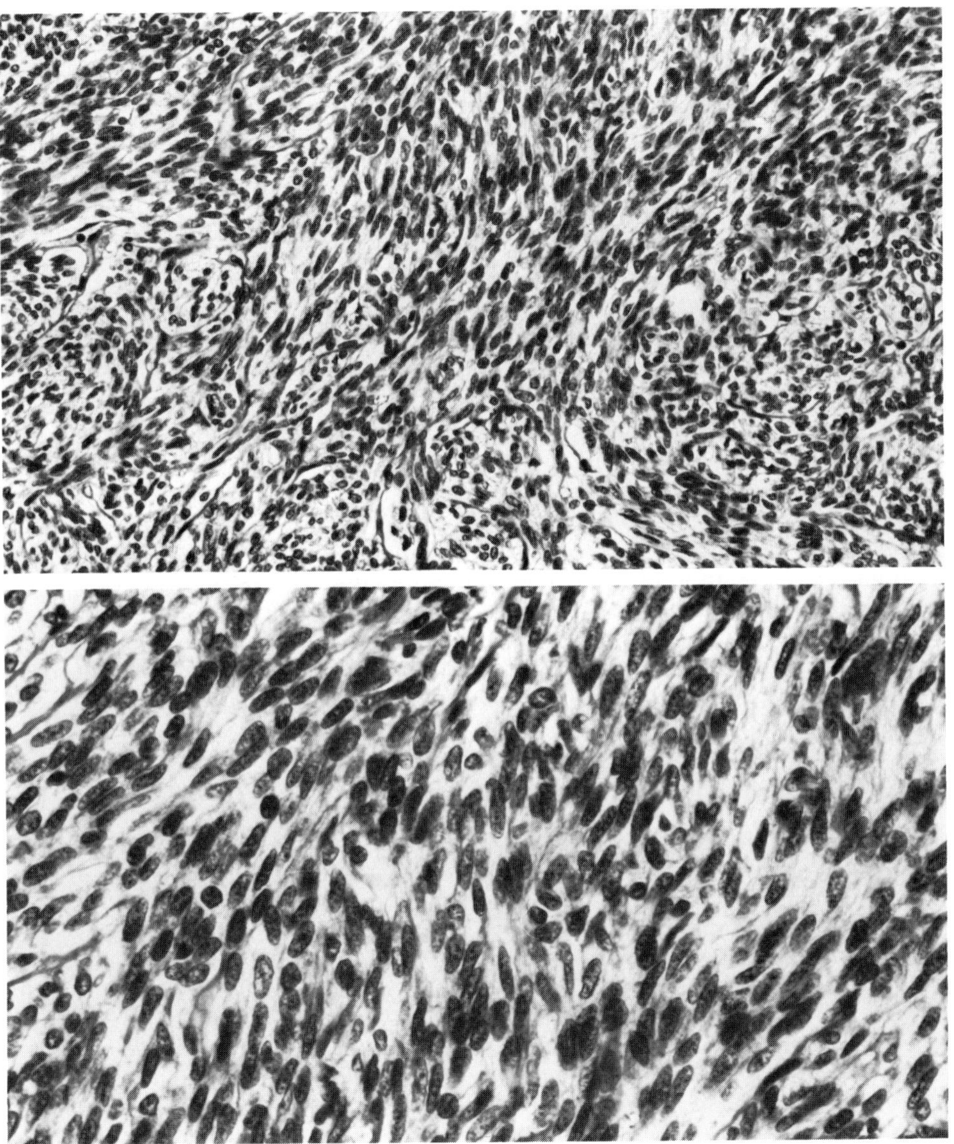

Figure 5–7. A spindled thymoma is characterized by sheets or fascicles of epithelial cells with elongated nuclei. The nuclear chromatin is diffuse and nucleoli are not prominent. (*Top*, H & E ×100; *bottom*, H & E ×400.)

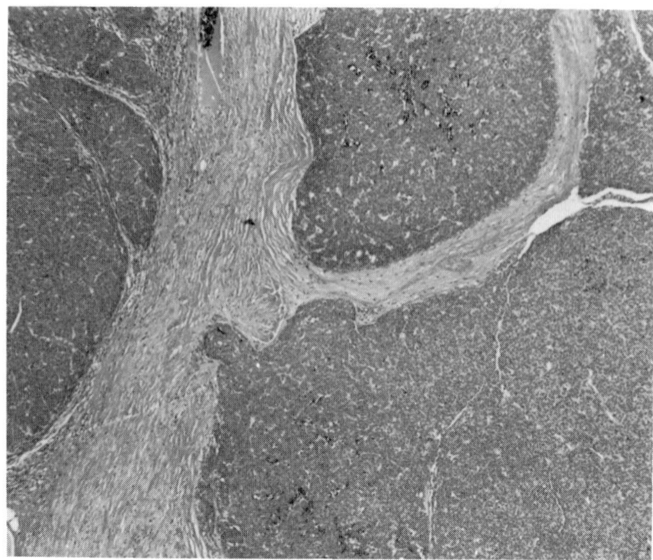

Figure 5–8. This photograph of a lymphocytic thymoma illustrates the broad fibrous bands that are commonly present in thymomas (H & E ×40).

settes (cells around small blood vessels) and may resemble carcinoid tumors. Gland-like formations may be found both within the tumor and within the capsule (Fig. 5–12). Foamy macrophages may be prominent (Fig. 5–13). Cystic thymomas may resemble thymic cysts with the tumor identifiable only focally within the cyst wall[74] (see Fig. 5–2, Fig. 5–14). Occasionally, papillary structures may be identified within the tumor.

Some investigators have given names to different histologic appearances. For example, Fukuda and colleagues have described a "microcytic" variant of thymoma that consists of round, vacuolated, "signet-ring"-like cells.[79] Pescarmona et al. describe the lymphocytic thymoma with medullary differentiation as "organoid" thymoma because of its resemblance to the normal thymus.[78] "Rhabdomyomatous" thymoma has prominent myoid cells.[80, 81]

Finally, germinal centers can be seen within the thymoma in about 6% of cases[70, 82] (Fig. 5–15). They are not necessarily associated with myasthenia gravis, unless the germinal centers are also present within the surrounding nonneoplastic thymus.[82]

Nuclear atypia (i.e., pleomorphism, hyperchromasia, and nucleolar prominence) was identified in 35% of thymomas in this author's series (see Fig. 5–5). The atypia may be identified in only one area of a large tumor or may be more extensive. The distinction between a thymoma with cellular atypia and a thymic carcinoma may be difficult (see later).

Some thymomas show prominent squamous differentiation (Fig. 5–16). Those with squamous differentiation are more likely to be invasive. In this author's series, about 10% of thymomas had areas of cytologically benign squamous differentiation (i.e., distinct cell borders, abundant eosinophilic cytoplasm, whorl formations, keratin pearls). Seventy percent of those thymomas with squamous differentiation were invasive (versus 35% of thymomas without squamous differentiation). Similar findings were reported by Kirchner et al.[83] and Shimosato et al.[84]

Kirchner et al. report a high association of squamous elements in thymomas with myasthenia gravis.[83] The present author could not confirm this finding: only 40% of such tumors were associated with myasthenia (versus 47% of thymomas without squamous differentiation). Kirchner and colleagues proposed the term well-differentiated thymic carcinoma for thymic epithelial cell tumors with squamous differentiation and "slight to moderate cytologic atypia."[83] In the present author's opinion, such a designation confuses the distinction between thymoma and thymic carcinoma (see later).

The number of lymphocytes often varies from one area to another. Frequently, a single tumor will have multiple histologic types ranging from lymphocytic to epithelial predominance. The shape of the epithelial cells commonly differs in different areas. The range of histologic features within a single tumor complicates attempts to classify them on this basis.

Text continued on page 83

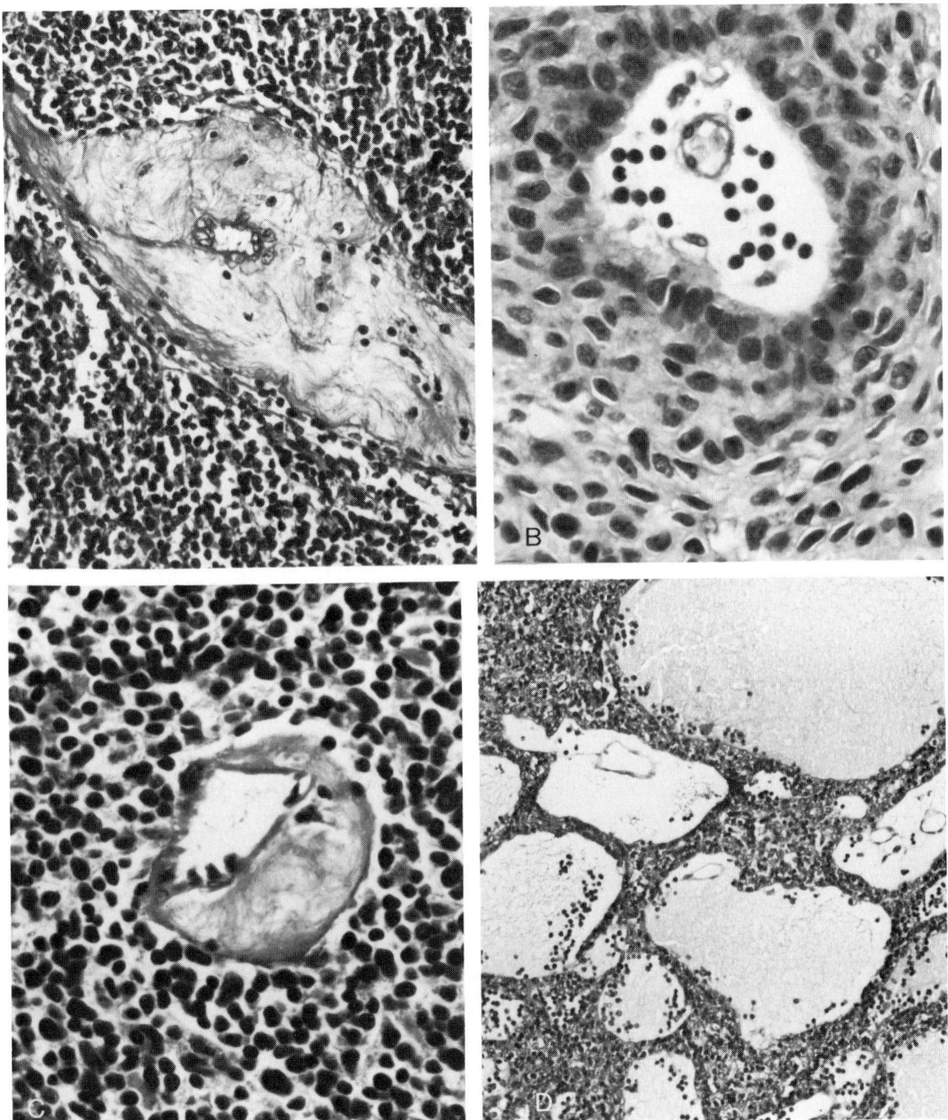

Figure 5–9. These photographs illustrate the perivascular space in thymomas. *A*, Lymphocytic thymoma with perivascular space containing loose, fibrillar material (H & E ×200). *B*, Epithelial thymoma with palisading cells around the perivascular space. A capillary is present within the space (H & E ×400). *C*, Lymphocytic thymoma with hyalinization of perivascular space (H & E ×400). *D*, Dilated perivascular spaces in a mixed lymphocytic and epithelial thymoma produce a cystic pattern (H & E ×100).

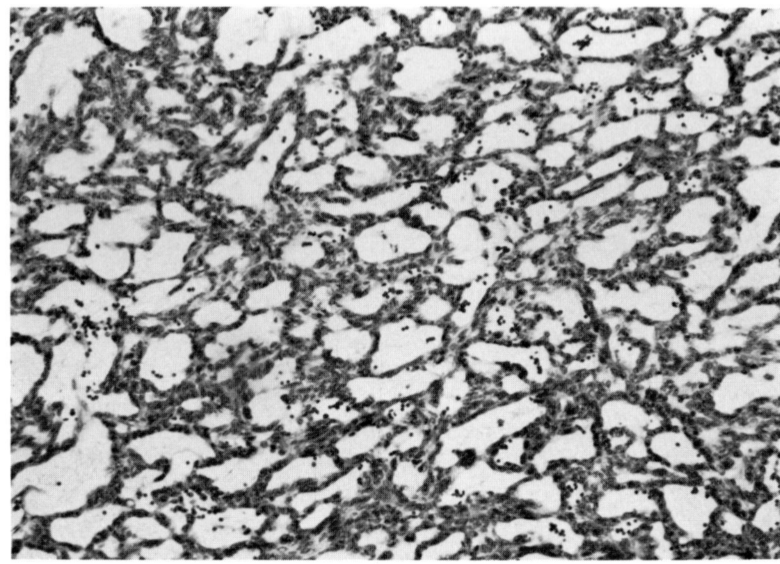

Figure 5–10. An epithelial thymoma with a reticular pattern. Many of the cyst-like structures represent dilated perivascular spaces (H & E ×100).

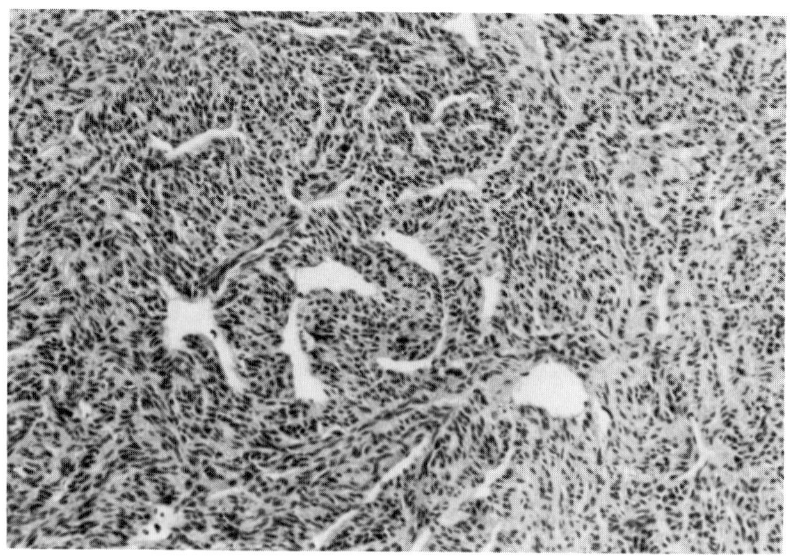

Figure 5–11. A spindled thymoma with "staghorn"-shaped vessels similar to a hemangiopericytoma (H & E ×100).

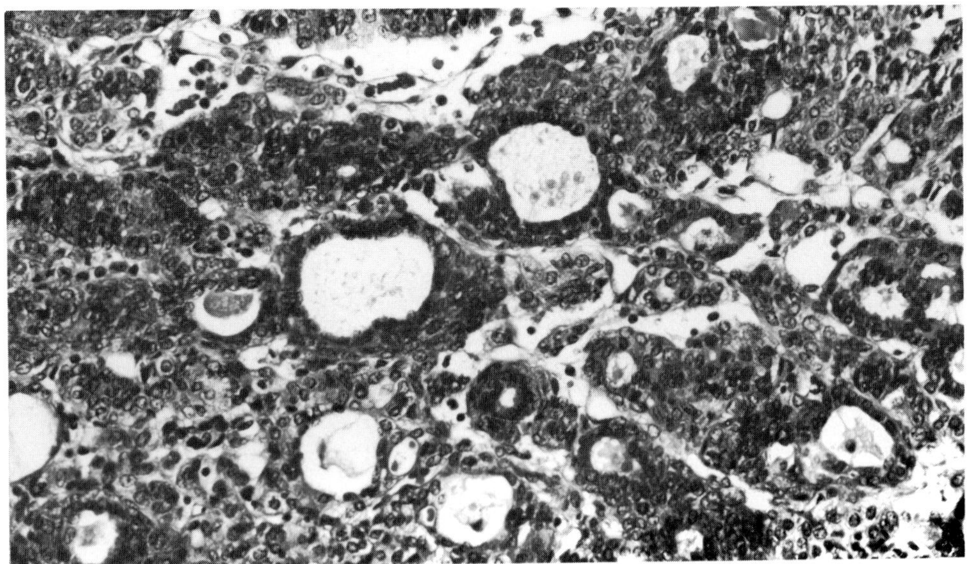

Figure 5–12. An epithelial thymoma with gland-like structures (H & E ×400).

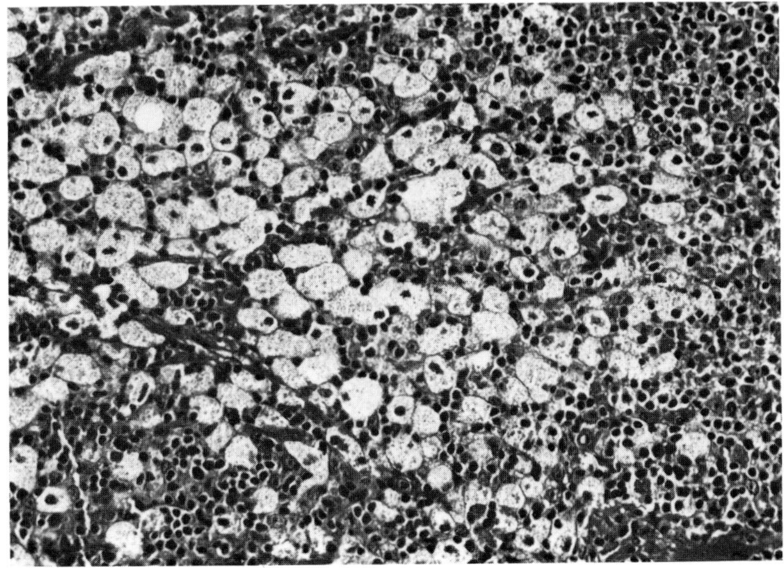

Figure 5–13. A lymphocytic thymoma with focally prominent foamy macrophages (H & E ×200).

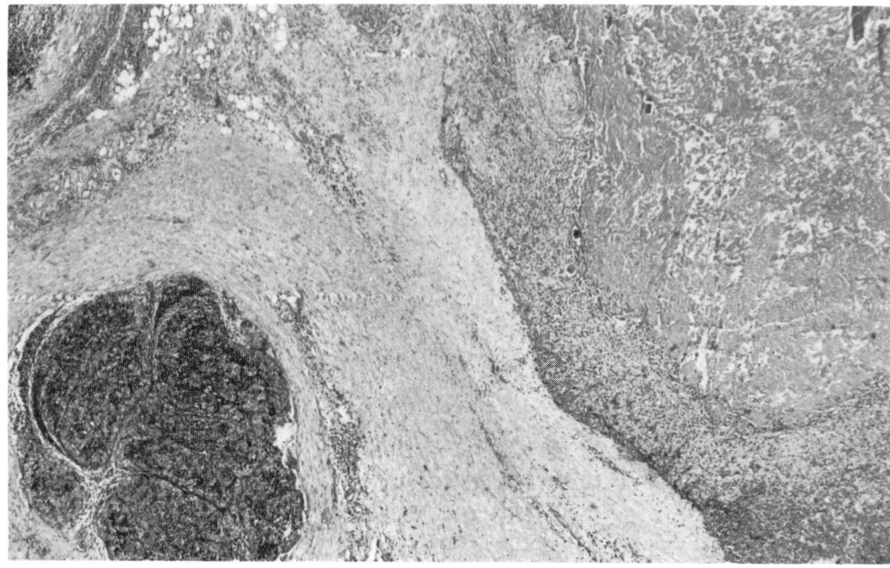

Figure 5–14. A cystic thymoma. Most of the tumor consists of degenerative debris, as shown on the right. Focal areas typical of a mixed lymphocytic and epithelial thymoma are evident, as shown at lower left (H & E ×100).

Table 5–6. "Histogenetic" Classification[89, 94, 149, 255]

Classification	Morphologic Features	Immunohistochemistry: *Epithelial Cell Phenotype*	Immunohistochemistry: *Lymphocyte Phenotype*
Cortical (polygonal cell)	Tumor cells morphologically similar to epithelial cells of normal thymic cortex (nuclei are round or oval with vesicular chromatin and one prominent nucleolus); variable numbers of lymphocytes	61% cortical phenotype, 2% medullary, 37% positive for antigens expressed by both cortical and medullary epithelial cells or negative for both	Predominantly immature phenotype (CD1+)
Mixed, common	Intermixed cortical and medullary cell types; variable number of lymphocytes	41% medullary, 59% both cortical and medullary (or neither)	Predominantly immature phenotype (CD1+)
Mixed, cortical predominant	Mixed thymoma with large areas containing cortical type cells; variable number of lymphocytes		
Mixed, medullary predominant	Mixed thymoma with a predominance of medullary type tumor cells; variable number of lymphocytes		
Medullary (spindled cell)	Tumor cells are spindle shaped; nucleus is fusiform with homogeneous chromatin that is more dense than in cortical type; fewer lymphocytes	41% medullary, 59% both cortical and medullary (or neither)	Tendency for fewer immature (CD1+) lymphocytes and more mature (CD1−) lymphocytes

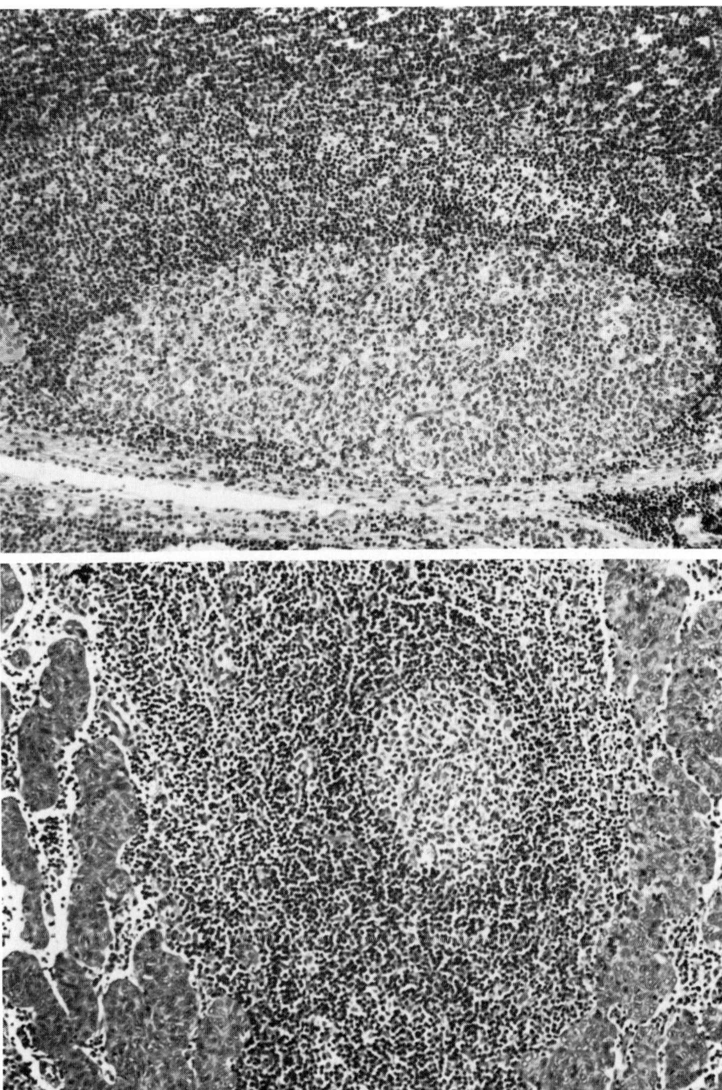

Figure 5–15. Germinal centers within thymomas. *Top*, A lymphocytic thymoma contains a germinal center in the subcapsular area (H & E ×100). *Bottom*, A mixed lymphocytic and epithelial thymoma contains a germinal center deep within the tumor (H & E ×100).

Nevertheless, certain correlations between clinical features and histopathologic appearance have been made. Patients with myasthenia gravis may have any type of thymoma, although in most studies, the spindled type is less common.[12, 14, 70, 85, 86] In contrast, most cases associated with pure red cell aplasia and hypogammaglobulinemia are of the spindled type.[14, 24, 70] In the adjacent thymus of patients with pure red cell aplasia, clusters of spindled epithelial cells have been described.[24] Unlike patients with myasthenia gravis, those with pure red cell aplasia have not had germinal centers in the adjacent thymus.

In the mid-1980s, Muller-Hermelink and colleagues proposed a histopathologic classification of thymomas based on morphologic similarities of the tumor cells to cortical or medullary thymic epithelium[87–89] (Table 5–6). They noted that medullary epithelial cells tend to be spindled in appearance. Therefore, they proposed the term medullary thymoma for those tumors composed of spindled epithelial cells (see Fig. 5–7). Similarly, they noted that cortical epithelial cells are polygonal with distinct central nucleoli. Thus, those thymomas composed of polygonal cells with distinct nucleoli are classified as "cortical" thymomas (Fig. 5–17). Tumors with both types of cells are classified as "mixed cortical and medullary" thymomas.

The basis of the cortical/medullary classifi-

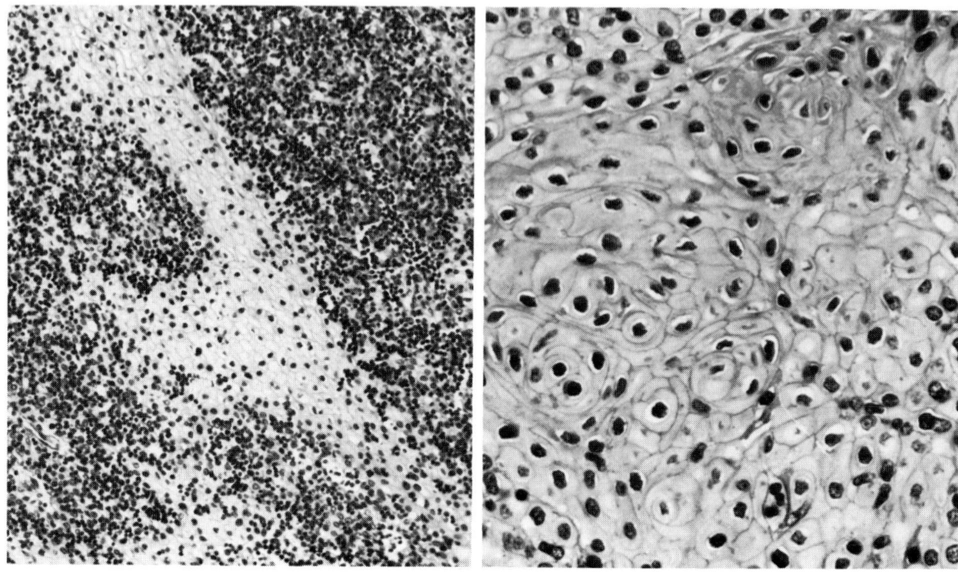

Figure 5–16. Predominantly epithelial thymoma with squamous differentiation. The epithelial cells have abundant eosinophilic cytoplasm and prominent cell borders. Whorls of squamous-appearing cells are evident (*Left,* H & E ×100; *Right,* H & E ×400).

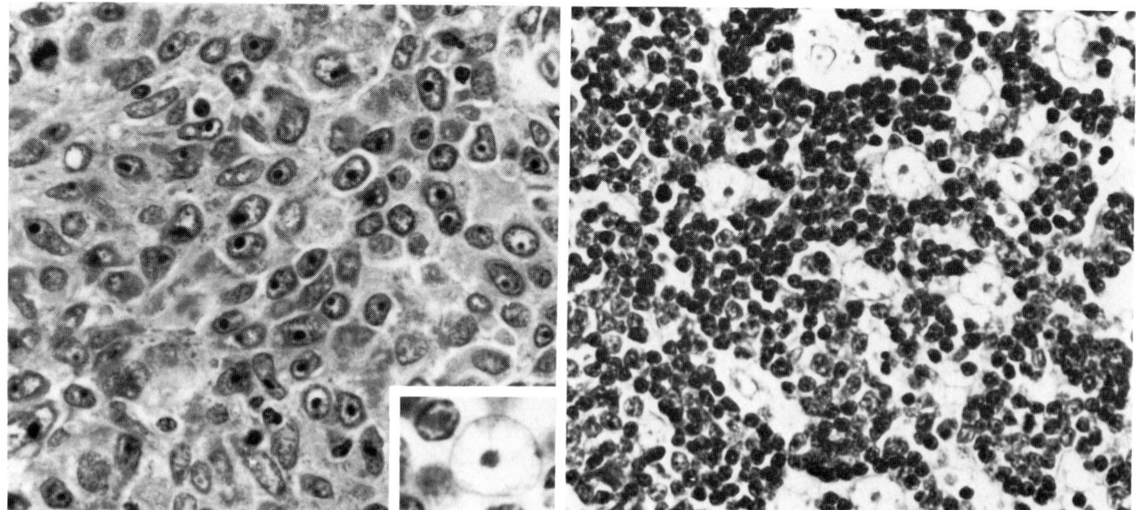

Figure 5–17. "Cortical" thymomas are characterized by epithelial cells resembling those in the thymic cortex. Morphologically, they have round-oval nuclei, vesicular chromatin, and prominent nucleoli. Such cells are present in the lymphocytic thymoma *(right)* and in the epithelial thymoma *(left)*. The *inset* of the left photograph is a cortical epithelial cell from normal thymus (H & E ×1000). (*Left* and *right,* H & E ×400.)

cation is the idea that tumors derived from cortical epithelial cells can be distinguished from those derived from medullary epithelial cells by histologic criteria. Immunohistochemical studies have used antibodies to cortical or medullary thymic epithelium on frozen sections.[83, 90–95, 95a] There is controversy about whether thymomas can be accurately classified immunologically as to origin from cortical or medullary epithelial cells. Most investigators report that many, if not most, thymomas contain epithelial cells of both phenotypes. Thus, a distinction between thymomas of cortical and medullary derivation may not be accurate.

Thymomas can also be phenotyped based on the associated lymphocytes. For example, cortical lymphocytes express CD1, whereas most medullary lymphocytes do not. The lymphocytic and mixed thymomas have lymphocytes with a cortical phenotype, whereas the predominantly epithelial and spindle cell thymomas tend to have phenotypically more mature lymphocytes.[87, 96–99] Similarly, "cortical" thymomas (many of which are rich in lymphocytes) tend to have more CD1-positive lymphocytes than "medullary" tumors do. Yet, the data based on epithelial cell morphology do not correlate well with an epithelial cell phenotype. Takacs and colleagues concluded that a thymoma's ability to induce phenotypic cortical T cells is independent of the epithelial cell phenotype.[100] Kraus and colleagues suggest that thymomas with immature epithelial cells (epithelial cells with a phenotype similar to that of fetal thymic epithelium) have lymphocytes with an immature phenotype.[101] Lymphocytes in a thymoma with phenotypically differentiated epithelial cells express a mature phenotype.

The evidence shows that thymomas derived from cortical or medullary epithelium cannot reliably be separated by histopathology or by immunophenotypic studies. A more straightforward classification based on epithelial cell morphology would divide thymomas descriptively into polygonal cell, spindle cell, and mixed categories.[94] However, many have concluded that a classification based on epithelial cell morphology is difficult and of limited clinical value.[70, 102, 103]

Whatever the classification system, the histopathology of thymomas is remarkable for its diversity among different tumors and within a single specimen. Certainly, any histologic classification based only on a biopsy could be misleading.

Frozen Sections

Intraoperative frozen sections on mediastinal tumors are notoriously difficult to interpret. In a retrospective study, Juttner and colleagues from Austria reported that only 28 of 76 malignant mediastinal tumors (37%) were correctly diagnosed on frozen sections.[104] The diagnosis was deferred in 35%, and an incorrect diagnosis was made in 28%. An incorrect diagnosis led to unnecessary, extended resections (including severing the phrenic nerve and/or resection of a pulmonary lobe) for lymphoma. The most common error was in the important distinction between lymphoma and malignant thymoma/thymic carcinoma.

In approaching a frozen section on a biopsy of a mediastinal tumor, one must have optimal communication with the surgeon as well as a good specimen and high-quality sections. The pathologist should know if the patient has myasthenia gravis, because a thymoma would then be more likely. Radiographic studies are useful. For example, extensive lymphadenopathy would be more compatible with lymphoma than with thymoma. The pathologist should know whether the surgeon finds the tumor to be resectable. If the lesion is unresectable, there may be no need for an immediate definitive diagnosis. Knowing that tumor is present in the biopsy may be sufficient information for the surgeon. Tissue should then be apportioned appropriately for routine sections, electron microscopy, and frozen section immunoperoxidase. If the surgeon needs to know whether or not to resect the mass, a more definitive diagnosis should be sought. The pathologist needs to have adequate tissue; multiple biopsies from different areas of the tumor may allow for a more accurate diagnosis. For example, a superficial biopsy consisting mostly of the tumor's fibrous capsule may be misleading.

Histologic clues such as fibrous bands, lobulation, prominent perivascular spaces, and medullary differentiation may be helpful, if present. Fibrous bands in a thymoma compartmentalize the tumor into relatively uniform lobules. In nodular sclerosing Hodgkin's disease and large-cell lymphoma with sclerosis, the fibrous bands are less orderly. Fibrosis is also a feature of sclerosing mediastinitis and radiation effect. Lymphocytic thymomas are easily misdiagnosed as lymphoma. Identification of the epithelial cell element can be difficult. Prominent perivascular spaces are a useful clue to a thymoma. Medullary differentiation is another feature of a thymoma that can be helpful, particularly on frozen sections. The epithelial cells may be more easily recognized adjacent to the fibrous trabeculae. Overstaining the frozen section with eosin accentuates the cytoplasm of the epithelial cells and may facilitate their recognition.[105]

Granulomatous inflammation may be associated with lymphomas (including Hodgkin's disease), seminoma, sarcoidosis, and infections (tuberculosis, histoplasmosis). Necrosis with a granulomatous response may also be present within a thymoma. Numerous eosinophils are uncommon in a thymoma and should raise the suspicion for Hodgkin's disease. In considering the diagnosis of spindle cell thymoma, one must also think about other spindle cell lesions, including mesothelioma, leiomyoma, neurofibroma, solitary fibrous tumor, and carcinoid.

Cytopathology

Cytologic techniques can be valuable preoperatively (see Chapter 1) and at the time of frozen section.[106–109] Intraoperative cytology can be a useful adjunct to the interpretation of frozen sections.[105, 110, 111] Smears from fine-needle aspiration biopsies or touch imprints are air-dried and stained with a rapid (less than 2-minute), modified Wright's stain (Diff-Quik, American Scientific Products, Columbia, MD). Smears can also be immediately fixed and stained with hematoxylin and eosin. If few cells are obtained on the touch imprint, a scrape preparation may be more useful.

Often, the dimorphic cell population (lymphocytes and epithelial cells) of a thymoma can be better appreciated on cytologic preparations than on frozen sections (Fig. 5–18). In lymphocytic thymomas, the epithelial cells can be best appreciated on imprints that are fixed and stained with hematoxylin and eosin. The predominantly epithelial tumors tend to have more cell clumping. Lymphomas tend to have noncohesive, individual cells, often with cytoplasmic fragments ("lymphoglandular bodies")[112] (see Chapter 6). The lymphoglandular bodies are best identified using the modified Wright's stain. The lymphoblastic lymphomas have monomorphic cells with scant cytoplasm and immature nuclear chromatin with or without nuclear convolutions. Seminomas form cohesive groups of cells with central round nucleoli (see Chapter 9). A "tigroid" or "striped" background of broken-up cytoplasm is characteristic of seminoma. Hodgkin's disease would have scattered large atypical cells

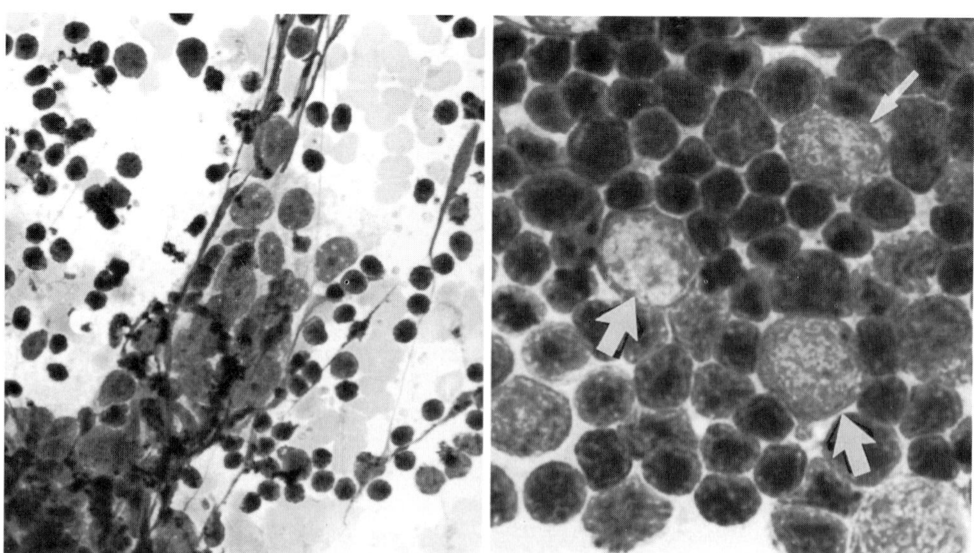

Figure 5–18. Cytologic features of thymoma. *Left,* Papanicolaou-stained fine needle aspirate demonstrates clumped epithelial cells and dispersed lymphocytes. Epithelial cell nuclei are slightly elongated. Some have prominent nucleoli. Histologic examination of the excised tumor demonstrated a predominantly epithelial thymoma of the spindled type (×400). *Right,* Diff-Quik–stained touch imprint of a lymphocytic thymoma. The larger epithelial cell nuclei *(arrows)* are readily distinguished from the lymphocytes that have more darkly staining chromatin. Occasional nucleoli in the epithelial cells can be appreciated (×1000).

with prominent nucleoli (Reed-Sternberg cells and variants) (see Chapter 6). Thymic carcinoma and metastatic carcinomas from other sites would have cohesive groups of pleomorphic cells with cytologic features of malignancy (see later). In combination with the frozen section and with some practice, touch imprints can add considerable confidence to a diagnosis.

Histochemistry

Histochemical stains may be helpful in the diagnosis of thymoma.[70, 113] Yet, in practice, they are rarely necessary. Epithelial or mixed lymphocytic and epithelial thymomas usually lack reticulin, except along the vessels and fibrous trabeculae. However, some thymomas have abundant reticulin fibers interspersed among the neoplastic cells.

The alcian blue/periodic acid-Schiff stain can identify mucin or glycogen. Mucin may be present, particularly within Hassall's corpuscles, as in normal thymus. Mucin may also be present within epithelial cells of occasional thymomas without Hassall's corpuscle formation. Glycogen may be demonstrated by its removal with diastase and by electron microscopy. Trichrome stains tend to accentuate the lobular nature of the tumor by highlighting the fibrous septa. Mast cells identified by metachromatic stains are present in most thymomas, particularly in fibrous septa, perivascular spaces, and areas of medullary differentiation. The argentaffin and argyrophil stains for neurosecretory granules are negative in thymoma.

Immunohistochemistry

Immunohistochemistry is most useful diagnostically in showing cytokeratin positivity in thymoma[77, 114] (Table 5–7). This distinguishes thymoma from lymphoma and from most, if not all, seminomas. Carcinoembryonic antigen, epithelial membrane antigen (EMA), Leu 7, and neuron-specific enolase are all variably present. The cytokeratins are a family of 19 different polypeptides. Different types of cytokeratin are expressed by different types of epithelial cells. In an immunohistochemical study, most thymic epithelial neoplasms contained cytokeratins 8, 13, 16, and 19.[115] Cytokeratin 18 was expressed to a greater extent in thymic carcinomas than in thymomas. Cytokeratin 13 was more often expressed in thymomas with polygonal cells than with spindled cells. In normal thymus, cytokeratins 8 and 19 identified all epithelial cells, whereas cytokeratins 6, 13, and 18 were present in epithelial subpopulations.

Table 5–7. Immunohistochemistry of Thymic Epithelial Cell Tumors

Antibody	Positive/ Total
Cytokeratin	49/52
Epithelial membrane antigen	37/48
Carcinoembryonic antigen	1/29*
Leu-7	40/50
Chromogranin	2/50†
Neuron-specific enolase (NSE)	12/35‡
LN3	7/12

*The one CEA-positive case was cytologically malignant and best classified as thymic carcinoma, undifferentiated type.
†In both of the positive cases, only rare chromogranin-positive cells were present.
‡In eight of these cases, only rare NSE-positive cells were present. In four cases, one of which was small cell carcinoma, NSE positivity was more extensive.
From Kornstein MJ, et al. Cortical versus medullary thymomas: a useful morphologic distinction? Hum Pathol 1988; 19:1335–1339.

EMA tends to stain areas of squamous differentiation and the epithelial cells around cystic spaces. Fukai and colleagues also report EMA staining of gland-like formations in thymomas.[116] These authors found EMA-positive thymomas to be more often invasive than EMA-negative tumors. Fukai et al. also report "much larger quantities" of EMA in thymic carcinoma than in thymomas.

The epithelial cells of thymomas are negative for S100 antigen. However, S100 is present in interdigitating reticulum cells in most cases.[117] Some S100-positive cells are Langerhans cells, which may be abundant.[101] Marx and colleagues reported some thymomas to be positive for neurofilament antigens on frozen sections.[118] Thymomas may have variable numbers of epithelial cells positive for p19, a protein isolated from the human T-cell lymphoma (leukemia) virus, which reacts with normal thymic epithelium.[93, 119, 120] Although one report found that invasive thymomas were less likely to have p19 reactivity than encapsulated tumors were,[119] this finding was not confirmed by others.[93, 120]

In this author's series, chromogranin was generally negative in all 30 cases tested, although rare positive cells were identified in two of the cases.[68] Strong chromogranin reactivity would favor the diagnosis of thymic carcinoid.

Most thymomas contain thymic hormones, including thymosins and thymulin. Hirokawa and colleagues reported that 80% of thymomas contain thymosin beta-1, and 89% contain thymosin beta-3.[92] Others report similar findings.[93, 121, 122]

Reports concerning expression of carcinoembryonic antigen (CEA) have been conflicting. Using a polyclonal antibody, Savino and colleagues found thymomas to express CEA strongly.[123] Using another polyclonal antibody, Giraud and colleagues found thymomas to have scattered CEA-positive cells.[93] In the present author's series, all thymomas were CEA-negative using a monoclonal antibody.[68] The different results most likely reflect the heterogeneity of different antibodies to CEA. Alpha-fetoprotein and vasopressin have also been identified in at least some thymomas.[93] Thymomas are variable with regard to human leukocyte antigen (HLA)-DR (class II major histocompatibility antigen) expression. Spindle cell (or "medullary") and epithelial thymomas tend to be HLA-DR negative, whereas lymphocyte-predominant tumors tend to be HLA-DR positive.[87, 100, 124–126] The problem with staining for HLA-DR is to separate reactivity of the epithelial cells from that of dendritic cells.

Many reports have examined the phenotype of the associated lymphocytes in thymomas.[87, 90, 96, 98, 99, 124, 126, 127] As discussed above, the lymphocytes are generally T cells. The lymphocytes in a thymoma may have a high rate of proliferation as demonstrated by labeling with Ki-67 antibody.[128] In lymphocytic and mixed thymomas, the lymphocytes usually express CD1 (Leu 6, T6), the surface antigen present on cortical lymphocytes in the normal thymus. With predominantly epithelial thymomas, however, the few lymphocytes present usually express a more mature phenotype (CD1− CD3+). Thymomas are often heterogeneous. Different areas of the same tumor often have lymphocytes with different phenotypes.[129] The same heterogeneity is true for the epithelial cell component.[93] Alterations in immunologic findings may occur with therapy. For example, pretreatment of the myasthenia patient with steroids may deplete the thymoma of cortical-type lymphocytes.[97] Investigators report no differences regarding the lymphocyte phenotype between thymomas from patients with and thymomas from patients without myasthenia gravis.[130]

Metastases from a thymoma frequently contain immature (CD1-positive) lymphocytes.[90, 99, 131] This can be a diagnostically helpful finding, because metastases from other epithelial tumors have only mature (CD1-negative) infiltrating lymphocytes.[90] Thymoma is the only human epithelial tumor known to contain T lymphocytes with a cortical phenotype. However, in mice, a virus-induced epithelial tumor of the salivary gland contains phenotypically immature lymphocytes.[132]

B cells may be present in a thymoma and may form germinal centers[70, 82] (see earlier). Some thymomas have abundant "asteroid" cells (i.e., dendritic-appearing cells labeling with B-cell marker CD20).[133, 134] One report found the asteroid cells to express both CD20 and cytokeratin.[133] CD20 has been reported to be expressed by follicular dendritic reticulum cells of germinal centers.[135] Perhaps the asteroid cells in thymomas represent dendritic cells, some of which have cytokeratin immunoreactivity.[136–138]

Immunoperoxidase studies of the extracellular matrix and basement membrane was reported by Mizuno and colleagues.[139] They found a diffuse network of fibers containing fibronectin and laminin in spindle cell thymomas. Polygonal cell thymomas contained fibronectin and laminin restricted to the septa, blood vessels, and perivascular spaces. Because spindle cell thymomas are less often invasive, the authors speculate that the distribution of fibronectin and laminin is related to the behavior of the tumor.

Molecular Pathology

To further analyze the lymphocytes in thymomas, investigators have studied DNA for evidence of gene rearrangements.[140, 141] No such rearrangements were identified using the Southern blotting technique with probes for the T-cell antigen receptor gene and immunoglobulin genes. Clonal lymphocytes show rearrangements of these genes when studied with this assay. Therefore, the lack of gene rearrangements is evidence that the lymphocytes within a thymoma are not neoplastic.

Electron Microscopy

Ultrastructural features of thymomas include prominent desmosomes and abundant tonofilaments[70, 142] (Fig. 5–19). The tonofilaments form bundles about 700 angstroms in width, and they may be over 2 μm in length. The tonofilaments insert into desmosomes

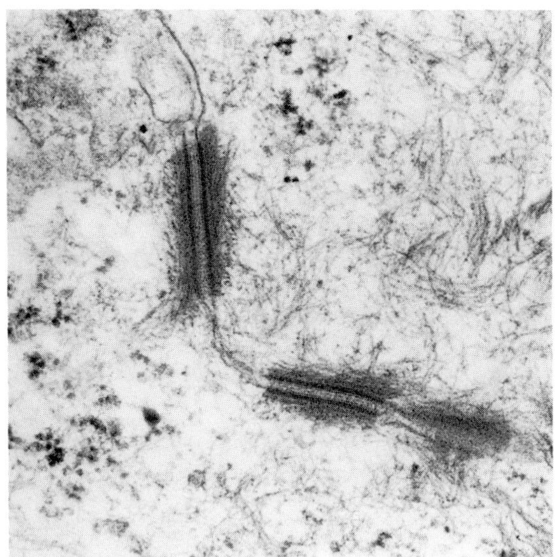

Figure 5–19. Electron micrograph demonstrating the well-formed intercellular junctions and abundant tonofilaments typical of a thymoma (×105,000).

that look like maculae adherents (thickened attachment plaques and a central dense line). The epithelial cells have elongated cytoplasmic processes. Basal lamina is present, especially where epithelial cells are next to vessels. It varies in width but is usually about 400 angstroms wide. The epithelial cell nuclei are usually oval and may be irregular in outline. Chromatin tends to concentrate beneath the nuclear membrane. Nucleoli may be inconspicuous. They may have an annular or solid shape; nucleolonema development may be identified. Cytoplasmic organelles are variable.

The lymphocyte element appears similar to that in the normal thymus.[70] Some lymphocytes show evidence of "activation" (i.e., less clumping of nuclear chromatin, prominent nucleoli, and prominent polyribosomes). Lymphocyte mitoses are common. Degenerated lymphocytes are found within macrophages and epithelial cells. The typical perivascular space is widened. It contains a central vessel surrounded by a space between the endothelial and epithelial laminae. Lymphocytes, histiocytes, plasma cells, red blood cells, and "scaffold cells" may be within the perivascular space. The latter attach to both the endothelial and epithelial laminae by means of attenuated process. These cells lack tonofilaments and desmosomes but have electron-dense cytoplasm containing numerous organelles.

Prognostic Factors

Once the diagnosis of thymoma is established, the most important histopathologic feature to recognize is the presence or absence of invasion. Clinicopathologic studies consistently have identified local invasion as an important prognostic factor (see Table 5–9). Traditionally, the distinction between invasive and noninvasive thymomas was made by the surgeon and was based on intraoperative findings.[85] If the tumor grossly involved adjacent mediastinal structures, it was determined to be invasive. One problem with this approach is the difficulty in distinguishing between adhesions and invasion. Adherence of the tumor to adjacent structures does not necessarily indicate invasion.

Bergh and colleagues published one of the first studies in which invasiveness was based on histologic findings.[143] Masaoka and colleagues revised the classification slightly.[144] As in prior studies based on gross findings, the presence of invasion was a significant prognostic factor. However, neither study attempted to show whether microscopic invasion into the mediastinal fat in a grossly encapsulated tumor was significant. A further confusing issue is that Masaoka et al. defined microscopic invasion as invasion "into" the capsule. This author's study found that only invasion "through" the capsule is significant[68] (Fig. 5–20). Table 5–8 summarizes several systems for staging thymoma.

The data concerning the importance of microscopic invasion are scant. With colleagues, this author identified nine patients with grossly encapsulated thymomas that were found to have microscopic invasion into the adjacent fat.[68] None received radiation therapy. Four of the nine had a local recurrence (9, 23, 50, and 84 months after diagnosis). In contrast, none of the 42 thymoma patients without microscopic invasion experienced relapse. Similarly, Wilkins and colleagues reported that four of six patients with microscopic invasion through the capsule developed recurrent disease (versus none of 45 patients without microscopic invasion).[76] On the other hand, Kuo and Lo found no recurrences among 10 thymomas with microscopic invasion, but median follow-up time was short (20 months).[145]

All clinicopathologic studies agree that invasiveness is an important prognostic factor for thymoma (Table 5–9). A major area of disagreement among these studies is the impor-

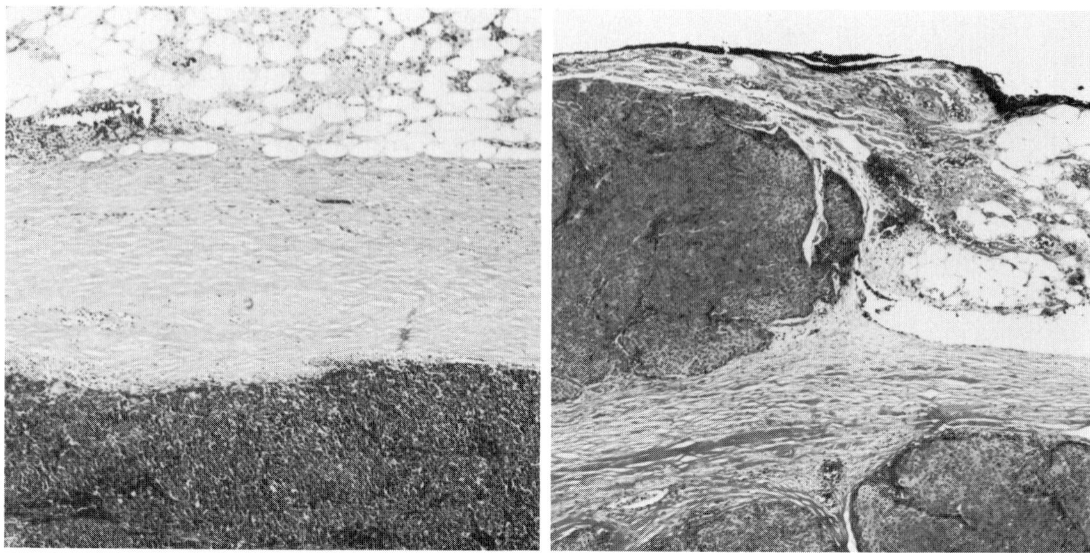

Figure 5–20. *Left,* A thick capsule surrounds this lymphocytic thymoma. *Right,* This epithelial thymoma has invasion through the capsule into the adjacent adipose tissue. The tumor approaches the inked resection margin (H & E ×100). (From Kornstein MJ. Controversies regarding the pathology of thymomas. *In* Rosen PP, Fechner RE, eds. Pathol Annu 1992; 27 [Part 2]:1–15.)

Table 5–8. Staging of Thymoma

Stage	Bergh et al.[143]	Masaoka et al.[144]	Verley and Hollmann[14]	Current*
I	Intact capsule or growth within the capsule	Macroscopically completely encapsulated and microscopically no capsular invasion	Grossly noninvasive a. Without adhesions b. With fibrous adhesions to mediastinal structures	Intact capsule or growth within the capsule
II	Pericapsular growth into the surrounding mediastinal fat tissue	1. Macroscopic invasion into surrounding fatty tissue or mediastinal pleura, *or* 2. Microscopic invasion into capsule	Localized (macroscopic) invasiveness (i.e., pericapsular growth into fat tissue or adjacent pleura or pericardium) a. Complete excision b. Incomplete excision	a. Microscopic invasion through capsule into adjacent mediastinal tissue b. Gross and microscopic invasion through capsule into surrounding fat or adjacent pleura or pericardium
III	Invasive growth into the surrounding organs, intrathoracic metastases, or both	Macroscopic invasion into neighboring organ (i.e., pericardium, great vessels, or lung)	Largely invasive tumor a. Invasion into surrounding organs and/or intrathoracic dissemination b. Lymphogenous or hematogenous metastasis	Invasion into surrounding structures (i.e., great vessels, lung)
IV		a. Pleural or pericardial dissemination b. Lymphogenous or hematogenous metastasis		a. Pleural or pericardial dissemination b. Lymphogenous or hematogenous metastases

*Synthesis of the three proposed staging systems.

tance of histopathologic classification. The traditional classification based on numbers of lymphocytes led to conflicting results. Some investigators reported the predominantly epithelial type to have the worst prognosis.[12, 14] Some found the mixed lymphocytic and epithelial type to have the worst prognosis.[85, 146] Lymphocytic and spindled types have been found by some to have better prognoses.[14, 147] In this author's study, mixed lymphocytic/epithelial tumors were statistically more likely to be invasive; lymphocytic and spindled thymomas were less likely. However, there was no independent significance to this classification in predicting relapse-free survival.[68] In contrast, invasion is consistently an important prognostic factor.

Concerning the cortical/medullary classification, most studies report that the cortical type has a worse prognosis, and the medullary type has a better one.[68, 75, 145, 148, 149, 149a] However, with one exception,[149a] all studies to date with multivariant statistical analyses have shown that invasion is the only significant, independent prognostic factor.[68, 75]

Some of the childhood thymomas have an aggressive, fatal course.[6, 9] In 1991, Ramon y Cajal and Suster reported a series of 10 thymic epithelial neoplasms in children from 1 to 16 years of age.[7] Three tumors were classified as thymic carcinoma (two small cell, one undifferentiated). These patients all died within 15 months. Two tumors had a spindle cell appearance with some cytologic atypia, mitoses (5 to 15 per high-power field), focal necrosis, and hemangiopericytoma-like areas. These two cases were described histologically as intermediate-grade. Both had metastasized (to the lung or bone). The other five cases were predominantly lymphocytic. One of the five was invasive. In four of these cases, the authors describe "unusual stromal features" (i.e., prominent fibrosis in and around the lobules). These five patients all did well. Pescarmona and colleagues reported five children (11 to 15 years) with thymoma, all of which were of the lymphocytic type.[8] All were grossly encapsulated, although two had microscopic capsular infiltration. All of the patients in the Pescarmona et al. series did well. Thus, children rarely develop thymic tumors, a subset of which are aggressive. Apparently, the aggressive tumors can be identified histologically.

Few studies investigating the usefulness of DNA flow cytometry[150] as a prognostic factor in thymomas have been reported. With this technique, cells are labeled with a DNA-binding fluorescent dye, such as propidium iodide.[151] Fluorescence is then detected using a flow cytometer. This assay measures DNA ploidy and can also determine the percentages of cells in the different phases of the cell cycle. Of four studies that have been done, aneuploidy *was* a significant prognostic factor in two[152, 153] and *was not* a significant prognostic factor in two.[154, 155] Each of these studies analyzed 25 to 40 cases. Larger studies are needed. In this author's experience, aneuploidy is more frequent in invasive tumors than in noninvasive ones.[155a] Similar findings have been reported by Kuo and Lo.[156] Thymic carcinomas are also frequently aneuploid. However, aneuploidy is unlikely to have prognostic significance independent of invasiveness and cytologic malignancy. Furthermore, Banez and colleagues reported artifactual near-diploid peaks in encapsulated lymphocytic thymomas that were studied from the paraffin-embedded tissue.[157]

Surgical Pathology Report

Important information on a thymoma in the surgical pathology report should include (1) correct diagnosis, which often requires immunoperoxidase studies and/or electron microscopy, (2) assessment of surgical margins, which requires "inking" the margins, and (3) determination of invasiveness, which may require multiple sections through the capsule. Additionally, the histologic appearance should be described, including the presence of such features as pleomorphism, mitoses, and atypia. Studies with retrospective reviews of histopathology have shown high rates of diagnostic error. In a series reported by Bretel, 33 of 161 tumors (20%) were incorrectly diagnosed as thymoma.[158] In the present author's series, the diagnosis was changed on review in 11% of cases, usually because of immunoperoxidase results. Thus, one should use immunoperoxidase studies to confirm the diagnosis if there is any uncertainty.

Prognosis and Therapy

Rates of relapse and survival are generally similar among the various clinicopathologic studies that have been published (Table 5–9). Zero to twelve percent of noninvasive thymomas recur. Twenty to thirty-three percent of invasive tumors recur, and 3 to 5% metastasize. Survival rates for patients with noninvasive tumors depend primarily on any accompanying diseases. Invasive thymomas are associated with 5-year survival rates of 50 to 80% (Fig. 5–21).

The optimal therapy for thymoma is complete excision.[159, 160] Some surgeons advocate radical procedures, if necessary, such as removal of portions of the superior vena cava with graft reconstruction.[161, 162] This contrasts with the management of lymphoma that requires only a surgical biopsy. Therefore, preoperative and/or intraoperative diagnosis is important. For completely excised noninvasive thymoma, no further therapy is indicated, in this author's opinion. Such tumors should rarely recur, especially if the capsule is carefully sectioned for evidence of microscopic invasion into the adjacent tissue. Some controversy exists, however; at least some authors advocate radiation therapy for all thymomas, whether invasive or not.[161, 163]

For completely excised thymoma with microscopically documented invasion through the capsule, radiation therapy is usually recommended. In a review of the literature, total resection without radiation resulted in a thoracic failure rate of 28% (20/72), whereas total resection with radiation therapy produced a thoracic failure rate of 5% (2/43).[15]

Table 5–9. Thymoma: Recurrence and Survival Rates Based on Selected Clinicopathologic Studies

First Author	No. of Cases (f/u)	Histologic Classification	Stage vs. Metastases and Local Recurrences	Survival
Lewis[12] 1987	283+ (46% MG) (40 yrs included in study)	25% epithelial 43% mixed 25% lymphocytic 6% spindled Thymic carcinoma excluded	32% of tumors grossly or microscopically invasive 5% of invasive tumors metastasized 12% of noninvasive tumors recurred 28% of invasive tumors recurred	5-yr survival: 67% overall 75% for noninvasive 50% for invasive Predominantly epithelial histologic type had lower survival Independent, adverse prognostic factors: 1. Invasion (most important) 2. Age <30 years 3. Any symptoms 4. Incomplete resection
Kornstein[15, 68] 1988	100 (78 with follow-up) (47% MG) (24 yrs included in study)	16% epithelial 34% mixed 31% lymphocytic 14% spindle 5% carcinoma 18% cortical 32% medullary 45% mixed cortical/medullary	58% of tumors grossly or microscopically invasive 3% of invasive tumors metastasized 0% of noninvasive tumors recurred 33% of invasive tumors recurred	5-yr survival: 70% overall (67% relapse-free survival) 67% for noninvasive (100% relapse-free survival) 86% for stage II (58% relapse-free survival) 69% for stage III (53% relapse-free survival) No effect of histology on relapse-free survival Independent, adverse prognostic factors: 1. Invasion 2. Incomplete resection Patients with MG had a significantly lower relapse rate

Table 5–9. Thymoma: Recurrence and Survival Rates Based on Selected Clinicopathologic Studies *Continued*

First Author	No. of Cases (f/u)	Histologic Classification	Stage vs. Metastases and Local Recurrences	Survival
Verley[14] 1985	200 (181 with follow-up) (52% MG) (27 years included in study)	33% epithelial (includes mixed and epithelial types) 30% lymphocytic 30% spindle/oval (regardless of lymphocytes) 7% undifferentiated epithelial (carcinoma)	33% grossly or microscopically invasive 7% of invasive tumors metastasized distantly 5% of noninvasive tumors recurred 28% of invasive tumors recurred	5-yr survival: 60% overall 85% for noninvasive 50% for invasive Undifferentiated epithelial type yielded worst survival Differentiated epithelial type worse survival than lymphocytic or spindled No effect of MG on survival Spindled and lymphocytic thymomas less likely to be invasive; when they were invasive, they behaved like epithelial thymoma
Maggi[85,86] 1986 & 1991	241 (234 with follow-up) (67% MG) (29 yrs included in study)	62% epithelial (includes mixed and epithelial types) 28% lymphocytic 7% spindle (regardless of lymphocytes) 3% carcinoma	45% grossly or microscopically invasive (according to Masaoka et al.) 2% of noninvasive tumors recurred 20% of invasive tumors recurred	5-yr survival: 81% overall 89% for noninvasive 71% for invasive (stage II or III) 59% for invasive with intrathoracic dissemination (stage IVa) Spindled, lymphocytic, and epithelial types all equal survival; undifferentiated tumors with poorer prognosis Higher survival in patients with MG, worse survival with other autoimmune disease Higher survival with complete resection than with subtotal resection or biopsy

MG, myasthenia gravis.

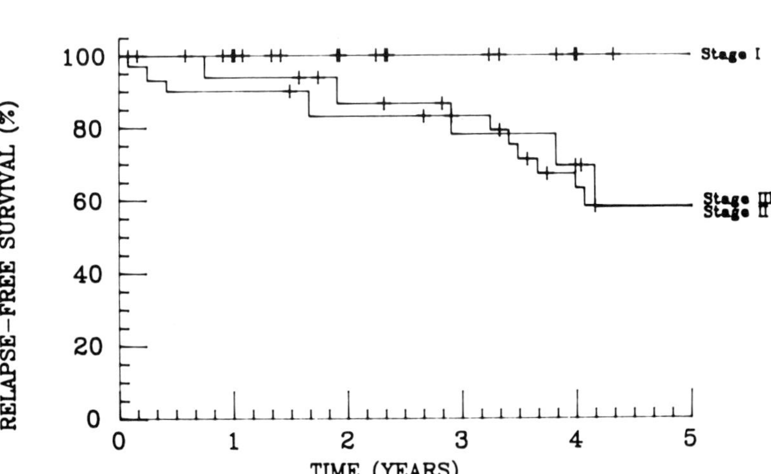

Figure 5–21. Thymoma: Percentage of relapse-free survival by stage. (Reprinted from Curran WJ Jr, Kornstein MJ, Brooks JJ, Turrisi AT III. Invasive thymoma: the role of mediastinal irradiation following complete or incomplete surgical resection. J Clin Oncol 1988; 6:1722–1727.)

For nonresectable thymoma, an unresolved issue is whether the tumor should be debulked or merely biopsied. In the present author's series, recurrence and survival rates were similar between patients undergoing biopsy and those having a subtotal resection when either procedure was followed by radiation therapy.[15] Similarly, a French multicenter study of 500 cases found no difference in prognosis between tumors that were biopsied and those that had undergone incomplete surgical treatment. The latter group had a higher morbidity rate.[164] Pollack et al. also found no statistically significant difference between the two groups.[146] However, Nakahara et al. report better survival rates in those patients undergoing subtotal resection than in those having a biopsy only.[161] Also, the radiation field can be smaller, if the tumor mass is reduced. Thus, the evidence is conflicting but seems to favor biopsy rather than debulking for nonresectable thymomas. Some authors advocate preoperative chemotherapy or radiotherapy for unresectable thymoma to improve resectability.[165, 166]

Postoperative radiation therapy and/or chemotherapy can be offered to the patient for palliation. Radiation therapy may prolong disease-free survival in patients with invasive thymoma.[15, 167] Doses up to and over 60 Gy have been recommended for long-term local control.[168] Thymomas often respond to chemotherapy.[169–171] One intergroup trial (Southwest Oncology Group and Southeastern Cancer Study Group) evaluated combination therapy with cisplatin, doxorubicin, and cyclophosphamide in patients with advanced thymoma.[172] Three complete and 11 partial remissions were obtained in 20 patients for a total response rate of 70%. The median duration of remission was 13 months. Three patients remained disease-free for over 2 years.

Local recurrences of thymoma can be managed surgically.[147, 173] Thymomas tend to recur locally and are usually slow growing; they may recur years after initial excision. Removal of a local recurrence can control the tumor for many more years. Combination chemotherapy and/or radiation may also be used in the treatment of locally recurrent or metastatic thymoma.[159, 160, 170, 174–176]

The response of associated syndromes to thymectomy is variable. Among patients with associated red blood cell aplasia, approximately one third will experience remission of the anemia after removal of the thymoma.[18, 24, 177] Few patients seem to recover from hypogammaglobulinemia.[18, 24, 32] Most studies indicate that myasthenia gravis patients with thymoma do not respond as well to thymectomy as do those without thymoma.[163, 173, 178] Slater et al. reported a 7% complete remission rate at 5 years for myasthenic patients after removal of a neoplastic thymus.[178] In contrast, myasthenia patients undergoing thymectomy without a tumor had a 40% 5-year complete remission rate. However, Levasseur and colleagues report that most myasthenic patients responded favorably to thymectomy, and the response rate was the same whether or not a thymoma was present.[18] Exacerbation of the myasthenia gravis may be associated with recurrence of the thymoma.[173] Resection of the recurrent tumor may alleviate the myasthenia symptoms.

THYMIC CARCINOMA

Clinical Features

Thymic carcinoma is a cytologically malignant anterior mediastinal tumor different from lymphoma, germ cell tumors, sarcoma, and metastases from other sites. In most cases, origin from the thymus can only be inferred, based on the tumor's anterior mediastinal location and absence of other primary lesions. A marker specific for neoplastic thymic epithelial cells has not been described.

Thymic carcinomas generally occur in older patients (Table 5–10). They are uncommonly associated with myasthenia gravis.[84, 89, 179–182] Some of the cases that have been reported in myasthenia gravis patients have been described as "well differentiated" and perhaps are better classified as epithelial thymomas[83, 183] (see later). Case studies have reported poorly differentiated thymic carcinomas in patients with aplastic anemia, Hashimoto's thyroiditis, and polymyositis.[184, 185] Most patients have symptoms attributable to the mediastinal mass.

Suster and Rosai reported the largest series of patients with thymic carcinoma in 1991.[182] They studied 60 patients with this diagnosis who were followed for at least 3 years or until the time of death. The patients ranged from 10 to 76 years of age and had a male-to-female ratio of 1.5:1. None had myasthenia gravis. Overall survival rates were 57%, 40%, and 33% at 1, 3, and 5 years, respectively. Thirty patients developed metastases, most commonly to lymph nodes (cervical and axillary), bone,

Table 5–10. Selected Clinicopathologic Studies of Thymic Carcinoma

First Author/Year	No. of Cases	Age Range/Mean	Male/ Female	Histologic Classification	Invasive/with Metastases	Survival
Shimosato[84] 1977	8	39–65/55	7/1	Squamous cell	7/3	2 died with tumor; 6 NED at 1–11 yrs
Snover[179] 1982	8	29–76/57	4/4	3 mixed small cell/squamous 2 basaloid 1 mucoepidermoid 1 clear cell 1 sarcomatoid	4/3	4 died with tumor; 1 alive w/metastases; 2 NED at 2 yrs (basaloid and mucoepidermoid)
Wick[180] 1982	20	4–72/48	14/6	11 lymphoepithelioma-like 2 spindling squamous 1 sarcomatoid 2 mixed small cell/squamous 4 small cell	19/13	15 died with tumor; average survival 20 mos; 1 NED at 43 mos
Kuo[181] 1990	13	19–64/40	9/4	2 undifferentiated 1 clear cell 2 mixed squamous/small cell 2 mixed adenosquamous/small cell 6 squamous	12/4	5 of 6 with squamous cell, NED; 6 of remaining 7 died with tumor (median survival 18 mos for nonsquamous cell)
Truong[189] 1990	13	30–74/54	7/6	7 squamous cell (6 with lymphoepithelioma-like component) 4 small cell 1 clear cell 1 adenosquamous	8/6	6 died with disease (3 small cell and 3 squamous); 4, NED
Suster[182] 1991	60	10–76/46	36/24	16 well-differentiated squamous 1 mucoepidermoid 3 basaloid 19 lymphoepithelioma-like 8 small cell 7 undifferentiated/ anaplastic 4 sarcomatoid 2 clear cell	34 of 43 invasive 30 of 60 with metastases	57% 1-yr survival 33% 5-yr survival 85% of patients with high-grade tumors died of disease versus 0% with low-grade tumors

NED, no evidence of disease.

lung, and liver. Thus, thymic carcinoma is a more aggressive disease than thymoma and has a greater risk of metastases.

Gross Pathology

Grossly, thymic carcinomas usually lack a well-defined capsule (Fig. 5–22). Areas of necrosis and hemorrhage are frequent within the gritty, gray-white tumor. Rarely, cystic changes are prominent (Fig. 5–23). Such cases may represent a carcinoma arising within a thymic cyst.[186, 187]

Histopathology

Microscopically, thymic carcinomas are characterized by a malignant appearance (i.e., high nuclear-to-cytoplasmic ratio, cellular pleomorphism, nucleoli, mitotic figures, necrosis). Occasionally, a carcinoma will appear to be arising within a thymoma[180–182, 188–190] (Fig. 5–24).

Thymic carcinoma has been subdivided into different histologic types[182] (Tables 5–10 and 5–11). Poorly differentiated squamous cell carcinomas have infiltrative tumor cells with large vesicular nuclei and prominent nucleoli. Evidence of squamous differentiation (eosinophilic cytoplasm, prominent cell borders, whorl formations, keratinization) may be present focally (Fig. 5–24). Glandular differentiation may also be identified and would make the diagnosis adenosquamous carcinoma[191] (Fig. 5–25). One case of a lymphoepithelioma-like thymic carcinoma had evidence of focal neuroblastoma.[192] The neuroblastoma element was documented by electron microscopy.

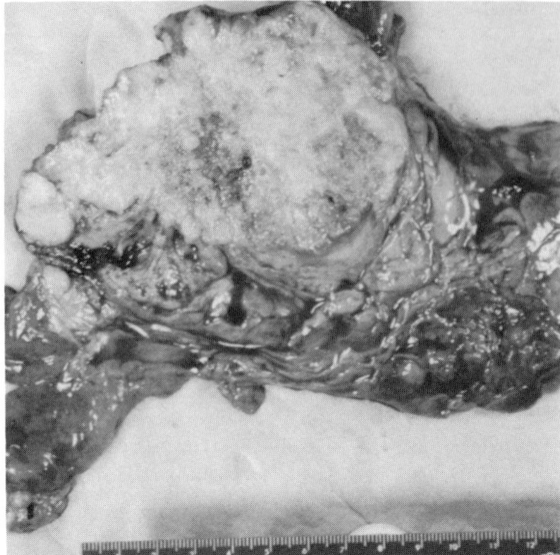

Figure 5–22. Thymic carcinoma, poorly differentiated squamous cell type. The tumor is a firm, tan mass with focal areas of hemorrhage and necrosis. The tumor does not have a well-defined capsule. The surrounding tissue is thymus.

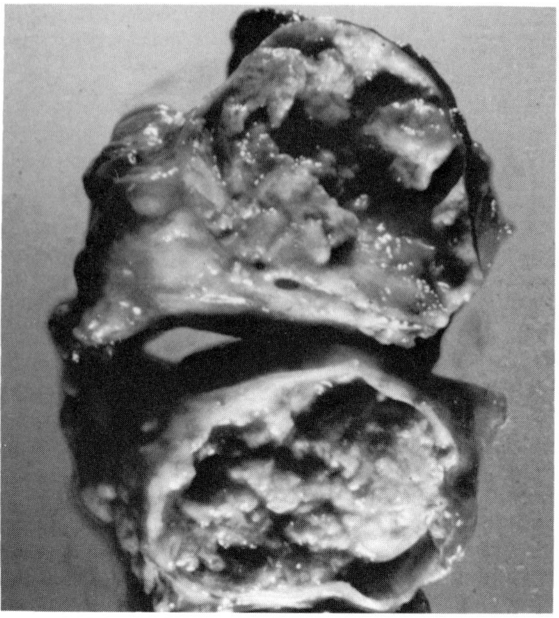

Figure 5–23. Cystic thymic carcinoma. The poorly differentiated squamous cell carcinoma appeared to arise within a thymic cyst.

Lymphoepithelioma-like carcinoma is characterized by large cells with indistinct borders and amphophilic cytoplasm, and it resembles the lymphoepithelioma of the nasopharynx (Fig. 5–26). The tumor cells have vesicular nuclei with prominent nucleoli. Mitoses are abundant. Necrosis is usually present. Glycogen may be present in small amounts. Reticulin is sparse and surrounds large clusters of tumor cells.[180] Many lymphoepithelioma-like carcinomas have foci of squamous differentiation and could be classified as poorly differentiated squamous cell carcinoma.

Well-differentiated squamous cell carcinoma is characterized by prominent lobular growth. Cells have an epidermoid appearance with eosinophilic cytoplasm and distinct cell borders (Fig. 5–27). The nuclear to cytoplasmic ratio is high. Necrosis is not a prominent feature.

Spindle cell carcinomas have been described under several terms, including sarcomatoid carcinoma, spindling squamous cell carcinoma, and carcinosarcoma.[179, 180, 182, 193] Sarcomatoid carcinoma is a biphasic tumor composed of closely packed, mitotically active,

Table 5–11. Thymic Carcinomas

Low Grade	High Grade
Well-differentiated squamous cell carcinoma	Poorly differentiated carcinoma
Basaloid carcinoma	Poorly differentiated squamous cell carcinoma*
Mucoepidermoid carcinoma	Lymphoepithelioma-like carcinoma
	Poorly differentiated adenosquamous carcinoma
	Small-cell carcinoma
	Clear-cell carcinoma
	Sarcomatoid carcinoma
	Anaplastic/undifferentiated carcinoma

*The terms poorly differentiated squamous cell carcinoma and lymphoepithelioma-like carcinoma are often used interchangeably.[180] The terms can be used to describe two patterns.[189] In poorly differentiated squamous tumors, the cell borders are distinct, and cells have eosinophilic cytoplasm. Focal keratinization may be present. In the lymphoepithelial pattern, cells grow as syncytial masses with ill-defined borders. The nuclei have more vesicular chromatin and more prominent nucleoli. In both types, necrosis and mitotic figures are prominent. The tumors infiltrate desmoplastic stroma as clusters or cords of cells with variable lymphocytic infiltrates. Most tumors show both patterns. The adenosquamous carcinoma representing a poorly differentiated squamous cell carcinoma with areas of glandular differentiation is included in the high-grade category because of the aggressive course of a case described by Truong and colleagues.[189]

Adapted from Suster S, Rosai J. Thymic carcinoma: a clinicopathologic study of 60 cases. Cancer 1991; 67:1025–1032.

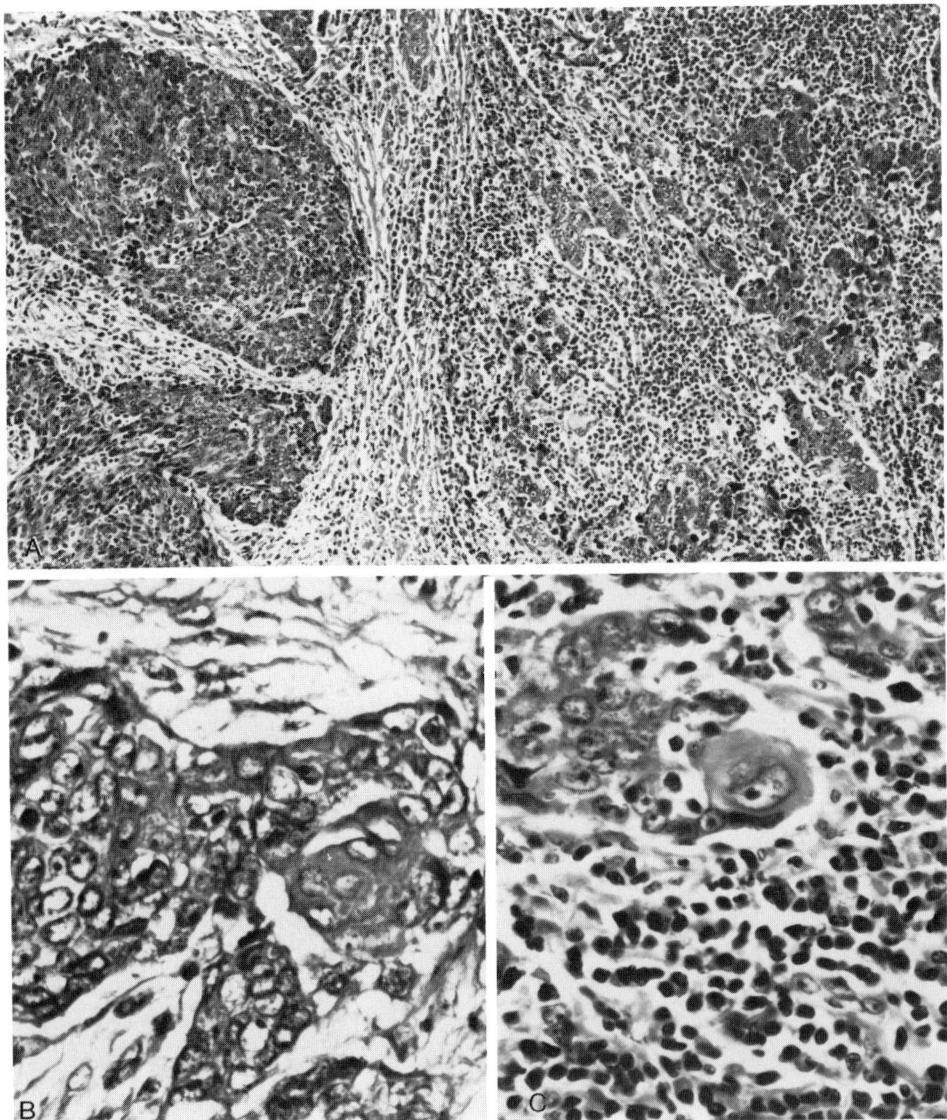

Figure 5–24. Poorly differentiated squamous cell carcinoma of the thymus appearing to arise within an epithelial thymoma. In *A*, the left side demonstrates features of an epithelial thymoma with a lobular growth pattern and perivascular spaces. On the right, the cells have infiltrative growth (H & E ×100). *B* and *C*, Note the malignant cytologic characteristics of the infiltrating cells (vesicular nuclei, prominent nucleoli). Focal keratinization indicates squamous differentiation (H & E ×400).

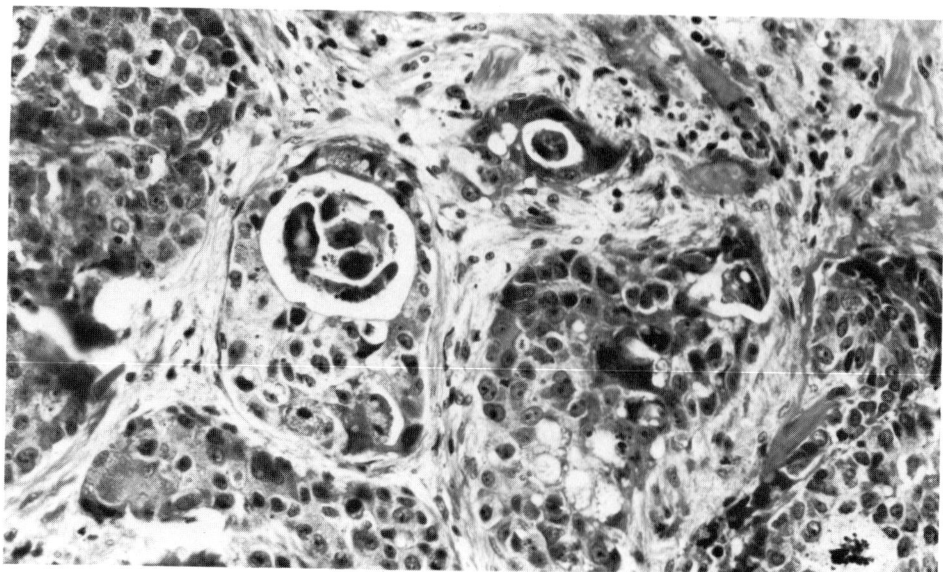

Figure 5–25. Adenosquamous carcinoma. Gland formation is identified within a poorly differentiated squamous cell carcinoma. A mucin stain was positive (H & E ×400).

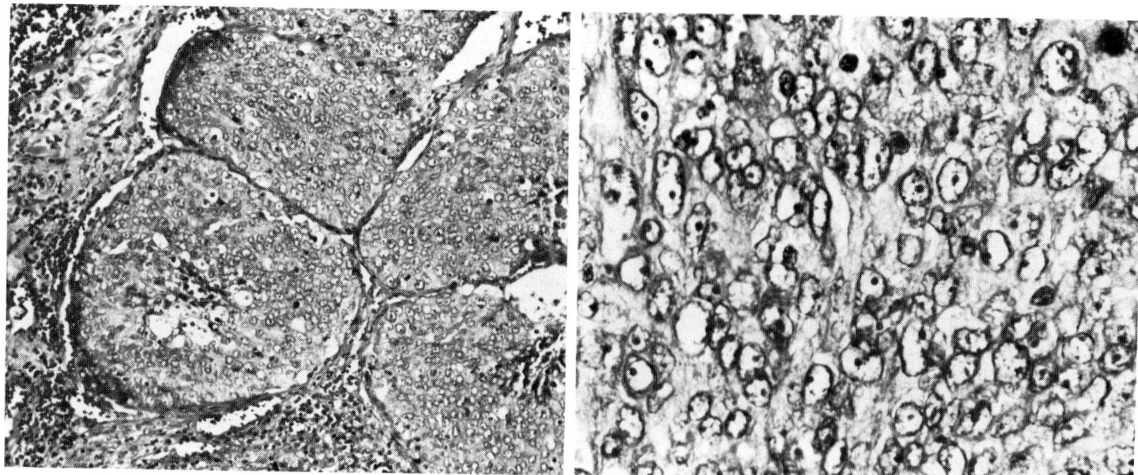

Figure 5–26. Lymphoepithelioma-like thymic carcinoma. *Left,* Note islands of tumor cells with central necrosis and lymphocytic infiltrate (×200). *Right,* The tumor cells have large, vesicular nuclei and prominent nucleoli (×400). (From Kornstein MJ. Controversies regarding the pathology of thymomas. *In* Rosen PP, Fechner RE, eds. Pathol Annu 1992; 27 [Part 2]:1–15.)

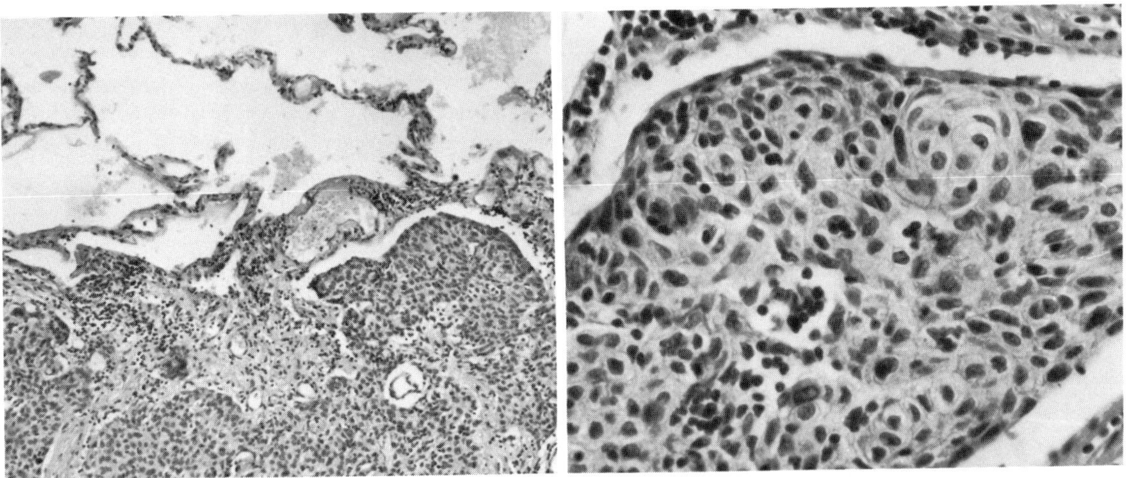

Figure 5–27. Well-differentiated squamous cell carcinoma invading lung. Epidermoid appearance and moderate nuclear atypia are evident. (H & E *Left*, ×100; *right*, ×400.)

elongated cells arranged in fascicles, admixed with a cytologically atypical epithelial cell element[179, 182] (Fig. 5–28, top). Identification of the spindled cell component as epithelial in origin is based on immunoreactivity for cytokeratin. In the case reported by Snover and colleagues, large, round, myoglobin-positive cells were scattered among the spindled cells.[179]

Spindling squamous cell carcinoma is composed of elongated tumor cells with a moderate amount of cytoplasm and distinct cell borders. Nuclear chromatin is coarse, nucleoli are prominent, and mitoses are frequent.[180]

A case report of a thymic carcinosarcoma describes a sarcomatous component of malignant-appearing cells with myoid differentiation (desmin and actin immunoreactivity).[194] In addition, a carcinomatous element was present that consisted of cohesive, cytologically malignant epithelial cells (immunoreactive for cytokeratin). At the periphery of the tumor, areas with the appearance of a spindle cell thymoma were found.

Anaplastic carcinoma has marked cellular pleomorphism, bizarre nuclei, and atypical mitoses (Fig. 5–28, bottom). The term undifferentiated carcinoma has been equated with the anaplastic type[182] and with the lymphoepithelioma-like type.[181]

Small-cell neuroendocrine carcinoma resembles small-cell carcinoma of other sites[195] (Fig. 5–29). These tumors contain monomorphic cells with scant cytoplasm and round-to-oval, hyperchromatic nuclei. Nucleoli are not prominent. Large areas of necrosis and numerous mitoses are common features. These tumors may have foci with features suggesting squamous differentiation where the tumor cells have more cytoplasm and larger nucleoli.

Other variations include: basaloid carcinoma, mucoepidermoid carcinoma, clear-cell carcinoma, and mixed small-cell undifferentiated squamous cell carcinoma.[179] Basaloid carcinoma is characterized by small, monomorphic cells with diffusely distributed nuclear chromatin, indistinct nucleoli, and high nuclear-to-cytoplasmic ratios[179] (Fig. 5–30). Tumor cells form nests or trabeculae with peripheral nuclear palisading. Cystic and gland-like spaces may be present. Foci of keratinizing squamous cells may be scattered through the tumor.

The mucoepidermoid carcinomas of the thymus are histologically similar to the low-grade mucoepidermoid tumor of salivary glands.[179, 196] These tumors have both squamous and glandular elements. They contain cells with abundant mucin. Squamous elements are less prominent. Mitoses are infrequent. Another typical salivary gland neoplasm, adenoid cystic carcinoma, has also been described in the anterior mediastinum.[179]

Clear-cell carcinoma contains tumor cells in clusters surrounded by fibrous stroma.[179, 182, 197, 198] Nuclei are oval to reniform with diffuse chromatin and single, central nucleoli. Most cells have clear or slightly granular cytoplasm. Some appear more eosinophilic. Periodic acid-Schiff staining is removed by diastase digestion. Oil red O, Sudan IV, methyl green-pyro-

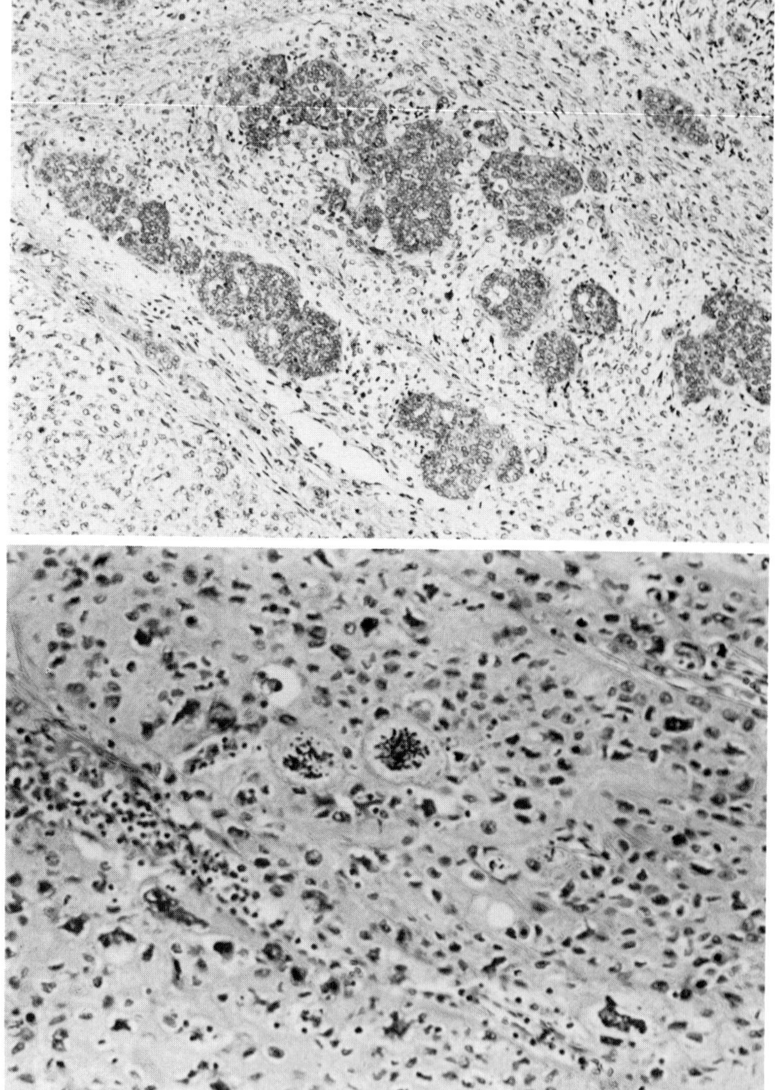

Figure 5–28. Uncommon high-grade thymic carcinomas. *Top*, Sarcomatoid carcinoma is a biphasic tumor with a cellular spindle cell component surrounding islands of atypical epithelial cells. Both elements stained positively for cytokeratin. *Bottom*, Anaplastic carcinoma is characterized by bizarre, pleomorphic cells with numerous mitoses. (From Suster S, Rosai J. Thymic carcinoma: a clinicopathologic study of 60 cases. Cancer 1991; 67:1025–1032.)

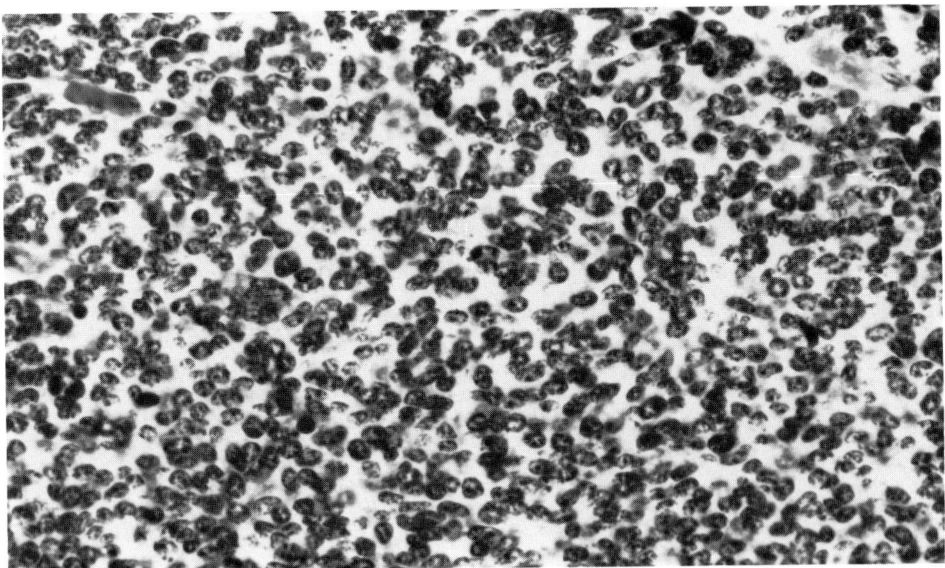

Figure 5–29. Small cell carcinoma has small cells with diffuse nuclear chromatin. This case is strongly positive for neuron-specific enolase. The patient died 7 months after diagnosis with widespread disease (H & E ×100).

nine, and mucicarmine stains are negative. Electron microscopy demonstrates broad cytoplasmic bundles of tonofilaments, some of which insert into maculae adherens. Basal lamina surrounds individual cells.

Prognostic Factors

Suster and Rosai divided thymic carcinoma into two histologic grades[182] (Table 5–11). High-grade carcinoma included those carcinomas classified as lymphoepithelioma-like, small-cell, clear-cell, sarcomatoid, and anaplastic. Low-grade malignancies included well-differentiated squamous carcinoma, mucoepidermoid carcinoma, and basaloid carcinoma. Eight-five percent of patients with high-grade malignancy died of tumor, as compared with 0% of patients with low-grade neoplasms. Adverse prognostic factors included poor circumscription, positive margins, absence of lobular growth patterns, nuclear atypia, necrosis, and high mitotic activity (greater than 10 mitoses per 10 high-power fields). The most important prognostic features were the histologic type of the tumor and its corresponding grade (high versus low).

Therapy

As with thymoma, the optimal therapy for thymic carcinoma is complete excision, when possible. Postoperative radiation therapy may help. In selected cases, chemotherapy may be a consideration for high-grade thymic carcinomas. These tumors may be responsive to cisplatin-based chemotherapy regimens.[199]

Comments

Several problems arise when the diagnosis of thymic carcinoma is contemplated. First, the differential diagnosis must be considered. Metastatic carcinoma to the mediastinum is much more common than thymic carcinoma. Therefore, other primary sites, such as lung, must be excluded. In some cases, one cannot determine whether the tumor is arising in the mediastinum and growing into the lung, or vice versa. If most of the tumor is in the lung, a lung primary tumor is generally the favored diagnosis. Shimosato and colleagues described histologic differences between squamous cell carcinomas arising in the thymus and those arising in the lung.[84] Thymic tumors have a more pronounced desmoplastic stromal response and less necrosis. Hassall's corpuscle–like keratin pearls strongly suggest thymic origin. Thymic squamous cell tumors lack the radial arrangement of cells at the periphery of nests. Such an arrangement is common in bronchogenic carcinoma. These histologic differences are rather subtle and probably do not allow for a definitive separation of thymic carcinoma from a lung primary tumor.

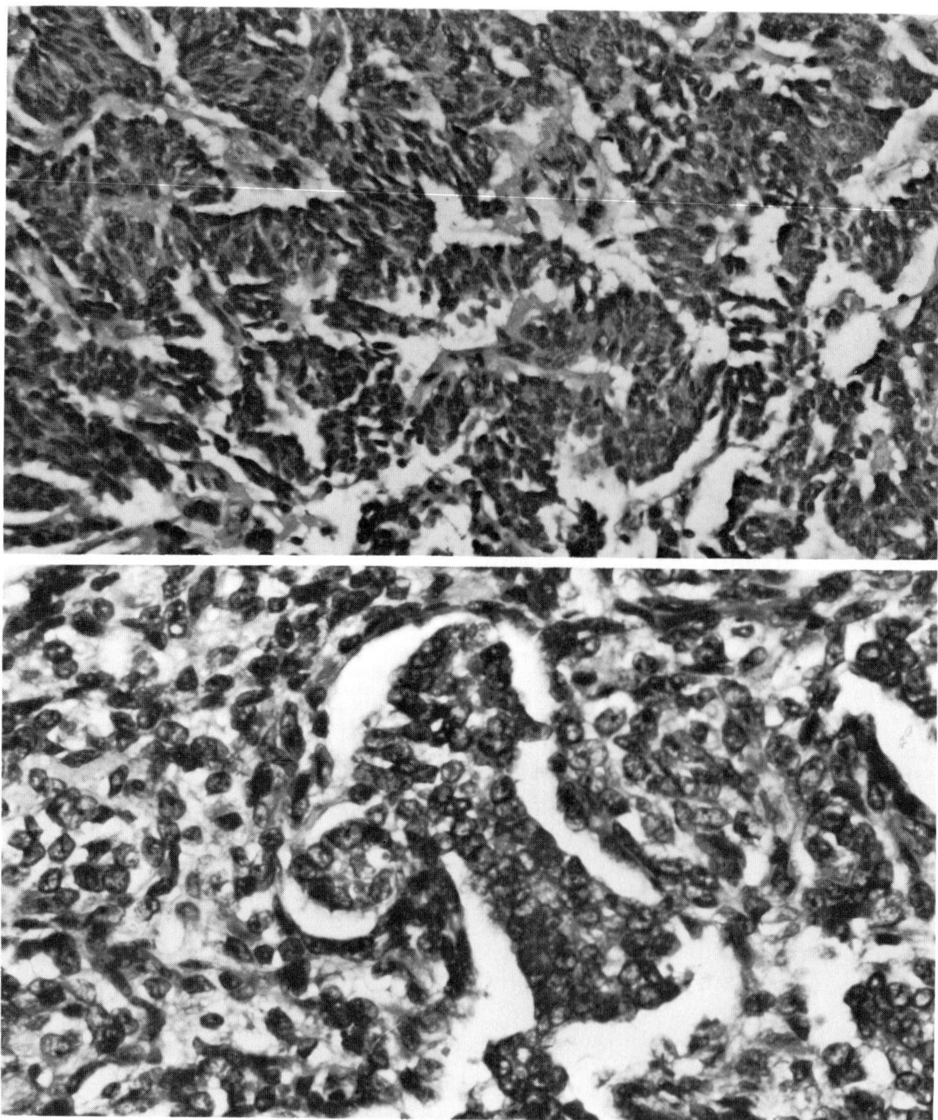

Figure 5–30. Basaloid carcinoma. Like small cell carcinoma, this tumor is composed of small cells with diffuse chromatin and scant cytoplasm. Cells are arranged in nests and trabeculae. Peripheral palisading of nuclei is characteristic (*top*, H & E ×100; *bottom*, H & E ×400).

Lymphomas and germ cell tumors must always be included within the differential diagnosis of a high-grade thymic carcinoma. Touch imprints may be helpful, particularly at the time of frozen section. Touch imprints of carcinoma typically have clusters of cytologically malignant cells (Fig. 5–31). (See the earlier discussion on thymomas.) Immunoperoxidase and/or electron microscopy may be necessary to differentiate epithelial thymic tumors from large-cell lymphomas and germ cell tumors.

Second, the dividing line between epithelial thymoma and thymic carcinoma is sometimes not clear-cut. In particular, there is overlap between epithelial thymoma and well-differentiated carcinoma. For example, some of the cases in the Shimosato et al. series[84] would be diagnosed by others as epithelial thymoma. A similar problem is evident in other descriptions.[83, 95a]

In practice, the distinction between an invasive thymoma and a well-differentiated carcinoma seems to be unimportant. Unlike the more aggressive thymic carcinomas, tumors described as well-differentiated carcinoma have a tendency for local recurrences rather than distant metastases. The long-term survival rate (approximately 70% at 10 years) for patients with this tumor is similar to that for patients with invasive thymoma.[182]

When the tumor is invasive, the patient should probably receive radiation therapy whether the tumor is called thymoma or thymic carcinoma. Therefore, the distinction between the two is usually not important to the management of the patient. In the completely encapsulated tumor, the presence of unequivocal cytologic malignancy might be an indication for radiation therapy. In these rare cases, there may be significant disagreements among different pathologists.

In contrast, lymphoepithelioma-like carcinoma, small-cell carcinoma, and other high-grade tumors of the thymus have a poor prognosis with a 10% 10-year survival rate.[180, 181] Recognition of these more aggressive types is important. In larger specimens, thorough sampling is necessary, because combinations of the various histologic types are frequently present in the same tumor.

Immunohistochemistry, electron microscopy, and DNA flow cytometry are generally not useful in distinguishing thymic carcinoma from metastases or in separating thymic carcinoma from thymoma. Yet, some differences have been described in immunohistochemical studies. For example, the infiltrating lymphocytes in thymic carcinoma are mature T cells (CD1-negative), whereas in thymomas they are frequently immature (CD1-positive).[99] However, some epithelial thymomas may have only the mature lymphocytes (Kornstein MJ, personal observations). One report found a difference in cytokeratin expression between lymphoepithelioma-like thymic carcinoma and thymoma, with the former having a greater percentage of cells positive for cytokeratin 18.[200] As noted previously, epithelial mem-

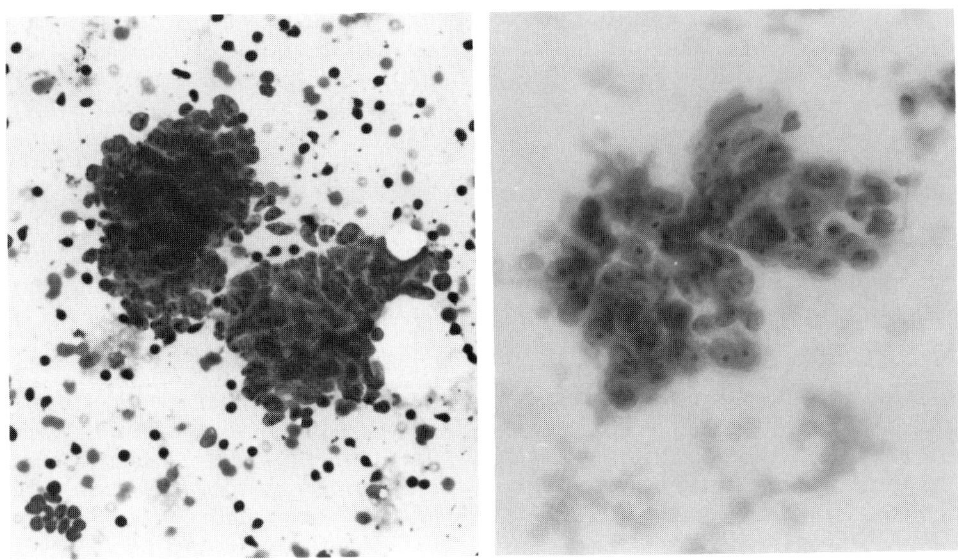

Figure 5–31. Touch imprint of lymphoepithelioma-like thymic carcinoma showing clumping of cells and marked atypia. (*Left,* H & E ×100; *right,* H & E ×1000.)

brane antigen may be more abundant in thymic carcinoma than in thymoma.[116, 189] According to Truong and colleagues, thymic carcinomas have more frequent immunoreactivity for carcinoembryonic antigen and B72.3.[189] However, only a few cells were labeled in the positive cases, and relatively few cases were studied.

By DNA analysis, thymic carcinomas are more likely to be aneuploid; however, this finding is not helpful in individual cases.[155a]

Another problem area is with tumors having neuroendocrine differentiation. Some authors include thymic carcinoid in the thymic carcinoma category (subtype: "neuroectodermal carcinoma").[89] Others reserve the diagnosis of neuroendocrine carcinoma for small-cell carcinoma.[195] In the present author's opinion, thymic carcinoid should be diagnosed as such and should not be included within the thymic carcinoma category.

THYMIC EPITHELIAL CELL TUMORS IN ANIMALS

In the animal literature, the term thymoma is often used for a lymphoma involving the thymus. For example, AKR mice are reported to develop a "thymoma."[201] However, the thymomas in these animals are in fact lymphomas and not epithelial tumors. Nevertheless, there are well-documented reports of spontaneously occurring thymic epithelial tumors in animals.[70, 202–210] These tumors are rare in domestic animals. Most of the cases in the literature are single case reports. The affected animals include cats, a rabbit, dogs, sheep, horses, cattle, and rodents. Most of the tumors are noninvasive and composed of ovoid or spindle cells with variable numbers of lymphocytes.[204] Reports of thymomas in animals with a myasthenia gravis–like illness have appeared.[70, 211]

In laboratory animals, spontaneously occurring thymomas are uncommon.[212] An exception is the *Mastomys natalensis*, an animal that has a high incidence of thymoma, particularly in females. Thymomas can be induced in mice by neonatal inoculation with polyoma virus.[213] Nearly 100% of BUF/Mna rats develop a spontaneous thymoma by 2 years of age.[214, 215] Histologically, these tumors usually are lymphocytic or mixed lymphocytic and epithelial. Cross-breeding experiments have related thymoma development to a single dominant gene in these animals.

PATHOGENESIS OF THYMIC EPITHELIAL TUMORS

There is considerable interest in the pathogenesis of thymic epithelial tumors. Two case reports from the United States have described thymic carcinoma (lymphoepithelioma-like type) containing Epstein-Barr virus (EBV).[216, 217] Investigators from Japan, Taiwan, and Hong Kong also reported individual cases of lymphoepithelioma-like carcinoma with EBV.[218–220] In addition, the Hong Kong group found EBV in two of eight "benign" thymomas (one from a myasthenia gravis patient, the other unassociated with myasthenia gravis). These authors report that three of five cases of thymic germinal center hyperplasia (four with myasthenia gravis) contained EBV.

Thymomas from patients in Hong Kong may contain EBV genomes more frequently than do thymomas from patients in some other countries.[218, 219, 221, 222] Studies from the United States, Europe, and Japan have not found EBV in thymomas or in thymuses with germinal center hyperplasia, even using the highly sensitive polymerase chain reaction.[219, 221, 222] Using in situ hybridization, one study from Taiwan found EBV in one of five lymphoepithelioma-like thymic carcinomas.[220] These authors did not find EBV in any of 21 thymomas. These results are similar to those reported in Western countries and conflict with other data from Hong Kong.[218] Reasons for the discrepancies are not clear but may include sampling problems and differences in patient populations. Larger studies are needed to clarify this issue.

Thymomas may be more common in the Far East. For example, studies from Hong Kong report that 38 to 48% of myasthenia gravis patients have a thymoma, compared with 10 to 28% of myasthenia gravis patients in the United States, Italy, and Japan.[223–228] Some authors have speculated that a high incidence of thymoma in Hong Kong may be related to the locally high incidence of undifferentiated carcinomas of the nasopharynx and salivary gland, both of which are associated with EBV.[218, 224, 229, 230]

Some evidence does link EBV to thymic tumors in Western countries. Perronne and colleagues from France found that 70% of patients (26/37) with "malignant" thymic tumors (invasive thymoma, thymic carcinoma, and lymphoma) had serologic immunoglobulin G (IgG) antibody to EBV early antigen.[231] This is a significantly higher percentage than the 38% of patients with benign thymoma.

However, these authors were unable to identify EBV by DNA hybridization in any of their specimens. Thus, there is evidence that some thymomas and thymic carcinomas represent another type of EBV-related tumor, particularly in some geographic areas.[232]

A second question concerning pathogenesis of thymic epithelial tumors is why thymomas are associated with myasthenia gravis. Investigators have reported acetylcholine receptor epitopes on tumor cells of thymomas.[233–237] Moreover, thymomas from myasthenia gravis patients express these epitopes more frequently than do thymomas from patients without myasthenia gravis. Marx and colleagues found anti-AChR immunoreactivity in 10 of 12 thymomas from patients with myasthenia gravis, compared with 2 of 6 thymomas from patients without myasthenia gravis.[233, 234] Cell lines were established from eight of the tumors and were also positive for acetylcholine receptor (AChR). Marx and colleagues isolated a protein, p153, that is present in most thymomas from myasthenia gravis patients and shares antigenic determinants with AChR of human muscle.[236, 238] These investigators propose that p153 is the sensitizing protein which leads to the autoimmune response to the AChR.

In addition, myasthenia gravis patients with thymoma frequently have serologic antibody to striated muscle.[228, 239] The striated muscle antibodies react with a myofibrillar protein, titin, and with thymic myoid cells.[240] Thymoma cells and skeletal muscle may share common epitopes.[241] For example, skeletal muscle is immunoreactive with a monoclonal antibody that labels a cytoplasmic epitope of the AChR.[242] This antibody also labels thymomas from myasthenia gravis patients. Thus, the thymoma could elicit the autoimmunity to the AChR and lead to the development of the antistriated muscle antibodies.

Marx and colleagues reported serologic antiaxon antibodies in 7 of 10 myasthenia gravis patients with thymoma, compared with 3 of 50 age-matched control subjects.[118] They also identified neurofilament antigens in some thymomas. Like the antistriated muscle antibodies, antibodies to neurofilament may result from aberrant protein expression by the thymoma.

These findings raise the possibility that the tumor may sensitize the patient to these antigens. Sensitization to AChR on the tumor could explain the association of thymoma with myasthenia gravis. Using Northern blots, Geuder et al. found no mRNA for AChR in thymomas.[243] Using the more sensitive polymerase chain reaction, Hara and colleagues found mRNA encoding for the alpha-subunit of the AChR in four thymomas and three thymuses affected by myasthenia gravis.[244] Yet, Siara and colleagues found no functional AChR in thymoma or thymus from myasthenia gravis patients.[245] Thus, the myasthenia gravis associated with thymoma may be initiated by an immune reaction against a tumor protein. The protein may be related to, or cross-reactive with, the AChR.

Several problems remain with the hypothesis that the thymoma elicits the sensitization. First, other groups of investigators must confirm the results concerning p153 that have been reported by Marx and colleagues. Second, the antibody against p153 does not induce experimental myasthenia gravis in laboratory animals.[237] Thus, it may not be important in the pathogenesis of human myasthenia gravis. Also, p153 is expressed on thymomas from patients without myasthenia gravis and on other tumors, including neuroblastoma. Why is p153 related to myasthenia gravis only when present on some thymic tumors? Finally, why do some patients develop myasthenia gravis years after excision of the thymoma?

The relationship between thymoma and other disorders (such as pure red cell aplasia and hypogammaglobulinemia) is even less clear.[24, 35] Experimental evidence suggests a role for the thymus in regulating myelopoiesis and erythropoiesis.[246, 247] Are there factors produced by some tumors that suppress hematopoietic precursors and/or B cells? Perhaps abnormalities of helper or suppressor T cells are involved.[25, 36] Perhaps the thymoma and associated disorders share a common etiology such as an as-yet-unidentified virus. At present, one can only speculate.

Little work has been reported on thymomas related to the subject of oncogenes and growth factors. One investigation described thymomas as having increased expression of RAS p21 protein compared with normal thymus.[248] Many thymomas express the receptor for epidermal growth factor.[93, 101] Rare cases of thymic epithelial tumors have been studied for cytogenetics but with no consistent findings.[249, 250] Retrovirus-like particles have been identified in normal thymus, thymus affected by myasthenia gravis, and thymomas by electron microscopy.[251, 252]

Finally, many authors have interpreted the immunohistochemical data as showing that some thymomas express a phenotype similar to that of fetal thymic epithelium.[90, 94, 102, 122] Perhaps thymomas are composed of immature epithelial cells capable of maturing into either cortical or medullary epithelium.[253] In most cases, there is a failure of differentiation. This would explain the frequent occurrence of both types of epithelium in most thymomas. A fetal phenotype of most thymomas would indicate that these tumors cannot be meaningfully classified as cortical or medullary. The derivation of thymic epithelium from a common stem cell would also contradict the belief that cortical epithelium and medullary epithelium derive from different embryonic cell layers (ectodermal and mesodermal, respectively).[77, 254]

Continuing research into thymic epithelial tumors may not just benefit the individual patient in terms of optimal therapy. Research may also provide clues to the workings of the normal thymus and to the etiology of autoimmune disorders such as myasthenia gravis.

SUMMARY

Tumors of the thymic epithelial cell include thymomas and thymic carcinomas. Thymomas are one of the most common neoplasms of the anterior mediastinum. They have been associated with numerous systemic disorders, most commonly with myasthenia gravis. Grossly, most thymomas are encapsulated, lobulated tumors. Histologically, they are characterized by a proliferation of cytologically bland epithelial cells admixed with a variable number of lymphocytes. On frozen section, lymphocytic thymoma may be difficult to differentiate from lymphoma. Touch imprints can be useful. For the final diagnosis, immunoperoxidase stains can support the diagnosis by demonstrating cytokeratin positivity of the epithelial cell. The most consistent prognostic factor is invasiveness beyond the tumor capsule. Noninvasive thymomas rarely recur, whereas the recurrence rate of invasive tumors is up to 33%. Approximately 5% of invasive thymomas metastasize.

Thymic carcinoma is a more aggressive neoplasm than thymoma and is characterized by cytologically malignant tumor cells. Patients with low-grade thymic carcinoma have long-term survival rates (70% at 10 years) similar to those of patients with invasive thymoma. In contrast, patients with high-grade thymic carcinomas have a poor prognosis (10% 10-year survival).

The subject of thymic epithelial tumors is controversial in several areas. Some investigators advocate classifying thymomas according to their histologic resemblance to cortical or medullary thymic epithelium. Another debate in the literature concerns the distinction between thymoma and well-differentiated thymic carcinoma—where to draw the line between these two entities. Fortunately, neither of these issues has great importance for patient management. There are few data to support differences in therapy based on histologic classification. Invasive thymoma and well-differentiated thymic carcinoma are treated similarly with complete excision (if possible) and postoperative radiation therapy. The importance of microscopic invasion of a thymoma through the capsule needs further study. Other areas of controversy relate to the pathogenesis of thymic epithelial tumors. The role of Epstein-Barr virus is unclear. The relationship of thymomas to myasthenia gravis also remains to be clearly explained.

REFERENCES

1. Lattes R. Thymoma and other tumors of the thymus: an analysis of 107 cases. Cancer 1962; 15:1224–1260.
2. Katz A, Lattes R. Granulomatous thymoma or Hodgkin's disease of thymus? A clinical and histologic study and a re-evaluation. Cancer 1969; 23:1–15.
3. Levine GD, Rosai J. Thymic hyperplasia and neoplasia: a review of current concepts. Hum Pathol 1978; 9:495–515.
4. Wick MR, Rosai J. Epithelial tumors. *In* Givel J-C, ed. Surgery of the Thymus. Berlin: Springer-Verlag, 1990:79–107.
5. Davis RD Jr, Oldham HN Jr, Sabiston DC Jr. Primary cysts and neoplasms of the mediastinum: recent changes in clinical presentation, methods of diagnosis, management, and results. Ann Thorac Surg 1987; 44:229–237.
6. Dehner LP, Martin SA, Sumner HW. Thymus related tumors and tumor-like lesions in childhood with rapid clinical progression and death. Hum Pathol 1977; 8:53–66.
7. Ramon Y, Cajal S, Suster S. Primary thymic epithelial neoplasms in children. Am J Surg Pathol 1991; 15:466–474.
8. Pescarmona E, Giardini R, Brisigotti M, Callea F, Pisacane A, Baroni CD. Thymoma in childhood: a clinicopathological study of five cases. Histopathology 1992; 21:65–68.
9. Kaplinsky C, Mor C, Cohen IJ, Goshen Y, Yaniv I, Jaber L, Stark B, Stern S, Zaizov R. Childhood malignant thymoma: clinical, therapeutic, immunohistochemical considerations. Pediatr Hematol Oncol 1993:261–268.
10. Rosai J. Mediastinum. *In* Ackerman's Surgical Pathology. St. Louis: CV Mosby, 1989:345–390.

11. Furman WL, Buckley PJ, Green AA, Stokes DC, Chien LT. Thymoma and myasthenia gravis in a 4 year old child: case report and review of the literature. Cancer 1985; 56:2703–2706.
12. Lewis JE, Wick MR, Scheithauer BW, Bernatz PE, Taylor WF. Thymoma: a clinicopathologic review. Cancer 1987; 60:2727–2743.
13. Hofmann W, Moller P, Manke H-G, Otto HF. Thymoma: a clinicopathologic study of 98 cases with special reference to three unusual cases. Pathol Res Pract 1985; 179:337–353.
14. Verley MM, Hollmann KH. Thymoma: a comparative study of clinical stages, histologic features, and survival in 200 cases. Cancer 1985; 55:1074–1086.
15. Curran WJ Jr, Kornstein MJ, Brooks JJ, Turrisi AT III. Invasive thymoma: the role of mediastinal irradiation following complete or incomplete surgical resection. J Clin Oncol 1988; 6:1722–1727.
16. Ackland SP, Bur ME, Adler SS, Robertson M, Baron JM. White blood cell aplasia associated with thymoma. Am J Clin Pathol 1988; 89:260–263.
17. Rothberg MS, Eisenbud L, Griboff S. Chronic mucocutaneous candidiasis-thymoma syndrome: a case report. Oral Surg Oral Med Oral Pathol 1989; 68:411–413.
18. Levasseur P, Menestrier M, Gaud C, Dartevelle P, Julia P, Rojas-Miranda A, Navajas M, Le-Brigand H, Merlier M. [Thymomas and associated diseases. Apropos of a series of 255 surgically treated thymomas]. Rev Mal Respir 1988; 5:173–178.
19. Chan PC, Lau CC, Cheng IK, Chan KW, Jones BM, Chan MK. Minimal change glomerulopathy in two patients after thymectomy. Singapore Med J 1990; 31:46–47.
20. Arntzenius AB, Bieger R. Disappearance of autoantibody-induced haemolysis after excision of a malignant thymoma. Neth J Med 1991; 38:117–121.
21. Ogawa M, Ueda S, Ohto M, Kono N, Itami J, Kondo Y, Yamamoto S. Minimal change nephrotic syndrome developed after non-surgical treatment of a thymoma [letter]. Clin Nephrol 1992; 38:171.
22. Ingenito GG, Berger JR, David NJ, Norenberg MD. Limbic encephalitis associated with thymoma. Neurology 1990; 40:382.
23. Ogawa M, Ueda S, Ohto M, Baba M, Yamaguchi Y, Kondo Y, Yamamoto S. Development of systemic lupus erythematosus after total resection of a thymoma and the adjacent thymic gland. J Rheumatol 1992; 19:1130–1132.
24. Masaoka A, Hashimoto T, Shibata K, Yamakawa Y, Nakamae K, Izuka M. Thymomas associated with pure red cell aplasia: histologic and follow-up studies. Cancer 1989; 64:1872–1878.
25. Sawai T, Tuchikawa K. Kaposi's sarcoma developed in a patient with a thymoma in the setting of excess numbers of CD8-positive cells in the peripheral blood. Arch Pathol Lab Med 1990; 114:611–613.
26. Mathieson PW, O'Neill JH, Durrant STS, Henderson SJ, Green PJ, Newsom-Davis J. Antibody-mediated pure neutrophil aplasia, recurrent myasthenia gravis and previous thymoma: case report and literature review. Q J Med 1990; 74:57–61.
27. Insler MS, Shelin RG. Sjögren's syndrome and thymoma. Am J Ophthalmol 1987; 104:90–91.
28. Tanaka F, Yoshitani M, Esaki H, Isobe J, Inoue R, Shiraki T, Uemura H. [A malignant thymoma combined with sarcoidosis.] Kyobu Geka 1990; 43:823–825.
29. Levasseur Ph, Menestrier M, Gaud C, Dartevelle Ph, Julia P, Rjojas-Miranda A, Le Brigand H, Merlier M. Thymomes et maladies auto-immunes. Rev Mal Respir 1986; 4:R12–R13.
30. Rosenow EC III, Hurley BT. Disorders of the thymus: a review. Arch Intern Med 1984; 144:763–770.
31. Bailey RO, Dunn HG, Rubin AM, Ritaccio AL. Myasthenia gravis with thymoma and pure red blood cell aplasia. Am J Clin Pathol 1988; 89:687–693.
32. Watts RG, Kelly DR. Fatal varicella infection in a child associated with thymoma and immunodeficiency (Good's syndrome). Med Pediatr Oncol 1990; 18:246–251.
33. Good RA. Agammaglobulinemia—a provocative experiment of nature. Bull Univ Minn Hosp 1954; 26:1–19.
34. Brasher GW, Howard PH Jr, Brindley GV Jr. Thymoma and hypogammaglobulinemia (Good's syndrome). Surg Clin North Am 1972; 52:429–438.
35. Cooper MD, Butler JL. Primary immunodeficiency diseases. *In* Paul WE, ed. Fundamental Immunology. New York: Raven Press, 1989:1033–1057.
36. Levinson AI, Hoxie JA, Kornstein MJ, Zembryki D, Matthews DM, Schreiber AD. Absence of the OKT4 epitope on blood T cells and thymus cells in a patient with thymoma, hypogammaglobulinemia, and red blood cell aplasia. J Allergy Clin Immunol 1985; 76:433–439.
37. Saito R, Isogami K, Fujimura S, Ookuda K. [OKT4 epitope deficiency in a patient with thymoma and hypogammaglobulinemia.] Nippon Kyobu Shikkan Gakkai Zasshi 1990; 28:1120–1124.
38. Shachor Y, Radnay J, Bernheim J, Rozenszajn A, Bruderman I, Klajman A, Steiner ZP. Malignant thymoma with peripheral blood lymphocytosis. Cancer 1988; 61:1222–1227.
39. Doll DC, Landreneau RJ, List AF. Malignant thymoma associated with peripheral T cell lymphocytosis. Med Pediatr Oncol 1991; 19:496–498.
40. Medeiros LJ, Bhagat SKM, Naylor P, Fowler D, Jaffe ES, Stetler-Stevenson M. Malignant thymoma associated with T-cell lymphocytosis: a case report with immunophenotypic and gene rearrangement analysis. Arch Pathol Lab Med 1993; 117:279–283.
41. Thomas J, de Wolf-Peeters C, Tricot G, Bekaert J, Broeckaert-van Orshoven A. T cell chronic lymphocytic leukemia in a patient with invasive thymoma in remission with chemotherapy. Cancer 1983; 52:313–317.
42. Macon WR, Rynalski TH, Swerdlow SH, Cousar JB. T cell lymphoblastic leukemia/lymphoma presenting in a recurrent thymoma. Mod Pathol 1991; 4:524–528.
42a. Friedman HD, Inman DA, Hutchison RE, Poiesz BJ. Concurrent invasive thymoma and T cell lymphoblastic lymphoma. Am J Clin Pathol 1994; 101:432–437.
43. Couture MM, Mountain CF. Thymoma. Semin Surg Oncol 1990; 6:110–114.
44. Gray GF, Gutowski WT. Thymoma: a clinicopathologic study of 54 cases. Am J Surg Pathol 1979; 3:235–249.
45. Monden Y, Uyama T, Kimura S, Taniki T. Extrathymic malignancy in patients with myasthenia gravis. Eur J Cancer 1991; 27:745–747.
46. Nemoto K, Ishikawa H, Ohnishi Y, Nakamura T, Ohsaki N. Hodgkin's disease accompanied with thymoma. Acta Pathol Jpn 1987; 37:1505–1512.
47. Skinnider LF, Alexander S. Concurrent thymoma and lymphoma: a report of two cases. Hum Pathol 1982; 13:163–166.

48. Souadjian JV, Silverstein MN, Titus JL. Thymoma and cancer. Cancer 1968; 22:1221.
49. Lindstrom FD, Williams RC, Brunning RD. Thymoma associated with multiple myeloma. Arch Intern Med 1968; 122:526.
50. Anderson V, Pedersen H. Thymoma and acute leukemia. Acta Med Scand 1967; 182:581.
51. Knowles DM. Thymoma and chronic myelogenous leukemia: a case report. Cancer 1976; 38:1414.
52. Buff DD, Greenberg SD, Leong P, Palumbo FS. Thymoma, pneumocystic carinii pneumonia, and AIDS. N Y State J Med 1988; 88:276–277.
53. Fukayama M, Maeda Y, Funata N, Koike M, Saito K, Sakai T, Ikeda T. Pulmonary and pleural thymoma. Diagnostic application of lymphocyte markers to the thymoma of unusual site. Am J Clin Pathol 1988; 89:617–621.
54. Green WR, Pressoir R, Gumbs RV, Warner O, Naab T, Qayumi M. Intrapulmonary thymoma. Arch Pathol Lab Med 1987; 111:1074–1076.
55. Martin JME, Randhawa G, Temple WJ. Cervical thymoma. Arch Pathol Lab Med 1986; 110:354–357.
56. Miller WT Jr, Gefter WB, Miller WT. Thymoma mimicking a thyroid mass. Radiology 1992; 184:75–76.
57. Tan A, Holdener GP, Hecht A, Gelfand C, Baker B. Malignant thymoma in an ectopic thymus: CT appearance. J Comput Assist Tomogr 1991; 15:842–844.
58. Vengrove MA, Schimmel M, Atkinson BF, Evans D, LiVolsi VA. Invasive cervical thymoma masquerading as a solitary thyroid nodule: report of a case studied by fine needle aspiration. Acta Cytol 1991; 35:431–433.
59. Chan JKC, Rosai J. Tumors of the neck showing thymic or related branchial pouch differentiation: a unifying concept. Hum Pathol 1991; 22:349–367.
60. James CL, Iyer PV, Leong AS-Y. Intrapulmonary thymoma. Histopathology 1992; 21:175–177.
61. Jansen JD, Johnson FE. Fatal ectopic thymoma. Ann Thorac Surg 1990; 50:469–470.
62. Damiani S, Filotico M, Eusebi V. Carcinoma of the thyroid showing thymoma-like features. Virchows Arch [A] 1991; 418:463–466.
63. Harach HR, Day ES, Franssila KO. Thyroid spindle-cell tumor with mucous cysts: an intrathyroid thymoma? Am J Surg Pathol 1985; 9:525–530.
64. Moran CA, Travis WD, Rosado-de-Christenson M, Koss MN, Rosai J. Thymomas presenting as pleural tumors: report of 8 cases. Am J Surg Pathol 1992; 16:138–144.
65. Asamura H, Morinaga S, Shimosato Y, Ono R, Naruke T. Thymoma displaying endobronchial polypoid growth. Chest 1988; 94:647–649.
66. Ichimanda M, Okada S, Kai T. [A case of invasive thymoma displaying endobronchial and endocaval polypoid growth.] Nippon Kyobu Geka Gakkai Zasshi 1991; 39:938–942.
67. Yokoi K, Miyazawa N, Mori K, Saito Y, Tominaga K, Suzuki K. [A case of invasive thymoma displaying endobronchial polypoid growth.] Nippon Kyobu Geka Gakkai Zasshi 1990; 28:529–534.
68. Kornstein MJ, Curran WJ Jr, Turrisi AT III, Brooks JJ. Cortical versus medullary thymomas: a useful morphologic distinction? Hum Pathol 1988; 19:1335–1339.
69. Wick MR, Nichols WC, Ingle JN, Bruckman JE, Okazaki H. Malignant, predominantly lymphocytic thymoma with central and peripheral nervous system metastases. Cancer 1981; 47:2036–2043.
70. Rosai J, Levine GD. Tumors of the Thymus. Washington, DC: Armed Forces Institute of Pathology, 1976:34–98.
71. Rosen VJ, Christiansen TW, Hughes RK. Metastatic thymoma presenting as a solitary pulmonary nodules. Cancer 1966; 19:527–532.
72. Knecht JW. Cancer in inguinal hernias. N Engl J Med 1990; 87:485–487.
73. Pescarmona E, Rosati S, Pisacane A, Rendina EA, Venuta F, Baroni CD. Microscopic thymoma: histological evidence of multifocal cortical and medullary origin. Histopathology 1992; 20:263–266.
74. Suster S, Rosai J. Cystic thymomas: a clinicopathologic study of ten cases. Cancer 1992; 69:92–97.
75. Pescarmona E, Rendina EA, Venuta F, D'Arcangelo E, Pagani M, Ricci C, Ruco LP, Baroni CD. Analysis of prognostic factors and clinicopathological staging of thymoma. Ann Thorac Surg 1990; 50:534–538.
76. Wilkins EW Jr, Grillo HC, Scannell G, Moncure AC, Mathisen DJ. Role of staging in prognosis and management of thymoma. Ann Thorac Surg 1991; 51:888–892.
77. Kornstein MJ. Immunopathology of the thymus: a review. Surg Pathol 1988; 1:249–272.
78. Pescarmona E, Pisacane A, Rendina EA, Ricci C, Ruco LP, Baroni CD. "Organoid" thymoma: a well-differentiated variant with distinctive clinicopathological features. Histopathology 1991; 18:161–164.
79. Fukuda T, Ohnishi Y, Emura I, Tachikawa S. Microcytic variant of thymoma: histological and immunohistochemical findings in two cases. Virchows Arch [A] 1992; 420:185–189.
80. Murakami S, Shamoto M, Miura K, Takeuchi J. A thymic tumor with massive proliferation of myoid cells. Acta Pathol Jpn 1984; 34:1375–1383.
81. Moran CA, Koss MN. Rhabdomyomatous thymoma. Am J Surg Pathol 1993; 17:633–636.
82. Kornstein MJ, Kay S. B cells in thymomas. Mod Pathol 1990; 3:61–63.
83. Kirchner T, Schalke B, Buchwald J, Ritter M, Marx A, Muller-Hermelink HK. Well-differentiated thymic carcinoma: an organotypical low-grade carcinoma with relationship to cortical thymoma. Am J Surg Pathol 1992; 16:1153–1169.
84. Shimosato Y, Kameya T, Nagai K, Suemasu K. Squamous cell carcinoma of the thymus: an analysis of 8 cases. Am J Surg Pathol 1977; 1:109–121.
85. Maggi G, Giaccone G, Donadio M, Cuffreda L, Dalesio O, Leria G, Trifiletti G, Casadio C, Palestro G, Mancuso M, Calciati A. Thymomas: a review of 169 cases, with particular reference to results of surgical treatment. Cancer 1986; 58:765–776.
86. Maggi G, Casadio C, Cavallo A, Cianci R, Molinatti M, Ruffini E. Thymoma: results of 241 operated cases. Ann Thorac Surg 1991; 51:152–156.
87. Muller-Hermelink HK, Marino M, Palestro G, Schumacher U, Kirchner T. Immunohistological evidences of cortical and medullary differentiation in thymoma. Virchows Arch [A] 1985; 408:143–161.
88. Muller-Hermelink HK, Marino M, Palestro G. Pathology of thymic epithelial tumors. *In* Muller-Hermelink HK, ed. The Human Thymus: Histophysiology and Pathology. Berlin: Springer-Verlag, 1986:207–268.
89. Marino M, Muller-Hermelink HK. Thymoma and thymic carcinoma: relation of thymoma epithelial cells to the cortical and medullary differentiation of thymus. Virchows Arch [A] 1985; 407:119–149.
90. Hofmann WJ, Pallesen G, Moller P, Kunze WP, Kayser K, Otto HF. Expression of cortical and medullary thymic epithelial antigens in thymomas. An immu-

nohistological study of 14 cases including a characterization of the lymphocytic compartment. Histopathology 1989; 14:447–463.
91. Takahashi T, Ueda R, Nishida K, Namikawa R, Fukami H, Matsuyama M, Masaoka A, Imaizumi M. Immunohistological analysis of thymic tumors with PE-35 monoclonal antibody reactive with medullary thymic epithelium. Cancer Res 1988; 48:1896–1903.
92. Hirokawa K, Utsuyama M, Moriizumi E, Hashimoto T, Masaoka A, Goldstein AL. Immunohistochemical studies in human thymomas. Localization of thymosin and various cell markers. Virchows Arch [B] 1988; 55:371–380.
93. Giraud F, Fabien N, Auger C, Girod C, Loire R, Monier JC. Human epithelial thymic tumours: heterogeneity in immunostaining of epithelial cell markers and thymic hormones. Thymus 1990; 15:15–29.
94. Fukai I, Masaoka A, Hashimoto T, Yamakawa Y, Mizuno T, Tanamura O, Hirokawa K, Ueda R. An immunohistologic study of the epithelial components of 81 cases of thymoma. Cancer 1992; 69:2463–2468.
95. Kodama T, Watanabe S, Sato Y, Shimosato Y, Miyazawa N. An immunohistochemical study of thymic epithelial tumors. I. Epithelial component. Am J Surg Pathol 1986; 10:26–33.
95a. Quintanilla-Martinez L, Wilkins EW Jr, Ferry J, Harris NL. Thymoma—morphologic subclassification correlates with invasiveness and immunohistologic features: A study of 122 cases. Hum Pathol 1993; 24:958–969.
96. Kornstein MJ, Hoxie JA, Levinson AI, Brooks JJ. Immunohistology of human thymomas. Arch Pathol Lab Med 1985; 109:460–463.
97. Willcox N, Schluep M, Ritter MA, Schuurman HJ, Newsom-Davis J, Christensson B. Myasthenic and nonmyasthenic thymoma. An expansion of a minor cortical epithelial cell subset. Am J Pathol 1987; 127:447–460.
98. Ito M, Taki T, Miyake M, Mitsuoka A. Lymphocyte subsets in human thymoma studied with monoclonal antibodies. Cancer 1988; 61:284–287.
99. Sato Y, Watanabe S, Mukai K, Kodama T, Upton MP, Goto M, Shimosato Y. An immunohistochemical study of thymic epithelial tumors. II. Lymphoid component. Am J Surg Pathol 1986; 10:862–870.
100. Takacs L, Savino W, Monostori E, Ando I, Bach J-F, Dardenne M. Cortical thymocyte differentiation in thymomas: an immunohistologic analysis of the pathologic microenvironment. J Immunol 1987; 138:687–698.
101. Kraus VB, Harden EA, Wittels B, Moore JO, Haynes BF. Demonstration of phenotypic abnormalities of thymic epithelium in thymoma including two cases with abundant Langerhans cells. Am J Pathol 1988; 132:552–562.
102. Kornstein MJ. Controversies regarding the pathology of thymomas. Pathol Annu 1992; 27:1–15.
103. Wick MR. Assessing the prognosis of thymomas. Ann Thorac Surg 1990; 50:521–522.
104. Juttner FM, Fellbaum C, Popper H, Arian K, Pinter H, Friehs G. Pitfalls in intraoperative frozen section histology of mediastinal neoplasms. Eur J Cardiothorac Surg 1990; 4:584–586.
105. Kraemer BB. Mediastinum. *In* Silva EG, Kraemer BB, eds. Intraoperative Pathologic Diagnosis: Frozen Section and Other Techniques. Baltimore: Williams & Wilkins, 1987:235–252.
106. Dahlgren S, Sandstedt B, Sundstrom C. Fine needle aspiration cytology of thymic tumors. Acta Cytol 1983; 27:1–6.
107. Bonfiglio TA, Dvoretsky PM, Piscioli F, dePapp EW, Patten SF, Jr. Fine needle aspiration biopsy in the evaluation of lymphoreticular tumors of the thorax. Acta Cytol 1985; 29:548–553.
108. Sherman ME, Black-Schaffer S. Diagnosis of thymoma by needle biopsy. Acta Cytol 1990; 34:63–68.
109. Blegvad S, Lippert H, Simper LB, Dybdahl H. Mediastinal tumours. A report of 129 cases. Scand J Thorac Cardiovasc Surg 1990; 24:39–42.
110. Wakely PE Jr, Frable WJ, Kornstein MJ. Role of intraoperative cytopathology in pediatric surgical pathology. Hum Pathol 1993; 24:311–315.
111. Mair S, Lash RH, Suskin D, Mendelsohn G. Intraoperative surgical specimen evaluation: frozen section analysis, cytologic examination, or both? Am J Clin Pathol 1991; 96:8–14.
112. Flanders E, Kornstein MJ, Wakely PE Jr, Kardos TF, Frable WJ. Lymphoglandular bodies in fine needle aspiration cytology. Am J Clin Pathol 1993; 99:566–569.
113. Henry K, Farrer-Brown G. Color Atlas of Thymus and Lymph Node Histopathology. Chicago: Year Book Medical, 1982:9–44.
114. Wick MR, Simpson RW, Niehans GA, Scheithauer BW. Anterior mediastinal tumors: a clinicopathologic study of 100 cases, with emphasis on immunohistochemical analysis. Prog Surg Pathol 1990; 11:79–119.
115. Fukai I, Masaoka A, Hashimoto T, Yamakawa Y, Mizuno T, Tanamura O. Cytokeratins in normal thymus and thymic epithelial tumors. Cancer 1993; 71:99–105.
116. Fukai I, Masaoka A, Hashimoto T, Yamakawa Y, Mizuno T, Tanamura O. The distribution of epithelial membrane antigen in thymic epithelial neoplasms. Cancer 1992; 70:2077–2081.
117. Lauriola L, Michetti F, Stolfi VM, Tallini G, Cocchia D. Detection by S-100 immunolabelling of interdigitating reticulum cells in human thymomas. Virchows Arch [B] 1984; 45:187–195.
118. Marx A, Kirchner T, Greiner A, Muller-Hermelink HK, Osborn M. Neurofilament epitopes in thymoma and antiaxonal autoantibodies in myasthenia gravis. Lancet 1992; 339:707–708.
119. Savino W, Berrih S, Dardenne M. Thymic epithelial antigen, acquired during ontogeny and defined by the anti-p19 monoclonal antibody, is lost in thymomas. Lab Invest 1984; 51:292–296.
120. Mokhtar N, Hsu S-M, Lad RP, Haynes BF, Jaffe ES. Thymoma: lymphoid and epithelial components mirror the phenotype of normal thymus. Hum Pathol 1984; 15:378–384.
121. Savino W, Manganella G, Verley JM, Wolff A, Berrih S, Levasseur P, Binet J-P, Dardenne M, Bach J-F. Thymoma epithelial cells secrete thymic hormone but do not express class II antigens of the major histocompatibility complex. J Clin Invest 1985; 76:1140–1146.
122. Haynes BF. The human thymic microenvironment. Adv Immunol 1984; 36:87–142.
123. Savino W, Durand D, Dardenne M. Immunohistochemical evidence for the expression of the carcinoembryonic antigen by human thymic epithelial cells in vitro and in neoplastic conditions. Am J Pathol 1985; 121:418–425.
124. Eimoto T, Kohichi T, Shirakusa T, Takeshita M, Okamura H, Naito H, Mitsui T, Kikuchi M. Heterogeneity of epithelial cells and reactive components in thymomas: an ultrastructural and immunohistochemical study. Ultrastruct Pathol 1986; 10:157–173.
125. Chilosi M, Iannucci AM, Pizzolo G, Menestrina F, Fiore-Donati L, Janossy G. Immunohistochemical

analysis of thymoma: evidence for medullary origin of epithelial cells. Am J Surg Pathol 1984; 8:309–318.
126. van der Kwast TH, van Vliet E, Cristen E, van Ewijk W, van der Heul RO. An immunohistologic study of the epithelial and lymphoid components of six thymomas. Hum Pathol 1985; 16:1001–1008.
127. Chan WC, Zaatari GS, Tabei S, Bibb M, Brynes RK. Thymoma: an immunohistochemical study. Am J Clin Pathol 1984; 82:160–166.
128. Chilosi M, Iannucci A, Menestrina F, Lestani M, Scarpa A, Bonetti F, Fiore-Donati L, Dipasquale B, Pizzolo G, Palestro G, Tridente G, Janossy G. Immunohistochemical evidence of active thymocyte proliferation in thymoma: its possible role in the pathogenesis of autoimmune diseases. Am J Pathol 1987; 128:464–470.
129. Palestro G, Geuna M, Novero D, Godio L, Ciccone G, Azzoni L. Immunophenotype of thymoma-associated lymphoid cell component of T-cell type. A new analytic procedure in keeping with structural heterogeneities. Virchows Arch [B] 1990; 59:297–304.
130. Ichikawa Y, Shimizu H, Yoshida M, Arimori S. Two-color flow cytometric analysis of thymic lymphocytes from patients with myasthenia gravis and/or thymoma. Clin Immunol Immunopathol 1992; 62:91–96.
131. Salter DM, Krajewski AS. Metastatic thymoma: a case report and immunohistological analysis. J Clin Pathol 1986; 39:275–278.
132. Harrod FA, Kettman JR. Transplantable polyoma virus-induced epitheliomas harbor immature T lymphocytes. Cell Immunol 1990; 125:29–41.
133. Chilosi M, Castelli P, Martignoni G, Pizzolo G, Montresor E, Facchetti F, Truini M, Mombello A, Lestani M, Scarpa A, Menestrina F. Neoplastic epithelial cells in a subset of human thymomas express the B cell–associated CD20 antigen. Am J Surg Pathol 1992; 16:988–997.
134. Taubenberger JK, Jaffe ES, Medeiros J. Thymoma with abundant L26-positive "asteroid" cells: a case report with an analysis of normal thymus and thymoma specimens. Arch Pathol Lab Med 1991; 115:1254–1257.
135. Zola H. The surface antigens of human B lymphocytes. Immunol Today 1987; 8:308–315.
136. Franke WW, Moll R. Cytoskeletal components of lymphoid organs. I. Synthesis of cytokeratins 8 and 18 and desmin in subpopulations of extrafollicular reticulum cells of human lymph nodes, tonsils, and spleen. Differentiation 1987; 36:145–163.
137. Iuzzolino P, Bontempini L. Keratin immunoreactivity in extrafollicular reticular cells of the lymph node. Am J Clin Pathol 1989; 91:239–240.
138. Doglioni C, Dell'Orto P, Zanetti G, Iuzzolino P, Coggi G, Viale G. Cytokeratin-immunoreactive cells of human lymph nodes and spleen in normal and pathological conditions: an immunocytochemical study. Virchows Arch [A] 1990; 416:479–490.
139. Mizuno T, Hashimoto T, Masaoka A. Distribution of fibronectin and laminin in human thymoma. Cancer 1990; 65:1367–1374.
140. Katzin WE, Fishleder AJ, Linden MD, Tubbs RR. Immunoglobulin and T-cell receptor genes in thymomas: genotypic evidence supporting the nonneoplastic nature of the lymphocytic component. Hum Pathol 1988; 19:323–328.
141. Scarpa A, Chilosi M, Capelli P, Bonetti F, Menestrina F, Zamboni G, Pizzolo G, Palestro G, Fiore-Donati L, Tridente G. Expression and gene rearrangement of the T-cell receptor in human thymomas. Virchows Arch [B] 1990; 58:235–239.
142. Hammond EH, Flinner RL. The diagnosis of thymoma: a review. Ultrastruct Pathol 1991; 15:419–438.
143. Bergh NP, Gatzinsky P, Larsson S, Lundin P, Ridell B. Tumors of the thymus and thymic region: I. Clinicopathological studies on thymomas. Ann Thorac Surg 1978; 25:91–98.
144. Masaoka A, Monden Y, Nakahara K, Tanioka T. Follow-up study of thymomas with special reference to their clinical stages. Cancer 1981; 48:2485–2492.
145. Kuo T-T, Lo S-K. Thymoma: a study of the pathologic classification of 71 cases with evaluation of the Muller-Hermelink system. Hum Pathol 1993; 24:766–771.
146. Pollack A, Komaki R, Cox JD, Ro JY, Oswald MJ, Shin DM, Putnam JB Jr. Thymoma: treatment and prognosis. Int J Radiat Oncol Biol Phys 1992; 23:1037–1043.
147. Kirschner PA. Reoperation for thymoma: report of 23 cases. Ann Thorac Surg 1990; 49:550–554.
148. Elert O, Buchwald J, Wolf K. Epithelial thymus tumors—therapy and prognosis. Thorac Cardiovasc Surg 1988; 36:109–113.
149. Kirchner T, Muller-Hermelink HK. New approaches to the diagnosis of thymic epithelial tumors. Prog Surg Pathol 1989; 10:167–189.
149a. Quintanilla-Martinez L, Wilkins EW Jr, Choi N, Efird J, Hug E, Harris NL. Thymoma: histologic classification is an independent prognostic factor. Cancer 1994; 74:606–617.
150. Koss LG, Czerniak B, Herz F, Wersto RP. Flow cytometric measurements of DNA and other cell components in human tumors: a critical appraisal. Hum Pathol 1989; 20:528–548.
151. Coon JS, Landay AL, Weinstein RS. Advances in flow cytometry for diagnostic pathology. Lab Invest 1987; 57:453–479.
152. Davies SE, Macartney JC, Camplejohn RS, Morris RW, Ring NP, Corrin B. DNA flow cytometry of thymomas. Histopathology 1989; 15:77–83.
153. Pollack A, El-Naggar AK, Cox JD, Ro JY, Sahin A, Komaki R. Thymoma: the prognostic significance of flow cytometric DNA analysis. Cancer 1992; 69:1702–1709.
154. Asamura H, Nakajima T, Mukai K, Noguchi M, Shimosato Y. Degree of malignancy of thymic epithelial tumors in terms of nuclear DNA content and nuclear area. An analysis of 39 cases. Am J Pathol 1988; 133:615–622.
155. Sauter ER, Sardi A, Hollier LH, Cooper ES, Bolton JS. Prognostic value of DNA flow cytometry in thymomas and thymic carcinomas. South Med J 1990; 83:656–659.
155a. Kenny-Moynihan MB, Gal AA, Kornstein MJ, DeRose PB, Cohen C. DNA flow cytometry in thymic neoplasms: A comparison between flow and image cytometry and correlation with clinical outcome. Mod Pathol 1994; 7:164A (abstract).
156. Kuo T-T, Lo S-K. DNA flow cytometric study of thymic epithelial tumors with evaluation of its usefulness in the pathologic classification. Hum Pathol 1993; 24:746–749.
157. Banez EI, Krishnan B, Ansari MQ, Carraway NP, McBride RA. False aneuploidy in benign tumors with a high lymphocyte content: a study of Warthin's tumor and benign thymoma. Hum Pathol 1992; 23:1244–1251.
158. Bretel J-J. Staging and preliminary results of the

thymic tumour study group. *In* Sarrazin R, Vrousos C, Vincent F, eds. Thymic Tumors. Basel: Karger, 1989:156–164.
159. Loehrer PJ. Thymomas: current experience and future directions in therapy. Drugs 1993; 45:477–487.
160. Cooper JD. Current therapy for thymoma. Chest 1993; 103(Suppl):334–336.
161. Nakahara K, Ohno K, Hashimoto J, Maeda H, Miyoshi S, Sakurai M, Monden Y, Kawashima Y. Thymoma: results with complete resection and adjuvant postoperative irradiation in 141 consecutive patients. J Thorac Cardiovasc Surg 1988; 95:1041–1047.
162. Chiou GTJ, Chen C-L, Wei J, Hwang W-S. Reconstruction of superior vena cava in invasive thymoma. Chest 1990; 97:502–503.
163. Rivner MH, Swift TR. Thymoma: diagnosis and management. Semin Neurol 1990; 10:83–88.
164. Dahan M, Gaillard J, Mary H, Renella-Coll J, Berjaud J. [Long-term survival of surgically treated lymphoepithelial thymomas.] Rev Mal Respir 1988; 5:159–165.
165. Mackintosh JF, Hawson GAT, Matar KS, Johnston NG. Initial chemotherapy followed by surgery in malignant thymoma. Aust N Z J Med 1989; 19:362–364.
166. Ribet M. Therapeutic strategies in inoperable thymomas: secondary resection after preoperative X-ray therapy. *In* Sarrazin R, Vrousos C, Vincent F, eds. Thymic Tumors. Basel: Karger, 1989:144–146.
167. Hanuida M, Morimoto M, Nishimura H, Kobayashi O, Yamanda T, Iida F. Adjuvant radiotherapy after complete resection of thymoma. Ann Thorac Surg 1992; 54:311–315.
168. Arriagada R, Bernal P, Le Chevalier T, Baldeyrou P, Bretel JJ. Therapeutic strategies in advanced epithelial thymic tumors: stages III and IV. *In* Sarrazin R, Vrousos C, Vincent F, eds. Thymic Tumors. Basel: Karger, 1989:125–133.
169. Fornasiero A, Daniele O, Ghiotto C, Piazza M, Fiore-Donati L, Calabro F, Rea F, Fiorentino MV. Chemotherapy for invasive thymoma: a 13 year experience. Cancer 1991; 68:30–33.
170. Kosmidis PA, Iliopoulos E, Pentea S. Combination chemotherapy with cyclophosphamide, adriamycin, and vincristine in malignant thymoma and myasthenia gravis. Cancer 1988; 61:1736–1740.
171. Fornasiero A, Daniele O, Ghiotto C, Sartori F, Rea F, Piazza M, Fiore-Donati L, Morandi PMV, Aversa SML, Paccagnella A, Pappagallo GO, Fiorentino MV. Chemotherapy for invasive thymoma. J Clin Oncol 1990; 8:1419–1423.
172. Loehrer PJ Sr, Perez CA, Roth LM, Greco A, Livingston RB, Einhorn LH. Chemotherapy for advanced thymoma. Preliminary results of an intergroup study. Ann Intern Med 1990; 113:520–524.
173. Ohmi M, Ohuchi M. Recurrent thymoma in patients with myasthenia gravis. Ann Thorac Surg 1990; 50:243–247.
174. Chahinian AP, Bhardwaj S, Meyer RJ, Jaffrey IS, Kirschner PA, Holland JF. Treatment of invasive or metastatic thymoma: report of eleven cases. Cancer 1981; 47:1752–1761.
175. Wakata N, Fujioka T, Nishina M, Kawamura Y, Kobayashi M, Kinoshita M. Myasthenia gravis and invasive thymoma: a 20-year experience. Eur Neurol 1993; 133:115–120.
176. Urgesi A, Monetti U, Rossi G, Ricardi U, Maggi G, Sannazzari GL. Aggressive treatment of intrathoracic recurrences of thymoma. Radiother Oncol 1992; 24:221–225.
177. Zeok JV, Todd EP, Dillon M, DeSimone P, Utley JR. The role of thymectomy in red cell aplasia. Ann Thorac Surg 1979; 28:257–260.
178. Slater G, Papatestas A, Genkins G, Kornfeld P, Horowitz SH, Bender A. Thymomas in patients with myasthenia gravis. Ann Surg 1978; 188:171–174.
179. Snover DC, Levine GD, Rosai J. Thymic carcinoma: five distinctive histological variants. Am J Surg Pathol 1982; 6:451–470.
180. Wick MR, Scheithauer BW, Weiland LH, Bernatz PE. Primary thymic carcinomas. Am J Surg Pathol 1982; 6:613–630.
181. Kuo T-T, Chang J-P, Lin F-J, Wu W-C, Chang C-H. Thymic carcinomas: histopathological varieties and immunohistochemical study. Am J Surg Pathol 1990; 14:24–34.
182. Suster S, Rosai J. Thymic carcinoma: a clinicopathologic study of 60 cases. Cancer 1991; 67:1025–1032.
183. Pescarmona E, Rosati S, Rendina EA, Venuta F, Baroni CD. Well differentiated thymic carcinoma: a clinicopathological study. Virchows Arch [A] 1992; 420:179–183.
184. Fong PH, Wee A, Chan HL, Tan YO. Primary thymic carcinoma and its association with dermatomyositis and pure red cell aplasia. Int J Dermatol 1992; 31:426–428.
185. Le Marc-hadour F, Ramos JM, Pasquier B, Pasquier D, Couderc P. Association d'un carcinome thymique, d'une thyroidite de Hashimoto et d'une polymyosite: une observation anatomoclinique avec donnees autopsiques. Ann Pathol 1989; 9:355–359.
186. Leong ASY, Brown JH. Malignant transformation in a thymic cyst. Am J Surg Pathol 1984; 8:471–475.
187. Katoh Y, Shimamura K, Kakudo K, Osamura RY, Tamaoki N. An autopsy case of a cystic variant of thymic carcinoma mimicking a thymic cyst. Virchows Arch [A] 1990; 417:85–87.
188. Morinaga S, Sato Y, Shimosato Y, Sinkai T, Tsuchiya R. Multiple thymic squamous cell carcinomas associated with mixed type thymoma. Am J Surg Pathol 1987; 11:982–988.
189. Truong LD, Mody DR, Cagle PT, Jackson-York GL, Schwartz MR, Wheeler TM. Thymic carcinoma: a clinicopathologic study of 13 cases. Am J Surg Pathol 1990; 14:151–166.
190. Hartmann CA, Roth C, Minck C, Niedobitek G. Thymic carcinoma. Report of five cases and review of the literature. J Cancer Res Clin Oncol 1990; 116:69–82.
191. Matsuno Y, Mukai K, Noguchi M, Sato Y, Shimosato Y. Histochemical and immunohistochemical evidence of glandular differentiation in thymic carcinoma. Acta Pathol Jpn 1989; 39:433–438.
192. Alguacil-Garcia A, Halliday WC. Thymic carcinoma with focal neuroblastoma differentiation. Am J Surg Pathol 1987; 11:474–479.
193. Walker AN, Mills SE, Fechner RE. Thymomas and thymic carcinomas. Semin Diagn Pathol 1990; 7:250–265.
194. Suarez Vilela D, Salas Valien JS, Gonzalez Moran MA, Izquierdo Garcia F, Riera Velasco JR. Thymic carcinosarcoma associated with a spindle cell thymoma: an immunohistochemical study. Histopathology 1992; 21:263–268.
195. Wick MR, Scheithauer BW. Oat-cell carcinoma of the thymus. Cancer 1982; 49:1652–1657.
196. Brightman I, Morgan JA, Kunze WP, Sheppard MN. Primary mucoepidermoid carcinoma of the thymus: a rare cause of mediastinal tumor. Thorac Cardiovasc Surg 1992; 40:90–91.

197. Wolfe JT, Wick MR, Banks PM, Scheithauer BW. Clear cell carcinoma of the thymus. Mayo Clin Proc 1983; 58:365–370.
198. Stephens M, Khalil J, Gibbs AR. Primary clear cell carcinoma of the thymus gland. Histopathology 1987; 11:763–765.
199. Weide LG, Ulbright TM, Loehrer PJ Sr, Williams SD. Thymic carcinoma: a distinct clinical entity responsive to chemotherapy. Cancer 1993; 71:1219–1223.
200. Savino W, Dardenne M. Immunohistochemical studies on a human thymic epithelial cell subset defined by the anti-cytokeratin 18 monoclonal antibody. Cell Tissue Res 1988; 254:225–231.
201. Warren W, Clark JP, Gardner E, Harris G, Cooper CS, Lawley PD. Chemical induction of thymomas in AKR mice: interaction of chemical carcinogens and endogenous murine leukemia viruses. Comparison of N-methyl-N-nitrosurea and methyl methanesulphonate. Mol Carcinog 1990; 3:126–133.
202. Parker GA, Casey HW. Thymoma in domestic animals. Vet Pathol 1976; 13:353–364.
203. Vos JH, Stolwijk J, Ramaekers FC, van Oosterhout IC, van den Ingh TS. The use of keratin antisera in the characterization of a feline thymoma. J Comp Pathol 1990; 102:71–77.
204. Simpson RM, Waters DJ, Gebhard DH, Casey HW. Massive thymoma with medullary differentiation in a dog. Vet Pathol 1992; 29:416–419.
205. Hitt ME, Shaw DP, Hogan PM, Lennon VA, Amann JF. Radiation treatment for thymoma in a dog. J Am Vet Med Assoc 1987; 190:1187–1190.
206. Furuoka H, Taniyama H, Matsui T, Takahashi T, Ichijo S, Ono T. Malignant thymoma with multiple metastases in a mare. Nippon Juigaku Zasshi [KRJ] 1987; 49:577–579.
207. Whiteley LO, Leininger JR, Wolf CB, Ames TR. Malignant squamous cell thymoma in a horse. Vet Pathol 1986; 23:627–629.
208. Kaspareit-Rittinghausen J, Deerberg F, Sommer R. Atypical epithelial thymomas in rats. Lab Anim 1989; 23:337–339.
209. Naylor DC, Krinke GJ, Ruefenacht HJ. Primary tumours of the thymus in the rat. J Comp Pathol 1988; 99:187–203.
210. Kostolich M, Panciera RJ. Thymoma in a domestic rabbit. Cornell Vet 1992; 82:125–129.
211. Scott-Moncrieff JC, Cook JR Jr, Lantz GC. Acquired myasthenia gravis in a cat with thymoma. J Am Vet Med Assoc 1990; 196:1291–1293.
212. Squire RA, Goodman DG, Valerio MG, Fredrickson T, Strandberg JD, Levitt MH, Lingeman CH, Harshbarger JC, Dawe CJ. Tumors: hemopoietic system. *In* Benirschke K, Garner FM, Jones TC, eds. Pathology of Laboratory Animals. New York: Springer-Verlag, 1978:1091–1125.
213. Hoot GP, Kettman JR. Primary polyoma virus-induced murine thymic epithelial tumors: a tumor model of thymus physiology. Am J Pathol 1989; 135:679–695.
214. Masuda A, Ohtsuka K, Matsuyama M. Establishment of functional epithelial cell lines from a rat thymoma and a rat thymus. In Vitro Cell Dev Biol 1990; 26:713–721.
215. Lu J, Sakai Y, Wajjawalku W, Isobe K-I, Saito M, Amo H, Kojima A, Utsumi KR, Takahashi M, Hiai H, Matsuyama M. Establishment of transplantable tumor lines and in vitro cell lines of malignant thymoma developed in a BUF/Mna rat. Jpn J Cancer Res 1992; 83:618–624.
216. Leyvraz S, Henle W, Chahinian AP, Perlmann C, Klein G, Gordon RE, Rosenblum M, Holland JF. Association of Epstein-Barr virus with thymic carcinoma. N Engl J Med 1985; 312:1296–1299.
217. Dimery IW, Lee JS, Blick M, Pearson G, Spitzer G, Hong WK. Association of the Epstein-Barr virus with lymphoepithelioma of the thymus. Cancer 1988; 61:2475–2480.
218. McGuire LJ, Huang DP, Teoh R, Arnold M, Wong K, Lee CK. Epstein-Barr virus genome in thymoma and thymic lymphoid hyperplasia. Am J Pathol 1988; 131:385–390.
219. Matsuno Y, Mukai K, Uhara H, Akao I, Furuya S, Sato Y, Hirohashi S, Shimosato Y. Detection of Epstein-Barr virus DNA in a Japanese case of lymphoepithelioma-like thymic carcinoma. Jpn J Cancer Res 1992; 83:127–130.
220. Wu T-C, Kuo T-T. Study of Epstein-Barr virus early RNA1 (EBER1) expression by in situ hybridization in thymic epithelial tumors of chinese patients in Taiwan. Hum Pathol 1993; 24:235–238.
221. Inghirami G, Chilosi M, Knowles DM. Western thymomas lack Epstein-Barr virus by Southern blotting analysis and by polymerase chain reaction. Am J Pathol 1990; 136:1429–1436.
222. Borisch B, Kirchner T, Marx A, Muller-Hermelink HK. Absence of the Epstein-Barr virus genome in the normal thymus, thymic epithelial tumors, thymic lymphoid hyperplasia in a European population. Virchows Arch [B] 1990; 59:359–365.
223. Yu YL, Hawkins BR, IP MS, Wong V, Woo E. Myasthenia gravis in Hong Kong Chinese. 1. Epidemiology and adult disease. Acta Neurol Scand 1992; 86:113–119.
224. Teoh R, McGuire L, Wong K, Chin D. Increased incidence of thymoma in Chinese myasthenia gravis: possible relationship with Epstein-Barr virus. Acta Neurol Scand 1989; 80:221–225.
225. Ferrari G, Lovaste MG. Epidemiology of myasthenia gravis in the province of Trento (northern Italy). Neuroepidemiology 1992; 11:135–142.
226. Monden Y, Nakahara K, Nanjo S, Fujii Y, Natsumara A, Masaoka A, Kawashima Y. Invasive thymoma with myasthenia gravis. Cancer 1984; 54:2513–2518.
227. Lisak RP, Barchi RL. Myasthenia Gravis. Philadelphia: WB Saunders, 1982:104–105.
228. Lanska DJ. Diagnosis of thymoma in myasthenics using anti-striated muscle antibodies: predictive value and gain in diagnostic certainty. Neurology 1991; 41:520–524.
229. Huang DP, Ng HK, Ho YH, Chan KM. Epstein-Barr virus (EBV)-associated undifferentiated carcinoma of the parotid gland. Histopathology 1988; 13:509–517.
230. Stewart JP, Arrand JR. Expression of the Epstein-Barr virus latent membrane protein in nasopharyngeal carcinoma biopsy specimens. Hum Pathol 1993; 24:239–242.
231. Perronne C, Ooka T, Decaussin G, De The G, Berrih-Aknin S, Verley JM. Antibodies to Epstein-Barr virus in 50 patients with thymic tumor [letter]. JAMA 1990; 264:570–571.
232. Smith RD. Epstein-Barr virus: a ubiquitous agent that can immortalize cells. Hum Pathol 1993; 24:233–234.
233. Marx A, Kirchner T, Hoppe F, O'Connor R, Schalke B, Tzartos S, Muller-Hermelink HK. Proteins with epitopes of the acetylcholine receptor in epithelial cell cultures of thymomas in myasthenia gravis. Am J Pathol 1989; 134:865–877.
234. Kirchner T, Tzartos S, Hoppe F, Schalke B, Wekerle

H, Muller-Hermelink HK. Pathogenesis of myasthenia gravis. Acetylcholine receptor-related antigenic determinants in tumor-free thymuses and thymic epithelial tumors. Am J Pathol 1988; 130:268–280.
235. Papadopoulos T, Kirchner T, Marx A, Muller-Hermelink HK. Primary cultures of human thymic epithelial tumors: morphological and immunocytochemical characterization. Virchows Arch [B] 1989; 56:363–370.
236. Marx A, O'Connor R, Geuder KI, Hoppe F, Schalke B, Tzartos S, Kalies I, Kirchner T, Muller-Hermelink HK. Characterization of a protein with an acetylcholine receptor epitope from myasthenia gravis–associated thymomas. Lab Invest 1990; 62:279–286.
237. Hohlfeld R. Myasthenia gravis and thymoma: paraneoplastic failure of neuromuscular transmission [editorial]. Lab Invest 1990; 62:241–243.
238. Marx A, O'Connor R, Tzartos S, Kalies I, Kirchner T, Muller-Hermelink HK. Acetylcholine receptor epitope in proteins of myasthenia gravis-associated thymomas and non-thymic tissues. Thymus 1989; 14:171–178.
239. Cikes N, Momoi MY, Williams CL, Howard FM Jr, Hoagland HC, Whittingham S, Lennon VA. Striational autoantibodies: quantitative detection by enzyme immunoassay in myasthenia gravis, thymoma, and recipients of D-penicillamine or allogeneic bone marrow. Mayo Clin Proc 1988; 63:474–481.
240. Williams CL, Hay JE, Huiatt TW, Lennon VA. Paraneoplastic IgG striational autoantibodies produced by clonal thymic B cells and in serum of patients with myasthenia gravis and thymoma react with titin. Lab Invest 1992; 66:331–336.
241. Dardenne M, Savino W, Bach JF. Thymomatous epithelial cells and skeletal muscle share a common epitope defined by a monoclonal antibody. Am J Pathol 1987; 126:194–198.
242. Marx A, Osborn M, Tzartos S, Geuder KI, Schalke B, Nix W, Kirchner T, Muller-Hermelink HK. A striational muscle antigen and myasthenia gravis–associated thymomas share an acetylcholine-receptor epitope. Dev Immunol 1992; 2:77–84.
243. Geuder KI, Marx A, Witzemann V, Schalke B, Kirchner T, Muller-Hermelink HK. Genomic organization and lack of transcription of the nicotinic acetylcholine receptor subunit genes in myasthenia gravis–associated thymoma. Lab Invest 1992; 66:452–458.
244. Hara Y, Ueno S, Uemichi T, Takahashi N, Yorifuji S, Fujii Y, Tarui S. Neoplastic epithelial cells express alpha-subunit of muscle nicotinic acetylcholine receptor in thymomas from patients with myasthenia gravis. FEBS Lett 1991; 279:137–140.
245. Siara J, Rudel R, Marx A. Absence of acetylcholine-induced current in epithelial cells from thymus glands and thymomas of myasthenia gravis patients. Neurology 1991; 41:128–131.
246. Sharkis SJ. The role of the thymus in erythropoiesis. Blood Cells 1984; 10:223–231.
247. Goodman JW, Shinpock SG. Thymic lymphocytes and haemopoiesis. Ann Immunol (Inst Pasteur) 1984; 135:268–302.
248. Mukai K, Sato Y, Hirohashi S, Shimosato Y. Expression of ras p21 protein by thymoma. Virchows Arch [B] 1990; 59:11–16.
249. Kubonishi I, Takehara N, Iwata J, Sonobe H, Ohtsuki Y, Abe T, Miyoshi I. Novel t(15:19) (q15; p13) chromosome abnormality in a thymic carcinoma. Cancer Res 1991; 51:3327–3328.
250. Kristoffersson U, Heim S, Mandahl N, Akerman M, Mitelman F. Multiple clonal chromosome aberrations in two thymomas. Cancer Genet Cytogenet 1989; 41:93–98.
251. Arimori S, Ichimura K, Tokunaga M, Morita K. Retrovirus-like particles in human thymomas. Tokai J Exp Clin Med 1990; 15:219–225.
252. Ono A, Saito H, Kondo S, Yoshimatsu H, Tsuchiya M. RNA tumor virus in human thymomas and thymus hyperplasia. Semin Surg Oncol 1985; 1:139–152.
253. Ring NP, Addis BJ. Thymoma: an integrated clinicopathological and immunohistochemical study. J Pathol 1986; 149:327–337.
254. Henry K. The thymus—what's new. Histopathology 1989; 14:537–548.
255. Muller-Hermelink HK, Marino M, Palestro G. Pathology of thymic epithelial tumors. *In* Muller-Hermelink HK, ed. Current Topics in Pathology: The Human Thymus. Berlin: Springer-Verlag, 1986:208–268.

Chapter

6

LYMPHOMAS (INCLUDING HODGKIN'S DISEASE) AND OTHER HEMATOLOGIC LESIONS

LYMPHOBLASTIC LYMPHOMA
- Clinical Features
- Histopathology
- Immunopathology
- Molecular Pathology
- DNA Ploidy and Cell Proliferation Indices
- Cytogenetics
- Cytochemistry
- Cytopathology
- Differential Diagnosis
- Prognosis and Therapy

LARGE-CELL LYMPHOMA OF THE MEDIASTINUM
- Clinical Features
- Histopathology
- Immunopathology
- Molecular Pathology
- DNA Ploidy and Cell Proliferation Indices
- Cytopathology
- Differential Diagnosis
- Prognosis and Therapy
- Pathogenesis

OTHER NON-HODGKIN'S LYMPHOMAS

MEDIASTINAL LYMPHOMAS IN ANIMALS

HODGKIN'S DISEASE
- Epidemiology
- Clinical Features
- Histopathology
- Immunopathology
- Molecular Pathology
- Cytopathology
- Pathogenesis
- Prognosis and Therapy

ANGIOFOLLICULAR LYMPHOID HYPERPLASIA (CASTLEMAN'S DISEASE)

HISTIOCYTOSIS X (LANGERHANS CELL HISTIOCYTOSIS)

MISCELLANEOUS HEMATOLOGIC LESIONS

SUMMARY

As discussed in Chapter 1, lymphomas (including both Hodgkin's and non-Hodgkin's types) account for approximately 20% of all anterior mediastinal masses. Among pediatric patients, the percentage is as high as 45%.[1]

Clinically, presentations range from patients who are asymptomatic to those in severe respiratory distress. When present, symptoms relate to the mediastinal location of the tumor and include cough, chest pain, dysphagia, and dyspnea. The superior vena cava syndrome may result from tumor compressing the superior vena cava and interfering with venous blood return from the head, neck, and upper extremities.[2] The tumor may obstruct the airway and must then be treated as a medical emergency.

Non-Hodgkin's lymphomas involve the mediastinum in about 20% of cases[3–5] and are limited to the mediastinum in less than 10%.[4,6] Approximately half of patients with lymphoma involving the mediastinum have signs or symptoms attributable to intrathoracic disease.[4]

Of 184 patients with non-Hodgkin's lymphoma, Lichtenstein et al. identified 17 teenage and adult patients (15 years old or older) who presented with symptoms related to a mediastinal mass.[6] Nine of the 17 had lymphoblastic lymphoma. Diffuse large-cell lymphoma was diagnosed in 6 patients, and diffuse small cleaved cell was identified in 2 cases. In another series of 215 non-Hodgkin's lymphomas, 12 patients had disease limited to the mediastinum.[4] Eight had diffuse large-cell lymphoma, and 4 had diffuse small cleaved cell. Other non-Hodgkin's types (e.g., follicular, small lymphocytic, intermediate lymphocytic, and small noncleaved cell lymphomas) uncommonly present as a mediastinal mass.[7]

LYMPHOBLASTIC LYMPHOMA

A connection between thymic tumors and leukemia has been recognized for the last 100 years.[8, 9] Magrath credits Ortner with the first description of such an association in 1890.[8] In 1916, Sternberg described mediastinal lymphomas that terminated in acute leukemia and called them "leukosarcoma."[10] Subsequently, the eponym "Sternberg sarcoma" was used for this entity.[11] In 1932, Cooke reported a series of nine boys with mediastinal tumors associated with acute leukemia.[12] In four of the cases, the discovery of the tumor because of clinical symptoms preceded the peripheral blood picture of acute leukemia. Cooke collected 74 additional cases from a review of the literature. Males were affected six times more frequently than females, and 90% of patients were under 30 years of age.

Similarly, in 1961, Webster reported that 11 of 15 children with lymphosarcoma of the thymus developed acute leukemia.[13] In comparison, leukemia developed in only 1 of 30 children with lymphosarcoma of other sites. The term lymphosarcoma was used to denote a tumor arising in lymphoid tissue distinct from Hodgkin's disease and reticulum cell sarcoma. Lymphosarcoma was subdivided into follicular, lymphocytic, and lymphoblastic types. Webster recognized the childhood mediastinal lymphomas as being of the lymphoblastic type ("lymphoblastoma").

With the use of the Rappaport classification for lymphoma in the 1960s, the term lymphosarcoma was eliminated.[9, 14, 15] The lymphoblastic type of lymphosarcoma was incorporated into the poorly differentiated lymphocytic lymphomas or into an "undifferentiated" category. The distinctive features of lymphoblastic lymphoma became obscured within these categories. With the advent of lymphocyte phenotyping in the 1970s and 1980s, this disorder received renewed attention. Smith and colleagues studied a lymph node from a child with mediastinal lymphoma.[16] Using a sheep red blood cell binding assay, these investigators reported the tumor to be of T-cell origin. In contrast, acute lymphoblastic leukemias without a mediastinal mass did not form sheep red blood cell rosettes and thus were apparently not of T-cell origin. In 1974, Kaplan and colleagues confirmed these results in a paper entitled "Childhood lymphoblastic lymphoma, a cancer of thymus-derived lymphocytes."[17]

In 1975, Barcos and Lukes described a tumor composed of primitive-appearing lymphoid cells with convoluted nuclei that had a predilection for the mediastinum in male adolescents.[18] This group of lymphomas is composed of immature lymphoid cells indistinguishable from acute lymphoblastic leukemia. These tumors had been classified as diffuse poorly differentiated lymphocytic, using the Rappaport system. Nathwani and colleagues found that nuclear convolutions did not identify a distinctive subset clinically.[19] They advocated the term lymphoblastic lymphoma. This designation was then included in the modified Rappaport classification.[20]

Thus, lymphoblastic lymphoma was "rediscovered" nearly a century after its first description. However, terminology remained confusing. For example, in the Kiel classification, lymphoblastic lymphomas were subdivided to include Burkitt's type and convoluted cell type.[21, 22] The convoluted cell type is equivalent to the lymphoblastic category in the modified Rappaport classification and in the National Cancer Institute Working Formulation.[20, 23] Finally, in a modification of the Kiel classification, Burkitt's lymphoma was placed in a different category from lymphoblastic lymphoma.[24, 25]

Clinical Features

Lymphoblastic lymphoma is now recognized as a distinct clinical-pathologic disorder with a characteristic age and sex distribution, morphology, phenotype, and course. Lymphoblastic lymphoma accounts for one third to one half of all non-Hodgkin's lymphomas (NHLs) in childhood.[26, 27] However, it may occur at any age and accounts for approximately 5% of NHLs in adults.[28] There is a bimodal age distribution, with the first peak at 16 years and the second peak above age 40.[29] In pediatric series, the median age is around 9 years.[26] The disease is approximately twice as common in males as in females.[29, 30] Depending on the series, 42 to 75% of patients have a mediastinal mass.

Most patients have disseminated disease at diagnosis.[27] Sites of involvement other than the mediastinum include the lymph nodes, bone marrow, central nervous system, head and neck, lung, liver, pleura, pericardium, peritoneum, skin, and gonad. Lymphoblastic lymphoma and acute lymphoblastic leukemia are closely related. The criteria to separate the two are arbitrary.[31] Patients are generally considered to have lymphoblastic lymphoma if the percentage of lymphoblasts in the bone marrow is less than 25%.[26] Others use the criteria of less than 10% lymphoblasts in the peripheral blood and absence of pancytopenia.[19, 32] Slater and colleagues found no difference in survival when patients with lymphoblastic lymphoma and acute lymphoblastic leukemia were treated with the same chemotherapy.[33] Patte and colleagues also reported no difference in survival between patients with less than 25% lymphoblasts in the bone marrow and those with more than 25%.[34]

Histopathology

Microscopically, lymphoblastic lymphoma is characterized by diffusely infiltrative, noncohesive cells[35, 36] (Fig. 6–1). Fibrosis is absent or scant. A "starry sky" pattern may be prominent from numerous tingible-body macrophages (the "stars") interspersed among the dark blue nuclei of the lymphoblasts. Crush artifact and necrosis may be extensive enough to obscure the diagnosis. The mitotic rate is high. On a mediastinal biopsy, residual thymic elements may be identified. Hassall's corpuscles should not be misconstrued as evidence for a thymoma. The malignant cells are usually "intermediate" in size (between small lymphocytic and large-cell lymphoma), or about 12 μm in diameter.[19] A large-cell variant also occurs.[27] Nuclear convolutions may be conspicuous. The nuclei have a delicate, fine chromatin pattern without prominent nucleoli.

The chromatin is best appreciated on Wright-stained cytologic preparations (touch imprints or fine-needle aspirates) that also show basophilic cytoplasm and occasional vacuoles (Fig. 6–2). The finely dispersed chromatin pattern is the single most useful feature that separates lymphoblastic from other lymphomas. The cells have scanty cytoplasm. The methyl green pyronin stain produces weak or absent cytoplasmic staining.[36]

Immunopathology

Immunologically, over 80% of lymphoblastic lymphomas are T-cell neoplasms as defined by

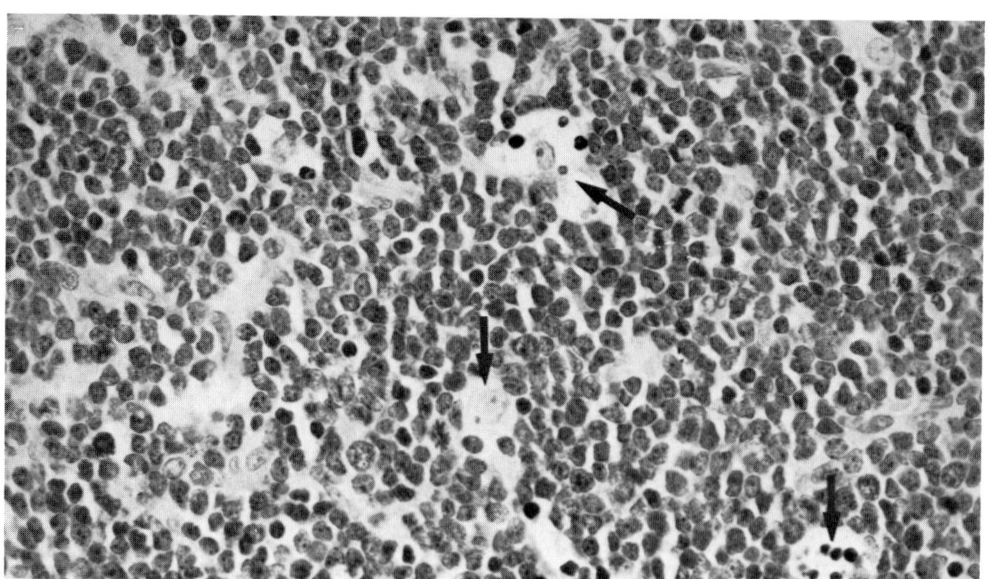

Figure 6–1. Lymphoblastic lymphoma. The tingible-body macrophages (*arrows*) create a "starry sky" appearance. The lymphoblasts are small-to-intermediate in size with diffuse chromatin and small nucleoli (H&E, ×400).

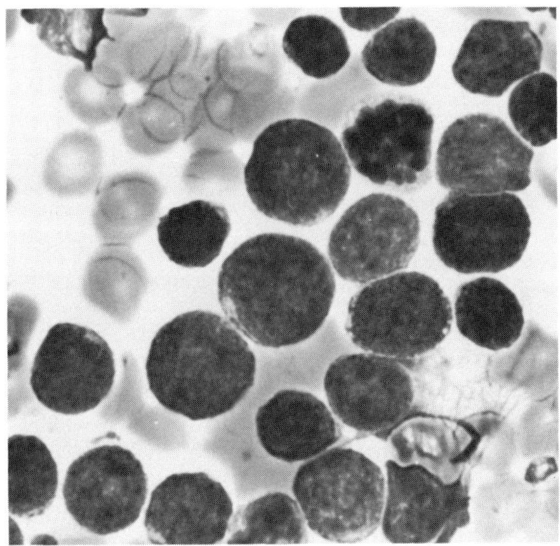

Figure 6–2. Modified Wright-stained (Diff-Quik) touch imprint of lymphoblastic lymphoma demonstrates diffuse nuclear chromatin. Some cells have small nucleoli. The scant cytoplasm has occasional small vacuoles (×1000).

expression of T-cell surface markers (most commonly CD7).[29, 37–39] (See Appendix for review of CD nomenclature.) In contrast, only 15% of acute lymphoblastic leukemias (ALLs) are T cell in origin.[37] In virtually every case of ALL and lymphoblastic lymphoma, the malignant cells are positive for terminal deoxynucleotidyl transferase (TDT).[40, 41] Lymphoblasts of both B-cell and T-cell origin express this marker within their nuclei.

T-cell ALL more often expresses an early thymocyte (precortical) phenotype (CD2 and CD7+; CD1,3,4,8−) than does lymphoblastic lymphoma[42] (Tables 6–1 and 6–2). Those cases of T-cell ALL or lymphoblastic lymphoma that express an intermediate thymocyte phenotype (CD1+; surface CD3−; positive for both CD4 and CD8) are most likely to have a mediastinal mass.[42] A mature T-cell phenotype (CD3+; CD4 and CD8 variably expressed on different cell populations) accounted for a greater percentage of lymphoblastic lymphomas than leukemias. Occasional cases of T-cell lymphoblastic lymphoma express CD10 (common acute lymphoblastic leukemia antigen, or CALLA). CD3, the antigen associated with the T-cell antigen receptor, is expressed in the cytoplasm of lymphoblastic cells with an early phenotype.[43] Only the more mature cases express surface CD3. Flow cytometry studies usually analyze only surface antigens; therefore, cells with cytoplasmic CD3 will not express CD3 by flow cytometry but will express CD3 by immunoperoxidase staining. Unusual cases of lymphoblastic lymphomas with biphenotypic features (T- and B-cell markers, T-cell and myeloid markers) have been described.[38, 44] Mediastinal lymphoblastic lymphomas nearly all have a T-cell origin. A rare case of mediastinal lymphoblastic lymphoma with an early B-cell phenotype has been reported.[45]

Sheibani and colleagues divided lymphoblastic lymphomas into five groups based on phenotype as detected by immunoperoxidase methods.[39] Thirty-three of thirty-six cases expressed T-cell antigens. Among these 33 cases, 22 expressed only T-cell antigens (group 1), and five expressed CD10 (CALLA) in addition to the T-cell markers (group 2). Six cases expressed natural killer cell antigens, CD16 and CD57 (group 3). Three cases expressed B-cell antigens (two immature, group 4; one mature, group 5). The percentage of patients with a mediastinal mass was highest (86%), and the ratio of males to females was greatest (10:1), in group 1.

In a study of 31 patients with T-cell lymphoblastic lymphoma, the stage of thymocyte differentiation did not affect relapse-free survival.[42] However, in a study of nine patients with T-cell lymphoblastic lymphoma, Yumura-Yagi and colleagues reported that the three patients who experienced relapse all had neoplastic cells corresponding to the earliest stage of T-cell differentiation.[46] Basing their reason-

Table 6–1. Phenotype of T-Cell Acute Lymphoblastic Leukemia (T-ALL) Versus Lymphoblastic Lymphoma (T-LL)[42*]

	Early (CD2, 5, 7)	Intermediate (CD1,2,5,7; 4 and 8)	Mature (CD2,3†,5,7; 4 or 8)	Total Number of Patients
T-ALL	34%‡	43%	23%	101
T-LL	6%	62%	32%	31

*Modified from reference 42.
†Surface CD3.
‡Percentage of cases with early phenotype.

Table 6–2. Phenotype of T Lymphoblastic Lymphoma*

	CD1	CD2	CD3	CD4	CD5	CD7	CD8	CD10	CD16	CD25	CD38	CD57	DR	TDT
#	31/68	50/68	13/16	36/68	60/70	37/38	26/68	16/61	6/33	1/33	20/47	5/33	25/60	44/46
%	46	74	81	53	86	97	38	26	18	3	42	15	42	96

= number of cases positive for antigen/total number of cases tested. % = percentage of cases that are positive.
Abbreviations: DR, HLA-DR; TDT, terminal deoxynucleotidyl transferase.
*Data from references 38, 39, 43, 44.

ing on this small number of patients, these authors suggest that T-cell lymphoblastic lymphoma with the early thymocyte phenotype may have a worse prognosis. However, another group of investigators reported three adult patients with "pre–T cell" lymphoblastic lymphoma (CD7+, CD2−, germ-line T-cell receptor genes) who all had an indolent course.[47] Two of the three cases were associated with Langerhans cell histiocytosis (histiocytosis X).

Numerous antibodies have been developed that are useful in immunoperoxidase studies using paraffin-embedded tissue.[48–53] These antibodies include the B-cell marker CD20 and T-cell markers CD43, CD45RO, polyclonal CD3, and OPD4.

Immunohistochemical studies of T-cell lymphoblastic lymphomas in paraffin-embedded tissue are summarized in Table 6–3.[52–64] Most T-cell lymphoblastic lymphomas express CD43 (Leu 22, MT1, L60). However, CD43 is not specific for T cells, because it also labels a B-cell subset, granulocytes, monocytes, macrophages, and megakaryocytes.[51] Many B-cell lymphomas, chronic lymphocytic leukemias, and acute leukemias (lymphoblastic and myeloid) express this antigen.[65–67] A polyclonal antibody to CD3 labels a high percentage of lymphoblastic lymphomas in formalin-fixed tissue.[52, 57] The sections must be treated with protease or other antigen retrieval methods before immunoperoxidase staining. Beta F1 is a monoclonal antibody to the beta chain of the T-cell antigen receptor. In paraffin-embedded sections, four of five T-cell lymphoblastic lymphomas reacted with this antibody.[54] None of 21 B-cell lymphomas reacted with beta F1.

CD45RO (UCHL1) is another monoclonal antibody that preferentially labels T cells.[58] It stains a smaller percentage of cases. OPD4 is a monoclonal antibody raised against a helper/inducer (CD4-positive) T-cell line. However, it does not distinguish between CD4- and CD8-positive neoplastic T cells in paraffin-embedded tissue sections. OPD4 has not yet been studied extensively but so far appears to label only a minority of T-cell lymphoblastic lymphomas.[55, 59]

Table 6–3. Immunohistochemistry of T-Lymphoblastic Lymphoma in Paraffin-Embedded Tissue: Literature Review (Primarily Using Formalin-Fixed Tissue)*

	CD43†	CD45RO	Polyclonal CD3	OPD4	Beta F1
#	29/36	19/32	13/13	1/5	4/5
%	81	59	100	20	80

= number of cases positive for antigen/total number of cases tested. % = percentage of cases that are positive.
*Data from references 52–64.
†CD43 includes the antibodies L60, MT1, and Leu 22. B5 fixative produced more intense staining than did formalin for CD43 (MT1).

Molecular Pathology

Molecular genetic studies have demonstrated rearrangement of the T-cell antigen receptor genes in most cases of T-cell lymphoblastic lymphoma.[9, 68, 69] The T-cell receptor is a heterodimer composed of two covalently linked polypeptide chains (see Chapter 3). A T cell has receptors with either alpha/beta chains or gamma/delta chains. Monoclonal antibodies have been developed that are specific for the alpha/beta or gamma/delta receptors. Most thymic and peripheral T lymphocytes express the alpha/beta receptor. Less than 5% express the gamma/delta type. CD3 is associated with both types of receptor.

In a study of 22 T-cell lymphoblastic lymphomas, Picker and colleagues noted a discordance between expression of CD3 and the alpha/beta T-cell receptor (as determined by immunoreactivity with the beta F1 antibody in frozen sections) in nine cases (40%).[70] These authors interpreted their findings as evidence of an aberrant phenotype. In another study of 15 lymphoblastic lymphomas that expressed the antigen receptor (CD3+), 13 (87%) expressed the alpha/beta type.[71] In contrast, only one third of 15 T-cell acute lymphoblastic leukemias expressed the alpha/beta receptor. The remaining cases had the gamma/delta receptor.

In a study of 18 T-cell lymphoblastic lymphomas, Falini and colleagues identified three cases that expressed the gamma/delta receptor as demonstrated by immunocytochemical studies.[72] All three cases had a thymic cortical phenotype (positive for CD1, 3, 5, and 7). All had rearrangements of the beta and gamma chain genes; two also had immunoglobulin heavy gene rearrangements. Thus, T-cell lymphoblastic lymphoma usually derives from the alpha/beta T cell; however, occasional cases appear to originate from a subset of thymic lymphocytes that express the gamma/delta receptor. T-cell acute lymphoblastic leukemias more often derive from the gamma/delta cells.

At the DNA level, T-cell receptor genes code for each of the four chains (alpha, beta, gamma, and delta) (see Chapter 3). Like the immunoglobulin genes, the T-cell receptor genes must rearrange to produce an RNA message for a functional protein. In ontogeny, rearrangement of the beta chain gene precedes expression of surface CD2, surface CD5, and cytoplasmic CD3.[73] However, CD7 expression occurs before or concurrently with the beta rearrangement. Those T-cell lymphoblastic malignancies with a prothymocyte phenotype (CD7+, CD1−, CD3−) usually have germ line configurations for the beta chain gene of the antigen receptor.[73–77] T-cell lymphoblastic lymphomas with a more mature phenotype (positive for CD1, CD4, CD8, and/or CD3) have beta chain gene rearrangements.[75, 78]

In addition to the beta rearrangements, T-cell malignancies commonly have rearrangements within the alpha, delta, and gamma chain loci.[79] The delta and gamma chain genes rearrange before the other T-cell receptor genes.[79–81] Thus, delta or gamma rearrangements may be present in lymphoblastic malignancies having an early ("prothymocyte") phenotype.[9] Those T-cell lymphoblastic lymphomas with more mature T-cell phenotypes may have rearrangements of all T-cell receptor genes, including the alpha, beta, gamma, and delta chains.[73, 79] Surprisingly, immunoglobulin heavy chain gene rearrangements occur in 7 to 25% of T-cell lymphoblastic lymphomas and leukemias.[9, 69, 72, 82, 83]

Similarly, T-cell antigen receptor rearrangements are common among precursor B cell–derived lymphoblastic lymphomas and leukemias. The percentages range from 20% of precursor B-cell lymphoblastic lymphomas and leukemias having a beta chain rearrangement to 80% with a delta chain rearrangement.[9] This finding highlights the fact that immunoglobulin and T-cell antigen receptor gene rearrangements are not lineage-restricted.

DNA Ploidy and Cell Proliferation Indices

DNA flow cytometry has been reported in few cases of lymphoblastic lymphoma. In one report, 13 of 15 cases were diploid.[44] The remaining two were near-diploid, having DNA content within 10% of normal (DNA indices of 1.1 and 0.9). Intermediate proliferation indices (percentage of cells in S, G2, and M phases of the cell cycle) were obtained. The prognostic significance of ploidy and S phase for lymphoblastic lymphoma is not established. Surprisingly, in childhood acute lymphoblastic leukemia, aneuploidy (DNA index greater than 1.16) is a favorable prognostic factor.[84]

Another measure of cell proliferation is expression of Ki-67, a nuclear antigen present in S, G1, G2, and M phases of the cell cycle, but absent in G0.[85] Weiss and colleagues studied expression of this antigen by frozen section immunoperoxidase staining of 33 cases of T-cell lymphoblastic lymphoma/acute lymphoblastic leukemia.[85] In these cases, an average of 46% of cells expressed Ki-67. Like the S phase, the percentage of cells positive for Ki-67 generally correlated with histologic grade. Small noncleaved (Burkitt's and non-Burkitt's) lymphomas had the highest percentage (about 80%). Small lymphocytic lymphoma/chronic lymphocytic leukemia had the lowest (11%). T-cell lymphoblastic malignancies had a percentage similar to that of large-cell lymphomas. Other investigators have obtained similar results.[86, 87]

Cytogenetics

Cytogenetic studies have demonstrated abnormalities in 94% of T-cell lymphoblastic lymphomas.[9] Thirty to fifty percent of the abnormalities include a breakpoint at 14q11, 7q34–36, or 7p15. The T-cell receptor alpha and delta genes are on chromosome 14, band q11. The beta and gamma genes have been mapped to bands q34–36 and p15, respectively, on chromosome 7. Thus, it is not surprising that T-cell malignancies commonly have karyotypes with abnormalities at these sites.

Cytochemistry

Cytochemistry in lymphoblastic lymphoma is significant for focal ("dot-like") acid phosphatase activity within the region of the Golgi apparatus in most cases.[88] Acid phosphatase activity is much higher in T cells than in B cells. Therefore, it labels T-cell lymphoblastic lymphomas and leukemias more than it does B-cell disease. However, positivity can also be present in erythroblasts and myeloblasts. With the immunologic studies now available, cytochemistry is rarely necessary for the characterization of lymphoblastic lymphoma.

Cytopathology

In many patients, diagnostic cellular material can most easily be obtained by fine-needle aspiration biopsy. Lymphoblastic lymphoma has a typical clinical presentation and characteristic cytologic appearance. It also has a characteristic immunophenotype with TDT positivity. When a child or adolescent has mediastinal lymphadenopathy and airway obstruction, obtaining a surgical biopsy is fraught with danger.[2, 89, 90] Instead, a percutaneous fine-needle aspiration biopsy can provide diagnostic material with minimal discomfort and little risk to the patient.[44, 91] Usually, the aspirate can be performed at the bedside on palpable lymph nodes in the cervical, axillary, or supraclavicular areas. If no lymph nodes can be palpated, the aspiration biopsy can be performed with computed tomography (CT) guidance. If present, pleural fluid can also be used to obtain cells for diagnosis.[92]

Air-dried smears of the aspirate are stained with a modified Wright preparation (Diff-Quik). Fragments of tissue obtained through the needle can be embedded in paraffin and stained with hematoxylin and eosin. Microscopic examination of the smears reveals a monotonous population of immature-appearing lymphoid cells (Fig. 6–2). Cytoplasmic fragments ("lymphoglandular bodies"[93]) may be present. Mitoses are frequent. Marker studies can be performed on aspirated material using flow cytometry and/or immunoperoxidase. Gene rearrangement studies can also be obtained but are rarely needed for diagnosis. On the basis of clinical presentation, cytologic appearance, and immunologic data, a diagnosis of lymphoblastic lymphoma can be made quickly and with confidence.[91, 94] If necessary, the patient can then receive radiation therapy and/or chemotherapy promptly to relieve the airway obstruction.

Differential Diagnosis

The differential diagnosis includes follicular and/or diffuse small cleaved cell lymphomas and small noncleaved cell (Burkitt's or non-Burkitt's) lymphomas. Clinical presentation together with histopathology and immunologic studies usually can clearly distinguish these entities. Follicular center cell lymphomas generally affect an older population. Marker studies would demonstrate a mature B-cell phenotype. Small noncleaved cell lymphomas (Burkitt's and non-Burkitt's) are uncommon above the diaphragm. In contrast to the lymphoblastic type, small noncleaved cell lymphomas have clumped nuclear chromatin, prominent nucleoli, and strong cytoplasmic positivity with the methyl green pyronin histochemical stain. These tumors have a B-cell phenotype and are TDT-negative.

Lymphocytic thymoma and true thymic hyperplasia must be considered in the differential diagnosis. In these entities, an immunoperoxidase stain for cytokeratin should demonstrate epithelial cells throughout the lesion. Similarly, mediastinal small-cell carcinoma should be positive for cytokeratin and neuron-specific enolase. This type of neoplasm appears more cohesive and has nuclear molding. Acute myeloid leukemia (or granulocytic sarcoma) may rarely produce a mediastinal mass (see later). Cytochemical and immunologic studies would establish a diagnosis. Confident distinction from other small round cell tumors of childhood may be difficult on morphologic grounds alone and generally requires immunophenotyping.

Prognosis and Therapy

The survival of patients with lymphoblastic lymphoma has improved dramatically over the last 20 years (Table 6–4). In a retrospective study of lymphoblastic lymphoma from 1976, Nathwani and colleagues reported a median survival of 8 months.[19] Early therapeutic pro-

Table 6–4. Summary of Clinicopathologic Studies of Lymphoblastic Lymphoma

First Author/Year	No. of Patients	Age Range	Male-to-Female Ratio	% with Mediastinal Mass	Survival
Nathwani, 1976[19]	30	1–75 (median 16)	1.7:1	50%	8 mos median survival (82% developed leukemia)
Nathwani, 1981[35]	95	4–84 (median 30)	2.5:1	42%	17 mos median survival (53% developed leukemia)
Griffith, 1987[27]	106	1 mo–19 yrs (median 7 yrs)	2.1:1	64%	30 mos median disease-free survival
Coleman, 1986[32]	44	Over 16 yrs	3:1	75%	56% 3-yr survival
Hvizdala, 1988[95]	76	11 mos–19 years (median 8 yrs)	2.5:1	67%	62% 3-yr survival
Patte, 1992[34]	84	10 mos–16 years (median 9 yrs)	1.5:1	71%	75% 3-yr survival (81% for patients with mediastinal disease and "negative" bone marrow)

tocols with chemotherapy and local radiation therapy produced complete remissions but had a high incidence of fatal relapse in the bone marrow, central nervous system, and gonads.[31] More aggressive chemotherapy regimens, including central nervous system prophylaxis, have resulted in much improved results. Long-term disease-free survival rates of 60 to 80% can be achieved in children.[31, 34, 95]

In adults, the prognosis is not quite as good. Coleman and colleagues reported a 56% 3-year disease-free survival rate in a series of 44 adult patients treated with aggressive chemotherapy and central nervous system prophylaxis.[32] Autologous bone marrow transplantation may further improve survival in adult patients.[96] Tumor burden at the time of diagnosis is the most consistent prognostic factor.[31] Specific adverse prognostic factors include bone marrow or central nervous system involvement, elevated initial serum lactate dehydrogenase (LDH) concentration of > 300 IU/L (normal < 200), age over 30 years, leukocyte count greater than 50 × 10^9/L, and failure to achieve a prompt complete remission.[31–33]

LARGE-CELL LYMPHOMA OF THE MEDIASTINUM

The clinical and pathologic features of large-cell lymphoma of the mediastinum have been better defined in recent years[97–112] (Table 6–5).

Clinical Features

The largest series of large-cell lymphomas of the mediastinum included 60 cases and was published in 1986 by Perrone and colleagues.[105] These investigators found a predominance of young adults and of women. Eighty-five percent of the patients were younger than 35 years; there were 43 females and 17 males. Seventy-three per cent of the patients had disease localized to the thoracic cavity at presentation. Symptoms at presentation usually related to the enlarging mass and included the superior vena cava syndrome, cough, shortness of breath, and chest pain. Five of the sixty patients were asymptomatic and had a mediastinal mass on a routine chest radiograph. Not all series have shown a predominance of females.[111]

An older patient population with mediastinal lymphoma has also been described.[102] The older patients are more often male and more likely to have lymphomas with immunoblastic morphology. Most patients with mediastinal large-cell lymphoma do not have superficial lymphadenopathy.[105, 106, 111] When advanced, the disease has a tendency to infiltrate the kidney. Involvement of the bone marrow and central nervous system is uncommon.

Histopathology

Histologically, mediastinal large-cell lymphomas typically are sclerotic. The fibrosis may

Table 6–5. Mediastinal Large-Cell Lymphoma: Summary of Studies

First Author/Year	No. of Patients	Male-to-Female Ratio	Age (yrs)	% Localized	Recurrences/Prognostic Factors
Perrone/1986[105]	60	17:43 (72% female)	10–63 (median 25)	73%	42% recurred (1–19 mos after diagnosis) **Poor prognostic factors:** age <25, extrathoracic disease, incomplete initial response to therapy (latter two interdependent) **Favorable prognostic factors:** greater degree of sclerosis (related to initial response to therapy)
Jacobson/1988[103]	30	10:20 (67% female)	15–71 (median 34)	73%	20% recurred (all within 14 mos) **Poor prognostic factor:** bulky mediastinal mass (at least 10 cm in diameter on chest radiograph) **Favorable prognostic factor:** more aggressive chemotherapy (dose intensity score >80%)
Todeschini/1990[106]	21	6:15 (71% female)	15–42 (median 30)	61%	61% complete remission Among patients treated more aggressively, 13 of 15 (87%) achieved complete remission; relapse-free survival curve for these 13 shows a plateau at 90%; median follow-up is 39 mos
Kirn/1993[111]	57	30:27 (47% female)	Median 30	*	53% complete response 54% relapsed (2–28 months after diagnosis) **Poor prognostic factors:** pleural effusion, extranodal disease, positive post-therapy gallium scan

*56 of the 57 patients had disease restricted to sites above the diaphragm.

be "compartmentalizing" with "hooks" of collagen around groups of tumor cells[105] (Fig. 6–3). Some cases have broad bands of fibrosis. Another pattern has fine interstitial fibrosis surrounding individual tumor cells. Most cases are morphologically classified as follicular center cell lymphomas, either large cleaved or large noncleaved cell.[102, 105] Nuclei are often multilobated. Frequently, the lymphoma is difficult to classify, because the tumor cells are smaller than most large-cell lymphomas. Depending at least partly on what fixative is used, the cytoplasm varies from clear to eosinophilic. Formalin fixation produces a more prominent clear cytoplasm.[105]

Depending on the series, 20 to 70% of primary mediastinal large-cell lymphomas have immunoblastic morphology.[101, 102, 105, 110, 111] Twelve percent of cases in the Perrone series were composed of monomorphous large cells with round-to-oval nuclei and prominent central nucleoli (termed B-immunoblastic sarcoma in the Lukes-Collins classification). Twenty-two percent of cases could be classified as "T-immunoblastic sarcoma." These tumors are composed of markedly pleomorphic large cells with prominent nucleoli, abundant cytoplasm, and well-defined cell borders. Some of these may represent what has later been described as "Ki-1 large-cell anaplastic lymphoma" (see later).

Residual thymic structures are commonly identified. Persistent thymic tissue may form epithelial-lined cysts.[105] Invasion of blood vessels is often prominent.

There is some variation among different reports on the distinctiveness of histologic features. Not all mediastinal lymphomas have sclerosis. Percentages of mediastinal lymphomas that have sclerosis range from 38 to 100%, depending on the report.[4, 97, 102, 105, 113] Series of large-cell lymphomas with sclerosis indicate a predilection for the mediastinum and, to a lesser extent, the retroperitoneum.[114, 115]

Also, not all mediastinal non-Hodgkin's, nonlymphoblastic lymphomas are large-cell. Four of twelve in the Levitt study were classified as diffuse small cleaved cell (some with sclerosis).[4] Only three out of eight in Moller et al.'s series were large cell; the remainder were composed of small-to-medium-sized tumor cells.[104] Seven out of the eight patients in this

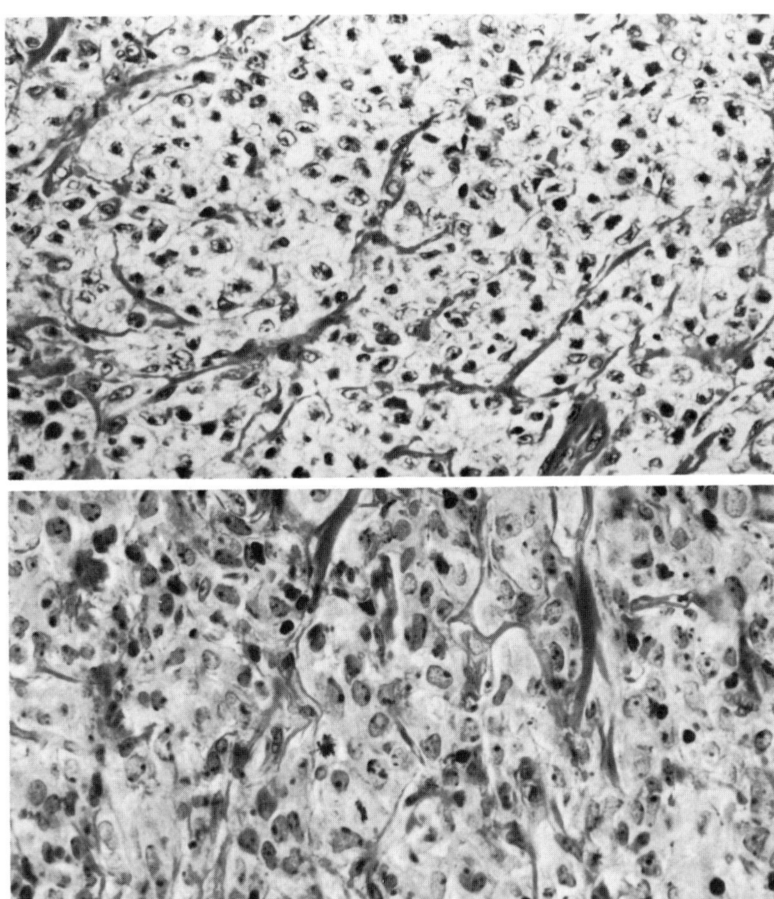

Figure 6–3. Mediastinal large cell lymphoma. "Compartmentalizing" fibrosis and large neoplastic cells are shown. The clear cytoplasm is more evident in formalin-fixed tissue (*top*) than when B5 fixative is used (*bottom*) (H&E, ×400).

study had progressive disease despite therapy and regardless of the histology, so it is not clear that the size of the cell in itself has any significance.

In another series, all mediastinal lymphomas were described as large-cell.[102] Because of the variability in cell size and apparent insignificance of cell size on prognosis, Moller and colleagues prefer the designation mediastinal clear cell lymphoma.[116] Stein and Dallenbach prefer the term primary mediastinal B-cell lymphoma.[117] Differences among the studies probably relate to how cases were selected and/or variations in criteria and interpretation by the authors.

Immunopathology

Immunohistochemical studies have demonstrated leukocyte common antigen in 141 of 142 cases of mediastinal nonlymphoblastic non-Hodgkin's lymphomas.[97–99, 102, 104, 105] Epithelial membrane antigen and cytokeratin have been absent in all cases tested.[97, 105, 109, 110] However, entrapped thymic epithelium is cytokeratin-positive and must be distinguished from tumor. Even if not obvious on routine sections, thymic epithelium frequently becomes apparent with an immunoperoxidase stain for cytokeratin.

Despite the marked predominance of T cells in the thymus, most series find that nearly all large-cell lymphomas of the mediastinum express B-cell markers, most commonly CD19 and CD20.[97, 98, 102, 104, 111] (See appendix for review of CD nomenclature.) CD20 is particularly useful, because it can be demonstrated in formalin- or B5-fixed, paraffin-embedded tissue using the L26 antibody. Staining with CD20 is weaker in Bouins'- or Zenker's-fixed tissues and in decalcified tissues.[51] CD20 is relatively specific for B-cell lymphomas; few T-cell neoplasms (less than 5%) express this antigen.[48, 49, 118, 119] CD20 is absent in nonhematologic neoplasms.[48, 54]

In immunohistochemical studies using paraffin-embedded tissue, 22 of 23 mediastinal large-cell lymphomas demonstrated CD20.[108–110] Only 1 of 39 was positive for CD43 (not the same case that lacked CD20), and 1 of 37 stained for CD45RO (Table 6–6).

LN1 (CDw75) and MB2 are additional B-cell markers for paraffin-embedded tissue that are less useful.[60, 109] LN1 reacts primarily with mature, surface immunoglobulin–positive B cells, particularly those in the germinal centers. Normal erythrocytes and 10 to 15% of peripheral blood T cells also express this antigen. The antibody works better in tissues fixed in B5 than in formalin. Overall, it identifies about 75% of B-cell lymphomas, and it labels 5 to 10% of T-cell neoplasms. LN1 has wide cross-reactivity with nonhematopoietic tissues.[51] LN1 labeled 10 of 15 mediastinal large-cell lymphomas.[109]

MB2 identifies normal B cells and some macrophages. It also labels nonhematopoietic tissues and neoplasms, including most Ewing's sarcomas and peripheral neuroectodermal tumors.[54, 60, 120] MB2 stained 12 of 15 mediastinal large-cell lymphomas.[109]

Immunophenotyping studies on frozen sections of mediastinal large-cell lymphomas have shown some unusual features. Despite reactivity with pan–B cell marker CD20, at least half the cases fail to demonstrate immunoglobulin.[102, 104, 110] In contrast, only 25% of all large-cell lymphomas are immunoglobulin-negative.[102] Using an immunoperoxidase assay on frozen sections, Moller and colleagues compared the phenotype of 12 mediastinal large-cell lymphomas with 46 follicular center cell lymphomas[116] (Table 6–7).

The mediastinal lymphomas were significantly more likely to express CD11c. They were less likely to express CD10 and CD21. CD11c (p150,95) belongs to a family of leukocyte adhesion proteins.[51, 121] These are glycoprotein heterodimers expressed on the cell surface that are important in cell-cell interactions. CD11c also functions as complement receptor for C3bi. This antigen is expressed on granulocytes, monocytes, and macrophages. On lymphoid cells, it is a marker of cell activation, and can be expressed on transformed B cells and T cells. CD11c is present on sinusoidal B cells in lymph nodes and is absent on follicular center cells. In addition to the mediastinal lymphomas, it labels hairy cell leukemia, some B-cell chronic lymphocytic leukemias, some T-cell lymphomas, and occasional lymphomas of uncertain lineage.[116, 122]

CD10 is known as the common acute lymphoblastic leukemia antigen (CALLA).[51, 116] It is expressed at an early stage of B-cell development and then later re-expressed by follicular center B cells. CD10 is expressed by hematopoietic precursor cells in the bone marrow. It is present on granulocytes, fibroblasts, and cells of the renal tubules and glomeruli. CD10 is present on most acute lymphoblastic leukemias and lymphoid blast crises of chronic myelogenous leukemia. CD10 may be expressed by T-cell acute lymphoblastic leukemia and lymphoblastic lymphoma, Burkitt's lymphoma, follicular lymphoma, and multiple myeloma.

CD21 (B2,OKB7) is the type 2 complement receptor on B cells.[51, 121] It is the receptor for C3d and for the Epstein-Barr virus. It is expressed on surface immunoglobulin–positive B cells and is lost after cell activation. CD21 is present on most B cells in the peripheral blood and lymphoid tissue. The follicular dendritic cells of germinal centers strongly express CD21; the dendritic pattern of staining ob-

Table 6–6. Phenotype of Mediastinal Large-Cell Lymphoma in Paraffin-Embedded Sections*

	CD45	CD20	CD43	CD45RO	CDw75	MB2†
#	24/24	22/23	1/39	1/37	10/15	12/15
%	100	96	3	3	67	80

= number of cases positive for antigen/total number of cases tested; % = percentage of cases that are positive.
*Data from references 108–110.
†MB2 does not have a CD designation.

Table 6–7. Phenotypic Comparison of Mediastinal Large-Cell Lymphoma with Follicular Center Cell Lymphoma (as Determined by the Immunoperoxidase Assay on Frozen Sections)*

Antigen	No. of Positive Cases/Total Tested (% Positive)	
	Mediastinal Large-Cell Lymphoma	*Extramediastinal Follicular Center Cell Lymphoma*
CD5	0/11 (0%)	5/46 (11%)
CD10	0/12 (0%)	19/45 (42%)
CD11c	5/10 (50%)	5/43 (12%)
CD19	12/12 (100%)	44/46 (96%)
CD20	11/12 (92%)	45/45 (100%)
CD21	0/12 (0%)	14/42 (33%)
CD22	12/12 (100%)	43/46 (93%)
CD30	0/12 (0%)	0/43 (0%)
CD38	2/12 (17%)	13/45 (29%)

*Modified from reference 116.

scures the evaluation of germinal center B cells. CD21 is present on most B-cell chronic lymphocytic leukemias and follicular lymphomas, some large-cell lymphomas, some lymphoblastic lymphomas, and occasional T-cell neoplasms.

When they do express immunoglobulin, mediastinal large-cell lymphomas frequently demonstrate IgG or IgA.[102] Frequent expression of plasma cell antigen PC-1 has led to speculation that these lymphoma cells correspond to a late step of B-cell differentiation.[104] The lack of immunoglobulin expression is unexplained. These tumors may arise from thymic B cells, which are negative for CD21 (but positive for surface immunoglobulin).[108] Also, the adhesion receptor profile of thymic B-cell lymphoma is similar to that of normal medullary B cells.[123]

Not all mediastinal large-cell lymphomas need have the same origin. Those which express immunoglobulin may originate from follicular center cells and arise from mediastinal lymph nodes. Indeed, tumors in older patients are predominantly immunoglobulin-positive, more often immunoblastic in morphology, and occur more often in males. The tumors in younger patients tend to be immunoglobulin-negative and have a predilection for females. Perhaps this latter group of tumors arises in the thymus.[102]

Molecular Pathology

Genotypic analysis has demonstrated immunoglobulin gene rearrangements in 13 of 14 cases.[99, 102, 110] This is additional evidence of a B-cell origin for these neoplasms.

DNA Ploidy and Cell Proliferation Indices

Flow cytometry data for DNA analysis[124] have not been reported in any of the series of mediastinal lymphomas. For non-Hodgkin's lymphomas in general, aneuploidy occurs in 37% of cases.[125] The low-grade lymphomas are aneuploid less often than are the high-grade lymphomas.[126, 127] However, aneuploidy is not a consistent prognostic factor. T-cell lymphomas may be less commonly aneuploid than B-cell lymphomas are.[128, 129]

The proliferative activity of a lymphoma as assessed by the flow cytometric determination of cells in S phase correlates with histologic grade[130] and has been reported to be a significant prognostic factor.[127, 131, 132] In a study by Bauer et al., 50 large-cell lymphomas were analyzed for DNA content by flow cytometry using paraffin-embedded, formalin-fixed tissue.[131] High proliferative activity as defined by less than 80% of cells in G0G1 was the single most important adverse prognostic factor and was independent of other factors (performance status and stage of disease). Paraffin-embedded tissue is suboptimal, especially for measurement of cell cycle phases.[133] Fresh or frozen tissue is preferable. Nevertheless, proliferative activity is a logical correlate of tumor aggressiveness in lymphomas. As noted earlier, S phase correlates with the histologic grade of the lymphoma.[126, 134] Ploidy and S phase analysis can also be performed using computerized image analysis on Feulgen-stained material.[135]

Another measure of proliferative activity is immunoreactivity for Ki-67[86, 136] (see earlier). In one study of 8 mediastinal large-cell lymphomas, Ki-67 was present in 4 to 50% of tumor cell nuclei.[7] It had no correlation with clinical parameters. In general, most studies show a correlation between the percentage of cells demonstrating Ki-67 and the grade of the lymphoma.[137] Among intermediate- and high-grade lymphomas (including those with mediastinal involvement), poorer survival has been associated with Ki-67 labeling exceeding 60%.[7, 138] However, not all studies agree with this finding.[139]

Antibodies to proliferating cell nuclear antigen (PCNA), or cyclin, also label proliferating cells and may be used in paraffin-embedded, formalin-fixed tissue.[136, 140–142] In a study of 140 non-Hodgkin's lymphomas, Klemi and colleagues correlated the presence of more than 50% PCNA-positive cells with high S phase and high histologic grade.[141] Tumors with a high PCNA expression and high S phase had a poorer prognosis. Large, prospective studies of uniformly treated patients are needed to meaningfully evaluate these measures of cell proliferation as prognostic factors.

Cytopathology

Fine needle aspiration and touch imprints can help in narrowing the differential diagnosis at the time of frozen sections.[143, 144] Non-Hodgkin's lymphomas, in general, are characterized cytologically by the presence of

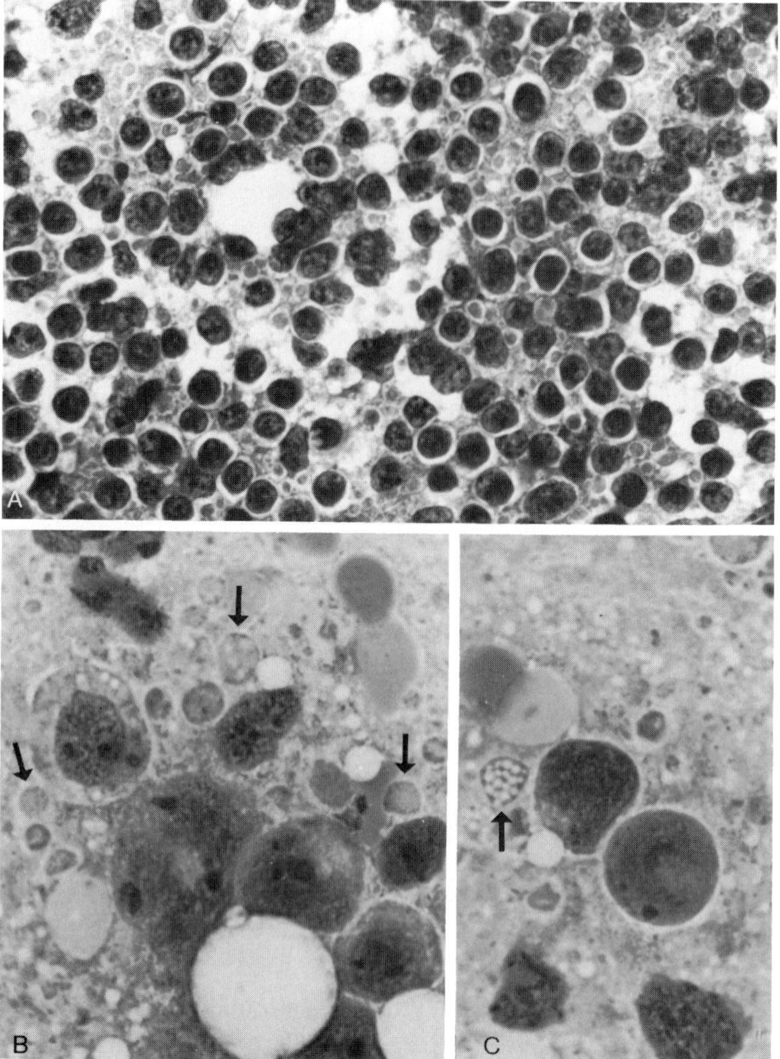

FIGURE 6–4. Touch imprints of large-cell lymphoma demonstrate individual, large cells. Numerous cytoplasmic fragments (known as lymphoglandular bodies) are present (*arrows*) in the Diff-Quik stained material. (*A,* Alcohol-fixed, H&E, stain, ×200; *B* and *C,* air-dried, Diff-Quik, ×1000.)

predominantly individual cells instead of the cohesive clusters associated with epithelial malignancy[145] (Fig. 6–4). Numerous lymphoglandular bodies (> 10 per high-power field) are another clue to the diagnosis of a lymphoma.[93]

In some mediastinal large-cell lymphomas, fine azurophilic granules have been identified in the cytoplasm of neoplastic cells.[110] Bizarre cells with prominent nucleoli may represent carcinoma, Hodgkin's disease, or a non-Hodgkin's lymphoma. Mitotic figures and tingible body macrophages along with a monomorphic cell population are features of a high-grade lymphoma. Germ cell tumors must also be considered. Immunologic studies can be performed on smears or cytospin preparations of a fine-needle aspirate to confirm a diagnosis.[146, 147]

Differential Diagnosis

The differential diagnosis includes thymoma, thymic carcinoma, metastatic carcinoma, and germ cell tumors. Immunoperoxidase studies for lymphoid markers help to establish the diagnosis of lymphoma and to exclude these other entities. Other types of lymphoma, including Hodgkin's disease, should be considered. Hodgkin's disease is characterized by inflammatory cells (eosinophils, neutrophils, plasma cells, small lymphocytes), which are usually absent in mediastinal large-cell lymphoma. Anaplastic large-cell lymphoma has larger and more bizarre cells than the typical mediastinal B-cell lymphoma. Strong expression of CD30 (Ki-1) is typical of this entity (see later).

Prognosis and Therapy

The prognosis of mediastinal large-cell lymphoma appears to be similar to the prognosis of large-cell lymphoma of other sites[103] (see Table 6–5). A complete remission rate of 80% was reported for patients presenting with "predominantly" mediastinal large-cell lymphoma and treated with cyclophosphamide, doxorubicin, vincristine, and prednisone (CHOP) chemotherapy and consolidation radiation therapy. The relapse-free survival rate at 5 years was 59%. Another report of 57 patients treated with varied chemotherapy and radiation therapy regimens described a 45% 5-year freedom-from-relapse rate.[111] The presence of a pleural effusion, large size of tumor, and involvement of two or more extranodal sites are significant adverse prognostic factors.[103, 111] A greater degree of sclerosis has been weakly correlated with better survival.[105] Immunoblastic morphology and age less than 25 years have been reported as adverse prognostic factors in one report but not in another.[105, 111]

A recent study from Italy obtained a high rate of complete remission using more aggressive chemotherapy: methotrexate with leucovorin, doxorubicin, cyclophosphamide, vincristine, prednisone, bleomycin (MACOP-B) or methotrexate, bleomycin, doxorubicin, cyclophosphamide, vincristine, and dexamethasone (M-BACOD).[106] Using these regimens, 90% of patients who achieve complete remission may be cured.

Pathogenesis

The pathogenesis of mediastinal large-cell lymphoma is as unclear as that of most other lymphomas. The thymus does contain B cells in the medulla.[148] Authors have speculated that the mediastinal lymphomas arise from intrathymic B cells.[97, 149] One report described abnormalities of the c-myc oncogene in three of six cases of mediastinal large-cell lymphoma.[150] These authors did not find bcl-2 gene rearrangements (associated with 85% of follicular lymphomas and 30% of large-cell lymphomas) or Epstein-Barr virus DNA sequences within these tumors using Southern blot hybridization.

OTHER NON-HODGKIN'S LYMPHOMAS

Isaacson et al. have reported a low-grade lymphoma of the thymus that histologically resembles the lymphomas in mucosa-associated lymphoid tissue (MALT)[149] (Fig. 6–5). These tumors had reactive germinal centers with a surrounding infiltrate of monotypic "centrocyte-like" B cells that infiltrated Hassall's cor-

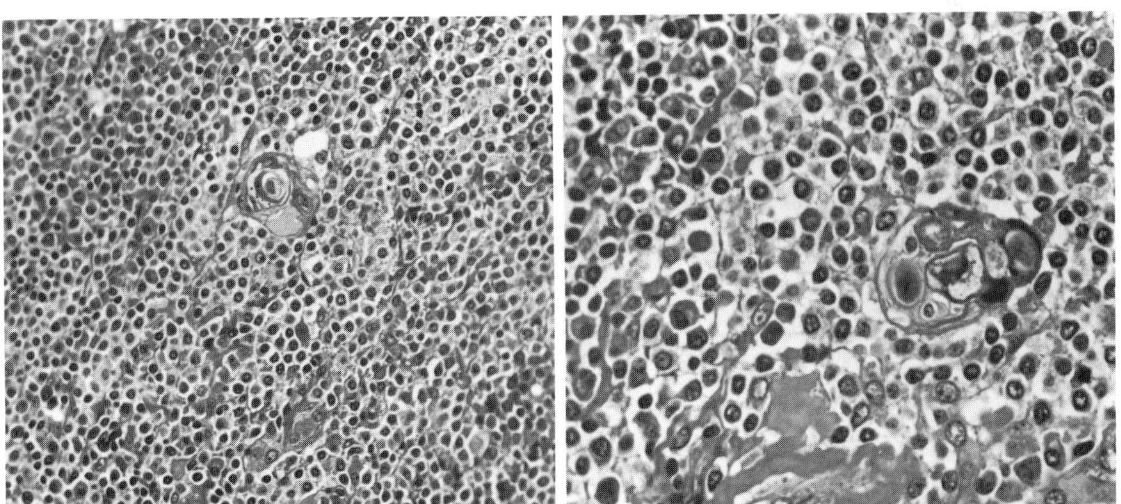

Figure 6–5. Low-grade B cell lymphoma of mucosa-associated lymphoid tissue involving the thymus. These photographs are from one of the two reported cases of this entity.[151] The dense population of small lymphoid cells with clear-to-eosinophilic cytoplasm and distinct cell borders surrounds and infiltrates Hassall's corpuscles. (H&E, *Left*, ×100; *Right*, ×400.) (From Takagi N, Nakamura S, Yamamoto K, et al. Malignant lymphoma of mucosa-associated lymphoid tissue arising in the thymus of a patient with Sjögren's syndrome. Cancer 1992; 1347–1355.)

puscles to form "lymphoepithelial lesions." These lymphoepithelial lesions resembled the myoepithelial structures seen in lymphomas arising in salivary glands. Takagi and colleagues reported a similar-appearing case in a patient with Sjögren's syndrome.[151] According to Nakagawa et al., the patient reported by Isaacson's group also had Sjögren's syndrome.[110] Many of the MALT lymphomas are indistinguishable from monocytoid B-cell lymphoma and appear to be the same entity.

Suster described a mediastinal large-cell lymphoma with a distinctive histologic pattern.[152] The tumors consisted of lymphoid tissue with prominent germinal centers. In the interfollicular areas were clusters of large atypical cells. The large cells also penetrated the germinal centers (Fig. 6–6). The patients (two male, one female) ranged in age from 36 to 70 years. All had disease confined to the mediastinum. After total surgical excision followed by radiation therapy, all patients were alive without relapse up to 22 years after the original diagnosis.

Various T-cell lymphomas other than the lymphoblastic type may involve the mediastinum. Head and colleagues described two children with a malignancy resembling adult T-cell leukemia/lymphoma.[153] These patients had skin rash, hepatosplenogemaly, and lymphadenopathy. They had leukemia characterized by lymphoid cells with irregular nuclei and a mature T-cell phenotype. Both patients died within 1 year of presentation. Unlike the adults, the children had mediastinal masses and were seronegative for human T-cell leukemia/lymphoma virus (HTLV-1). Adult T-cell leukemia/lymphoma affects adults (older than

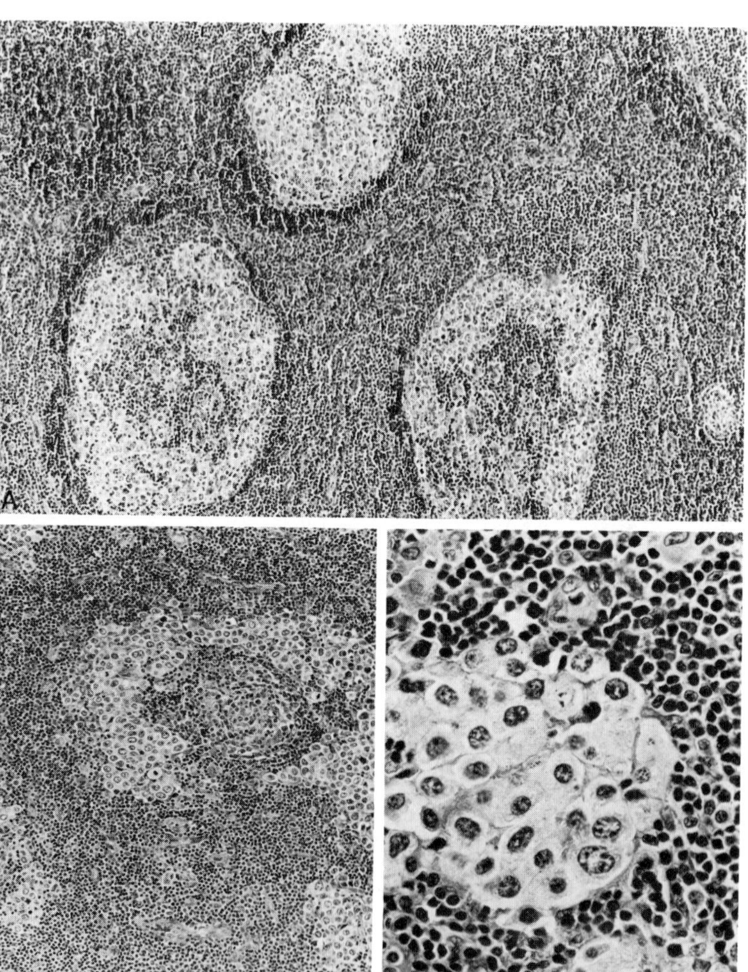

Figure 6–6. Large-cell lymphoma of mediastinum with tropism for germinal centers. *A*, Replacement of follicles by neoplastic cells (H&E, ×40). *B*, Neoplastic cells are distributed around a germinal center (H&E, ×100). *C*, Neoplastic cells have clear cytoplasm and well-defined cell borders (H&E, ×400). (From Suster S. Large cell lymphoma of the mediastinum with marked tropism for germinal centers. Cancer 1990; 69:2910–2916.)

16 years) and is characterized by peripheral lymphadenopathy, leukemic dissemination, skin involvement, hepatosplenomegaly, and hypercalcemia.[154–156] The tumor is composed of pleomorphic malignant cells with a mature T-cell phenotype. The lesion is associated with HTLV-1 infection and has an aggressive course. The mediastinum is not typically involved.

In the 1980s, Ki-1 large-cell anaplastic lymphoma was defined as a clinicopathologic entity.[117, 157–160] Mediastinal involvement may occur, most commonly when the disease is disseminated. It is a type of lymphoma characterized by large, pleomorphic cells that express the Ki-1 (CD30) antigen. The cells have bizarre nuclei, prominent nucleoli, and abundant cytoplasm (Fig. 6–7). Multinucleated tumor cells are often present. The mitotic rate is high. The tumor cells tend to spread within the sinusoids of lymph nodes. Capsular thickening and parenchymal fibrosis are common.[161] The fibrosis ranges from fibrillary to dense and sclerotic. Microscopically, the tumors may resemble carcinoma, melanoma, or Hodgkin's disease. This resemblance leads to frequent misdiagnosis.

Patients range from 3 months to 78 years of age.[117, 162] Most patients are between 8 and 30 years old. A second peak in incidence occurs in later adulthood. The male-to-female ratio is 1.6:1. Most patients (82%) present with peripheral lymphadenopathy. Extranodal disease was identified in 42% of patients, with the skin being the most common site.[117] Bone marrow involvement is uncommon. Some patients have "secondary" anaplastic large-cell lymphomas. These are tumors that occur with or subsequent to another type of lymphoma. The original tumor may be a T- or B-cell lymphoma, or Hodgkin's disease (particularly the lymphocyte predominant type).[117]

Marker studies demonstrate that 77% of tumors have a T-cell phenotype, 13% have a B-cell phenotype, and 10% are indeterminate.[162] Gene rearrangement studies usually confirm the immunohistochemical findings.[163] Most cases demonstrate epithelial membrane antigen (EMA).[117] Up to 40% of cases are negative for CD45 (leukocyte common antigen, or LCA).[164] One must be cautious about misinterpreting these immunohistologic data (EMA+, LCA−) in favor of metastatic carcinoma. Additional B-cell and T-cell antigens must be studied to reach the correct diagnosis.

Recent studies have found that CD30-positive lymphomas are morphologically heterogeneous. In addition to the anaplastic large-cell type, CD30 is expressed by some more monomorphic large-cell lymphomas composed of smaller cells.[165]

Cytogenetic studies of CD30-positive anaplastic large-cell lymphomas have identified a recurring chromosomal abnormality: a translocation with a break in the long arm of chromosome 5 (q35), usually a reciprocal translo-

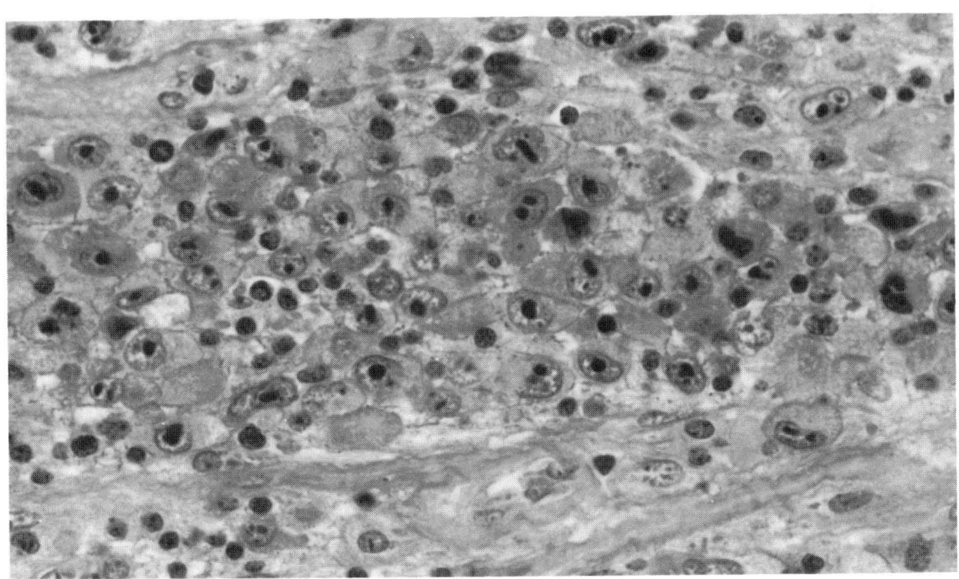

Figure 6–7. CD30 (Ki-1) positive, large-cell anaplastic lymphoma is characterized by large cells with prominent nucleoli, abundant cytoplasm, and distinct cell borders (H&E, ×400).

cation between chromosomes 2 and 5 [(t2;5)(p23;q35)].[161, 166, 167] Initial reports associated this translocation with malignant histiocytosis.[168] However, the cases reported as malignant histiocytosis may actually be anaplastic large-cell lymphomas.[117, 166] The 2:5 translocation appears to be associated only with the CD30+ lymphomas that have the anaplastic large cell morphology, and only with those of T-cell or indeterminate phenotype.

Whether the Ki-1 large-cell anaplastic lymphomas should be separated on clinicopathologic features from other large-cell lymphomas is controversial. Large, prospective studies of uniformly treated patients with thorough histologic, phenotypic, and cytogenetic analyses are needed. According to studies of small groups of patients, the prognosis in general seems similar to[105, 162, 165] or, in some reports, better than that for large-cell lymphoma.[161, 166] A study from The Netherlands found that intensively treated patients with large-cell anaplastic lymphoma had a significantly better survival than did patients with other types of T-cell lymphoma.[169] Younger age and skin involvement at presentation are favorable prognostic factors.[117, 165, 170, 171] Survival for 9 years without therapy has been reported.[172] However, in one study of Ki-1 positive lymphomas by Offit and colleagues, disease-free survival was relatively poor compared with overall survival because of a high relapse rate.[166]

CD30-positive, large-cell anaplastic lymphomas involve the mediastinum in 10 to 15% of cases.[158, 162, 173] Mediastinal involvement usually occurs when the disease is widely disseminated. In a study of 41 patients with Ki-1 positive large-cell lymphoma, two patients presented with a mediastinal mass.[165] In a study of 14 non-Hodgkin's lymphomas limited to the mediastinum, Nakagawa and colleagues identified five Ki-1 positive large-cell anaplastic lymphomas.[110] In contrast to the large-cell lymphomas with sclerosis, the large-cell anaplastic tumors did not express B-cell marker CD20. Two of the five demonstrated CD43. All were negative for CD15 (Leu M1). This series is unlike the other studies described earlier in which virtually all primary mediastinal large-cell lymphomas expressed a B-cell phenotype. Part of the reason for the discrepancy may involve geography. Japan has a higher proportion of lymphomas with a T-cell phenotype than does the United States or Europe.[174]

However, close examination of the published series from the United States is also enlightening. As noted earlier concerning Perrone's series of mediastinal large-cell lymphomas, 22% of cases were classified as immunoblastic T-cell by the Lukes-Collins classification.[105] Some of these cases might represent the CD30 anaplastic large-cell lymphoma. Complete phenotyping was not performed in this study. Also, in Waldron et al.'s series of 20 mediastinal large-cell lymphomas, nine patients (45%) had the immunoblastic T-cell morphology.[101] Studies performed on three of these nine patients demonstrated a T-cell phenotype. In two other series, 3 of 27 mediastinal large-cell lymphomas had a T-cell phenotype.[7] Thus, a proportion of mediastinal large-cell lymphomas have a T-cell phenotype. Some of these are the CD30-positive large-cell anaplastic type.

Most types of non-Hodgkin's lymphoma may involve mediastinal lymph nodes when disseminated. Jenkins and colleagues studied 81 lymphoma patients for radiographic evidence of intrathoracic disease.[175] They identified mediastinal and/or hilar lymphadenopathy in 1 of 11 patients with follicular lymphoma, 5 of 25 with well or moderately well differentiated lymphocytic lymphoma, 8 of 26 with diffuse poorly differentiated lymphocytic lymphoma, and 1 of 17 with large-cell lymphoma. In total, 21% of all patients with non-Hodgkin's lymphoma had mediastinal lymphadenopathy. In the absence of pulmonary or pleural disease, mediastinal lymphadenopathy did not affect the prognosis adversely. Small noncleaved cell lymphoma (Burkitt's and non-Burkitt's) infrequently involves the mediastinum.[176, 177] Unusual cases of primary mediastinal Burkitt's-like lymphoma have been reported.[7, 100]

MEDIASTINAL LYMPHOMAS IN ANIMALS

Lymphomas originating in the thymus are common in certain strains of mice and in domestic cats.[178] Histologically, these thymic lymphomas have a lymphoblastic morphology and originate from T cells. In cats, lymphomas are caused by oncornaviruses. In mice, strains have been developed that have high or low incidences of lymphomas. For example, AKR mice have a high risk of spontaneously developing a thymic lymphoma that is related to a retrovirus. With neonatal inoculation of retrovirus, 100% of the mice develop a thymic lymphoma at between 60 and 100 days of age.[179] Chemical carcinogens and radiation induce thymic lymphomas in AKR mice as well as in several other strains.[178] The development of the lymphoma within the thymus can be followed by examining the organ at different stages of tumor development.

HODGKIN'S DISEASE

Until the 1970s there was much confusion about mediastinal Hodgkin's disease. The eminent pathologist James Ewing wrote that thymic Hodgkin's disease originated from "reticulum cells of the thymus" and should be separated from other forms of Hodgkin's disease.[180] There was great difficulty in distinguishing thymic epithelial cells from the atypical mononuclear cells and Reed-Sternberg cells of Hodgkin's disease. "Granulomatous thymoma"[181] or "carcinoma of the thymus of granulomatous type"[182] were used as designations for what we now accept as Hodgkin's disease. The problem was clarified by clinical-pathologic correlation. Among patients presenting with isolated "granulomatous thymoma," a large number developed extrathoracic nodal metastases. The "metastases" were indistinguishable from Hodgkin's disease.[183–185]

Epidemiology

Hodgkin's disease accounts for 1% of all new cancers in the United States and other developed countries.[186, 187] It has a bimodal age distribution with a peak in the late 20s followed by a decline until age 45 years. The incidence then increases steadily with age. There are several differences between the disease affecting the younger patients and that affecting the older group.[188] The nodular sclerosis type is more frequent in the younger ages, whereas mixed cellularity is more common in the older group. Older patients are less likely to have a mediastinal mass. Mediastinal involvement occurs in 70% of patients younger than 40 years and in only 44% of those over age 60.[188]

Among the younger patients, the incidence varies geographically according to the level of economic development.[187, 189] In underdeveloped countries, a greater proportion of patients are children (younger than 15 years). Also, patients are more likely to present with symptomatic, advanced stage disease. The mixed cellularity histologic type is more common. With economic development, the incidence of Hodgkin's increases among young adults. In the United States and Europe, the risk of Hodgkin's disease in young adults increases with higher social class, as defined by education or occupation. Among lower socioeconomic groups in the United States, the "third world" epidemiologic pattern emerges.[190]

These data have led to the hypothesis that Hodgkin's disease may occur as a rare consequence of a common infection.[187] The risk increases if infection is delayed until adolescence or later. The epidemiology of Hodgkin's disease is similar to paralytic poliomyelitis in the prevaccine era, when early exposure to the virus was protective. For both, rates vary with economic status. This similarity (plus other clinical and histopathologic features) leads to speculation that the pathogenesis of Hodgkin's involves an infectious agent. Epstein-Barr virus is one candidate. Patients with Hodgkin's disease are more likely to have a history of infectious mononucleosis, a syndrome caused by Epstein-Barr virus.[191] Epstein-Barr virus has been demonstrated within affected lymph nodes from some Hodgkin's disease patients.[192] In particular, virtually all cases from underdeveloped countries appear to be associated with Epstein-Barr virus.[193, 194] (See later discussion on pathogenesis.)

Clinical Features

Most patients present with peripheral lymphadenopathy, usually in the cervical area.[195] Mediastinal lymph nodes are enlarged in approximately 60% of patients.[196, 197] However, only 3% of patients with Hodgkin's disease have disease limited to intrathoracic sites, usually the anterior mediastinum.[198] Fever and night sweats are present at the time of diagnosis in 25 to 30%. Fever, night sweats, and/or weight loss of greater than 10% of body weight in 6 months ("B" symptoms) are poor prognostic factors. Patients with B symptoms are more likely to have a mediastinal mass.[197] Extensive mediastinal disease (defined as mediastinal enlargement greater than one third of the chest diameter) is also an adverse prognostic factor.[199] In a series of children, mediastinal enlargement greater than or equal to one quarter of the chest diameter indicated a greater likelihood of intrathoracic relapse in patients treated only with radiation therapy.[197]

With isolated mediastinal Hodgkin's disease, the tumors are most often discovered on routine chest radiographs in asymptomatic patients.[183, 184] In other cases, chest pain, respiratory infections, dyspnea, or weight loss leads to the chest radiograph. Numbers of males and females are about equal.

The role of laparotomy for accurate staging of Hodgkin's disease is controversial.[200] Approximately one third of patients with clinical Ann Arbor stage I or II disease[201] (Table 6–8) will have unsuspected splenic involvement. Even CT cannot adequately visualize nodules of less than 1 cm. Its sensitivity in detecting splenic involvement has been reported as only 31%. Perhaps newer CT scanners and/or magnetic resonance imaging will be better. The indication for staging laparotomy is to determine the course of therapy.[202] For example, a clinical stage I or II patient might get radiation therapy alone. If intra-abdominal disease is discovered at surgery, the patient is then "upstaged," and chemotherapy would be used. Obviously, for the laparotomy to be of value, the pathologist must carefully examine the surgical specimens. In particular, the spleen must be grossly sectioned as thinly as possible (every 3 to 4 mm) to detect small nodules.

Hodgkin's disease tends to spread along contiguous areas.[196] In theory, mediastinal disease would spread first to supraclavicular, infraclavicular, or cervical nodes. Intra-abdominal disease would follow. (Mediastinal disease may spread to hilar lymph nodes prior to pulmonary involvement.) Thus, a patient with a mediastinal mass in the absence of lymphadenopathy would be unlikely to have intra-abdominal disease. Indeed, among 27 patients with disease clinically limited to intrathoracic sites, only 2 had occult splenic involvement at staging laporatomy.[198] Both patients with splenic disease had systemic symptoms. None of the 18 patients without systemic symptoms had intra-abdominal disease at staging laparotomy.

Table 6–8. Ann Arbor Staging System for Hodgkin's Disease*

Stage I: Involvement of a single lymph node region
Stage II: Involvement of two or more lymph node regions on the same side of the diaphragm
Stage III: Involvement of lymph node regions on both sides of the diaphragm (may include spleen)
Stage IV: Multiple or disseminated foci of involvement of extralymphatic organs or tissues (usually bone marrow or liver)

Extranodal disease contiguous with an adjacent involved lymph node is designated by the extent of lymph node involvement (IE, IIE, or IIIE)
Patients are further classified as either A or B according to the absence or presence of systemic symptoms (fever, night sweats, or weight loss greater than 10% of body weight)

*Data from references 195, 201.

Hodgkin's disease does occur in acquired immunodeficiency syndrome (AIDS) patients. However, whether Hodgkin's disease can be related to human immunodeficiency virus (HIV) infection is not clear.[203, 204] Both affect patients at a similar age. The incidence of Hodgkin's disease does not seem to be increased among AIDS patients. In contrast to non-Hodgkin's lymphomas, the incidence of Hodgkin's disease among young men has not increased since 1980.[204–207] The association between Hodgkin's disease and HIV infection may be coincidental. Hodgkin's disease is not a criterion for the diagnosis of AIDS.

Nevertheless, Hodgkin's disease in patients with HIV has certain clinical and pathologic features. Clinically, the disease usually presents at an advanced stage; as many as 90% are stage III or IV.[208–211] Bone marrow involvement is common. The histopathology of Hodgkin's disease in HIV-positive patients tends to include fewer reactive lymphocytes and less fibrosis.[210, 211] Most cases are classified as the mixed cellularity type.[208, 210, 212] Mediastinal involvement even in patients with the nodular sclerosing type is relatively uncommon. In one group of 13 HIV patients with nodular sclerosing Hodgkin's disease, only 2 had mediastinal disease.[209, 212] In patients with HIV infection, Hodgkin's disease has a more aggressive course with a poor response to chemotherapy.[210, 213–217]

Histopathology

The importance of histopathology is primarily for the diagnosis and staging of Hodgkin's disease. The histologic types correlate with biologic aggressiveness of the disease. However, with modern chemotherapy, the histologic subtypes do not appear to have prognostic significance.[202, 218] The Rye classification is useful in recognizing the spectrum of histopathology. Four types are described: nodular sclerosis, mixed cellularity, lymphocyte predominant, and lymphocyte depleted.

In the *nodular sclerosis* type of Hodgkin's disease, dense collagenous bands divide the tumor into nodules (Fig. 6–8). Lacunar cells are also characteristic. These cells are variants of Reed-Sternberg cells that have clear cytoplasm

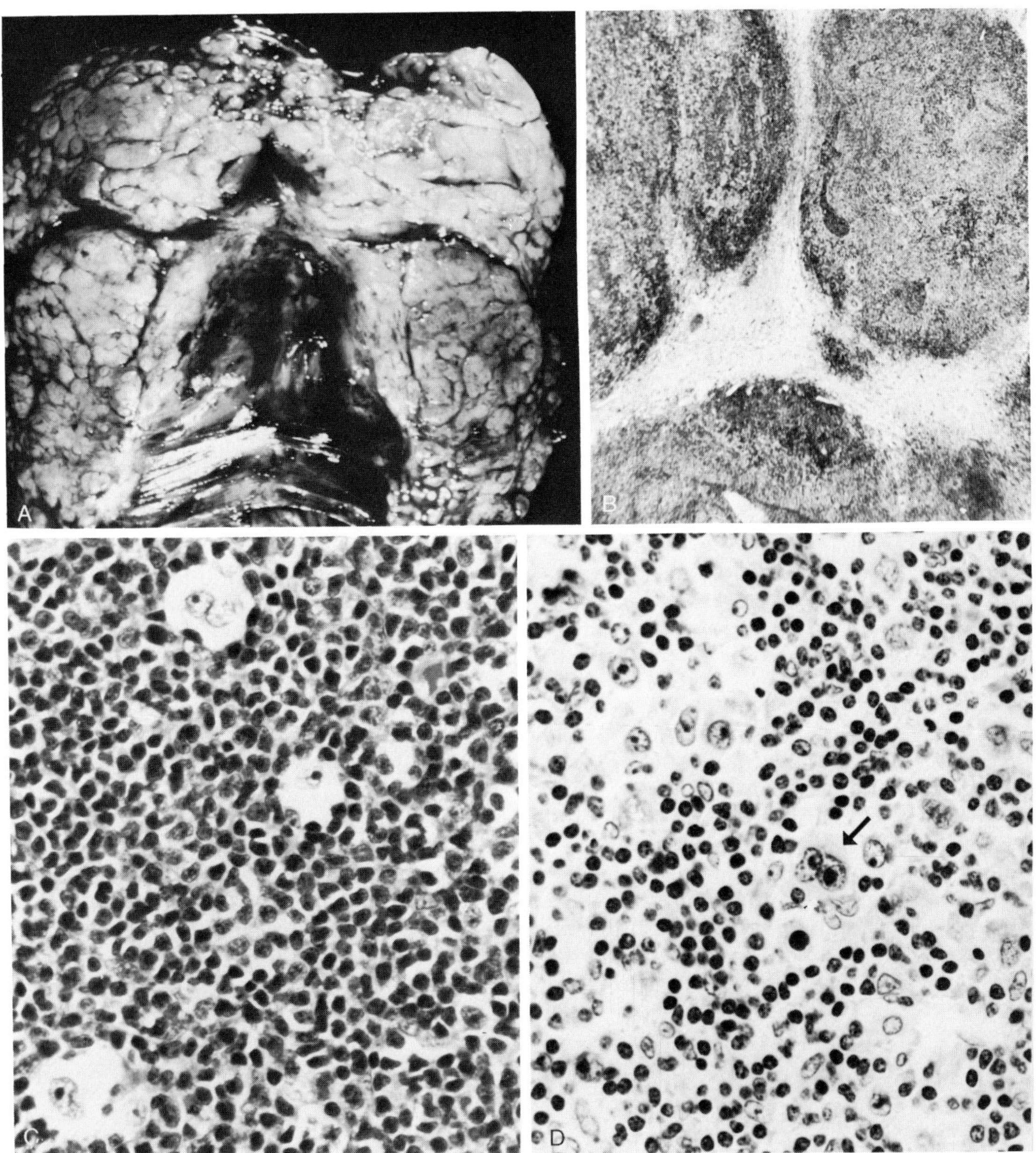

Figure 6–8. Nodular sclerosing Hodgkin's disease of the mediastinum. *A,* The nodularity can be appreciated in the gross photograph and simulates a thymoma. The tumor was resected along with the pericardium. *B,* Broad fibrous bands separate the tumor into nodules of lymphoid tissue (H&E, ×40). *C,* Lacunar cells are Reed-Sternberg cell variants that appear to be located within empty spaces (lacunae) (H&E, ×400). *D,* A Reed-Sternberg cell (*arrow*), atypical mononuclear cells, and a background of small lymphocytes are characteristic of Hodgkin's disease (H&E, ×400).

and polylobated nuclei. They appear to be within empty spaces, or lacunae, especially when formalin-fixed. As in all types of Hodgkin's disease, the "classic" Reed-Sternberg cell in the proper background is diagnostic. The classic Reed-Sternberg cell is a large cell with bilobed nucleus, pale chromatin, and prominent, eosinophilic nucleoli. Background cells include lymphocytes, eosinophils, plasma cells, histiocytes, and neutrophils. The cellularity of nodular sclerosing type is variable; some authors have described a cellular phase and a "lymphocyte depleted" phase. Investigators have tried to correlate histologic features with prognosis. MacLennan and colleagues found that those cases of nodular sclerosis with a greater percentage of anaplastic cells ("lymphocyte depleted" areas) had a poorer prognosis.[219] Others have not found such an association.[220]

Nodular sclerosing Hodgkin's disease in the mediastinum has the same general appearance as it does elsewhere. In addition, when the thymus is involved, there is a proliferation of thymic epithelium[183, 185] (Fig. 6–9). Sheets of thymic epithelial cells with formation of squamous lined cysts may be seen. Reed-Sternberg cells and variants often infiltrate the epithelium.

In the syncytial variant of nodular sclerosing Hodgkin's disease, sheets and cohesive clusters of large, malignant-appearing cells are present.[221, 222] The diagnosis is established by finding focal areas of typical nodular sclerosis and by demonstrating an appropriate phenotype. In a series of 18 cases of syncytial Hodgkin's reported by Strickler and colleagues, five were diagnosed on mediastinal biopsies.[221] In another series by Ben-Yehuda-Salz et al., all eight patients had mediastinal disease, and in most the mediastinal mass was "huge."[222]

Histologically, the differential diagnosis includes metastatic carcinoma, metastatic melanoma, germ cell tumors, thymic carcinoma, and large-cell lymphoma. Immunohistochemistry is useful. Cytokeratin expression would support a diagnosis of carcinoma or germ cell tumor (except seminoma, which is usually cytokeratin-negative). Melanomas are generally S100-positive. If immunohistochemical studies are equivocal, the distinction between syncytial Hodgkin's disease and large-cell lymphoma may be impossible.[223] In such cases, patients can be managed with the understanding that these two disorders may overlap and be indistinguishable.

The nodular sclerosis type of Hodgkin's disease is the most common variant, accounting for slightly more than 50% of cases in the United States.[207] It usually affects adolescents and young adults. Unlike other forms of Hodgkin's disease that have a preponderance of males, the nodular sclerosis type has a slight predilection for females (1.2:1). It has a high incidence of mediastinal involvement, and it is usually localized (stage I or II; see Table 6–1) at diagnosis.

In *lymphocyte predominant* Hodgkin's disease, the "L and H" (lymphohistiocytic) cells are characteristic.[224] These cells have pale cytoplasm, large polylobated ("twisted") nuclei, and small nucleoli (Fig. 6–10). Histiocytes are also present individually and in small clusters. The L and H cells and histiocytes produce a "moth-eaten" appearance. Classic Reed-Sternberg cells are rare. Epithelioid histiocytes and granulomata may be prominent. The growth pattern may be nodular or diffuse. Lymphocyte predominant Hodgkin's disease is uncommon in the mediastinum.[196, 224] In a series of 35 lymphocyte-predominant cases, Trudel and colleagues found three patients with mediastinal disease at presentation.[225] In one of the three, the mediastinum was the only site of disease. On a mediastinal biopsy, distinction from a thymoma can be difficult. Immunohistochemical studies for lymphoid markers and cytokeratin should be helpful. Unlike other

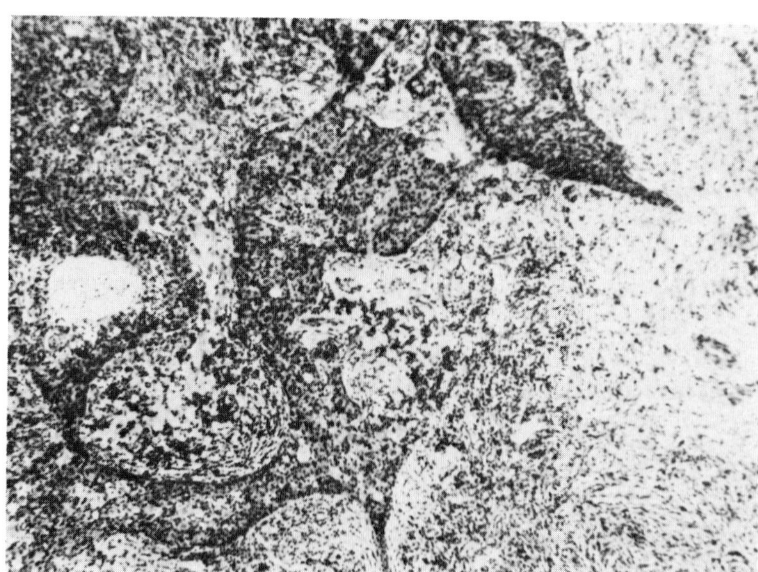

Figure 6–9. Epithelial proliferation, presumably of thymic origin, is illustrated in this case of nodular sclerosing Hodgkin's disease. A small cystic space within the epithelium can be seen on the left (H&E, ×100).

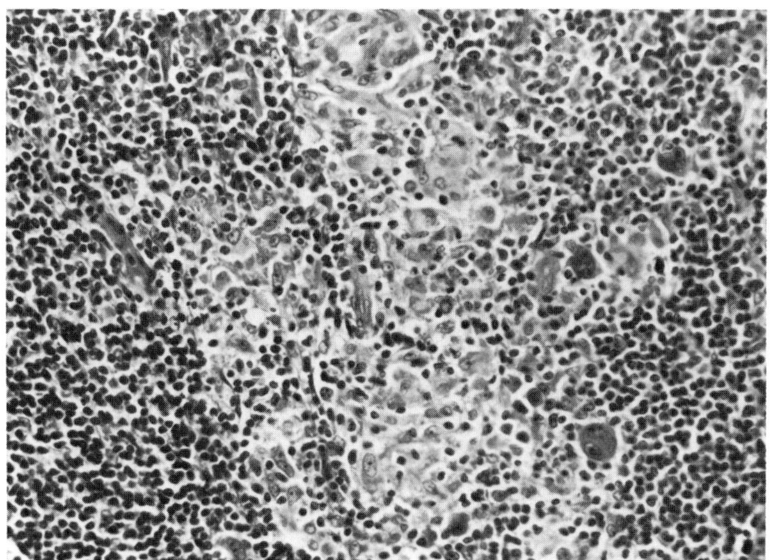

FIGURE 6–10. Mixed cellularity Hodgkin's disease. This photograph illustrates scattered Reed-Sternberg cell variants along with epithelioid histiocytes and lymphocytes. Fibrous bands are absent (H&E, ×200).

types of Hodgkin's disease, the lymphocyte predominant form has Reed-Sternberg cells that typically express B-cell marker CD20 and LCA. Reactivity for EMA is common. These cells usually do not express CD15 and CD30 (see later). B cells tend to predominate among the small lymphocytes. Small lymphocytic lymphoma would be another entity to consider. Demonstration that the small lymphocytes are monoclonal B cells would establish this diagnosis.

Lymphocyte predominant Hodgkin's disease accounts for about 5 to 10% of cases.[207] It occurs at virtually any age, with a median of 32 years.[225] Most cases are asymptomatic and present at an early stage. Lymphocyte predominant Hodgkin's disease is generally an indolent disease. However, relapses do occur, particularly for the nodular type. One study found that patients with nodular lymphocyte predominant disease had significantly more relapses than did those with diffuse lymphocyte predominant disease.[226]

Mixed cellularity is to some extent a diagnosis of exclusion. These are the cases that lack the fibrosis of nodular sclerosis. They contain too many Reed-Sternberg cells to be lymphocyte predominant. These cases have diffuse effacement of the lymph node by a polymorphous cell population with eosinophils, plasma cells, neutrophils, histiocytes, and lymphocytes (Fig. 6–11). Reed-Sternberg cells are easily detected. Mixed cellularity can closely resemble non-Hodgkin's lymphomas, particularly the peripheral T-cell type.[227] Immunohistologic studies can be helpful in supporting the diagnosis.

Mixed cellularity is second in frequency to nodular sclerosis, accounting for approximately one third of cases.[207] Compared to the nodular sclerosing type, mixed cellularity disease more often presents at an advanced stage and is more likely to be associated with systemic symptoms.[196] Mediastinal involvement is less common than with nodular sclerosing Hodgkin's disease. In one series, 37% of patients with mixed cellularity Hodgkin's disease had mediastinal disease, compared with 81% of patients with the nodular sclerosing type.[228]

Lymphocyte depleted Hodgkin's disease is controversial at the present time. As originally described, there were two types of lymphocyte depleted disease: diffuse fibrosis and reticular. The former is characterized by cellular depletion and abundant, "disorderly" fibrosis without collagenous bands. The reticular variant has a more cellular composition. In both forms, the Reed-Sternberg cells are the dominant cellular component.

The problem with lymphocyte depleted disease is in its distinction from non-Hodgkin's lymphoma (NHL). In a review of 39 cases from the National Institutes of Health diagnosed as lymphocyte depleted Hodgkin's disease from 1965 to 1975, only 25% were diagnosed as such in 1986.[220] Most were reclassified as nodular sclerosis. However, 25% of the cases were reclassified as NHL, usually of the large-cell immunoblastic variety. Similar findings have been reported by Mir and colleagues.[188] Among 11 cases originally diagnosed as lymphocyte depleted Hodgkin's disease, only 3 were accepted as such by a pathology review panel. Most were reclassified as either NHL or

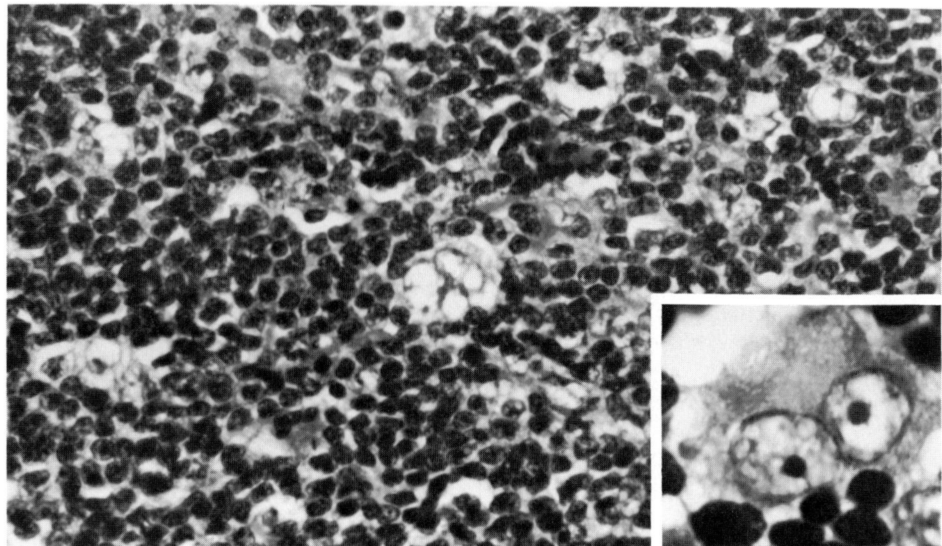

Figure 6–11. Lymphocyte-predominant Hodgkin's disease. As shown in the center of the photograph, the L/H ("popcorn") cell is large and has a convoluted nucleus, vesicular chromatin, and inapparent nucleolus. The background consists of mature lymphocytes (×400). *Inset,* One of the infrequent Reed-Sternberg cells in this type of Hodgkin's disease (H&E, ×1000).

nodular sclerosis Hodgkin's disease. The criteria most useful in distinguishing lymphocyte depleted Hodgkin's disease from NHL are the absence of atypia in the background lymphocytes and absence of a spectrum of atypical lymphoid cells. Immunophenotyping studies also are useful (see later). The inclusion of aggressive NHL within the lymphocyte depleted Hodgkin's disease category accounts for some of the poorer survival traditionally associated with this subtype.

Altered histologic appearances after therapy have been described.[229] Increased numbers of Reed-Sternberg cells and variants may make differentiation from non-Hodgkin's lymphoma difficult. Another problem is post-therapy fibrosis. After therapy for mediastinal Hodgkin's disease, a residual mass may appear on chest radiograph. Hyalinized, acellular scars may persist and cause space-occupying lesions. Inflammation and necrosis may be present.[230] Thymic cysts may also develop, particularly after radiation therapy.[231, 232] Histologic examination is required to exclude residual Hodgkin's disease by the absence of Reed-Sternberg cells and variants.

Immunopathology

Numerous immunohistochemistry studies have attempted to define a phenotype unique to Reed-Sternberg cells. Although Reed-Sternberg cells are characteristically positive for CD15 (Leu M1) and CD30 (Ki-1), these markers are also present on some NHLs.[233–236] Unfortunately, those NHLs that express CD15 and CD30 tend to be the T-cell lymphomas that mimic Hodgkin's disease morphologically. Also, Reed-Sternberg cells generally do not express CD45 leukocyte common antigen [LCA],[237] but again, this is true for many NHLs. Reed-Sternberg cells may also express a variety of other antigens.[237, 238] One study reported that 40% of Hodgkin's disease cases contain Reed-Sternberg cells that express one or more T-cell markers (including CD2, 3, 4, and 5) and that 18% of cases expressed one or more B-cell antigens (including CD20 and 22).[237] Lewis X antigen has been reported to be present on Reed-Sternberg cells and variants in 87% of Hodgkin's disease cases but only in 7% of peripheral T-cell lymphomas.[239] It can be demonstrated in paraffin-embedded tissue.

No single immunologic marker has yet been identified that is diagnostic of Reed-Sternberg cells. Nevertheless, immunologic studies may be useful. For example, a lymphoma that is labeled as a monoclonal B-cell neoplasm (positive for B-cell antigens and either kappa or lambda) should not be diagnosed as Hodgkin's disease. Similarly, a Hodgkin's-like lymphoma that is negative for CD15 and CD30 but positive for CD45 and other T-cell antigens is most likely a T-cell lymphoma.

Table 6–9 summarizes several studies that analyze the value of immunoperoxidase studies on paraffin-embedded tissue.[58, 61–64, 119, 233–235, 240–247] Note that fixatives vary. This variation in fixatives may account for some of the discrepancies among the studies. For example, LN1, LN2, and Leu M1 work best with B5,[119, 244] whereas BerH2 (an antibody against a formalin-resistant epitope of Ki-1, or CD30) works best with formalin.[244] The number of non-Hodgkin's lymphomas expressing the various markers depends on the distribution of histologic types studied. For example, the large-cell, pleomorphic T-cell lymphoma is more likely to express Leu M1 and Ber-H2 than other histologic types.

Molecular Pathology

The role of gene rearrangement studies in the diagnosis of Hodgkin's disease is not entirely clear at the present time. Rearranged immunoglobulin genes have been reported in Hodgkin's disease, particularly when Reed-Sternberg cells are enriched by density gradient centrifugation.[248–251] Often, the heavy chain gene is rearranged without a corresponding light chain. Rearrangements of the gene for the T-cell antigen receptor have also been reported,[249, 250] but questions about technical problems with these findings have been raised.[248] In many of these studies, it is possible that the gene rearrangements occur in the background inflammatory cells rather than in the Reed-Sternberg cells. Furthermore, because some T-cell lymphomas lack gene rearrangements, DNA analysis cannot discriminate reliably between Hodgkin's and non-Hodgkin's lymphomas.

Flow cytometry for DNA analysis has been applied to Hodgkin's disease. As expected, aneuploid cells can be identified, particularly when Reed-Sternberg cells are isolated, such as by multiparameter analysis with an antinucleolar antibody.[252] Multiple aneuploid peaks have been found in each of the 15 cases studied from deparaffinized tissue. The clinical significance of this finding is uncertain. In single-parameter studies, 11% of cases have been reported as aneuploid.[253, 254] Aneuploidy was not associated with any particular histology. One study found a trend toward better survival for patients with aneuploid tumors and low S phase.[254] However, the trend was not statistically significant. In contrast, Joensuu et al. found that S phase had significant, independent prognostic value.[253] In another report, S phase determination was useful in discriminating between Hodgkin's disease and peripheral T-cell lymphoma, because the latter had a significantly higher S phase fraction.[255]

Cytopathology

Cytologic techniques for mediastinal Hodgkin's disease are useful for both preoperative and intraoperative evaluations. Preoperatively, fine-needle aspiration biopsies (FNABs) can raise the suspicion of Hodgkin's disease and exclude other neoplasms such as metastatic carcinoma.[256–258] The FNAB can be performed while the patient undergoes CT to assure proper needle localization. Patients with mediastinal Hodgkin's disease frequently have palpable cervical lymph nodes that are more easily accessible to FNAB. Although a tissue diagnosis is recommended for initial diagnosis of Hodgkin's disease, FNAB can be of value in guiding the initial work-up of the patient, in staging patients, and in diagnosing recurrent disease. Intraoperatively, touch imprints can be used in conjunction with frozen sections. For both FNAB and touch imprints, air-dried smears with a modified Wright stain are easily prepared.

The cytologic features are what one would

Table 6–9. Immunohistochemistry of Hodgkin's Disease: Paraffin-Embedded Sections*

	CD15	CD20	CD30	CD43	CD45	CD45RA	CD45RO	CD74	CDw75	EMA	PNA
#	300/348	32/77	119/134	61/190	10/55	88/100	0/90	73/119	14/119	13/61	2/28
%	86	41	89	32	18	88	41	61	12	18	7

= number of positive cases/total number of cases stained. Only nodular sclerosing and mixed cellularity cases are included. Positivity refers to staining of the Reed-Sternberg cells and variants. % = percentage of cases that are positive.

Abbreviations: EMA, epithelial membrane antigen; PNA, peanut agglutinin.

Notes: Fixatives included: Bouin's, formol-saline, formalin, B5, Zenker's, and Bayley's. MT1 and L60 (Leu 22) are both CD43 antibodies.

*Data from references 58, 61–64, 119, 233–235, 240–245, 247.

expect based on histopathology (Fig. 6–12). Large, nucleolated, polylobated cells are identified on a background of inflammatory cells, including lymphocytes, plasma cells, eosinophils, and neutrophils. Granulomas are frequently present. The cellularity may be low in cases with abundant fibrosis. The differential diagnosis would include reactive or granulomatous lymphadenopathy (should lack atypical polylobated cells), non-Hodgkin's lymphoma (may be difficult to distinguish morphologically; immunologic studies can help), epithelial neoplasms (clusters of tumor cells), and germ cell tumors (large cells with abundant cytoplasm and prominent central nucleoli, and a lacy or "tigroid" background of stripped cytoplasm).

Pathogenesis

Hodgkin's disease is one of the most puzzling of human neoplasms. It is peculiar epidemiologically and histologically. As a consequence, numerous theories about the pathogenesis of Hodgkin's disease have been proposed. The origin of the Reed-Sternberg cell has been debated for decades, with every hematopoietic cell a candidate. Recent evidence suggests an activated ("transformed") lymphocyte.[259] As discussed earlier, this evidence includes the finding of lymphocyte surface markers and activation antigens on Reed-Sternberg cells and the reports of gene rearrangements. Some investigators report cases of Hodgkin's disease with a t(14:18) translocation involving the bcl-2 oncogene similar to follicular lymphoma.[260, 261] The debate on the origin of the Reed-Sternberg cell continues.[262]

The nodular lymphocyte predominant type of Hodgkin's disease appears to express a somewhat different phenotype.[245, 263] The L and H variants of Reed-Sternberg cells are more likely to express CD45 (LCA) and B-cell antigens (e.g., CD20) than are the Reed-Sternberg cells of other types of Hodgkin's disease. The nodular lymphocyte predominant type is also less likely to express CD15 (Leu M1). Thus, perhaps this type of Hodgkin's disease has a different pathogenesis than other types.

Epstein-Barr virus has been demonstrated in Reed-Sternberg cells and variants by in-situ DNA hybridization.[192, 264] In the United States, Italy, and France, most cases of mixed cellularity Hodgkin's disease have Epstein-Barr virus, whereas the nodular sclerosis type has Epstein-Barr virus infrequently.[193, 265, 266] In underdeveloped countries, virtually all cases have Epstein-Barr virus regardless of histologic type.[193, 194] Similarly, immunocompromised patients with Hodgkin's disease, including those with AIDS, usually have Epstein-Barr virus.[267, 268] Analysis of the terminal portions of the Epstein-Barr virus genomes has indicated monoclonality of the cells infected by Epstein-Barr virus.[264, 269] The infected cells express latent membrane protein (LMP-1), an Epstein-Barr virus gene product that acts as an oncogene in transformation assays.[270] The immunoperoxidase assay

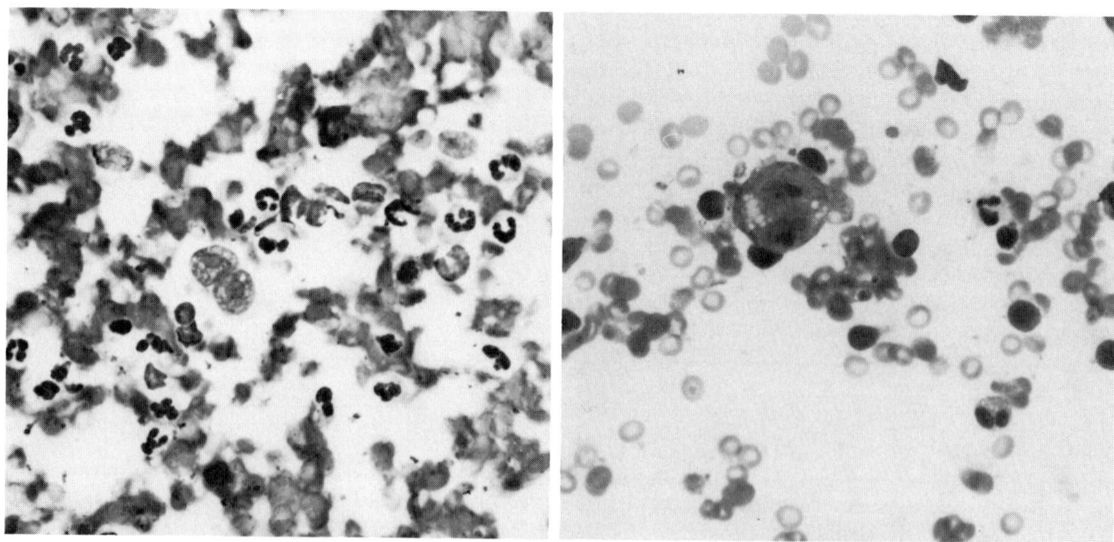

Figure 6–12. Fine-needle aspirate smears of Hodgkin's disease demonstrate bi-lobed Reed-Sternberg cells along with acute and chronic inflammatory cells (Diff-Quik stain, ×400).

for LMP-1 in paraffin-embedded tissue is virtually equal in sensitivity to in-situ DNA hybridization using biotinylated DNA probes.[266] Epstein-Barr virus may be related to the pathogenesis of Hodgkin's disease, or it may be a secondary phenomenon. Perhaps Epstein-Barr virus induces transformation of lymphocytes that then undergo additional chromosomal changes (similar to the model for Burkitt's lymphoma).

Prognosis and Therapy

Despite the confusion about the origin of Reed-Sternberg cells, nearly all patients (> 90%) with early stage Hodgkin's disease and the majority of those with advanced stage are curable.[202, 203] Nitrogen mustard, developed in the war-related research of the 1940s, was the first drug shown to have therapeutic activity. Modern combination chemotherapy began with nitrogen mustard, vincristine, procarbazine, and prednisone (MOPP) in the 1970s. Various modifications were introduced to lessen toxicity. A completely different combination—doxorubicin, bleomycin, vinblastine, and dacarbazine (ABVD)—was also developed. One study of patients with advanced disease had a better response rate with ABVD than with MOPP (81% vs. 69%) but no difference in overall survival. This remains an area of controversy. For early stage disease, radiation therapy appears to be as effective as chemotherapy. However, bulky mediastinal disease, even if localized, is a poor prognostic factor and is generally considered an indication for combined modality therapy.[197, 203] Bone marrow transplantation (autologous or allogeneic) has been tried for refractory Hodgkin's disease with some success.[202]

With the excellent cure rates now achievable, the long-term complications are getting more attention.[202, 203] Sterility may occur in both sexes with all therapeutic modalities. Patients treated with chemotherapy or combined-modality therapy have an increased risk of acute leukemia.[271] The incidence of leukemia peaks between 3 and 9 years after initial treatment. However, the risk of developing non-Hodgkin's lymphoma and nonhematologic neoplasms continues to increase with time. The histopathologic distinction between recurrent Hodgkin's disease and a secondary large-cell lymphoma can be difficult. Some monomorphic lymphomas developing in these patients have a phenotype similar to that of Reed-Sternberg cells and may not be a second neoplasm.[272]

ANGIOFOLLICULAR LYMPHOID HYPERPLASIA (CASTLEMAN'S DISEASE)

In a clinicopathologic exercise at the Massachusetts General Hospital published in 1954, Castleman discussed a case of hyperplasia of the mediastinal lymph nodes that had peculiar histologic features thought to resemble a thymoma.[273] In 1956, Castleman, Iverson, and Menendez described 13 such cases.[274] The series was expanded and combined with cases from the Pulmonary and Mediastinal Branch of the Armed Forces Institute of Pathology (AFIP) to reach a total of 81 patients in a 1972 report.[275] Because of the AFIP patients, this series is biased toward males and intrathoracic lesions compared with other reports[276–278] (Table 6–10).

Since then, the lesion has become known as Castleman's disease, or angiofollicular lymphoid hyperplasia. Other designations include giant lymph node hyperplasia and lymph node hamartoma. Another early series was collected by Flendrig and Schilling in the Netherlands, who designated the disorder "benign giant lymphoma."[279]

Angiofollicular lymphoid hyperplasia may form tumors up to 25 cm in diameter and occurs at virtually any site in the body.[278] Intrathoracic locations are common. In Castleman's original series, more than half of the cases were along the tracheobronchial tree.[274] Only two of the lesions were in the mid-anterior mediastinum. Two cases had been misdiagnosed and previously reported as ectopic thymomas. (One was located beneath the pleura at the root of the left lung; the other was close to the trachea.) Karcher and colleagues reported a case of Castleman's disease involving the thymus.[282] Virmani et al. reported an intrapericardial tumor adherent to both atria.[283] Another case arose in an intercostal space of the chest wall.[284] Other extranodal locations include muscle, larynx, vulva, and cranium.[285]

Histologically, angiofollicular lymphoid hyperplasia has been divided into two types.[275] The hyaline vascular variant has germinal centers and a prominent, hyalinized vascular proliferation (Fig. 6–13). The follicles often have radially penetrating capillaries surrounded by collagenous hyalinization. Concentrically lay-

Table 6–10. Castleman's Disease: Summary of Studies

First Author/Year	No. of Patients	Age	No. of Mediastinal Cases	Type	Localized or Multicentric	Associated Findings
Keller/1972[275]*	81	8–66	70 (86%) *Mediastinal location* Anterior-superior: 25 (36% of the mediastinal cases) Hilum: 24 (34%) Middle: 3 (4%) Posterior: 15 (21%) Unspecified: 3 (4%)	74 hyaline vascular; 7 plasma cell	Localized	Fever, anemia, hyperglobulinemia
Frizzera/1988[278]	46	12–69 (median 33)	24 (52%) Anterior mediastinum in 16 of the 24 mediastinal cases (67%) Other locations: abdomen 12 (26%) peripheral node 7 (15%) misc. (including extranodal) 3 (7%)	Hyaline vascular	Localized	10% with systemic symptoms or laboratory abnormalities (anemia, high ESR, hyperglobulinemia)
Frizzera/1989[278]	32	8–62 (median 22)	12 (38%) (all anterior) Other locations: abdomen 18 (56%) peripheral node 2 (6%) extranodal 0 (0%)	Plasma cell	Localized	67% with systemic symptoms (fever, weight loss, fatigue), 90% with anemia, 80% with hyperglobulinemia
Baruch/1991[276]	6	1–77	2	2 hyaline vascular; 1 plasma cell; 3 mixed	4 localized; 2 multicentric	—
Salisbury/1990[277]	13†	5–13	5 (2 at hilum)	Not reported	Localized	Anemia, fever, growth failure, recurrent infections

*This series includes 35 cases from the Massachusetts General Hospital (including those from the original 1956 series) and 46 from the Armed Forces Institute of Pathology (AFIP). Only intrathoracic lesions were included in the material from the AFIP.
†This series is a literature review of pediatric patients only.

ered ("onion skin") mantle zones are prominent. The mantle zones may assume a squamoid appearance. Some follicles have an atrophic ("burned out") appearance. With a hyalinized center surrounded by squamoid, concentric mantle zones, the follicles resemble Hassall's corpuscles. Some cases have extensive mantle zones surrounding the small germinal centers. Adjacent follicles may become confluent, forming geographic areas of small lymphocytes without apparent germinal centers.

Between the follicles, extensive capillary proliferation effaces the lymphoid sinuses. The cells in the interfollicular areas are predominantly lymphocytes. Immunoblasts, plasma cells, and eosinophils are also present. Fibrosis may be prominent in the interfollicular areas, particularly around central vessels. Histologically, the calcifications may be seen in hyalinized follicles or within fibrotic areas in the interfollicular zones.[275, 280]

Frizzera has emphasized that the combination of abnormal germinal centers and hypervascular interfollicular areas should be relied on for the diagnosis of hyaline vascular Castleman's disease.[278] Either finding alone is less useful. The characteristic germinal center changes may occur in otherwise unremarkable reactive lymph nodes as a manifestation of germinal center involution. Similar changes may occur in angioimmunoblastic lymphadenopathy and in patients with HIV infection. Hypervascularity is common in any reactive lymph node.

The hyaline vascular type has been associated with vascular neoplasia. Gerald and colleagues reported seven cases of hyaline vascular Castleman's disease associated with vascular

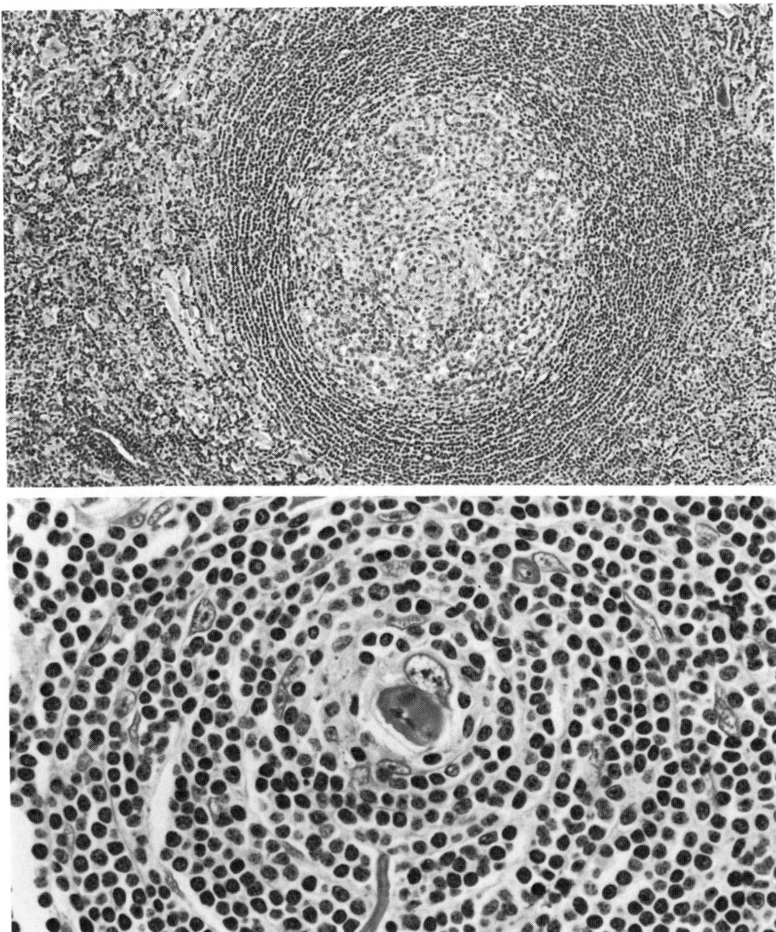

FIGURE 6–13. Angiofollicular lymphoid hyperplasia, hyaline vascular variant. *Top,* A germinal center with concentric layers of mantle zone lymphocytes is surrounded by numerous small capillaries (×100). *Bottom,* In the midportion of this photograph, an atrophic, hyalinized germinal center resembles a Hassall's corpuscle. A hyalinized vessel is at bottom center (H&E, ×400).

neoplastic elements.[281] The latter seemed to arise from interfollicular areas and was composed of fascicles of spindled, oval, and epithelioid cells. Some cells formed well-defined lumina with or without red blood cells. One of the seven cases was a mediastinal mass. Others were located in the retroperitoneum or kidney.

The plasma cell type of Castleman's disease is less common. It accounts for about 10 to 20% of all cases.[275, 278] It is characterized by solid sheets of mature plasma cells in the interfollicular areas (Fig. 6–14). The germinal centers are normal to large in size without the penetrating vessels. Prominent vascularity of the interfollicular area is not characteristic. In occasional cases, features of both the plasma cell and hyaline vascular types are present in the same lesion.

Over the years since Castleman described the lesion, the same histologic appearance has been noted in lymph nodes from a wide variety of patients, including those with HIV-1 infection, Wiskott-Aldrich syndrome, Kaposi's sarcoma, and rheumatoid arthritis.[278, 285–288] Similar changes have been noted in lymph nodes draining sites of carcinoma or lymphoma.[285, 289] Hodgkin's disease has been described in lymph node biopsies also showing features of Castleman's disease.[285, 290, 291] In most of the above associations, the lymph nodes resemble the plasma cell variant of Castleman's disease. In some patients, no associated disease can be identified, and a diagnosis of Castleman's disease is appropriate. In the presence of other disorders, the lymph nodes are best described as reactive follicular hyperplasia showing "Castleman's-like changes."

Localized and systemic ("multicentric") forms of Castleman's disease are now recognized.[285, 292, 293] With regard to the localized form, either histologic variant can occur in pa-

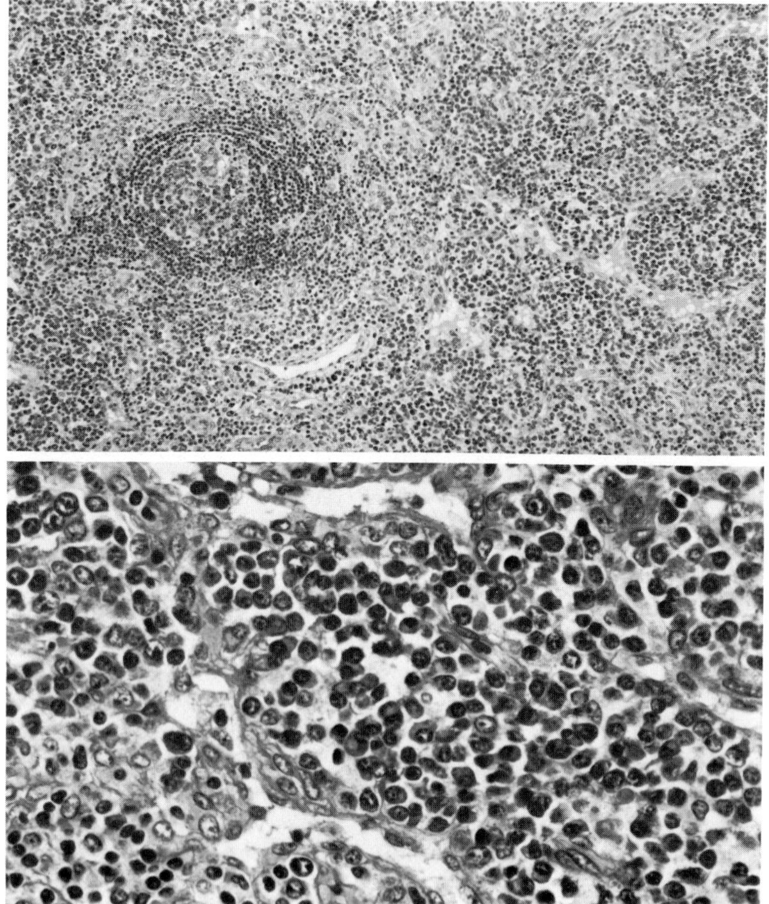

Figure 6–14. Angiofollicular lymphoid hyperplasia, plasma cell variant. *Top,* Germinal center is at left. The interfollicular area is expanded (×100). *Bottom,* The interfollicular area contains sheets of mature plasma cells (×400).

tients of any age; the male-to-female ratio is about equal.[275, 294] Median age is in the third decade of life. Clinically, the hyaline vascular type is usually asymptomatic.[275] If present, symptoms generally relate to the location of the tumor. Intrathoracic lesions may present with respiratory tract infection, cough, dyspnea, hemoptysis, back pain, and chest pain.[275, 278, 295] Recurrent pleural effusions may be a problem.[275, 296] Less than 10% of patients have consitutional symptoms or laboratory abnormalities such as anemia or hypergammaglobulinemia.[275, 278]

Radiographically, the hyaline vascular type shows enhancement following intravenous injection of contrast medium.[280] This is presumably related to the marked vascularity of the lesion. This enhancement is best demonstrated by angiography. Calcifications may be apparent on plain films or by CT.

In contrast to the hyaline vascular variant, the plasma cell lesions are associated with systemic symptoms in 67% of patients.[278] Hematologic abnormalities occur in approximately 50% of patients.[275] In addition to anemia, patients may have a wide variety of clinical and serologic findings. These abnormalities include fever, splenomegaly, elevated sedimentation rate, hypoalbuminemia, hyperglobulinemia, leukocytosis, and thrombocytosis. Growth failure, nephrotic syndrome, peripheral neuropathy, and amyloidosis are other associations.[278, 285, 297, 298] The anemia is typically microcytic and hypochromic; it does not respond to iron supplements or erythropoietin.[299] Serologic anti-erythropoietin antibodies have been reported.[300] The abnormalities often resolve within 60 days of mass resection.[275]

The plasma cell variant is less likely to involve the mediastinum than the hyaline vascular type is. In Frizzera's series, 56% of plasma cell type tumors were within the abdomen, usually in the small bowel mesentery.[278] Peripheral node involvement is uncommon, and extranodal disease is rare.

Some cases of the plasma cell variant have light chain restriction as judged by immunoperoxidase stains on paraffin-embedded tissue. Hall and colleagues reported that three of five cases had sheets of plasma cells staining only for IgA and lambda light chain.[301] Two of these cases had clonal immunoglobulin heavy chain gene rearrangements. A third case with heavy chain rearrangements had a polyclonal staining pattern by immunohistochemistry. Radaszkiewicz and colleagues found monoclonal plasma cells in 7 of 18 cases of the plasma cell type of Castleman's disease.[302] All expressed the lambda light chain. Two had generalized lymphadenopathy. Those with monoclonal plasma cells did not experience progression to generalized disease. The light chain restricted plasma cells appear to represent a form of benign monoclonal gammopathy. However, longer periods of follow-up are needed. The clinical significance of light chain restriction and/or gene rearrangements is not known.

For both types of localized Castleman's disease, complete excision is curative in almost all cases. Recurrences are rare. For the hyaline vascular type, profuse bleeding may be encountered by the surgeon during the excision.[275] Systemic symptoms may respond to radiation therapy when the mass is unresectable.[303, 304] However, the radiation does not usually result in complete disappearance of the mass.

The systemic form of Castleman's disease tends to occur in males (2.5:1 male-to-female ratio) during late adulthood.[285, 292, 305] These patients have systemic symptoms, hepatosplenomegaly, and hypergammaglobulinemia. Lymphadenopathy is prominent, especially in peripheral areas. In contrast to the localized form, less than 10% of patients have mediastinal involvement. In a series of 16 patients with multicentric angiofollicular lymphoid hyperplasia, only 1 had a large mediastinal mass.[306] Many cases of multicentric Castleman's disease have been associated with Kaposi's sarcoma.[278, 307, 308] These cases have been elderly patients who have no evidence of AIDS.

In multicentric disease, the plasma cell type occurs four times more frequently than the hyaline vascular variant.[306] Using the Southern blotting technique, Hanson and colleagues demonstrated rearrangements for the immunoglobulin heavy chain gene in three of four cases.[309] Two of the three cases also had rearrangements of the T-cell antigen receptor beta chain gene. None of four localized tumors had gene rearrangements. Multicentric disease can behave aggressively. Ten of sixteen patients died of the disease, with a median survival of 26 months.[306] Two of the patients developed a non-Hodgkin's lymphoma.

Multicentric Castleman's disease has been associated with numerous laboratory findings (anemia, elevated erythrocyte sedimentation rate, hypergammaglobulinemia) and clinical findings (e.g., peripheral neuropathy, Evan's syndrome, and myelofibrosis).[278, 297] Multicentric disease is often associated with osteosclerotic myeloma (in contast to the usual osteolytic type) and the POEMS syndrome.[278, 310] The POEMS syndrome involves polyneuropathy, organomegaly (hepatosplenomegaly, lymphadenopathy), endocrinopathy (diabetes mellitus, gynecomastia, amenorrhea), M proteins, and skin manifestations (pigmentation, sclerosis, hypertricosis, hemangiomas). Two case reports describe patients with multicentric disease who developed a solitary plasmacytoma.[311, 312]

In some patients, the distinction between localized and multicentric forms is not clear.[285] In the localized disease, "satellite" nodules may occur adjacent to the main mass. Also, some of the "localized" cases have splenomegaly and peripheral lymphadenopathy. Finally, some of the patients with multicentric disease may initially present with only one site of involvement. Nevertheless, in most cases, the localized and multicentric forms are markedly different. The localized form involves younger patients (median age 20 years vs. 57 years for multicentric disease) with a local tumor curable by excision. Any systemic symptoms resolve with removal of the tumor. In contrast, the multicentric disease involves widespread lymphadenopathy and more severe symptoms. It is an aggressive disease that is associated with infections and a greater risk of malignancy. Responses to chemotherapy have been reported.[313]

Some evidence suggests that interleukin-6 (IL-6) may be involved in the pathogenesis of Castleman's disease. IL-6 is a cytokine that induces maturation of B cells into antibody-producing cells.[314] It also induces production of acute phase proteins by hepatocytes. IL-6 is produced by a variety of cell types, including B and T lymphocytes, monocytes, fibroblasts, keratinocytes, and endothelial cells. In 1989, Yabuhara and colleagues found that supernatant from cultures of a case of Castleman's disease had B-cell differentiation factor activity, a characteristic now attributed to IL-6.[315] The patient had localized mediastinal involvement with systemic symptoms. Histologically, the mass had features of both types of Castleman's disease.

In the same year, Yoshizaki et al. reported elevated serum IL-6 levels in two patients, one with localized mediastinal disease with systemic symptoms and the other with multicentric disease.[316] Other cytokines were not elevated. After excision of the localized tumor, the IL-6 level returned to normal. Microscopically, the affected lymph nodes had features of the hyaline vascular variant (hyperplastic follicles, vascular proliferation with hyalinization). Plasma cells were numerous. Immunohistochemical studies demonstrated IL-6 in the follicles of the two lymph nodes with Castleman's disease but not in two normal nodes.

Additional evidence implicating IL-6 in Castleman's disease was published in 1991. Leger-Revet and colleagues studied eight lymph nodes affected with Castleman's disease.[317] Using in situ hybridization, they found high levels of IL-6 gene expression in the follicles of two lymph nodes from localized Castleman's disease patients having systemic symptoms. Other cytokines (IL-1 alpha and beta) were not identified. No IL-6 gene expression was found in the follicles of two patients with localized disease but without systemic symptoms or in the nodes of five patients with multicentric disease. In the interfollicular areas of all the lymph nodes affected with Castleman's disease, cells expressing the IL-6 gene were located outside sinuses near blood vessels and plasma cells. In the normal lymph nodes, cells expressing the IL-6 gene were present only inside the sinuses. Similar differences in the distribution of interfollicular cells were noted using in-situ hybridization for IL-1 (alpha and beta) genes.

An animal model further supports a role for IL-6. Genetically manipulated mice with dysregulated expression of IL-6 developed anemia, transient granulocytosis, polyclonal hypergammaglobulinemia, splenomegaly, and peripheral lymphadenopathy.[318] Microscopic examination of the lymph nodes revealed atretic follicles with almost complete replacement of the nodes by mature plasma cells. Some of the clinical and microscopic features of this syndrome resemble multicentric Castleman's disease.

Thus, IL-6 appears to be involved in the pathogenesis of Castleman's disease. Excess IL-6 may explain many of the systemic manifestations, including anemia, hypergammaglobulinemia, and autoimmune phenomena. However, some questions remain. It is unknown why IL-6 production is increased. Also, the studies do not clearly distinguish between the two variants of Castleman's disease. Finally, there are conflicting data on IL-6 in multicentric disease.

Undoubtedly, additional factors must be involved. As in any lymphoproliferative disorder, Epstein-Barr virus has been implicated in some cases. Two patients have been described with apparent Epstein-Barr virus infections.[275, 319] Hanson and colleagues found the Epstein-Barr virus genome in lymph nodes from two of four patients with multicentric disease.[309] The significance of Epstein-Barr virus in these cases is not known.

Perhaps some regulatory abnormality of the immune system occurs. However, no consistent immunologic defect has been defined.[303, 320, 321] Most investigators favor the hypothesis that localized Castleman's disease is a reactive process.[278] Some evidence has suggested the idea of a lymphoid hamartoma. This evidence includes the occasional extranodal location and an association with an angiolipomatous component. It is unclear whether the two variants are different stages of the same process or two different entities altogether.

Multicentric Castleman's disease appears to represent a disorder that is unrelated to the localized form, particularly the hyaline vascular variant. Frizzera has hypothesized that multicentric Castleman's disease is a plasma cell lesion derived from B lymphocytes that traffic to lymph nodes.[285] Polyclonal plasma cells circulate to peripheral lymph nodes, spleen, and bone marrow. Monoclonal plasma cell proliferations may develop at any of these sites.

HISTIOCYTOSIS X (LANGERHANS CELL HISTIOCYTOSIS)

Histiocytosis X is a rare cause of a mediastinal mass. Because it is now known to be a lesion of the Langerhans cell, the term Langerhans cell histiocytosis is more accurate.[322] Siegal and colleagues reported four patients aged 2 months to 8 years with histiocytosis X that presented as a mediastinal mass.[323] One of the masses was encapsulated; the other three were locally infiltrative. Only the patient with the encapsulated tumor had evidence of extrathoracic disease (i.e., multiple lytic and osteosclerotic bone lesions). Histologically, the mediastinal masses were similar to histiocytosis X in other sites. Histiocytoid cells with folded, grooved nuclei were present in large sheets. Eosinophils were prominent, as were scattered multinucleated giant cells. In the two cases studied by immunoperoxidase staining, S100 (a marker for Langerhans cells) was strongly expressed. Adjacent thymus was unremarkable. Patients were treated with chemotherapy or radiation. All were alive and well from 3 to 14 years after diagnosis. Nakata and colleagues described a similar patient, a 15-month-old child who presented with histiocytosis X as a mediastinal mass.[324] This patient subsequently developed skin and bone lesions but responded to chemotherapy.

Mediastinal masses have also been described in children who present with disseminated disease.[325–327] After therapy, air-filled cysts may develop within the mediastinal mass.[326, 327] With further therapy, the cysts resolve.

Focal involvement of the thymus by histiocytosis X has been reported in a study of two patients with myasthenia gravis[328] (Fig. 6–15). In both patients, the thymus was grossly normal in shape. Palpation of the thymus in one case led to the identification of four nodules (each 4 to 8 mm in diameter with two nodules in each lobe). Histologically, the nodules contained large cells with grooved nuclei. The cells expressed S100. Electron microscopy showed that they contained the Birbeck granules characteristic of Langerhans cells. Another case report describes a myasthenic patient with thymic follicular hyperplasia. Within the thymus, a single nodule, 4 mm in diameter, was identified. The histologic diagnosis of histiocytosis X was supported by immunoperoxidase studies demonstrating S100 expression in the large cells of the nodule.[329]

With disseminated disease, histiocytosis X infiltrates the interlobular connective tissue of the thymus.[330] In addition, accumulation of histiocytosis X cells within the medulla has been described.[331]

Histiocytosis X may be associated with other neoplasms, including Hodgkin's disease, non-Hodgkin's lymphoma, acute leukemia, and carcinoma.[47, 332] Two cases have been reported in association with adult lymphoblastic lymphoma of a pre–T cell ("prethymic") phenotype.[47]

The differential diagnosis of thymic histio-

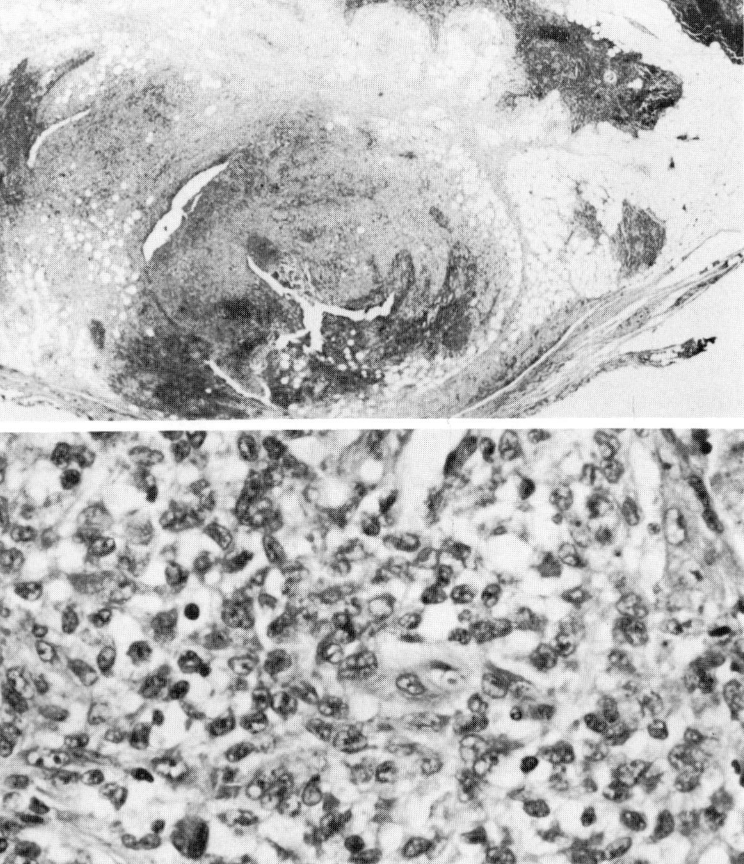

Figure 6–15. Histiocytosis X of the thymus removed from a patient with myasthenia gravis. *Top,* Central area is one of four nodules (4 to 8 mm in diameter) that were palpated within the thymus. Residual thymic tissue is present at the periphery (H&E, ×40). *Bottom,* The nodule contains sheets of Langerhans cells with characteristic grooved nuclei and indistinct cell outlines (H&E, ×400). Eosinophils were also noted. Electron microscopy revealed Birbeck granules. (This case was reported by Bramwell and Burns.[328])

cytosis X includes Hodgkin's disease, non-Hodgkin's lymphoma, and thymoma. The Reed-Sternberg cells and variants of Hodgkin's disease are absent in histiocytosis X. However, the eosinophils, lymphocytes, and histiocytes would raise the suspicion of Hodgkin's disease as well as of non-Hodgkin's lymphomas. Immunoperoxidase stains can confirm a diagnosis of histiocytosis X by demonstrating S100 expression in the majority of large cells. CD1 is another marker of Langerhans cells that is expressed in histiocytosis X (but is useful only in frozen sections). Of course, neither marker is specific for histiocytosis X. In particular, CD1 also labels lymphocytes of the thymic cortex. Also, Langerhans cells may be present normally in the thymus. Thus, the finding of S100-positive, CD1-positive Langerhans cells does not necessarily support a diagnosis of histiocytosis X, unless the histologic appearance is appropriate. Sheets of large cells with bland nuclei may resemble thymoma. However, the grooved nuclei are characteristic of histiocytosis X, and the tumor cells should not express cytokeratin.

Another lesion to consider in the differential diagnosis was described by Halicek and Rosai as "histioeosinophilic granuloma."[333] These lesions histiologically resemble histiocytosis X except that they are located in the capsule or septa of the thymus. No infiltration of the thymic parenchyma was noted. Immunoperoxidase studies demonstrated no staining for S100. Clinical correlation indicated that these lesions occurred only in myasthenia gravis patients who had had a diagnostic pneumomediastinum approximately 1 week prior to thymectomy (see Chapter 4).

Histiocytosis X is usually a disorder of children and young adults. It may occur in a localized form (eosinophilic granuloma) or as a multisystemic disease.[334] Bones are the most common site of involvement. A predilection for skin, lymph nodes, spleen, lung, liver, and bone marrow has also been noted.[334–336]

Langerhans cells are dendritic cells that are typically found in the epidermis.[337] Like other types of dendritic cells, they are believed to derive from monocytes originating in the bone marrow. The Langerhans cells in histiocytosis X have a characteristic phenotype.[333, 338] Most express vimentin, S100, CD1, LN2, LN3, CD4, CD11c, and CD14. They do not express CD15, CD30, and CD45. Normal Langerhans cells lack CD11 and CD14.

The pathogenesis of histiocytosis X is unknown. Many cases may be reactive rather than neoplastic.[334] One study documented monoclonality.[334a] Abnormalities of T-cell function have been described.[339–341] Interestingly, grossly uninvolved thymus in patients with histiocytosis X shows changes similar to those associated with congenital immunodeficiency. Hamoudi and colleagues studied the thymus at autopsy in 32 children with histiocytosis X.[342] In four cases, the thymus showed loss of normal lobular architecture. Corticomedullary differentiation and Hassall's corpuscles were absent. These glands resembled those associated with primary immunodeficiencies These patients all died of infection within 5 months of diagnosis and most likely did have a congenital immunodeficiency. Twenty-three patients had a thymus similar to that just described but with a histiocytic infiltrate. The infiltrate was adjacent to the thymic lobules or within large clefts. The remaining five patients had thymic involution with marked depletion of cortical lymphocytes, intact architecture, and normal Hassall's corpuscles. The dysplastic-appearing glands in some histiocytosis X patients suggest an underlying immunodeficiency. Others have also described a dysmorphic thymus with absent Hassall's corpuscles in patients with disseminated disease.[331, 343]

The disorder has a variable course. Certain clinical parameters, including age less than 2 years at diagnosis, are adverse prognostic factors. Morphologic features do not appear to distinguish indolent from aggressive disease. Ben-Ezra and colleagues described malignant histiocytosis X as a clinicopathologic entity characterized by atypical, malignant-appearing Langerhans cells and an aggressive clinical course.[344] The patients all had disseminated disease. Two of seven had thymic involvement. However, the morphologic criteria of malignancy did not always correlate with an aggressive clinical course, and not all patients with an aggressive course had malignant morphology. The entity could be defined only retrospectively.[337]

MISCELLANEOUS HEMATOLOGIC LESIONS

Cases have been reported of plasmacytomas involving the mediastinum.[345–347] The tumors were in the upper mediastinum or hilar area. In the report by Davis and colleagues, the plasmacytoma caused a superior vena cava syndrome.[347]

Rarely, a granulocytic sarcoma (chloroma)

causes an anterior mediastinal mass.[348–350] Cases in which a granulocytic sarcoma encased the heart have also been described.[351, 352] Immunoperoxidase studies are useful in identifying granulocytic sarcoma. For example, in paraffin-embedded tissue, CD68 (KP-1) identifies approximately 50% of acute myeloid leukemias and is not expressed in acute lymphoblastic leukemia.[353] CD43 is less specific but stains about 90% of acute leukemias (both myeloid and lymphoid). A histochemical stain for chloroacetate esterase can be performed in paraffin-embedded tissue. The enzyme is present in myeloid cells beginning at the promyelocyte stage of differentiation.[354] Hairy cell leukemia may also produce significant mediastinal lymphadenopathy.[355]

SUMMARY

Lymphomas of several histologic types may present as a mediastinal mass. Lymphoblastic lymphoma is most common in the pediatric and young adult age groups, and the majority of patients have a mediastinal mass. The lesions consist of a diffuse infiltrate of immature lymphoid cells. Those cases associated with a mediastinal mass usually have a T cell phenotype. Large cell lymphoma of the mediastinum most commonly affects young adult women. Histologically, prominent fibrosis is typical. These lymphomas usually have a B cell phenotype. Hodgkin's disease may produce an isolated mediastinal mass, although usually peripheral lymphadenopathy is also present. Most cases of mediastinal Hodgkin's disease are the nodular sclerosis histologic type. Immunoperoxidase studies may be useful, although no single marker is specific for this lesion. The differential diagnosis of mediastinal lymphomas includes thymoma, thymic carcinoma, metastatic carcinoma, and germ cell tumors. Cytopathology may be helpful in preoperative or intraoperative diagnosis.

Angiofollicular lymphoid hyperplasia, or Castleman's disease, may be localized or widespread. The localized form may produce an isolated mediastinal mass, usually along the tracheobronchial tree, in a patient of any age. Histologically, hyaline-vascular and plasma cell types have been described. The former is more likely to involve the mediastinum and is less likely to be associated with systemic symptoms. The systemic form of Castleman's disease has a male predilection and occurs in older adults. Mediastinal involvement is infrequent.

Several cases have been described of histiocytosis X, presenting as a mediastinal mass or focally involving the thymus. Case reports of mediastinal plasmacytomas and granulocytic sarcomas have been published.

REFERENCES

1. Mullen B, Richardson JD. Primary anterior mediastinal tumors in children and adults. Ann Thorac Surg 1986; 42:338–345.
2. Yellin A, Mandel M, Rechavi G, Neuman Y, Ramot B, Lieberman Y. Superior vena cava syndrome associated with lymphoma. Am J Dis Child 1992; 146:1060–1063.
3. Patchefsky AS, Brodovsky HS, Menduke H, Southard M, Brooks J, Nicklas D, Hoch WS. Non-Hodgkin's lymphomas: a clinicopathologic study of 293 cases. Cancer 1974; 34:1173–1186.
4. Levitt LJ, Aisenberg AC, Harris NL, Linggood RM, Poppema S. Primary non-Hodgkin's lymphoma of the mediastinum. Cancer 1982; 50:2486–2492.
5. Strickler JG, Kurtin PJ. Mediastinal lymphoma. Semin Diagn Pathol 1991; 8:2–13.
6. Lichtenstein A, Levine A, Taylor CR, Boswell W, Rossman S, Feinstein D, Lukes RJ. Primary mediastinal lymphoma in adults. Am J Med 1980; 68:509–514.
7. Payne CM, Grogan TM, Spier CM. Lymphomas of the mediastinum. Ultrastruct Pathol 1991; 15:439–474.
8. Magrath I. Historical perspective: the origins of modern concepts of biology and management. *In* Magrath I, ed. The Non-Hodgkin's Lymphomas. Baltimore: Williams & Wilkins, 1990:15–28.
9. Knowles DM. Lymphoblastic lymphoma. *In* Knowles DM, ed. Neoplastic Hematopathology. Baltimore: Williams & Wilkins, 1992:715–747.
10. Sternberg C. Leukosarkomatose und myeloblastenleukamie. Beitr Path Anat Allg Path 1916; 61:75–100.
11. Otto HF. Tumours of the thymus and their nomenclature. Virchows Arch [A] 1991; 419:257–260.
12. Cooke JV. Mediastinal tumor in acute leukemia: a clinical and roentgenologic study. Am J Dis Child 1932; 44:1153–1177.
13. Webster R. Lymphosarcoma of the thymus: its relation to acute lymphatic leukemia. Med J Aust 1961; 48:582–586.
14. Rappaport H. Tumors of the hematopoietic system. *In* Atlas of Tumor Pathology. Washington, D.C.: Armed Forces Institute of Pathology, 1966.
15. Rappaport H, Winter WJ, Hicks EB. Follicular lymphoma: a reevaluation of its position in the scheme of malignant lymphoma, based on a survey of 253 cases. Cancer 1956; 9:792–821.
16. Smith JL, Barker CR, Clein GP, Collins RD. Characterisation of malignant mediastinal lymphoid neoplasm (Sternberg sarcoma) as thymic in origin. Lancet 1973; 1:74–77.
17. Kaplan J, Mastrangelo R, Peterson WD Jr. Childhood lymphoblastic lymphoma, a cancer of thymus-derived lymphocytes. Cancer Res 1974; 34:521–525.
18. Barcos MP, Lukes RJ. Malignant lymphoma of convoluted lymphocytes: a new entity of possible T cell type. *In* Sinks LF, Godden JO, eds. Conflicts in Childhood Cancer: An Evaluation of Current Management. New York: Alan R. Liss, 1975:147–178.

19. Nathwani BN, Kim H, Rappaport H. Malignant lymphoma, lymphoblastic. Cancer 1976; 38:964–983.
20. Jaffe ES. An overview of the classification of non-Hodgkin's lymphomas. *In* Jaffe ES, ed. Surgical Pathology of the Lymph Nodes and Related Organs. Philadelphia: WB Saunders, 1985:135–145.
21. Gerard-Marchant R, Hamlin I, Lennert K, Rilke F, Stansfeld AG, van Unnik JAM. Classification of non-Hodgkin's lymphoma. Lancet 1974; 2:406–408.
22. Mazza P, Bertini M, Mazza S, Lauria F, Pileri S, Rivano MT, Baccarani M, Ricci P, Fiacchini M, Vitolo U, Canta M, Paolino W, Zinzani PL, Poletti G, Verlicchi F, Gherlinzoni F, Tura S. Lymphoblastic lymphoma in adolescents and adults: clinical, pathological, and prognostic evaluation. Eur J Cancer Clin Oncol 1986; 22:1503–1510.
23. Rosenberg SA. National Cancer Institute sponsored study of classifications of non-Hodgkin's lymphomas: summary and description of a working formulation for clinical usage. Cancer 1982; 2112:2112–2135.
24. Stansfeld AG, Diebold J, Kapanci Y, Kelenyi G, Lennert K, Mioduszewska O, Noel H, Rilke F, Sundstrom C, van Unnik JAM, Wright DH. Updated Kiel classification for lymphomas. Lancet 1988; 1:293–294.
25. Nathwani BN, Brynes RK, Lincoln T, Hansmann ML. Classifications of non-Hodgkin's lymphomas. *In* Knowles DM, ed. Neoplastic Hematopathology. Baltimore: Williams & Wilkins, 1992:555–601.
26. Murphy SB. Classification, staging and end results of treatment of childhood non-Hodgkin's lymphomas: dissimilarities from lymphomas in adults. Semin Oncol 1980; 7:332–339.
27. Griffith RC, Kelly DR, Nathwani BN, Shuster JJ, Murphy SB, Hvizdala E, Sullivan MP, Berard CW. A morphologic study of childhood lymphoma of the lymphoblastic type: the pediatric oncology group experience. Cancer 1987; 59:1126–1131.
28. Simon R, Durrleman S, Hoppe RT, Bonadonna G, Bloomfield CD, Rudders RA, Cheson BD, Berard CW. The non-Hodgkin's lymphoma pathologic classification project: long term follow-up of 1153 patients with non-Hodgkin's lymphomas. Ann Intern Med 1988; 109:939–945.
29. Picozzi VJ Jr, Coleman CN. Lymphoblastic lymphoma. Semin Oncol 1990; 17:96–103.
30. Hausner RJ, Rosas-Uribe A, Wickstrum DA, Smith PC. Non-Hodgkin's lymphoma in the first two decades of life: a pathological study of 30 cases. Cancer 1977; 40:1533–1547.
31. Sandlund J, Magrath I. Lymphoblastic lymphoma. *In* Magrath IT, ed. The Non-Hodgkin's Lymphomas. Baltimore: Williams & Wilkins, 1990:240–255.
32. Coleman CN, Picozzi VJ Jr, Cox RS, McWhirter K, Weiss LM, Cohen JR, Yu K-P, Rosenberg SA. Treatment of lymphoblastic lymphoma in adults. J Clin Oncol 1986; 4:1628–1637.
33. Slater DE, Mertelsmann R, Koziner B, Higgins C, McKenzie S, Schauer P, Gee T, Straus D, Kempin S, Arlin Z, Clarkson BD. Lymphoblastic lymphoma in adults. J Clin Oncol 1986; 3:57–67.
34. Patte C, Kalifa C, Flamant F, Hartmann O, Brugieres L, Valteau-Couanet D, Bayle C, Gaillaud J-M, Lemerle J. Results of the LMT81 protocol, a modified LSA2L2 protocol with high dose methotrexate, on 84 children with non-B-cell (lymphoblastic) lymphoma. Med Pediatr Oncol 1992; 20:105–113.
35. Nathwani BN, Diamond LW, Winberg CD, Kim H, Bearman RM, Glick JH, Jones SE, Gams RA, Nissen NI, Rappaport H. Lymphoblastic lymphoma: a clinicopathologic of 95 patients. Cancer 1981; 48:2347.
36. Lukes RJ, Collins RD. Tumors of the Hematopoietic System. Washington, D.C.: Armed Forces Institute of Pathology, 1992:52–63.
37. Foon KA, Todd RF III. Immunologic classification of leukemia and lymphoma. Blood 1986; 68:1–31.
38. Weiss LM, Bindl JM, Picozzi VJ, Link MP, Warnke RA. Lymphoblastic lymphoma: an immunophenotype study of 26 cases with comparison to T cell acute lymphoblastic leukemia. Blood 1986; 67:474–478.
39. Sheibani K, Nathwani BN, Winberg CD, Burke JS, Swartz WG, Blayney D, van de Velde S, Hill LR. Antigenically defined subgroups of lymphoblastic lymphoma: relationship to clinical presentation and biologic behavior. Cancer 1987; 60:183–190.
40. Murphy S, Jaffe ES. Terminal transferase activity and lymphoblastic neoplasms. N Engl J Med 1984; 311:1373–1374.
41. Kung PC, Long JC, McCaffrey RP, Ratliff RL, Harrison TA, Baltimore D. Terminal deoxynucleotidyl transferase in the diagnosis of leukemia and malignant lymphoma. Am J Med 1978; 64:788–794.
42. Crist WM, Shuster JJ, Falletta J, Pullen DJ, Berard CW, Vietti TJ, Alvarado CS, Roper MA, Prasthofer E, Grossi CE. Clinical features and outcome in childhood T-cell leukemia-lymphoma according to stage of thymocyte differentiation: a pediatric oncology group study. Blood 1988; 72:1891–1897.
43. Mori N, Oka K, Yoda Y, Abe T, Kojima M. Leu-4 (CD3) antigen expression in the neoplastic cells from T-ALL and T-lymphoblastic lymphoma. Am J Clin Pathol 1988; 90:244–249.
44. Jacobs JC, Katz RL, Shabb N, El-Naggar A, Ordonez NG, Pugh W. Fine needle aspiration of lymphoblastic lymphoma: a multiparameter diagnostic approach. Acta Cytol 1992; 36:887–894.
45. Sander CA, Jaffe ES, Gebhardt FC, Yano T, Medeiros LJ. Mediastinal lymphoblastic lymphoma with an immature B cell immunophenotype. Am J Surg Pathol 1992; 16:300–305.
46. Yumura-Yagi K, Ishihara S, Hara J, Murata M, Izumi Y, Tawa A, Sato A, Matsumoto Y, Kozaiwa K, Nishida M, Kawa-Ha K. Poor prognosis of mediastinal non-Hodgkin's lymphoma with an immature phenotype of CD2+, CD7 (or CD5)+, CD3−, CD4−, and CD8−. Cancer 1989; 63:671–674.
47. Quintanilla-Martinez L, Zukerberg LR, Harris NL. Prethymic adult lymphoblastic lymphoma: a clinicopathologic and immunohistochemical analysis. Am J Surg Pathol 1992; 16:1075–1084.
48. Norton AJ, Isaacson PG. Lymphoma phenotyping in formalin-fixed and paraffin wax-embedded tissues: II. Profiles of reactivity in the various tumour types. Histopathology 1989; 14:557–579.
49. Segal GH, Stoler MH, Fishleder AJ, Tubbs RR. Reliable and cost-effective paraffin section immunohistology of lymphoproliferative disorders. Am J Surg Pathol 1991; 15:1034–1041.
50. Linder J. Antibodies marking paraffin-embedded leukocytes: status report 1991. Am J Clin Pathol 1991; 95:607–608.
51. Knowles DM, Chadburn A, Inghirami G. Immunophenotypic markers useful in the diagnosis and classification of hematopoietic neoplasms. *In* Knowles DM, ed. Neoplastic Hematopathology. Baltimore: Williams & Wilkins, 1992:73–167.
52. Cabecadas JM, Isaacson PG. Phenotyping of T-cell lymphomas in paraffin sections—which antibodies? Histopathology 1991; 19:419–424.
53. Norton AJ, Isaacson PG. An immunohistochemical study of T cell lymphomas using monoclonal and

polyclonal antibodies effective in routinely fixed wax embedded tissues. Histopathology 1986; 10:1243–1260.
54. Krajewski AS, Myskow MW, Salter DM, Cunningham DS, Ramage EF. Diagnosis of T-cell lymphoma using beta F1, anti–T cell receptor beta chain antibody. Histopathology 1989; 15:239–247.
55. Yoshimo T, Mukuzono H, Aoki H, Takahashi K, Takeuchi T, Kubonishi I, Ohtsuki Y, Motoi M, Akagi T. A novel monoclonal antibody (OPD4) recognizing a helper/inducer T cell subset. Am J Pathol 1989; 134:1339–1346.
56. Said JW, Stoll PN, Shintaku P, Bindl JM, Butmarc JR, Pinkus GS. Leu-22: a preferential marker for T-lymphocytes in paraffin sections: staining profile in T- and B-cell lymphomas, Hodgkin's disease, other lymphoproliferative disorders, myeloproliferative diseases, and various neoplastic processes. Am J Clin Pathol 1989; 91:542–549.
57. Davey FR, Gatter KC, Ralfkiaer E, Pulford KA, Krissansen GW, Mason DY. Immunophenotyping of non-Hodgkin's lymphomas using a panel of antibodies on paraffin-embedded tissues. Am J Pathol 1987; 129:54–63.
58. Norton AJ, Ramsay AD, Smith SH, Beverley PCL, Isaacson PG. Monoclonal antibody (UCHL1) that recognises normal and neoplastic T cells in routinely fixed tissues. J Clin Pathol 1986; 39:399–405.
59. Chadburn A, Husain S, Knowles DM. Monoclonal antibody OPD4 detects neoplastic T cells but does not distinguish between CD4 and CD8 neoplastic T cells in paraffin tissue sections. Hum Pathol 1992; 23:940–947.
60. Poppema S, Hollema H, Visser L, Vos H. Monoclonal antibodies (MT1, MT2, MB1, MB2, MB3) reactive with leukocyte subsets in paraffin embedded tissue sections. Am J Pathol 1987; 127:418–429.
61. Andrade RE, Wick MR, Frizzera G, Gajl-Paczalska KJ. Immunophenotyping of hematopoietic malignancies in paraffin sections. Hum Pathol 1988; 19:394–402.
62. Ng CS, Chan JKC, Hui PK, Lo STH. Monoclonal antibodies reactive with normal and neoplastic T cells in paraffin sections. Hum Pathol 1988; 19:295–303.
63. Linder J, Ye Y, Harrington DS, Armitage JO, Weisenburger DD. Monoclonal antibodies marking T lymphocytes in paraffin-embedded tissue. Am J Pathol 1987; 127:1–8.
64. Wieczorek R, Buck D, Bindl J, Knowles DM. Monoclonal antibody Leu-22 (L60) permits the demonstration of some neoplastic T cells in routinely fixed and paraffin-embedded tissue sections. Hum Pathol 1988; 19:1434–1443.
65. Contos MJ, Kornstein MJ, Innes DI, Ben-Ezra J. CD43 expression in low grade lymphoproliferative disorders. Mod Pathol 1992; 5:631–633.
66. Segal GH, Stoler MH, Tubbs RR. The "CD43 only" phenotype: an aberrant, nonspecific immunophenotype requiring comprehensive analysis for lineage resolution. Am J Clin Pathol 1992; 97:861–865.
67. Macon WR, Casey TT, Kinney MC, Collins RD, Cousar JB. Leu-22 (L60): a more sensitive marker than UCHL1 for peripheral T-cell lymphomas, particularly large-cell types. Am J Clin Pathol 1991; 95:696–701.
68. Knowles DM. Immunophenotypic and antigen receptor gene rearrangement analysis in T cell neoplasia. Am J Pathol 1989; 134:761–785.
69. Knowles DM, Pelicci P-G, Dalla-Favera R. T-cell receptor beta chain gene rearrangements. Hum Pathol 1986; 17:546–551.
70. Picker LJ, Brenner MB, Weiss LM, Smith SD, Warnke RA. Discordant expression of CD3 and T-cell receptor beta-chain antigens in T-lineage lymphomas. Am J Pathol 1987; 129:434–440.
71. Gouttefangeas C, Bensussan A, Boumsell L. Study of the CD3-associated T-cell receptors reveals further differences between T-cell acute lymphoblastic lymphoma and leukemia. Blood 1990; 75:931–934.
72. Falini B, Flenghi L, Fagioli M, Martelli MF, Pileri S, Grignani F, Beltrami A, Novero D, Pelicci P-G. T-lymphoblastic lymphomas expressing the non-disulfide-linked form of the T-cell receptor gamma/delta: characterization with monoclonal antibodies and genotypic analysis. Blood 1989; 74:2501–2507.
73. Pittaluga S, Uppenkamp M, Cossman J. Development of T3/T cell receptor gene expression in human pre-T neoplasms. Blood 1987; 69:1062–1067.
74. Kneba M, Bolz I, Bergholz M, Batge R, Nauck M, Nitsche R, Krieger G. Clinical characteristics of high-grade lymphomas with immune genes in germline configuration. Cancer 1991; 67:603–609.
75. Williams ME, Innes DJ Jr, Borowitz MJ, Lovell MA, Swerdlow SH, Hurtubise PE, Brynes RK, Chan WC, Byrne GE Jr, Whitcomb CC, Thomas CY IV. Immunoglobulin and T cell receptor gene rearrangements in human lymphoma and leukemia. Blood 1987; 69:79–86.
76. Miwa H, Konishi H, Kobayashi N, Kita K, Shirakawa S, Shimizu A, Honjo T, Hatanaka M. The T-cell receptor gene rearrangements in T-lineage tumors without OKT3,4,6,8 markers. J Mol Cell Immunol 1987; 3:37–42.
77. Pittaluga S, Raffeld M, Lipford EH, Cossman J. 3A1 (CD7) expression precedes Tbeta gene rearrangements in precursor T (lymphoblastic) neoplasms. Blood 1986; 68:134–139.
78. Vezzoni P, Cairo G, Pozzi MR, Bardella L, Schiaffonati L, Giardini R, Rilke F, Delia D, Biunno I. The contribution of molecular biology in the diagnosis of human lymphomas. Diagn Immunol 1986; 4:247–252.
79. Dyer MJS. T-cell receptor delta/alpha rearrangements in lymphoid neoplasms. Blood 1989; 74:1073–1083.
80. Pardoll DM, Kruisbeek AM, Fowlkes BJ, Coligan JE, Schwartz RH. The unfolding story of T cell receptor gamma. FASEB J 1987; 1:103–109.
81. Born W, Rathbun G, Tucker P, Marrack P, Kappler J. Synchronized rearrangement of T-cell gamma and beta chain genes in fetal thymocyte development. Science 1986; 234:479–484.
82. Sheibani K, Wu A, Ben-Ezra J, Stroup R, Rappaport H, Winberg C. Rearrangement of k-chain and T-cell receptor beta-chain genes in malignant lymphomas of "T-cell" phenotype. Am J Pathol 1987; 129:201–207.
83. Liang R, Chan V, Chan TK, Chiu E, Todd D. Rearrangement of immunoglobulin, T-cell receptor, and bcl-2 genes in malignant lymphomas in Hong Kong. Cancer 1990; 66:1743–1747.
84. Trueworthy R, Shuster J, Look T, Crist W, Borowitz M, Carroll A, Frankel L, Harris M, Wagner H, Haggard M, Mosijczuk A, Pullen J, Steuber P, Land V. Ploidy of lymphoblasts is the strongest predictor of treatment outcome in B-progenitor cell acute lymphoblastic leukemia of childhood: a pediatric oncology group study. J Clin Oncol 1992; 10:606–613.
85. Weiss LM, Strickler JG, Medeiros LJ, Gerdes J, Stein H, Warnke RA. Proliferative rates of non-Hodgkin's lymphomas as assessed by Ki-67 antibody. Hum Pathol 1987; 18:1155–1159.

86. Houmand A, Abrahamsen B, Tinggaard Pedersen N. Relevance of Ki-67 expression in the classification of non-Hodgkin's lymphomas: a morphometric and double-immunostaining study. Histopathology 1992; 20:13–20.
87. Schwartz BR, Pinkus G, Bacus S, Toder M, Weinberg DS. Cell proliferation in non-Hodgkin's lymphomas: digital image analysis of Ki-67 antibody staining. Am J Pathol 1989; 134:327–336.
88. Sun T, Li C-Y, Yam LT. Atlas of Cytochemistry and Immunochemistry of Hematologic Neoplasms. Chicago: American Society of Clinical Pathologists Press, 1985:26–27.
89. Halpern S, Chatten J, Meadows AT, Byrd R, Lange B. Anterior mediastinal masses: anesthesia hazards and other problems. J Pediatr 1983; 102:407–410.
90. Azarow KS, Pearl RH, Zurcher R, Edwards FH, Cohen AJ. Primary mediastinal masses: a comparison of adult and pediatric populations. J Thorac Cardiovasc Surg 1993; 106:67–72.
91. Kardos TF, Sprague RI, Wakely PE Jr, Frable WJ. Fine needle aspiration biopsy of lymphoblastic lymphoma and leukemia: a clinical and immunologic study. Cancer 1987; 60:2448–2453.
92. Mitchell CD, Gordon I, Chessells JM. Clinical, haematological, and radiological features in T-cell lymphoblastic malignancy in childhood. Clin Radiol 1986; 37:257–261.
93. Flanders E, Kornstein MJ, Wakely PE Jr, Kardos TF, Frable WJ. Lymphoglandular bodies in fine needle aspiration cytology. Am J Clin Pathol 1993; 99:566–569.
94. Kardos TF, Maygarden SM, Blumberg AK, Wakely PE Jr, Frable WJ. Fine needle aspiration biopsy in the management of children and young adults with peripheral lymphadenopathy. Cancer 1989; 63:703–707.
95. Hvizdala EV, Berard C, Calihan T, Falletta J, Sabio H, Shuster JJ, Sullivan M, Wharam MD. Lymphoblastic lymphoma in children—a randomized trial comparing LSA2-L2 with the A-COP+ therapeutic regimen: a pediatric oncology group study. J Clin Oncol 1988; 6:26–33.
96. Baro J, Richard C, Sierra J, Garcia-Conde J, Larana JC, Roscha E, Solano C, Caballero D, Carrera D, Leon A, Zuazu J, Martinez F, Domingo A, Hernandez F, Marin P, Iriondo A, Montserrat E, Conde E. Autologous bone marrow transplantation in 22 adult patients with lymphoblastic lymphoma responsive to conventional dose chemotherapy. Bone Marrow Transplant 1992; 10:33–38.
97. Addis B, Isaacson PG. Large cell lymphoma of the mediastinum: a B cell tumour of probable thymic origin. Histopathology 1986; 10:379–390.
98. Menestrina F, Chilosi M, Bonetti F, Lestani M, Scarpa A, Novelli P, Doglioni C, Todeschini G, Ambrosetti A, Fiore-Donati L. Mediastinal large-cell lymphoma of B-type, with sclerosis: histopathological and immunohistochemical study of eight cases. Histopathology 1986; 10:589–600.
99. Scarpa A, Bonetti F, Menestrina F, Menegazzi M, Chilosi M, Lestani M, Bovolenta C, Zamboni G, Fiore-Donati L. Mediastinal large-cell lymphoma with sclerosis: genotypic analysis establishes its B cell nature. Virchows Arch [A] 1987; 412:17–21.
100. Trump DL, Mann RB. Diffuse large cell and undifferentiated lymphomas with prominent mediastinal involvement. Cancer 1982; 50:277–282.
101. Waldron JA Jr, Dohring EJ, Farber LR. Primary large cell lymphomas of the mediastinum: an analysis of 20 cases. Semin Diagn Pathol 1985; 2:281–295.
102. Lamarre L, Jacobson JO, Aisenberg AC, Harris NL. Primary large cell lymphoma of the mediastinum: a histologic and immunophenotypic study of 29 cases. Am J Surg Pathol 1989; 13:730–739.
103. Jacobson JO, Aisenberg AC, Lamarre L, Willett CG, Linggood RM, Miketic LM, Harris NL. Mediastinal large cell lymphoma: an uncommon subset of adult lymphoma curable with combined modality therapy. Cancer 1988; 62:1893–1898.
104. Moller P, Moldenhauer G, Mombutg F, Lammler B, Eberlein-Gonska M, Kiesel S, Dorken B. Mediastinal lymphoma of clear cell type is a tumor corresponding to terminal steps of B cell differentiation. Blood 1989; 69:1087–1095.
105. Perrone T, Frizzera G, Rosai J. Mediastinal diffuse large-cell lymphoma with sclerosis. Am J Surg Pathol 1986; 10:176–191.
106. Todeschini G, Ambrosetti V, Meneghini V, Pizzolo G, Menestrina F, Chilosi M, Benedetti F, Veneri D, Cetto GL, Perona G. Mediastinal large-B-cell lymphoma with sclerosis: a clinical study of 21 patients. J Clin Oncol 1990; 8:804–808.
107. Lavabre-Bertrand T, Donadio D, Fegeux N, Jessueld D, Taib J, Charlier D, Rousset T, Emberger J-M, Baldet P, Navarro M. A study of 15 cases of primary mediastinal lymphoma of B-cell type. Cancer 1992; 69:2561–2566.
108. Davis RE, Dorfman RF, Warnke RA. Primary large cell lymphoma of the thymus: a diffuse B-cell neoplasm presenting as primary mediastinal lymphoma. Hum Pathol 1990; 21:1262–1268.
109. Al-Sharabati M, Chittal S, Duga-Neulat I, Laurent G, Mazerolles C, Al-Saati T, Brousset P, Delsol G. Primary anterior mediastinal B-cell lymphoma: a clinicopathologic and immunohistochemical study of 16 cases. Cancer 1991; 67:2579–2587.
110. Nakagawa A, Nakamura S, Koshikawa T, Nakayama A, Nagasaka T, Motoori T, Kojima M, Hosomura Y, Ueda R, Mori S, Asai J, Suchi T. Clinicopathologic study of primary mediastinal non-lymphoblastic non-Hodgkin's lymphomas among the Japanese. Acta Pathol Jpn 1993; 43:44–54.
111. Kirn D, Mauch P, Shaffer K, Pinkus G, Shipp MA, Kaplan WD, Tung N, Wheeler C, Beard CJ, Canellos GP, Shulman LN. Large-cell and immunoblastic lymphoma of the mediastinum: prognostic features and treatment outcome in 57 patients. J Clin Oncol 1993; 11:1136–1143.
112. Bertini M, Orsucci L, Vitolo U, Levis A, Todeschini G, Meneghini V, Novero D, Tarella C, Gallo E, Luxi G, Pizzuti M, Novarino A, Urgesi A, Resegotti L. Stage II large B cell lymphoma with sclerosis treated with MACOP-B. Ann Oncol 1991; 2:733–737.
113. Yousem SA, Weiss LM, Warnke RA. Primary mediastinal non-Hodgkin's lymphomas: a morphologic and immunologic study of 19 cases. Am J Clin Pathol 1985; 83:676–680.
114. Ree HJ, Leone LA, Crowley JP. Sclerosis in diffuse histiocytic lymphoma: a clinicopathologic study. Cancer 1982; 49:1636–1648.
115. Miller JB, Variakojis D, Bitran JD, Sweet DL, Kinzie JJ, Golomb HM, Ultmann JE. Diffuse histiocytic lymphoma with sclerosis: a clinicopathologic entity frequently causing superior venacaval obstruction. Cancer 1981; 47:748–756.
116. Moller P, Matthei-Maurer DU, Hofmann WJ, Dorken B, Moldenhauer G. Immunophenotypic similarities of mediastinal clear cell lymphoma and sinusoidal (monocytoid) B cells. Int J Cancer 1989; 43:10–16.
117. Stein H, Dallenbach F. Diffuse large cell lymphomas

of B and T cell type. *In* Knowles DM, ed. Neoplastic Hematopathology. Baltimore: Williams & Wilkins, 1992:675–714.

118. Cartun RW, Coles FB, Pastuszak WT. Utilization of monoclonal antibody L26 in the identification and confirmation of B-cell lymphomas: a sensitive and specific marker applicable to formalin- and B5-fixed, paraffin-embedded tissues. Am J Pathol 1987; 129:415–421.
119. Linder J, Ye Y, Armitage JO, Weisenburger DD. Monoclonal antibodies marking B-cell non-Hodgkin's lymphoma in paraffin-embedded tissue. Mod Pathol 1988; 1:29–34.
120. Kahn HJ, Thorner PS. Monoclonal antibody MB2: a potential marker for Ewing's sarcoma and primitive neuroectodermal tumor. Pediatr Pathol 1989; 9:153–162.
121. Shevach EM. Accessory molecules. *In* Paul WE, ed. Fundamental Immunology. New York: Raven Press, 1989:413–441.
122. Weiss LM, Picker LJ, Copenhaver CM, Warnke RA, Sklar J. Large cell hematolymphoid neoplasms of uncertain lineage. Hum Pathol 1988; 29:967–973.
123. Eichelmann A, Koretz K, Mechtersheimer G, Moller P. Adhesion receptor profile of thymic B cell lymphoma. Am J Pathol 1992; 141:729–741.
124. Coon JS, Landay AL, Weinstein RS. Advances in flow cytometry for diagnostic pathology. Lab Invest 1987; 57:453–479.
125. Wain SL, Braylan RC, Borowitz MJ. Correlation of monoclonal antibody phenotyping and cellular DNA content in non-Hodgkin's lymphoma. Cancer 1987; 60:2403–2411.
126. Juneia SK, Cooper IA, Hodgson GS, Wolf MM, Ding JC, Ironside PNJ, Thomas RJS, Parkin JD. DNA ploidy patterns and cytokinetics of non-Hodgkin's lymphoma. J Clin Pathol 1986; 39:987–992.
127. Jalkanen S, Joensuu H, Klemi P. Prognostic value of lymphocyte homing receptor and S phase fraction in non-Hodgkin's lymphoma. Blood 1990; 75:1549–1556.
128. Egerter DA, Said JW, Epling S, Lee S. DNA content of T-cell lymphomas: a flow cytometric analysis. Am J Pathol 1988; 130:326–334.
129. O'Brien CJ, Holgate C, Quirke P, Stuart NSA, Ellis IO, Elston CW, Jones EL, Bird CC. Correlation of morphology, immunophenotype, and flow cytometry with remission induction and survival in high grade non-Hodgkin's lymphoma. J Pathol 1989; 158:31–39.
130. Diamond LW, Nathwani BN, Rappaport H. Flow cytometry in the diagnosis and classification of malignant lymphoma and leukemia. Cancer 1982; 50:1122–1135.
131. Bauer KD, Merkel DE, Winter JN, Hauck WW, Marder RJ, Wallemark CB, Williams TJ, Variakojis D. Prognostic implications of ploidy and proliferative activity in diffuse large cell lymphomas. Cancer Res 1986; 46:3173.
132. Joensuu H, Alanen K, Klemi PJ. Prognosis of lymphoma from a fine-needle aspirate. Eur J Cancer 1993; 29A:29–33.
133. Zalupski MM, Maciorowski Z, Ryan JR, Ensley JF, Hussein ME, Sundareson AS, Baker LH. DNA content parameters of paraffin-embedded soft tissue sarcomas: optimization of retrieval technique and comparison to fresh tissue. Cytometry 1993; 14:327–333.
134. Christensson B, Tribukait B, Linder I, Ullman B, Biberfeld P. Cell proliferation and DNA content in non-Hodgkin's lymphoma: flow cytometry in relation to lymphoma classification. Cancer 1986; 58:1295–1304.
135. Vuckovic J, Dubravcic M, Matthews JM, Wickramasinghe SN, Dominis M, Jaksic B. Prognostic value of cytophotometric analysis of DNA in lymph node aspirates from patients with non-Hodgkin's lymphoma. J Clin Pathol 1990; 43:626–629.
136. Crocker J. Proliferation indices in malignant lymphomas. Clin Exp Immunol 1989; 77:299–308.
137. Grogan TM, Miller TP. New biologic markers in non-Hodgkin's lymphomas. Hematol Oncol Clin North Am 1991; 5:925–933.
138. Grogan TM, Lippman SM, Spier CM, Slymen DJ, Rybski JA, Rangel CS, Richter LC, Miller TP. Independent prognostic significance of nuclear proliferation antigen in diffuse large cell lymphomas as determined by the monoclonal antibody Ki-67. Blood 1988; 71:1157–1160.
139. Hall PA, Richards MA, Gregory WM, D'Ardenne AJ, Lister TA, Stansfeld AG. The prognostic value of Ki67 immunostaining in non-Hodgkin's lymphoma. J Pathol 1988; 154:223–235.
140. Kamel OW, LeBrun DP, Davis RE, Berry GJ, Warnke RA. Growth fraction estimation of malignant lymphomas in formalin-fixed paraffin embedded tissue using anti-PCNA/cyclin 19A2. Am J Pathol 1991; 138:1471–1477.
141. Klemi PJ, Alanen K, Jalkanen S, Joensuu H. Proliferating cell nuclear antigen (PCNA) as a prognostic factor in non-Hodgkin's lymphoma. Br J Cancer 1992; 66:739–743.
142. Woods AL, Hall PA, Shepherd NA, Hanby AM, Waseem NH, Lane DP, Levison DA. The assessment of proliferating cell nuclear antigen (PCNA) immunostaining in primary gastrointestinal lymphomas and its relationship to histological grade, S+G2+M phase fraction (flow cytometric analysis) and prognosis. Histopathology 1991; 19:21–27.
143. Wakely PE Jr, Frable WJ, Kornstein MJ. Role of intraoperative cytopathology in pediatric surgical pathology. Hum Pathol 1993; 24:311–315.
144. Kraemer BB. Mediastinum. *In* Silva EG, Kraemer BB, eds. Intraoperative Pathologic Diagnosis: Frozen Section and Other Techniques. Baltimore: Williams & Wilkins, 1987:235–252.
145. Frable WJ, Kardos TF. Fine needle aspiration biopsy: applications in the diagnosis of lymphoproliferative diseases. Am J Surg Pathol 1989; 12(Suppl 1):62–72.
146. Oertel J, Oertel B, Kastner M, Lobeck H, Huhn D. The value of immunocytochemical staining of lymph node aspirates in diagnostic cytology. Br J Haematol 1988; 70:307–316.
147. Tani E, Christensson B, Porwit A, Skoog L. Immunocytochemical analysis and cytomorphologic diagnosis on fine needle aspirates of lymphoproliferative disease. Acta Cytol 1988; 32:209–215.
148. Hofmann WJ, Momburg F, Moller P, Otto HF. Intra- and extrathymic B cells in physiologic and pathologic conditions: immunohistochemical study on normal thymus and lymphofollicular hyperplasia of the thymus. Virchows Arch [A] 1988; 412:431–442.
149. Isaacson PG, Chan JKC, Tang C, Addis BJ. Low-grade B-cell lymphoma of mucosa-associated lymphoid tissue arising in the thymus: a thymic lymphoma mimicking myoepithelial sialadenitis. Am J Surg Pathol 1990; 14:342–351.
150. Scarpa A, Borgato L, Chilosi M, Capelli P, Menestrina F, Bonetti F, Zamboni G, Pizzolo G, Hirohashi S, Fiore-Donati L. Evidence of c-myc gene abnormalities in mediastinal large B-cell lymphoma of young adult age. Blood 1991; 78:780–788.
151. Takagi N, Nakamura S, Yamamoto K, Kunishima K,

Takagi I, Suyama M, Shinoda M, Sugiura T, Oyama A, Suzuki H, Koshikawa T, Kontani K, Ueda R, Takahashi T, Ariyoshi Y, Suchi T. Malignant lymphoma of mucosa-associated lymphoid tissue arising in the thymus of a patient with Sjögren's syndrome. Cancer 1992; 69:1347–1355.
152. Suster S. Large cell lymphoma of the mediastinum with marked tropism for germinal centers. Cancer 1992; 69:2910–2916.
153. Head DR, Kjeldsberg CR, Kadin ME, Pick T, Bybee B, Longbotham J, Shumski E. Childhood T cell malignancy resembling adult T cell leukemia/lymphoma. Hematol Pathol 1987; 1:15–25.
154. Jaffe ES, Blattner WA, Blayney DW, Bunn PA Jr, Cossman J, Robert-Guroff M, Gallo RC. The pathologic spectrum of adult T-cell leukemia/lymphoma in the United States: human T-cell leukemia/lymphoma virus–associated lymphoid malignancies. Am J Surg Pathol 1984; 8:263–275.
155. Foucar K, Carroll TJ, Tannous R, Peterson L, Goeken JA, Binion S, Gajl-Peczalska J, Kadin ME, Yokoyama WM. Nonendemic adult T-cell leukemia/lymphoma in the United States: report of two cases and review of the literature. Am J Clin Pathol 1985; 83:18–26.
156. Ehrlich GD, Poiesz BJ. Clinical and molecular parameters of HTLV-1 infection. Clin Lab Med 1988; 8:65–84.
157. Kadin ME, Sako D, Berliner N, Franklin W, Woda B, Borowitz M, Ireland K, Schweid A, Herzong P, Lange B, Dorfman R. Childhood Ki-1 lymphoma presenting with skin lesions and peripheral lymphadenopathy. Blood 1986; 68:1042–1049.
158. Tashiro K, Kikuchi M, Takeshita M, Yoshida T, Oshima K. Clinicopathological study of Ki-1 positive lymphomas. Pathol Res Pract 1989; 185:461–467.
159. Stein H, Mason DY, Gerdes J, O'Connor N, Wainscoat J, Pallesen G, Getter K, Falini B, Delsol G, Lemke H, Schwarting R, Lennert K. The expression of the Hodgkin's disease associated antigen Ki-1 in reactive and neoplastic lymphoid tissue: evidence that Reed-Sternberg cells and histiocytic malignancies are derived from activated lymphoid cells. Blood 1985; 66:848–858.
160. Agnarsson BA, Kadin ME. Ki-1 positive large cell lymphoma: a morphologic and immunologic study of 19 cases. Am J Surg Pathol 1988; 124:264–274.
161. Bitter MA, Franklin WA, Larson RA, McKeithan TW, Rubin CM, Le Beau MM, Stephens JK, Vardiman JW. Morphology in Ki-1(CD30)–positive non-Hodgkin's lymphoma is correlated with clinical features and the presence of a unique chromosomal abnormality, t(2;5) (p23;q35). Am J Surg Pathol 1990; 14:305–316.
162. Greer JP, Kinney MC, Collins RD, Salhany KE, Wolff SN, Hainsworth JD, Flexner JM, Stein RS. Clinical features of 31 patients with Ki-1 anaplastic large cell lymphoma. J Clin Oncol 1991; 9:539–547.
163. Penny RJ, Blaustein JC, Longtine JA, Pinkus GS. Ki-1 positive large cell lymphomas, a heterogenous group of neoplasms: morphologic, immunophenotypic, genotypic, and clinical features of 24 cases. Cancer 1991; 682:362–373.
164. Falini B, Pileri S, Stein H, Dieneman D, Dallenbach F, Delsol G, Minelli O, Poggi S, Martelli MF, Pallesen G, Palestro G. Variable expression of leucocyte-common (CD45) antigen in CD30 (Ki1)–positive anaplastic large cell lymphoma: implications for the differential diagnosis between lymphoid and nonlymphoid malignancies. Hum Pathol 1990; 21:624–629.
165. Chott A, Kaserer K, Augustin I, Vesely M, Heinz R, Oehlinger W, Hanak H, Radaszkiewicz T. Ki-1 positive large cell lymphoma: a clinicopathologic study of 41 cases. Am J Surg Pathol 1990; 14:439–448.
166. Offit K, Ladanyi M, Gangi MD, Ebrahim SAD, Filippa D, Chaganti RSK. Ki-1 antigen expression defines a favorable clinical subset of non-B cell non-Hodgkin's lymphoma. Leukemia 1990; 4:625–630.
167. Le Beau MM, Bitter MA, Larson RA, Doane LA, Ellis ED, Franklin WA, Rubin CM, Kadin ME, Vardiman JW. The t(2;5) (p23;q35): a recurring chromosomal abnormality in Ki-1 positive anaplastic large cell lymphoma. Leukemia 1989; 3:866–870.
168. Benz-Lemoine E, Brizard A, Huret J, Babin P, Guilhot F, Couet D, Tanzer J. Malignant histiocytosis: a specific t(2:5) (p23:q35) translocation? Review of the literature. Blood 1988; 72:1045–1047.
169. de Bruin PC, Noorduyn AL, van der Valk P, van Heerde P, van Diest PJ, van de Sandt MM, Ossenkoppele GJ, Meijer CJLM. Noncutaneous T-cell lymphomas: recognition of a lymphoma type (large cell anaplastic) with a relatively favorable prognosis. Cancer 1993; 71:2604–2612.
170. Chan JKC, Ng CS, Hui PK, Leung TW, Lo ESF, Lau WH, McGuire LJ. Anaplastic large cell Ki-1 lymphoma: delineation of two morphological types. Histopathology 1989; 15:11–34.
171. Beljaards RC, Kaudewitz P, Berti E, Gianotti R, Neumann C, Rosso R, Paulli M, Meijer CJLM, Willemze R. Primary cutaneous CD30-positive large cell lymphoma: definition of a new type of cutaneous lymphoma with a favorable prognosis: a European multicenter study of 47 patients. Cancer 1993; 71:2097–2104.
172. Salhany KE, Collins RD, Greer JP, Kinney MC. Long-term survival in Ki-1 lymphoma. Cancer 1991; 67:516–522.
173. Nakamura S, Takagi N, Kojima M, Motoori T, Kitoh K, Osada H, Suzuki H, Ogura M, Kurita S, Oyama A, Ueda R, Takahashi T, Suchi T. Clinicopathologic study of large cell anaplastic lymphoma (Ki-1-positive large cell lymphoma) among the Japanese. Cancer 1991; 68:118–129.
174. Kadin ME, Berard CW, Nanba CW, Wakasa H. Lymphoproliferative diseases in Japan and Western countries. Hum Pathol 1983; 14:745–772.
175. Jenkins PF, Ward MJ, Davies P, Fletcher J. Non-Hodgkin's lymphoma, chronic lymphatic leukemia and the lung. Br J Dis Chest 1981; 75:22–30.
176. Lee S-H, Su I-J, Chen R-L, Lin K-S, Lin D-T, Chuu W-M. A pathologic study of childhood lymphoma in Taiwan with special reference to peripheral T-cell lymphoma and the association with Epstein-Barr viral infection. Cancer 1991; 68:1954–1962.
177. Magrath IT, Jain V, Jaffe ES. Small noncleaved cell lymphoma. *In* Knowles DM, ed. Neoplastic Hematopathology. Baltimore: Williams & Wilkins, 1992:749–772.
178. Squire RA, Goodman DG, Valerio MG, Fredrickson T, Strandberg JD, Levitt MH, Lingeman CH, Harshbarger JC, Dawe CJ. Tumors: hemopoietic system. *In* Benirschke K, Garner FM, Jones TC, eds. Pathology of Laboratory Animals. New York: Springer-Verlag, 1978:1091–1125.
179. Hays EF, Bristol GC, McDougall S, Klotz JL, Kronenberg M. Development of lymphoma in the thymus of AKR mice treated with lymphomagenic virus SL 3-3. Cancer Res 1989; 49:4225–4230.
180. Ewing J. The thymus and its tumors: report of three cases of thymoma. Surg Gynecol Obstet 1916; 22:461–472.
181. Lattes R. Thymoma and other tumors of the thymus: an analysis of 107 cases. Cancer 1962; 15:1224–1260.

182. Lowenhaupt E, Brown R. Carcinoma of the thymus of granulomatous type: a clinical and pathological study. Cancer 1951; 4:1193–1209.
183. Keller AR, Castleman B. Hodgkin's disease of the thymus gland. Cancer 1974; 33:1615–1623.
184. Katz A, Lattes R. Granulomatous thymoma or Hodgkin's disease of thymus? A clinical and histologic study and a re-evaluation. Cancer 1969; 23:1–15.
185. Fechner RE. Hodgkin's disease of the thymus. Cancer 1969; 23:16–23.
186. Gutensohn N, Cole P. Epidemiology of Hodgkin's disease. Semin Oncol 1980; 7:92–101.
187. Mueller NE. The epidemiology of Hodgkin's disease. *In* Selby P, McElwain TJ, eds. Hodgkin's disease. Oxford: Blackwell Scientific Publications, 1987:68–94.
188. Mir R, Anderson J, Strauchen J, Nissen NI, Cooper R, Rafla S, Canellos GP, Bloomfield CD, Gottlieb AJ, Peterson B, Marcos M. Hodgkin's disease in patients 60 years of age or older. Cancer 1993; 71:1857–1866.
189. Olweny CLM, Ziegler J, Berard CW, Templeton AC. Adult Hodgkin's disease in Uganda. Cancer 1971; 27:1295–1301.
190. Hu E, Hufford S, Lukes R, Bernstein-Singer M, Sobel G, Gill P, Pinter-Brown L, Rarick M, Rosen P, Brynes R, Nathwani B, Feinstein D, Levine A. Third-World Hodgkin's disease at Los Angeles County-University of Southern California Medical Center. J Clin Oncol 1988; 6:1285–1292.
191. Gutensohn N, Cole P. Childhood social environment and Hodgkin's disease. N Engl J Med 1981; 304:135–140.
192. Weiss LM, Movahed LA, Warnke RA, Sklar J. Detection of Epstein-Barr viral genomes in Reed-Sternberg cells of Hodgkin's disease. N Engl J Med 1989; 320:502–506.
193. Ambinder RF, Browning PJ, Lorenzana I, Leventhal BG, Cosenza H, Mann RB, MacMahon EME, Medina R, Cardona V, Grufferman S, Olshan A, Levin A, Petersen EA, Blattner W, Levine PH. Epstein-Barr virus and childhood Hodgkin's disease in Honduras and the United States. Blood 1993; 81:462–467.
194. Chang KL, Albujar PF, Chen Y-Y, Johnson RM, Weiss LM. High prevalence of Epstein-Barr virus in the Reed-Sternberg cells of Hodgkin's disease occurring in Peru. Blood 1993; 81:496–501.
195. Selby P, McElwain TJ. Clinical features of Hodgkin's disease. *In* Selby P, McElwain TJ, eds. Hodgkin's disease. Oxford: Blackwell Scientific Publications, 1987:94–125.
196. Kaplan HS. Hodgkin's Disease. Cambridge, MA: Harvard University Press, 1972:1–14.
197. Maity A, Goldwein JW, Lange B, D'Angio GJ. Mediastinal masses in children with Hodgkin's disease: an analysis of the Children's Hospital of Philadelphia and the Hospital of the University of Pennsylvania experience. Cancer 1992; 69:2755–2760.
198. Johnson DW, Hoppe RT, Cox RS, Rosenberg SA, Kaplan HS. Hodgkin's disease limited to intrathoracic sites. Cancer 1983; 52:8–13.
199. Mauch P, Goodman R, Hellman S. The significance of mediastinal involvement in early stage Hodgkin's disease. Cancer 1978; 42:1039–1045.
200. Delaney TF, Glatstein E. Updates 1: The role of the staging laparotomy in the management of Hodgkin's disease. *In* DeVita VT Jr, Hellman S, Rosenberg SA, eds. Cancer: Principles and Practice of Oncology. Philadelphia: JB Lippincott, 1987:1–14.
201. Hellman S, Jaffe ES, DeVita VT Jr. Hodgkin's disease. *In* DeVita VT Jr, Hellman S, Rosenberg SA, eds. Cancer: Principles and Practice of Oncology. Philadelphia: JB Lippincott, 1989:1696–1740.
202. Urba WJ, Longo DL. Hodgkin's disease. N Engl J Med 1992; 326:678–687.
203. Wiernik PH. Updates Volume 2 Number 8: Chemotherapy of Hodgkin's disease. *In* DeVita VT Jr, Hellman S, Rosenberg SA, eds. Cancer: Principles and Practice of Oncology. Philadelphia: JB Lippincott, 1988:1–12.
204. Knowles DM, Chadburn A. Lymphadenopathy and the lymphoid neoplasms associated with the acquired immune deficiency syndrome (AIDS). *In* Knowles DM, ed. Neoplastic Hematopathology. Baltimore: Williams & Wilkins, 1992:773–835.
205. Kristal AR, Burnett WS, Nasca PC, Mikl J. Changes in the epidemiology of non-Hodgkin's lymphoma associated with epidemic human immunodeficiency virus (HIV) infection. Am J Epidemiol 1988; 128:711–718.
206. Ahmed T, Wormser GP, Stahl RE, Mamtani R, Cimino J, Glasser M, Mittelman A, Friedland M, Arlin Z. Malignant lymphomas in a population at risk for acquired immunodeficiency syndrome. Cancer 1987; 60:719–723.
207. Glaser SL, Swartz WG. Time trends in Hodgkin's disease incidence: the role of diagnostic accuracy. Cancer 1990; 66:2196–2204.
208. Knowles DM, Chamulak GA, Subar M, Burke JS, Dugan M, Wernz J, Slywotzky C, Pelicci P-G, Dalla-Favera R, Raphael B. Lymphoid neoplasia associated with the acquired immunodeficiency syndrome (AIDS). Ann Intern Med 1988; 108:744–753.
209. Lowenthal DA, Straus DJ, Campbell SW, Gold JWM, Clarkson BD, Koziner B. AIDS-related lymphoid neoplasia: the Memorial Hospital experience. Cancer 1988; 61:2325–2337.
210. Ree HJ, Strauchen JA, Khan AA, Gold JE, Crowley JP, Kahn H, Zalusky R. Human immunodeficiency virus-associated Hodgkin's disease: clinicopathologic studies of 24 cases and preponderance of mixed cellularity type characterized by the occurrence of fibrohistiocytoid stromal cells. Cancer 1991; 67:1614–1621.
211. Pelstring RJ, Zellmer RB, Sulak LE, Banks PM, Clare N. Hodgkin's disease in association with human immunodeficiency virus infection: pathologic and immunologic features. Cancer 1991; 67:1865–1873.
212. Serrano M, Bellas C, Campo E, Ribera J, Martin C, Rubio R, Ruiz C, Ocana I, Buzon L, Yebra M, Font M, Martinez MA. Hodgkin's disease in patients with antibodies to human immunodeficiency virus: a study of 22 patients. Cancer 1990; 65:2248–2254.
213. Unger PD, Strauchen JA. Hodgkin's disease in AIDS complex patients: report of four cases and tissue immunologic marker studies. Cancer 1986; 58:821–825.
214. Alfonso PG, Sanudo KEF, Carretero JM, Galindo RC, Altozano JG, Gomez LP, Manga GP. Hodgkin's disease in HIV-infected patients. Biomed Pharmacother 1988; 42:321–325.
215. Robert NJ, Schneiderman H. Hodgkin's disease and the acquired immunodeficiency syndrome. Ann Intern Med 1984; 101:142–143.
216. Scheib RG, Siegel RS. Atypical Hodgkin's disease and the acquired immunodeficiency syndrome [Letter]. Ann Intern Med 1985; 102:554.
217. Schoeppel SL, Hoppe RT, Dorfman RF, Horning SJ, Collier AC, Chew TG, Weiss LM. Hodgkin's disease in homosexual men with generalized lymphadenopathy. Ann Intern Med 1985; 102:68–70.
218. Sloane JP. Histopathology of Hodgkin's disease. *In* Selby P, McElwain TJ, eds. Hodgkin's Disease. Oxford: Blackwell Scientific Publications, 1987:4–30.
219. MacLennan KA, Bennett MH, Tu A, Hudson BV, Easterling J, Hudson GV, Jelliffe AM. Relationship of

histopathologic features to survival and relapse in nodular sclerosing Hodgkin's disease: a study of 1659 patients. Cancer 1989; 64:1686–1693.
220. Kant JA, Hubbard SM, Longo DL, Simon RM, DeVita VT Jr, Jaffe ES. The pathologic and clinical heterogeneity of lymphocyte-depleted Hodgkin's disease. J Clin Oncol 1986; 4:284–294.
221. Strickler JG, Michie SA, Warnke RA, Dorfman RF. The "syncytial variant" of nodular sclerosing Hodgkin's disease. Am J Surg Pathol 1986; 10:470–477.
222. Ben-Yehuda-Salz D, Ben-Yehuda A, Polliack A, Ron N, Okon E. Syncytial variant of nodular sclerosing Hodgkin's disease. Cancer 1990; 65:1167–1172.
223. Frizzera G. The distinction of Hodgkin's disease from anaplastic large cell lymphoma. Semin Diagn Pathol 1992; 9:291–296.
224. Poppema S. Lymphocyte-predominance Hodgkin's disease. Semin Diagn Pathol 1992; 9:257–264.
225. Trudel MA, Krikorian JG, Neiman RS. Lymphocyte predominance Hodgkin's disease: a clinicopathologic reassessment. Cancer 1987; 59:99–106.
226. Regula DP, Hoppe RT, Weiss LM. Nodular and diffuse types of lymphocyte predominance Hodgkin's disease. N Engl J Med 1988; 318: 214–219.
227. Butler JJ. The histologic diagnosis of Hodgkin's disease. Semin Diagn Pathol 1992; 9:252–256.
228. Kadin ME, Glatstein E, Dorfman RF. Clinicopathologic studies of 117 untreated patients subjected to laparotomy for the staging of Hodgkin's disease. Cancer 1971; 27:1277–1294.
229. Grogan TM. Hodgkin's disease. *In* Jaffe ES, ed. Surgical Pathology of the Lymph Nodes and Related Organs. Philadelphia: WB Saunders, 1985:86–134.
230. Durkin W, Durant J. Benign mass lesions after therapy for Hodgkin's disease. Arch Intern Med 1979; 139:333–336.
231. Baron RL, Sagel SS, Baglan RJ. Thymic cysts following radiation therapy for Hodgkin's disease. Radiology 1981; 141:593–597.
232. Murray JA, Parker AC. Mediastinal Hodgkin's disease and thymic cysts. Chest 1984; 71:282–284.
233. Kornstein MJ, Bonner H, Gee B, Cohen R, Brooks JJ. Leu M1 and S100 in Hodgkin's disease and non-Hodgkin's lymphomas. Am J Clin Pathol 1986; 85:433–437.
234. Hsu S-M, Jaffe ES. Leu M1 and peanut agglutinin stain the neoplastic cells of Hodgkin's disease. Am J Clin Pathol 1984; 82:29–32.
235. Pinkus GS, Thomas P, Said JW. Leu M1—a marker for Reed-Sternberg cells in Hodgkin's disease. Am J Pathol 1985; 119:244–252.
236. Kadin ME, Muramoto L, Said J. Expression of T-cell antigens on Reed-Sternberg cells in a subset of patients with nodular sclerosing and mixed cellularity Hodgkin's disease. Am J Pathol 1988; 130:345–353.
237. Agnarsson B, Kadin ME. The immunophenotype of Reed-Sternberg cells: a study of 50 cases of Hodgkin's disease using fixed frozen tissues. Cancer 1989; 63:2083–2087.
238. Zukerberg LR, Collins AB, Ferry JA, Harris NL. Coexpression of CD15 and CD20 by Reed-Sternberg cells in Hodgkin's disease. Am J Pathol 1991; 139:475–483.
239. Ree HJ, Teplitz C, Khan A. The Lewis X antigen: a new paraffin section marker for Reed-Sternberg cells. Cancer 1991; 6738:1338–1346.
240. Chittal SM, Caveriviere P, Schwarting R, Gerdes J, Al Saati T, Rigal-Huguet F, Stein H, Delsol G. Monoclonal antibodies in the diagnosis of Hodgkin's disease: the search for a rational panel. Am J Surg Pathol 1988; 12:9–21.
241. Frierson HF Jr, Innes DJ Jr. Sensitivity of anti-Leu-M1 as a marker in Hodgkin's disease. Arch Pathol Lab Med 1985; 109:1024–1028.
242. Dorfman RF, Gatter KC, Pulford KAF, Mason DY. An evaluation of the utility of anti-granulocyte and anti-leukocyte monoclonal antibodies in the diagnosis of Hodgkin's disease. Am J Pathol 1986; 123:508–509.
243. Sherrod AE, Felder B, Levy N, Epstein A, Marder R, Lukes RJ, Taylor CR. Immunohistologic identification of phenotypic antigens associated with Hodgkin and Reed-Sternberg cells: a paraffin section study. Cancer 1986; 57:2135–2140.
244. Ree HJ, Neiman RS, Martin AW, Dallenbach F, Stein H. Paraffin section markers for Reed-Sternberg cells: a comparative study of peanut agglutinin, Leu-M1, LN-2, and Ber-H2. Cancer 1989; 63:2030–2036.
245. Pinkus GS, Said JW. Hodgkin's disease, lymphocyte predominance type, nodular—further evidence for a B cell derivation: L and H variants of Reed-Sternberg cells express L26, a pan–B cell marker. Am J Pathol 1988; 133:211–217.
246. Clark JR, Williams ME, Swerdlow SH. Detection of B- and T-cells in paraffin-embedded tissue sections: diagnostic utility of commercially obtained 4KB5 and UCHL1. Am J Clin Pathol 1990; 93:58–69.
247. Strickler JG, Weiss LM, Copenhaver CM, Bindl J, McDaid R, Buck D, Warnke R. Monoclonal antibodies reactive in routinely processed tissue sections of malignant lymphoma, with emphasis on T cell lymphomas. Hum Pathol 1987; 18:808–814.
248. Sundeen J, Lipford E, Uppenkamp M, Sussman E, Wahl L, Raffeld M, Cossman J. Rearranged antigen receptor genes in Hodgkin's disease. Blood 1987; 70:96–103.
249. Griesser H, Feller AC, Mak TW, Lennert K. Clonal rearrangements of T-cell receptor and immunoglobulin genes and immunophenotypic antigen expression in different subclasses of Hodgkin's disease. Int J Cancer 1987; 40:157–160.
250. Herbst H, Tippelmann G, Anagnostopoulos I, Gerdes J, Schwarting R, Boehm T, Pileri S, Jones DB, Stein H. Immunoglobulin and T-cell receptor gene rearrangements in Hodgkin's disease and Ki-1-positive anaplastic large cell lymphoma: dissociation between phenotype and genotype. Leuk Res 1989; 13:103–116.
251. Weiss LM, Strickler JG, Hu E, Warnke RA, Sklar J. Immunoglobulin gene rearrangements in Hodgkin's disease. Hum Pathol 1986; 17:1009–1014.
252. Anastasi J, Bauer KD, Variakojis D. DNA aneuploidy in Hodgkin's disease: a multiparameter flow-cytometric analysis with cytologic correlation. Am J Pathol 1987; 128:573–582.
253. Joensuu H, Klemi PJ, Korkeila E. Prognostic value of DNA ploidy and proliferative activity in Hodgkin's disease. Am J Clin Pathol 1988; 90:670–673.
254. Morgan KG, Quirke P, O'Brien CJ, Bird CC. Hodgkin's disease: a flow cytometric study. J Clin Pathol 1988; 41:365–369.
255. Osborne BM, Uthman MO, Butler JJ, McLaughlin P. Differentiation of T-cell lymphoma from Hodgkin's disease: mitotic rate and S-phase analysis. Am J Clin Pathol 1990; 93:227–232.
256. Kardos TF, Vinson JH, Behm FG, Frable WJ, O'Dowd GJ. Hodgkin's disease: diagnosis by fine needle aspiration biopsy. Am J Clin Pathol 1986; 86:286–291.
257. Dmitrovsky E, Martin SE, Krudy AG, Chu EW, Jaffe ES, Longo DL, Young RC. Lymph node aspiration in the management of Hodgkin's disease. J Clin Oncol 1986; 4:306–310.

258. Das DK, Gupta SK, Datta BN, Sharma SC. Fine needle aspiration cytodiagnosis of Hodgkin's disease and its subtypes. I. Scope and limitations. Acta Cytol 1990; 34:329–336.
259. Jaffe ES. The elusive Reed-Sternberg cell [Editorial]. N Engl J Med 1989; 320:529–531.
260. Gupta RK, Whelan JS, Lister TA, Young BD, Bodmer JG. Direct sequence analysis of the t(14:18) chromosomal translocation in Hodgkin's disease. Blood 1992; 79:2084–2088.
261. Reid AH, Cunningham RE, Frizzera G, O'Leary TJ. Bcl-2 rearrangement in Hodgkin's disease: results of polymerase chain reaction, flow cytometry, and sequencing on formalin-fixed, paraffin-embedded tissue. Am J Pathol 1993; 142:395–402.
262. Hsu S-M. The never-ending controversies in Hodgkin's disease [Letter]. Blood 1990; 75:1742–1744.
263. Timens W, Visser L, Poppema S. Nodular lymphocyte predominance type of Hodgkin's disease is a germinal center lymphoma. Lab Invest 1986; 54:457–461.
264. Weiss LM, Strickler JG, Warnke RA, Purtilo DT, Sklar J. Epstein-Barr viral DNA in tissues of Hodgkin's disease. Am J Pathol 1987; 129:86–91.
265. Carbone A, Gloghini A, Zanette I, Canal B, Rizzo A, Volpe R. Co-expression of Epstein-Barr virus latent membrane protein and vimentin in "aggressive" histological subtypes of Hodgkin's disease. Virchows Arch [A] 1993; 422:39–45.
266. Delsol G, Brousset P, Chittal S, Rigal-Hugue F. Correlation of the expression of Epstein-Barr virus latent membrane protein and in situ hybridization with biotinylated BamHi-W probes in Hodgkin's disease. Am J Pathol 1992; 140:247–253.
267. Boyle MJ, Vasak E, Tshucchnigg M, Turner JJ, Sculley T, Penny R, Cooper DA, Tindall B, Sewell WA. Subtypes of Epstein-Barr virus (EBV) in Hodgkin's disease: association between B-type EBV and immunocompromise. Blood 1993; 81:468–474.
268. Herndier BG, Sanchez HC, Chang KL, Chen Y-Y, Weiss LM. High prevalence of Epstein-Barr virus in the Reed-Sternberg cells of HIV-associated Hodgkin's disease. Am J Pathol 1993; 142:1073–1079.
269. Anagnostopoulos I, Herbst H, Niedobitek G, Stein H. Demonstration of monoclonal EBV genomes in Hodgkin's disease and Ki-1-positive anaplastic large cell lymphoma by combined Southern blot and in situ hybridization. Blood 1989; 74:810–816.
270. Straus SE, Cohen JI, Tosato G, Meier J. Epstein-Barr virus infections: biology, pathogenesis, and management. Ann Intern Med 1993; 118:45–58.
271. Pedersen-Bjergaard J, Larsen SO. Incidence of acute nonlymphocytic leukemia, preleukemia, and acute myeloproliferative syndrome up to 10 years after treatment of Hodgkin's disease. N Engl J Med 1982; 307:965–971.
272. Casey TT, Cousar JB, Mangum M, Williams ME, Lee JT, Greer JP, Collins RD. Monomorphic lymphomas arising in patients with Hodgkin's disease: correlation of morphologic, immunophenotypic, and molecular genetic findings in 12 cases. Am J Pathol 1990; 136:81–94.
273. Castleman B. Pathological discussion, case records of the Massachusetts General Hospital, Case 40011. N Engl J Med 1954; 250:26–30.
274. Castleman B, Iverson L, Menendez VP. Localized mediastinal lymph node hyperplasia resembling thymoma. Cancer 1956; 9:822–830.
275. Keller AR, Hochholzer L, Castleman B. Hyaline-vascular and plasma cell types of giant lymph node hyperplasia of the mediastinum and other locations. Cancer 1972; 29:670–683.
276. Baruch Y, Ben Arie Y, Kerner H, Lorber M, Best LA, Gershoni Baruch R. Giant lymph node hyperplasia (Castleman's disease): a clinical study of eight patients. Postgrad Med J 1991; 67:366–370.
277. Salisbury JR. Castleman's disease in childhood and adolescence: report of a case and review of literature. Pediatr Pathol 1990; 10:609–615.
278. Frizzera G. Castleman's disease and related disorders. Semin Diagn Pathol 1988; 5:346–364.
279. Schillings PHM, Flendrig JA. Benign giant lymphoma, the morphological aspects [Abstract]. Folia Med Neerl 1969; 12:119–120.
280. Samuels TH, Hamilton PA, Ngan B. Mediastinal Castleman's disease: demonstration with computed tomography and angiography. Can Assoc Radiol J 1990; 41:380–383.
281. Gerald W, Kostianovsky M, Rosai J. Development of vascular neoplasia in Castleman's disease: report of seven cases. Am J Surg Pathol 1990; 14:603–614.
282. Karcher DS, Pearson CE, Butler WM, Hurwitz MA, Cassell PF. Giant lymph node hyperplasia involving the thymus with associated nephrotic syndrome and myelofibrosis. Am J Clin Pathol 1981; 77:100–104.
283. Virmani R, Bewtra C, McAllister HA, Schulte RD. Intrapericardial giant lymph node hyperplasia. Am J Surg Pathol 1982; 6:475–481.
284. Matsuda H, Mori M, Yasumoto K, Sugimachi K. Angiofollicular lymph node hyperplasia arising from the intercostal space. Thorax 1988; 43:337–338.
285. Frizzera G. Castleman's disease: more questions than answers. Hum Pathol 1985; 16:202–205.
286. Lachant NA, Sun NCJ, Leong LA, Oseas RS, Prince HE. Multicentric angiofollicular lymph node hyperplasia (Castleman's disease) followed by Kaposi's sarcoma in two homosexual males with the acquired immunodeficiency syndrome (AIDS). Am J Clin Pathol 1985; 83:27–33.
287. Diebold J, Marche C, Audoin J, Aubert JP, le Tourneau A, Bouton C, Reynes M, Wizniak J, Capron F, Tricottet V. Lymph node modification in patients with the acquired immunodeficiency syndrome (AIDS) or with AIDS related complex (ARC). Pathol Res Pract 1985; 180:590–611.
288. Lowenthal DA, Filippa DA, Richardson ME, Bertoni M, Straus DJ. Generalized lymphadenopathy with morphologic features of Castleman's disease in an HIV-positive man. Cancer 1987; 60:2454–2458.
289. Buijs L, Wijermans PW, van Groningen K, Gerrits WB, Kluin P, Haak HL. Hyaline-vascular type Castleman's disease with concomitant malignant B-cell lymphoma. Acta Haematol 1992; 87:160–162.
290. Maheswaran PR, Ramsay AD, Norton AJ, Roche WR. Hodgkin's disease presenting with the histological features of Castleman's disease. Histopathology 1991; 18:249–253.
291. Harris NL. Pathological discussion, Case 39-1990, Case records of the Massachusetts General Hospital. N Engl J Med 1990; 13:895–908.
292. Kessler E. Multicentric giant lymph node hyperplasia: a report of seven cases. Cancer 1985; 56:2446–2451.
293. Gaba A, Stein RS, Sweet DL, Variakojis D. Multicentric giant lymph node hyperplasia. Am J Clin Pathol 1978; 69:86–90.
294. Hunt SJ, Anderson WD. Giant lymph node hyperplasia of the hyaline vascular type with plasmacytoid T-cells and presentation in infancy. Am J Clin Pathol 1989; 91:344–347.
295. Ozkan H, Tolunay S, Gozu O, Ozer ZG. Giant lym-

phoid hamartoma of mediastinum (Castleman's disease). Thorac Cardiovasc Surg 1990; 38:321–323.

296. Awotedu AA, Otulana BA, Ukoli CO. Giant lymph node hyperplasia of the lung (Castleman's disease) associated with recurrent pleural effusion. Thorax 1990; 45:775–776.
297. Marsh JH, Colbourn DS, Donovan V, Staszewski H. Systemic Castleman's disease in association with Evan's syndrome and vitiligo. Med Pediatr Oncol 1990; 18:169–172.
298. Chan WC, Hargreaves H, Keller J. Giant lymph node hyperplasia with unusual clinicopathologic features. Cancer 1984; 53:2135–2139.
299. Mito M, Takahashi M, Suda T, Yagisawa K, Shinada S, Moriyama Y, Shibata A. Thrombocytosis and erythropoietin-unresponsive anemia in patients with Castleman's disease. Am J Hematol 1991; 36:77–78.
300. Steinberg JJ, Huang PL, Ljubich P, Lee Huang S. Anti-erythropoietin antibodies in hyperviscosity syndrome associated with giant lymph node hyperplasia (GLNH; Castleman's disease). Br J Haematol 1990; 74:543–544.
301. Hall PA, Donaghy M, Cotter FE, Stansfeld AG, Levison DA. An immunohistological and genotypic study of the plasma cell form of Castleman's disease. Histopathology 1989; 14:333–346.
302. Radaszkiewicz T, Hansmann M-L, Lennert K. Monoclonality and polyclonality of plasma cells in Castleman's disease of the plasma cell variant. Histopathology 1989; 14:11–24.
303. Massey GV, Kornstein MJ, Wahl D, Huang XL, McCrady CW, Carchman RA. Angiofollicular lymph node hyperplasia (Castleman's disease) in an adolescent female: clinical and immunologic findings. Cancer 1991; 68:1365–1372.
304. Sethi T, Joshi K, Sharma SC, Gupta BD. Radiation therapy in the management of giant lymph node hyperplasia. Br J Radiol 1990; 63:648–650.
305. Frizzera G, Massarelli G, Banks PM, Rosai J. A systemic lymphoproliferative disorder with morphologic features of Castleman's disease: pathological findings in 15 patients. Am J Surg Pathol 1983; 7:211–231.
306. Weisenburger DD, Nathwani BN, Winberg CD, Rappaport H. Multicentric angiofollicular lymph node hyperplasia: a clinicopathologic study of 16 cases. Hum Pathol 1985; 16:162–172.
307. Chen KTK. Multicentric Castleman's disease and Kaposi's sarcoma. Am J Surg Pathol 1984; 8:287–293.
308. Dickson D, Ben-Ezra JM, Reed J, Flax H, Janis R. Multicentric giant lymph node hyperplasia, Kaposi's sarcoma, and lymphoma. Arch Pathol Lab Med 1985; 9:1013–1018.
309. Hanson CA, Frizzera G, Patton DF, Peterson BA, McClain KL, Gajl-Peczalska KJ, Kersey JH. Clonal rearrangement for immunoglobulin and T-cell receptor genes in systemic Castleman's disease: association with Epstein-Barr virus. Am J Pathol 1988; 131:84–91.
310. Bosco J, Pathmanathan R. POEMS syndrome, osteosclerotic myeloma and Castleman's disease: a case report. Aust N Z J Med 1991; 21:454–456.
311. Gould SJ, Diss T, Isaacson PG. Multicentric Castleman's disease in association with a solitary plasmacytoma: a case report. Histopathology 1990; 17:135–140.
312. Rolon PG, Audouin J, Diebold J, Rolon PA, Gonzalez A. Multicentric angiofollicular lymph node hyperplasia associated with a solitary osteolytic costal IgG lambda myeloma. Pathol Res Pract 1989; 185:468–475.
313. Pavlidis NA, Skopouli FN, Bai MC, Bourantas CL. A successfully treated case of multicentric angiofollicular hyperplasia with oral chemotherapy (Castleman's disease). Med Pediatr Oncol 1990; 18:333–335.
314. Kishimoto T. The biology of interleukin-6. Blood 1989; 74:1–10.
315. Yabuhara A, Yanagiwawa M, Murata T, Kawai H, Komiyama A, Akjabane T, Itoh M, Ishii E, Fujimoto J, Hata J-I. Giant lymph node hyperplasia (Castleman's disease) with spontaneous production of high levels of B-cell differentiation factor activity. Cancer 1989; 63:260–265.
316. Yoshizaki K, Matsuda T, Nishimoto N, Kuritani T, Taeho L, Aozasa K, Nakahata T, Kawai H, Tagoh H, Komori T, Kishimoto S, Hirano T, Kishimoto T. Pathogenic significance of interleukin-6 (IL-6/BSF-2) in Castleman's disease. Blood 1989; 74:1360–1367.
317. Leger Ravet MB, Peuchmaur M, Devergne O, Audouin J, Raphael M, Van Damme J, Galanaud P, Diebold J, Emilie D. Interleukin-6 gene expression in Castleman's disease. Blood 1991; 78:2923–2930.
318. Brandt SJ, Bodine DM, Dunbar CE, Nienhuis AW. Dysregulated interleukin 6 expression produces a syndrome resembling Castleman's disease in mice. J Clin Invest 1990; 86:592–599.
319. Weisenburger DD, DeGowin RL, Gibson DP, Armitage JO. Remission of giant lymph node hyperplasia with anemia after radiotherapy. Cancer 1979; 44:457–462.
320. Carbone A, Manconi R, Volpe R, Poletti A, de Paoli P, Tirelli U, Santini G. Immunohistochemical, enzyme histochemical, and immunologic features of giant lymph node hyperplasia of the hyaline-vascular type. Cancer 1986; 58:908–916.
321. Ruco LP, Gearing AJ, Pigott R, Pomponi D, Burgio VL, Cafolla A, Baiocchini A, Baroni CD. Expression of ICAM-1, VCAM-1 and ELAM-1 in angiofollicular lymph node hyperplasia (Castleman's disease): evidence for dysplasia of follicular dendritic reticulum cells. Histopathology 1991; 19:523–528.
322. Gonzalez CL, Jaffe ES. The histiocytoses: clinical presentation and differential diagnosis. Oncology 1990; 4:47–60.
323. Siegal GP, Dehner LP, Rosai J. Histiocytosis X (Langerhans' cell granulomatosis) of the thymus: a clinicopathologic study of four childhood cases. Am J Surg Pathol 1985; 9:117–124.
324. Nakata H, Suzuki H, Sato Y, Kawahara H, Horie A. Histiocytosis X with anterior mediastinal mass as its initial manifestation. Pediatr Radiol 1982; 12:84–85.
325. Odagiri K, Nishihira K, Hatekeyama S, Kobayashi K. Anterior mediastinal masses with calcifications on CT in children with histiocytosis-X (Langerhans cell histiocytosis). Pediatr Radiol 1991; 21:550–551.
326. Abramson SJ, Berdon WE, Reilly BJ, Kuhn JP. Cavitation of anterior mediastinal masses in children with histiocytosis-X: report of four cases with radiographic, pathologic findings and clinical follow up. Pediatr Radiol 1987; 17:10–14.
327. Eftekhari F, Shirkhoda A, Cangir A. Cavitation of a mediastinal mass following chemotherapy for histiocytosis-X: CT demonstration. J Comput Assist Tomogr 1986; 10:130–132.
328. Bramwell NH, Burns BF. Histiocytosis X of the thymus in association with myasthenia gravis. Am J Clin Pathol 1986; 86:224–227.
329. Pescarmona E, Rendina EA, Ricci C, Baroni CD. Histiocytosis X and lymphoid follicular hyperplasia of the thymus in myasthenia gravis. Histopathology 1989; 14:465–470.
330. Jaffe R. Pathology of Histiocytosis X. Perspect Pediatr Pathol 1987; 9:4–47.

331. Bove KE, Hurtubise P, Wong KY. Thymus in untreated systemic histiocytosis-X. Pediatr Pathol 1985; 4:99–115.
332. Egeler RM, Neglia JP, Puccetti DM, Brennan CA, Nesbit ME. Association of Langerhans cell histiocytosis with malignant neoplasms. Cancer 1993; 71:865–873.
333. Halicek F, Rosai J. Histioeosinophilic granulomas in the thymuses of 29 myasthenic patients: a complication of pneumomediastinum. Hum Pathol 1984; 15:1137–1144.
334. Favara BE, McCarthy RC, Mierau GW. Histiocytosis X. Hum Pathol 1983; 14:663–676.
334a. Willman CL, Busque L, Griffith BB, Favara BE, McClain KL, Duncan MH, Gilliland DG. Langerhans' cell histiocytosis (histiocytosis X)—a clonal proliferative disease. N Engl J Med 1994; 331:191–193.
335. Williams JW, Dorfman RF. Lymphadenopathy as the initial manifestation of histiocytosis X. Am J Surg Pathol 1979; 3:405–421.
336. Favara BE, Jaffe R. Pathology of Langerhans cell histiocytosis. Hematol Oncol Clin North Am 1987; 1:75–97.
337. Ben-Ezra JM, Koo CH. Langerhans' cell histiocytosis and malignancies of the M-PIRE system. Am J Clin Pathol 1993; 99:464–471.
338. Azumi N, Sheibani K, Swartz WG, Stroup RM, Rappaport H. Antigenic phenotypic of Langerhans cell histiocytosis: an immunohistochemical study demonstrating the value of LN2, LN3, and vimentin. Hum Pathol 1988; 19:1376–1382.
339. Consolini R, Cini P, Cei B, Botonne E. Thymic dysfunction in histiocytosis-X. Am J Pediatr Hematol Oncol 1987; 9:146–148.
340. Newton WA Jr, Hamoudi AB, Shannon BT. Role of the thymus in histiocytosis-X. Hematol Oncol Clin North Am 1987; 1:63–74.
341. Leikin SL. Immunobiology of histiocytosis X. Hematol Oncol Clin North Am 1987; 1:49–61.
342. Hamoudi AB, Newton WA Jr, Mancer K, Penn GM. Thymic changes in histiocytosis. Am J Clin Pathol 1982; 77:169–173.
343. Leikin S, Puruganan G, Frankel A, Steerman R, Chandra R. Immunologic parameters in histiocytosis-X. Cancer 1973; 32:796–802.
344. Ben-Ezra J, Bailey A, Azumi N, Delsol G, Stroup R, Sheibani K, Rappaport H. Malignant histiocytosis X: a distinct clinicopathologic entity. Cancer 1991: 68:1050–1060.
345. Muller C, Chantelot JM, Kemeny JL, Terrioux P, de Saint-Florent G, Blanchon F. Plasmocytome du mediastin. Un nouveau cas. Rev Pneumol Clin 1988; 44:39–42.
346. Niwa K, Tanaka T, Mori H, Takahashi M. Extramedullary plasmacytoma of the mediastinum. Jpn J Clin Oncol 1987; 17:95–100.
347. Davis SR, King HS, Le Roux I, Bolding E. Superior vena cava syndrome caused by an intrathoracic plasmacytoma. Cancer 1991; 68:1376–1379.
348. Kubonishi I, Ohtsuki Y, Machida K, Agatsuma Y, Tukuoka H, Iwata K, Miyoshi I. Granulocytic sarcoma presenting as a mediastinal tumor. Am J Clin Pathol 1984; 82:730–734.
349. Bannerjee D, Silva E. Mediastinal mass with acute leukemia myeloblastoma masquerading as lymphoblastic lymphoma. Arch Pathol Lab Med 1981; 105:126–129.
350. Neiman RS, Barcos M, Berard C, Bonner H, Mann R, Rydell RE, Bennett JM. Granulocytic sarcoma: a clinicopathologic study of 61 biopsied cases. Cancer 1981; 48:1426–1437.
351. Voller H, Dingerkus H, Albrecht A, Hennig L, Stein H, Schroder R. Mediastinal-chlorom mit rechtsherzbeteiligung: seltene ursache eines vena-cava-superiorsyndroms. Dtsch Med Wochenschr 1993; 118:416–420.
352. Tillawi IS, Variakojis D. Refractory right ventricular failure due to granulocytic sarcoma. Arch Pathol Lab Med 1990; 114:983–985.
353. Kurec AS, Cruz VE, Barrett D, Mason DY, Davey FD. Immunophenotyping of acute leukemias using paraffin-embedded tissue sections. Am J Clin Pathol 1993; 93:502–509.
354. Litz CE, Brunning RD. Acute myeloid leukemias. *In* Knowles DM, ed. Neoplastic Hematopathology. Baltimore: Williams & Wilkins, 1992:1315–1349.
355. Raz I, Or R, Okon E, Leizerowitz R, Polliack A. Hairy cell leukemia: report of an unusual case with hepatomegaly due to a large vascular tumor of the liver, mediastinal mass and pleural effusion containing hairy cells. Acta Haematol 1984; 71:393–399.

Chapter

7 METASTASES

METASTASES FROM LUNG
METASTASES FROM EXTRATHORACIC SITES
METASTASES FROM UNKNOWN PRIMARY TUMOR
IMMUNOPEROXIDASE
SUMMARY

Metastases to the mediastinal lymph nodes originate most commonly from carcinomas of the lung and less frequently from tumors of the esophagus and of extrathoracic sites[1] (Table 7–1).

METASTASES FROM LUNG

In one study of patients with primary lung carcinoma undergoing mediastinoscopy, 48% had evidence of mediastinal spread.[2] The percentage was similar for all histologic types except well-differentiated squamous cell carcinoma. Mediastinal disease was present in 70% of cases of adenocarcinoma, large-cell undifferentiated, and small-cell types but in only 16% of cases of well-differentiated squamous cell carcinoma.

Recent reports have studied mediastinal metastases from lung carcinomas to evaluate the usefulness of radiographic imaging techniques. In a series of 143 consecutive patients with non–small cell carcinoma, McLoud and colleagues reported 42 (29%) with histologically documented nodal metastases diagnosed by mediastinoscopy or thoracotomy.[3] Seely et al. found mediastinal metastases in 22 of 96 patients (23%) with T_1 bronchogenic carcinoma (tumors less than 3 cm in diameter not invading the visceral pleura).[4] Computed tomography and magnetic resonance imaging detect mediastinal lymph node enlargement.[5] However, large lymph nodes may be benign, and even small lymph nodes may contain metastases. Thus, these imaging modalities are relatively insensitive and nonspecific in detecting metastatic disease.[3, 6] Therefore, histologic assessment of mediastinal lymph nodes is usually considered necessary for staging purposes.

Because of crossover lymphatic drainage, the primary tumor may be in the lung that is contralateral to the mediastinal lymph node.[7] Mediastinal lymph node involvement in carcinoma of the lung is an adverse prognostic factor and is considered at least stage III disease.[2, 7] Involvement of only peribronchial or hilar lymph nodes may constitute stage II or III depending on location and local extent of the tumor.[7] Contralateral hilar lymph node involvement also means stage III.

METASTASES FROM EXTRATHORACIC SITES

Metastases to the mediastinum from extrathoracic, nonhematopoietic neoplasms are uncommon. When present, they most likely represent spread from primary tumors of the gastrointestinal tract, genitourinary tract, and breast[1, 8–10] (Table 7–1). Among extrathoracic tumors with mediastinal metastases on chest radiographs, common primary sites include the kidney, testis, colon and rectum, ovary, prostate, breast, bladder, and stomach. Less frequently, other tumors, including malignant melanoma and sarcomas, metastasize to this area.[11, 12] For a melanoma presenting as a mediastinal mass, determination of the primary site may be impossible.[13] Perhaps rare melano-

Table 7–1. Most Common Extrathoracic Primary Sites of Tumors That Metastasize to the Mediastinum

Mediastinal Metastases Diagnosed by Mediastinoscopy: Extrathoracic Primary Sites[8, 10]	Mediastinal Metastases Diagnosed Radiographically: Extrathoracic Primary Sites[9, 11]
Breast (10)*	Kidney (28)†
Kidney (4)	Testis (12)
Stomach (4)	Colon/rectum (6)
Prostate (4)	Ovary (5)
Thyroid (3)	Prostate (4)
Rectum (2)	Breast (3)
Melanoma (2)	Bladder (3)
Pancreas (1)	Stomach (3)
Ovary (1)	Miscellaneous‡

*In parentheses is the number of patients with tumors of that particular primary site.

†Renal cell carcinomas accounted for 50% of the extrathoracic primary tumors in the study of Mahon and Libshitz versus 12% in the study of McLoud et al.[9, 11] The higher percentage in the first study reflects a special interest in metastatic renal cell carcinoma at the M. D. Anderson Cancer Center.

‡These series included two cases of melanoma and one or two tumors of the following primary sites: thyroid, larynx, nasopharynx/nasal cavity, lingual tonsil, tongue, bladder, cervix uteri, and corpus uteri. Other reports document mediastinal metastases from mesothelioma (pleural and peritoneal), hepatocellular carcinoma, and osteosarcoma.[12, 14, 15, 37]

mas are primary to the mediastinum. Alternatively, a primary cutaneous melanoma may regress after metastasizing. Hepatocellular carcinoma metastatic to the mediastinum has also been reported.[14, 15]

Two studies have addressed mediastinal metastases diagnosed by mediastinoscopy[8, 10] (Table 7–1). Metastases from carcinomas of the lung have exceeded those from extrathoracic primary tumors by a 12:1 ratio.[10] The most common extrathoracic primary sites were breast, prostate, gastrointestinal tract (stomach and colon/rectum), kidney, and thyroid.

Extrathoracic metastases most commonly involve the middle mediastinum, particularly the right paratracheal nodes.[9, 11] Other lymph node groups may be affected, including those of the pulmonary hila, anterior and posterior mediastinum, subcarinal area, and diaphragmatic region. Metastatic disease from extrathoracic primary tumors may affect bilateral hilar nodes. Subdiaphragmatic malignancies may disseminate to the mediastinum via the thoracic duct and/or the lymphatics of the posterior mediastinum.[9] As stated by Heinemann and colleagues, "all lymphatics join in the mediastinum."[8] Therefore, metastases from all body regions may involve this area.

Carcinomas of the thyroid (including papillary and medullary types) may disseminate to mediastinal lymph nodes, particularly those in the upper mediastinum.[16, 17] The metastasis may be significantly larger than the primary tumor. Thus, the patient may present with mediastinal metastases from an occult thyroid carcinoma. The mediastinal metastasis may undergo cystic degeneration and simulate a mediastinal cyst.[18]

In one series, about 5% of patients with a first recurrence of breast carcinoma had mediastinal involvement.[19] Disease limited to the mediastinum was found in only 1% of patients. Metastases to internal mammary lymph nodes usually represent spread from a breast primary tumor.[1]

In an autopsy study of patients with prostatic carcinoma metastatic to lymph nodes, Saitoh et al. found 5% of cases with mediastinal (nonhilar) node involvement and 41% with disease in pulmonary hilar lymph nodes.[20] Among patients initially presenting with carcinoma of the prostate, approximately 1% have mediastinal lymphadenopathy.[21] On occasion, a patient will present with a mediastinal mass that, when resected, is discovered to be a metastasis from a prostatic primary tumor[22–24] (Fig. 7–1).

In gastrointestinal malignancies, mediastinal lymphadenopathy is uncommon.[25, 26] It generally occurs in patients with known advanced disease or symptoms related to the abdominal tumor. A case report describes a patient with a history of rectal carcinoma who developed metastatic disease limited to the mediastinum.[26] At autopsy, the mediastinal mass encased the trachea, esophagus, and great vessels. No residual tumor was present below the diaphragm.

METASTASES FROM UNKNOWN PRIMARY TUMOR

Some patients have metastatic disease from an unknown primary tumor. When metastatic disease is found in the mediastinum, the unknown primary tumor usually is found in the lung. The problem of an unknown primary tumor has been studied from a therapeutic perspective. In 1986, Greco and colleagues described 71 patients with advanced poorly differentiated carcinoma of unknown primary site.[27] Patients were included in the study if they had been diagnosed with poorly differentiated carcinoma or poorly differentiated adenocarcinoma. Diagnoses were made by light

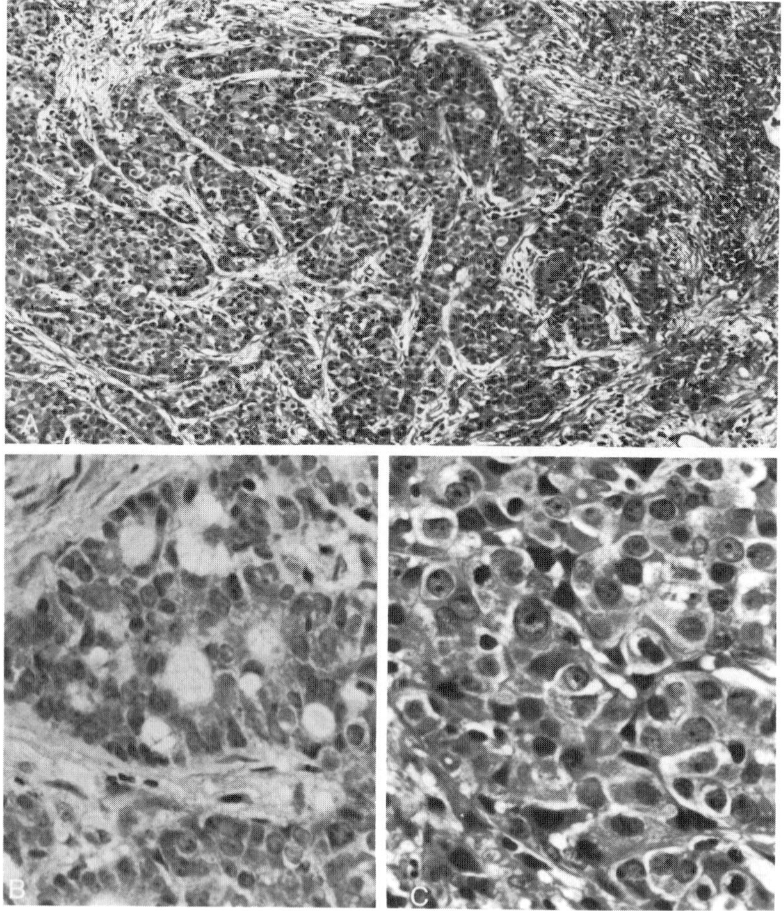

Figure 7–1. *A–C,* Photomicrographs of an enlarged mediastinal lymph node removed from a 61-year-old male by mediastinoscopy. The pattern of growth with islands and trabeculae of tumor cells having eosinophilic cytoplasm suggested the possibility of a carcinoid tumor. Immunoperoxidase studies, however, demonstrated negative chromogranin. Furthermore, the tumor was positive for prostate-specific antigen and prostate-specific acid phosphatase. On questioning the patient, the surgeon discovered that the patient had a previous diagnosis of prostate carcinoma. The prominent nucleoli (*C*) are characteristic of metastatic carcinoma but not usually seen in carcinoid tumors. (*A,* H&E, ×100; *B,* ×400; *C,* ×1000.)

microscopy. Twenty-one patients had mediastinal involvement.

The authors speculated that the patients had unrecognized extragonadal germ cell tumors. Therefore, 62 were treated with intensive cisplatin-based combination chemotherapy of the type used for germ cell tumors. Fifteen patients of the sixty-two (24%) had complete responses, and nine of them were free of tumor more than 8 years after therapy.[28] A later report confirmed the finding that a subgroup of patients diagnosed with poorly differentiated carcinoma is potentially curable with chemotherapy.[29]

IMMUNOPEROXIDASE

In another article, Greco and colleagues described the results of immunoperoxidase staining on tumors from 87 patients reported to have poorly differentiated carcinoma of unknown primary site.[30] Most of these patients had received intensive chemotherapy; a 28% complete response rate was obtained. Twelve patients, or half of the complete responders, were long-term survivors. Using a limited number of immunoperoxidase stains, the authors changed the diagnosis in 14 cases. The revised diagnoses included lymphoma (4), melanoma (8), prostate carcinoma (1), and yolk sac tumor (1). All four of the lymphoma patients were complete responders and long-term survivors. Among the melanoma cases, three of the seven patients given chemotherapy had complete responses and were long-term survivors. Eleven of forty-nine patients (22%) with poorly differentiated carcinoma confirmed by immunoperoxidase staining responded completely.

These authors emphasize the value of immunoperoxidase stains on tumors that are morphologically poorly differentiated.[28] In particular, cytokeratin positivity supports a diagnosis of carcinoma. Immunoreactivity for CD45 (leukocyte common antigen) supports the diagnosis of lymphoma. CD20 (L26) is also useful because it labels most B-cell lymphomas

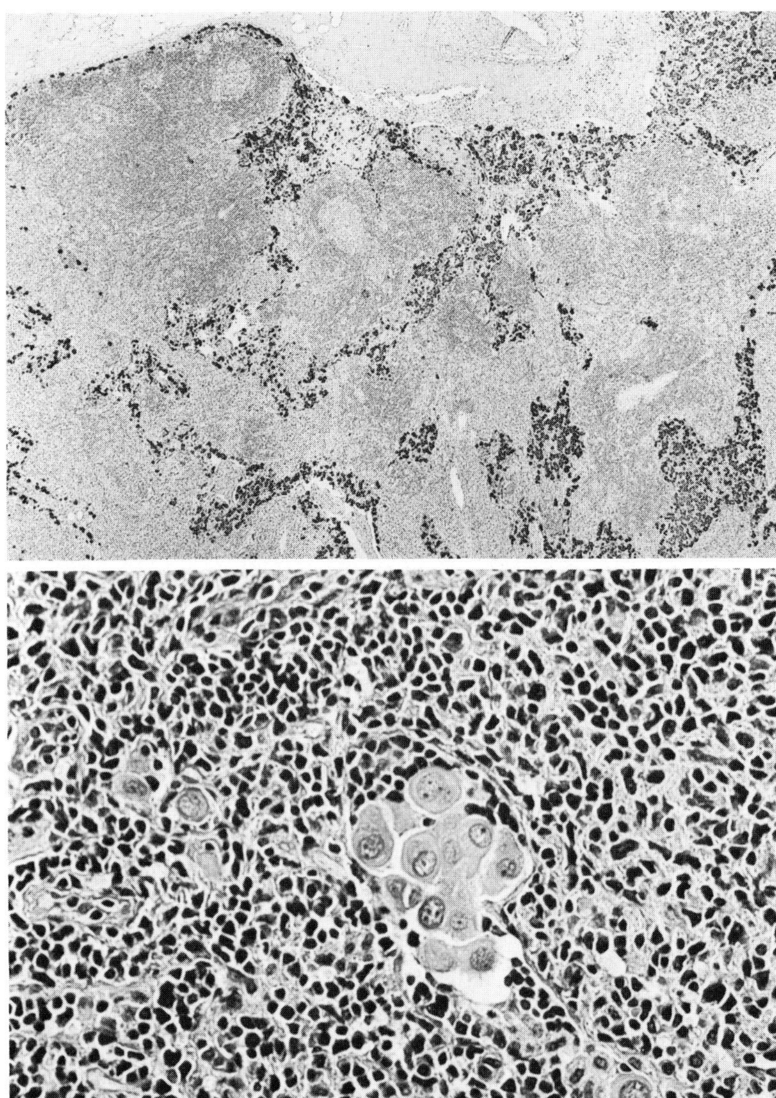

Figure 7–2. Mesothelial cells in mediastinal lymph node. *Top*, Immunoperoxidase stain for cytokeratin demonstrates immunoreactivity within the sinuses of a mediastinal lymph node (×40). *Bottom*, Clusters of epithelioid cells have the microscopic features (including prominent intercellular spaces) of mesothelial cells. However, the possibility of metastatic carcinoma or mesothelioma must be considered (H&E, ×400). (From Brooks JSJ. Mesothelial cell inclusions in mediastinal lymph nodes mimicking metastatic carcinoma. Am J Clin Pathol 1990; 93:741–748.)

in paraffin-embedded tissue. CD30 helps to identify large-cell anaplastic lymphomas, a tumor easily misdiagnosed on light microscopy (see Chapter 6). Melanoma is typically negative for cytokeratin and positive for S100.[31] HMB-45 is another marker for melanoma that is more specific than S100. Markers for germ cell tumors include placental alkaline phosphatase, alpha-fetoprotein, and human chorionic gonadotropin. Not all are specific, however (see Chapter 9).

Several antibodies are useful in determining the origin of metastatic carcinoma.[22, 32] These include prostate-specific antigen and acid phosphatase for prostate carcinoma, gross cystic disease fluid protein (GCDFP-15) for breast carcinoma, and thyroglobulin for thyroid carcinoma. Thus, before one concludes that a patient has a poorly differentiated carcinoma of unknown primary site in the mediastinum (or elsewhere), immunoperoxidase studies should be performed.

In addition to those patients with lymphomas, other subgroups in the Greco et al. studies have responded favorably to chemotherapy. One such subgroup includes those with germ cell tumors. Some germ cell tumors in young men can be suspected on the basis of abnormalities of chromosome 12 or elevations of serum markers (human chorionic gonadotropin or alpha-fetoprotein).[33, 34] (See Chapter 9.) These patients have responded well to cisplatin-based therapy. Characteristic cytogenetic abnormalities are also associated with peripheral neuroectodermal tumor, Ewing's sarcoma, and some lymphomas.[33] Thus, karyotypic analysis can be of value in the diagnosis of histologically "undifferentiated" mediastinal neoplasms.

Another subgroup includes those with poorly differentiated carcinomas showing neuroendocrine differentiation as defined by dense core granules on electron microscopy or chromogranin immunoreactivity. Three of twenty-nine such patients had disease predominantly involving the mediastinum.[35] Six of twenty-three evaluable patients receiving cisplatin-based combination chemotherapy achieved a complete response, whereas another twelve had a partial response lasting 3 to 15 months (overall response rate 78%). Four of the complete responders had long-term disease-free survival. The nonresponders had a median survival of 11 months.

Many patients with a poorly differentiated carcinoma predominantly involving the mediastinum should be considered to have a thymic carcinoma rather than a metastasis from an unknown primary site. Some of these tumors respond to chemotherapy (see Chapter 5). Surprisingly, thymic carcinoma is not considered a diagnostic entity in the studies by Greco and colleagues.

Mesothelial cells in mediastinal lymph nodes may mimic metastatic carcinoma. Brooks and colleagues reported two patients who had been misdiagnosed as having metastatic carcinoma.[36] The mediastinal lymph nodes contained epithelioid-appearing cells within the sinuses (Fig. 7–2). By immunoperoxidase stains, these cells were strongly positive for cytokeratin, but negative for carcinoembryonic antigen and CD15 (Leu M1). Ultrastructurally, the cells had slender microvilli typical of mesothelial cells. Extensive work-up and follow-up of up to 3 years failed to identify a primary tumor. Nevertheless, the authors recommended that any patient with this finding on mediastinal lymph node biopsy be evaluated for possible primary tumors. Immunohistochemistry and electron microscopy should also be performed. In particular, the possibility of metastatic malignant mesothelioma must be considered. Rarely, patients with peritoneal or pleural mesotheliomas present with mediastinal lymphadenopathy.[37]

SUMMARY

The most common primary tumor that metastasizes to mediastinal lymph nodes is carcinoma of the lung. Mediastinal metastases from extrathoracic tumors may originate from any region of the body. The most frequent are the breast, gastrointestinal tract, and genitourinary tract. In the absence of a primary lesion, thymic carcinoma and germ cell tumors must be considered. Immunoperoxidase stains are often helpful in determining the origin of a metastatic tumor.

REFERENCES

1. McLoud TC, Meyer JE. Mediastinal metastases. Radiol Clin North Am 1982; 20:453–468.
2. Goldberg EM, Shapiro CM, Glicksman AS. Mediastinoscopy for assessing mediastinal spread in clinical staging of lung carcinoma. Semin Oncol 1974; 1:205–215.
3. McLoud TC, Bourgouin PM, Greenberg RW, Kosiuk JP, Templeton PA, Shepard JO, Moore EH, Wain JC, Mathisen DJ, Grillo HC. Bronchogenic carcinoma: analysis of staging in the mediastinum with CT by correlative lymph node mapping and sampling. Radiology 1992; 182:319–323.
4. Seely JM, Mayo JR, Miller RR, Muller NL. T1 lung cancer: prevalence of mediastinal nodal metastases and diagnostic accuracy of CT. Radiology 1993; 186:129–132.
5. Kaplan DK. Mediastinal lymph node metastases in lung cancer: is size a valid criterion? Thorax 1992; 47:332–333.
6. Medina Gallardo JF, Borderas Naranjo F, Torres Cansino M, Rodriguez-Panadero F. Validity of enlarge mediastinal nodes as markers of involvement by non–small cell lung cancer. Am Rev Respir Dis 1992; 146:1210–1212.
7. Minna JD, Pass H, Glatstein E, Ihde DC. Cancer of the lung. *In* DeVita VT Jr, Hellman S, Rosenberg SA, eds. Cancer: Principles and Practice of Oncology. Philadelphia: JB Lippincott, 1989:591–705.
8. Heinemann M, Wacha H, Rosenthal R. [Mediastinal metastases of extrathoracic tumors—important findings in mediastinoscopy]. Chirurg 1986; 57:560–564.
9. Mahon TG, Libshitz HI. Mediastinal metastases of infradiaphgramatic malignancies. Eur J Radiol 1992; 15:130–134.
10. Welsh LW, Chinnici JC, Welsh JJ, Huck GF. Mediastinoscopy for extrathoracic malignancies. Ann Otol Rhinol Laryngol 1982; 91:659–665.
11. McLoud TC, Kalisher L, Stark P, Greene R. Intrathoracic lymph node metastases from extrathoracic neoplasms. AJR 1978; 131:403–407.
12. van Zanten TE, Golding RP, Taets ven Amerongen AH. Osteosarcoma with calcific mediastinal lymphadenopathy. Pediatr Radiol 1987; 17:258–259.
13. Feldman L, Kricun ME. Malignant melanoma presenting as a mediastinal mass. JAMA 1979; 241:396–397.
14. Yamashita R, Takahashi M, Kosugi M, Kobayashi C, Annen Y. [A case of metastatic hepatocellular carcinoma of the superior mediastinum]. Nippon Kyobu Geka Gakkai Zasshi 1993; 41:709–713.
15. Nakagawa K, Nakahara K, Ohno K, Matsumura A, Kawashima Y. [Mediastinal dissection of hepatocellular carcinoma with bilateral hilar and mediastinal lymph node metastasis]. Kyobu Geka 1989; 42:857–860.
16. Dralle H, Damm I, Scheumann GFW, Kotzerke J, Kupsch E. Frequency and significance of cervicome-

diastinal lymph node metastases in medullary thyroid carcinoma: results of a compartment-oriented microdissection method. Henry Ford Hosp Med J 1992; 40:264–267.
17. Ahuja S, Ernst H, Lenz K. Papillary thyroid carcinoma: occurrence and types of lymph node metastases. J Endocrinol Invest 1991; 14:543–549.
18. Okumura M, Yasumitsu T, Kotake Y, Ohta M, Ohshima S, Miyauchi A. [Three cases of occult thyroid cancer with mediastinal lymph node metastasis manifesting as a mediastinal cyst]. Nippon Kyobu Geka Gakkai Zasshi 1990; 38:2307–2313.
19. Kamby C, Vejborg I, Kristensen B, Olsen LO, Mouridsen HT. Metastatic pattern in recurrent breast cancer: special reference to intrathoracic recurrences. Cancer 1988; 62:2226–2233.
20. Saitoh H, Yoshida K-I, Uchijima Y, Kobayashi N, Suwata J, Kamata S. Two different lymph node metastatic patterns of a prostatic cancer. Cancer 1990; 65:1843–1846.
21. Lindell MM, Doubleday LC, von Eschenbach AC, Libshitz HI. Mediastinal metastases from prostatic carcinoma. J Urol 1982; 128:331–334.
22. Cho KR, Epstein JE. Metastatic prostatic carcinoma to supradiaphragmatic lymph nodes: a clinicopathologic and immunohistochemical study. Am J Surg Pathol 1997; 11:457–463.
23. Makhija M. Metastatic prostatic carcinoma presenting as an anterior mediastinal mass on gallium imaging. Clin Nucl Med 1991; 16:923–925.
24. Park Y, Oster MW, Olarte MR. Prostatic cancer with an unusual presentation: polymyositis and mediastinal adenopathy. Cancer 1981; 48:1262–1264.
25. Libson E, Bloom RA, Halperin I, Peretz T, Husband JE. Mediastinal lymph node metastases from gastrointestinal carcinoma. Cancer 1987; 59:1490–1493.
26. Satur CM, Gebitekin C, Da Costa PE, Saunders NR. Recurrence of rectal carcinoma in the mediastinum. South Med J 1993; 86:697–698.
27. Greco FA, Vaughn WK, Hainsworth JD. Advanced poorly differentiated carcinoma of unknown primary site: recognition of a treatable syndrome. Ann Intern Med 1986; 104:547–553.
28. Hainsworth JD, Greco FA. Treatment of patients with cancer of unknown primary site. N Engl J Med 1993; 329:257–263.
29. Hainsworth JD, Johnson DH, Greco FA. Cisplatin-based combination chemotherapy in the treatment of poorly differentiated carcinoma and poorly differentiated adenocarcinoma of unknown primary site: results of a 12 year experience. J Clin Oncol 1992; 10:912–922.
30. Hainsworth JD, Wright EP, Johnson DH, Davis BW, Greco FA. Poorly differentiated carcinoma of unknown primary site: clinical usefulness of immunoperoxidase staining. J Clin Oncol 1991; 9:1931–1938.
31. Gown AM, Vogel AM, Hoak D, Gough F, McNutt MA. Monoclonal antibodies specific for melanocytic tumors distinguish subpopulations of melanocytes. Am J Pathol 1986; 123:195–203.
32. Yazdi HM, Dardick I. Determination of the primary site. *In* Diagnostic Immunocytochemistry and Electron Microscopy. New York: Igaku-Shoin, 1992:236–290.
33. Motzer RJ, Rodriguez E, Reuter VE, Samaniego F. Genetic analysis as aid in diagnosis of patients with midline carcinoma of uncertain histologies. J Natl Cancer Inst 1991; 83:341–346.
34. Richardson RL, Schoumacher RA, Fer MF, Hande K, Forbes JT, Oldham RK, Greco FA. The unrecognized extragonadal germ cell cancer syndrome. Ann Intern Med 1981; 94:181–186.
35. Hainsworth JD, Johnson DH, Greco FA. Poorly differentiated neuroendocrine carcinoma of unknown primary site. Ann Intern Med 1988; 109:364–371.
36. Brooks JSJ, LiVolsi VA, Pietra GG. Mesothelial cell inclusions in mediastinal lymph nodes mimicking metastatic carcinoma. Am J Clin Pathol 1990; 93:741–748.
37. Sussman J, Rosai J. Lymph node metastasis as the initial manifestation of malignant mesothelioma: report of six cases. Am J Surg Pathol 1990; 14:819–828.

Chapter

8

INFECTIOUS AND INFLAMMATORY CONDITIONS

GRANULOMATOUS LYMPHADENOPATHY
- Tuberculosis
- Histoplasmosis
- Sarcoidosis
- Silicosis

ACUTE MEDIASTINITIS
SCLEROSING MEDIASTINITIS
SUMMARY

GRANULOMATOUS LYMPHADENOPATHY

Granulomatous inflammation is a common explanation for non-neoplastic mediastinal lymphadenopathy. When an organism can be identified, granulomatous lymphadenopathy in the mediastinum is usually caused by tuberculosis or endemic fungi such as histoplasmosis.[1] The granulomas may result in an adherent mass of lymph nodes that can compress adjacent structures.[1] The granulomas also can induce an inflammatory reaction leading to sclerosing mediastinitis. All of the mediastinal structures, including the trachea, superior vena cava, pericardium, and esophagus, may be involved by either the granulomatous or the sclerosing process.

Tuberculosis

In cases of tuberculosis, hilar or mediastinal lymphadenopathy with focal pulmonary disease is considered a primary infection. Lymphadenopathy in the absence of lung disease may represent an occult pulmonary focus that cannot be visualized. Alternatively, the disease may represent reactivation in a previously infected lymph node.[2] Mediastinal lymph node involvement in tuberculosis is more common in children than in adults.[3–5] One explanation is that adults have acquired resistance that tends to confine the organisms to the site of infection. Tuberculous mediastinal lymphadenopathy is common in patients with impaired resistance from the acquired immunodeficiency syndrome (AIDS).[6] Non-European immigrant groups in the United Kingdom have also been reported as more likely to have involvement of mediastinal lymph nodes.[5, 7]

One third of patients with isolated mediastinal tuberculosis are asymptomatic.[4] When present, symptoms include fever, anorexia, malaise, and weight loss. The disease may be unilateral or bilateral.[5] Hilar, paratracheal, and subcarinal lymph nodes are most commonly affected.[3, 4] When the disease is unilateral, right-sided involvement predominates.[3, 5] The right-sided predominance is understandable, because the right paratracheal lymph nodes drain the entire right lung and left lower lung. Also, pulmonary tuberculosis more often involves the right lung than the left.[3]

Histologically, caseating granulomas are characteristic (Fig. 8–1). Confluent granulomas with irregularly shaped areas of necrosis are surrounded by epithelioid histiocytes, giant cells, lymphocytes, plasma cells, and fibroblasts. Hyalinization and calcification are common. The diagnosis of tuberculosis re-

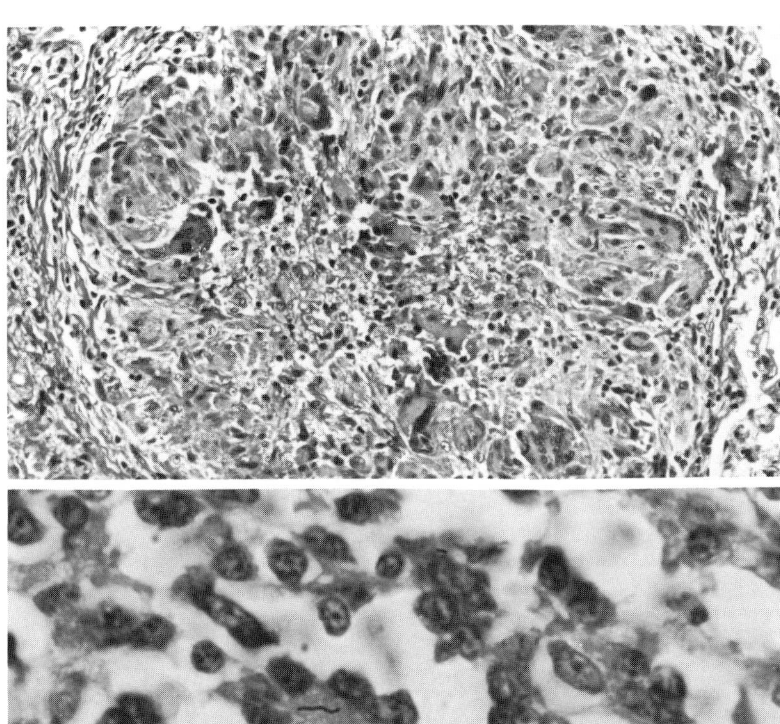

Figure 8–1. Mediastinal lymph node with caseating granulomas from tuberculosis. *Top,* Epithelioid histiocytes and giant cells surround areas of necrosis (H&E, ×200). *Bottom,* Acid-fast bacillus (*arrow*) is identified within a giant cell (Ziehl-Neelson stain, ×1000).

quires identification of beaded, rod-shaped, acid-fast bacilli using the Ziehl-Neelsen or Fite stain.[8] The bacilli are most often identified at the periphery of the necrotic areas within the epithelioid cells. The number of bacilli varies with the patient's immune status, age of the lesion, and previous therapy. Failure to identify the acid-fast bacilli does not exclude the diagnosis of tuberculosis. On computed tomography, areas of low density within the lymph nodes correspond to the caseous necrosis.[3]

Serious complications may result from compression of mediastinal structures such as the superior vena cava and pericardium.[2] Extrinsic compression of the esophagus or spread of infection into this organ may produce dysphagia.

Histoplasmosis

Histoplasmosis is clinically and pathologically similar to tuberculosis.[2] In endemic areas (such as the Mississippi and Ohio river valleys in the United States), almost all inhabitants are infected at some time in their lives, and it is the most common cause of granulomatous mediastinal infection.[9] Most acute infections are asymptomatic. Patients may present with cough, chest pain, fever, dyspnea, weight loss, dysphagia, or hemoptysis. Like tuberculosis, histoplasmosis may present as mediastinal lymphadenopathy, most often in the right paratracheal region.[6, 10–12] Cystic degeneration and calcification are common.

The involved lymph nodes are generally larger than the lung lesions and consist of confluent granulomas with central areas of caseous necrosis.[8] The necrosis is surrounded by epithelioid cells with occasional multinucleated giant cells. Fibrosis is typically present in the peripheral areas. Complete calcification of both lung and lymph node lesions usually occurs in 3 to 6 months. *Histoplasma capsulatum* can be visualized using the Grocott or Gomori silver stain; the tissue may have to be decalcified first. The organisms are oval yeast forms,

2 to 5 μm long. Budding may be present. The histoplasmin skin test and serologic titers (by complement fixation) may aid diagnosis. As in tuberculosis, adjacent mediastinal structures may be involved. Between 5% and 13% of patients with histoplasmosis have esophageal involvement, particularly in the subcarinal region.[13] Other less frequent causes of caseating granulomas in mediastinal lymph nodes include coccidioidomycosis, blastomycosis, and cryptococcosis.[2, 8]

Sarcoidosis

Mediastinal lymphadenopathy is a common manifestation of sarcoidosis, an idiopathic granulomatous disease. The disorder primarily affects adults, but has a wide age range. In the United States, sarcoidosis occurs more commonly among blacks.[14, 15] A female preponderance has been noted. In one series of sarcoidosis patients with intrathoracic lymphadenopathy, 97% of cases had bilateral hilar lymphadenopathy.[16] Seventy-five percent had lymphadenopathy in the right paratracheal or aortopulmonic window areas. In 20%, the subcarinal or anterior mediastinal lymph nodes were enlarged.

Histologically, sarcoidosis is characterized by monotonous-appearing, noncaseating granulomas[14, 17] (Fig. 8–2). All granulomas appear to be at the same stage of development. Each consists of a compact, circumscribed collection of epithelioid histiocytes and multinucleated giant cells (of the Langhans or foreign body type) with few lymphocytes and plasma cells. Any residual lymph node tissue typically shows little evidence of immune stimulation. Germinal centers appear small, and immunoblasts are absent. In the central areas of the granulomas, focal necrosis may be present.[14] However, extensive caseating necrosis is not characteristic. The granulomas tend to coalesce. Hyalinization may be seen.

Various cytoplasmic inclusions have been described in lymph nodes affected by sarcoidosis.[14] Schaumann bodies are laminated ("conchoidal"), basophilic structures with an outer calcified shell enclosing refractile crystalline material. Asteroid bodies are star-shaped, refractile structures within a cytoplasmic vacuole (Fig. 8–2). The inclusions may be seen in other granulomatous diseases and therefore are not specific to sarcoidosis. Polarizable crystalline material may be present within giant cells, in Schaumann bodies, and as small ovoid bodies.[18, 19] The material is predominantly calcium oxalate and is also a nonspecific finding.

Another type of inclusion is the Hamazaki-Wesenberg body, also known as the "yellow-brown" body[20, 21] (Fig. 8–2). These are round-to-oval structures 1 to 15 μm in length. On sections stained with hematoxylin and eosin, they are pale yellow-brown. The appearance of budding-like forms suggests yeast, particularly *Candida* or *Histoplasma*. Furthermore, the bodies appear black with Grocott's methanamine silver stain for fungi and red with periodic acid–Schiff. Unlike yeast, however, the bodies are usually within the sinusoids of lymph nodes, rather than within the granulomas. They are unassociated with inflammation, fibrosis, or necrosis. Also unlike yeasts, these bodies are pale red with the Ziehl-Neelsen stain for acid-fast bacilli and black with the Fontana-Masson silver stain. These structures are believed to represent lipofuchsin pigment. Although they have been found in lymph nodes from many patients with sarcoidosis, they have also been observed in a variety of other conditions. The pathologist should be familiar with Hamazaki-Wesenberg bodies to avoid confusion with a fungal infection.

The histopathologic distinction of sarcoidosis from other granulomatous processes may not be possible.[14] Some patients with tuberculosis do not develop the typical extensive caseation.[22] Such lymph nodes are histologically indistinguishable from sarcoidosis. Only the presence of occasional acid-fast bacilli or the subsequent development of classic tuberculosis permit the correct diagnosis. "Sarcoid-type" granulomas may also be associated with lymphomas, including Hodgkin's disease, and with metastatic carcinomas. Foreign material can elicit a granulomatous reaction that may simulate sarcoidosis.

Silicosis

Sclerohyaline nodules identical to those that occur in the lungs of patients with silicosis may be found in extrapulmonary sites, particularly hilar and mediastinal lymph nodes (Fig. 8–3). Slavin and colleagues identified three stages in the evolution of these nodules.[23] Most patients have occupational exposure (e.g., as coal miners or sandblasters). The initial lesion consists of an aggregate of histiocytes sometimes admixed with lymphocytes, plasma cells, and neutrophils. Giant cells are infrequent. Necrosis within the nodules can be extensive. In the

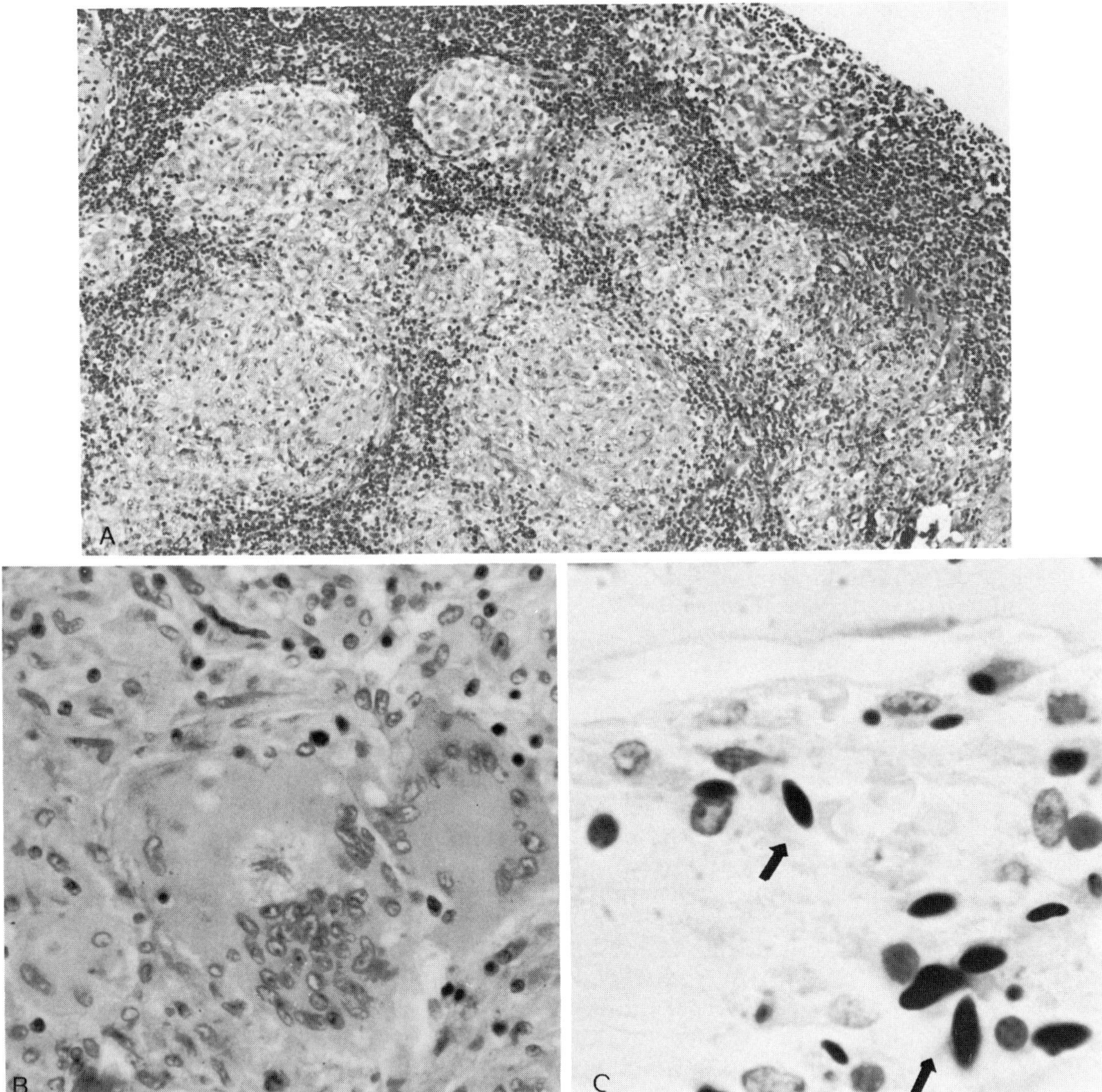

Figure 8–2. *A*, Mediastinal lymph node from a patient with sarcoidosis demonstrates noncaseating granulomas (H&E, ×100). *B*, Asteroid body is present within a multinucleated giant cell (H&E, ×400). *C*, Hamazaki-Wesenberg bodies (*arrows*) are shown within the subcapsular lymph node of a patient with sarcoidosis (Ziehl-Neelson stain, H&E, ×1000).

next stage, histiocytes and fibroblasts predominate. Thickened collagen fibers are also evident. In the final stage, the nodules are larger and nearly acellular. The collagen bundles appear thickened in the center and normal at the periphery. The nodules evolve into amorphous, hyalinized masses. Fibrosis can extend through the lymph node capsule to involve the adipose tissue of the mediastinum.[24] Calcification at the periphery of the node creates an "eggshell" pattern on radiographs.[24, 25] Silica can be observed under polarized light in all stages. The silica particles are bluish-white, 1 to 2 μm long, needle-shaped crystals, usually within the cytoplasm of histiocytes.

Some of the nodules have silica admixed with other minerals and anthracotic carbon pigment ("anthrasilicosis"). Carbon itself is relatively inert and does not tend to elicit a fibrous reaction.[26] It is commonly seen within sinus histiocytes of mediastinal lymph nodes. The presence of anthracotic pigment helps to distinguish histiocytes from metastatic carcinoma.[27]

All of the stages of silicotic nodule development may be seen in lymph nodes.[23] The nod-

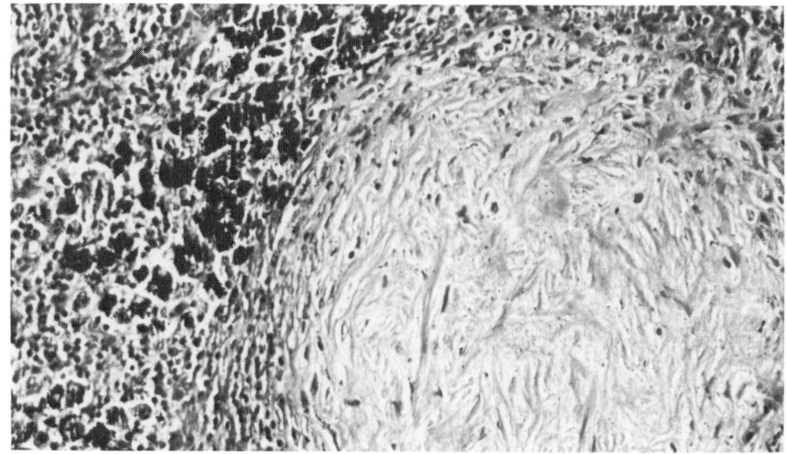

Figure 8–3. Anthrasilicotic nodule within a mediastinal lymph node from a patient with silicosis. The nodule (on right) is composed of dense fibrous tissue. Anthracotic pigment is present both within the nodule and within histiocytes of the lymph node (left) (H&E, ×200).

ules form in the sinusoids and cause compression of adjacent follicles. The nodules must be distinguished from granulomas caused by fungi and mycobacteria, particularly because there is a high incidence of infections with these organisms in silicosis. In the developing silicotic nodules, histiocytes have a "smudged" appearance and are not epithelioid. Giant cells are uncommon and not of the Langhans type. Fibrinoid rather than caseous necrosis is found. Collagen shows the characteristic changes. When completely sclerosed, the silicotic nodules look like old granulomas from infection or sarcoidosis. A thickened lymph node capsule and nodules with necrosis but no cellular reaction are typical of old silicosis.[24] Even at this stage, birefringent silica particles can be seen under polarized light. The presence of silica can be confirmed by energy-dispersive microanalysis of the nodal tissue.

ACUTE MEDIASTINITIS

Acute mediastinitis may result from esophageal perforation, or as a result of spread from infections of the neck, lung, pleura, vertebrae, or retroperitoneum.[28] Infection of median sternotomy wounds may develop after cardiothoracic surgery.[29] Mediastinal abscess may occur as a sequela of penetrating injury or esophageal perforation due to an ingested foreign body.[30] Mediastinal actinomycosis (usually as a result of contiguous spread from the lungs) has been reported.[31]

SCLEROSING MEDIASTINITIS

Fibrous tissue may proliferate within the mediastinum as a consequence of infection, usually histoplasmosis. Mediastinal granuloma overlaps with sclerosing mediastinitis. The former is characterized predominantly by caseating granulomas, whereas the latter has predominantly fibrous tissue.[1] Cases with predominantly fibrous tissue appear to be in a later stage of the disease process.

In some patients, no infectious etiology is apparent. Such patients may have an aggressive, lethal proliferation of fibrous tissue involving the mediastinum and, in particular, the pulmonary hilar region.[32, 33] This disorder may be associated with other idiopathic fibrosing lesions, including retroperitoneal fibrosis.[8, 34] The relationship between sclerosing mediastinitis and these other disorders is not clear. In a 1980 review, Eggleston stated that sclerosing mediastinitis occurs almost exclusively as a result of *Histoplasma* infection.[35] Yet the other fibrosing lesions have not been related to *Histoplasma*. They have no clear etiology. Eggleston has speculated that the histologic similarities between sclerosing mediastinitis and other idiopathic fibrosing lesions suggest a common mechanism of sclerosis, "perhaps on an immunologic basis."[35]

A case report by Drut suggests that some cases of sclerosing mediastinitis may have an immunologic component.[33] Drut reported a 9-year-old patient with systemic vasculitis and sclerosing mediastinitis diagnosed at autopsy. The mediastinum was encased by dense sclerotic tissue. A necrotizing lymphoplasmacytic vasculitis was identified within the sclerotic mediastinal tissue and the spleen. Granulomatous lymphadenitis was not identified, although small caseating granulomas were present within fibrous tissue near the lung. Stains for fungi and bacilli were negative. The patient also had granulomatous glomerulone-

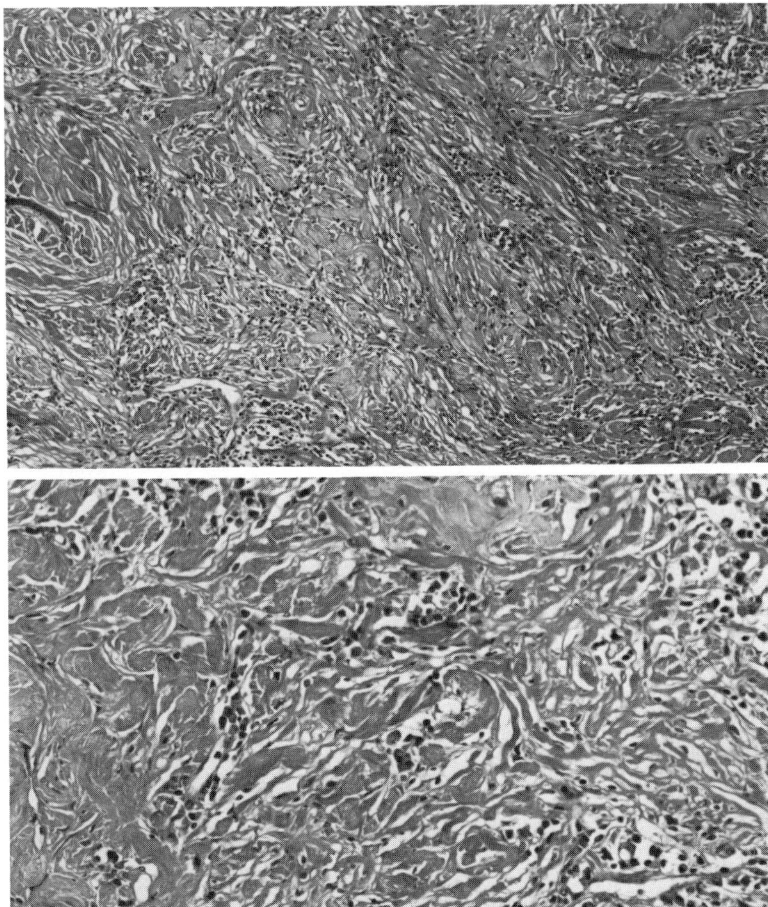

Figure 8–4. Sclerosing mediastinitis in a 20-year-old female admitted to the hospital with a 3-day history of hemoptysis. Tissue from the mediastinum and adjacent lung is replaced by dense, hyalinized sclerosis. Occasional lymphocytes, histiocytes, and plasma cells are also present. No granulomas were identified. Stains and cultures for fungi were negative. (H&E, *top*, ×40; *bottom*, ×100.)

phritis; the sclerosing mediastinitis may have been related to the systemic vasculitis and may have had an immunologic pathogenesis.

Patients with sclerosing mediastinitis may be asymptomatic and present with a mediastinal mass, usually in the region of the tracheal bifurcation or pulmonary hila. The mass may extend into surrounding structures. Symptoms generally depend on the extent to which adjacent structures are involved. Patients may have progressive dyspnea related to occlusion of major pulmonary arteries, hemoptysis, pleuritic chest pain, or dysphagia. Although rare, sclerosing mediastinitis is the most common benign cause of the superior vena cava syndrome.[35]

Microscopically, the mass is composed of dense hyalinized fibrous tissue with plasma cells and lymphocytes[35–37] (Fig. 8–4). Caseating granulomas and calcifications may be present. Adjacent to the granulomas, the hyalinized material forms concentric rings. In other areas, the sclerosis is more disordered. The hyaline material surrounds arteries and nerves. It may infiltrate and replace the walls of bronchi and veins, including the superior vena cava. Associated venous thrombosis is common. Calcifications, bone, and bone marrow may be present within the sclerotic tissue (Fig. 8–5). Arteriolar obliteration by intimal hyperplasia and medial thickening has been described.[36, 37]

Organisms are difficult to demonstrate, and cultures are usually negative. Silver stains demonstrated *Histoplasma* in 9 of 20 resected specimens in the series by Mathisen and Grillo.[38] The stains and cultures frequently are negative despite elevated serologic titers. In the series by Urschel and colleagues, *Histoplasma* was identified by silver stain and culture in 2 of 22 patients with sclerosing mediastinitis.[37] An additional 10 had increasing *Histoplasma* titers. Rare cases of mediastinal fibrosis have been attributed to tuberculosis and *Aspergillus*.[9, 39]

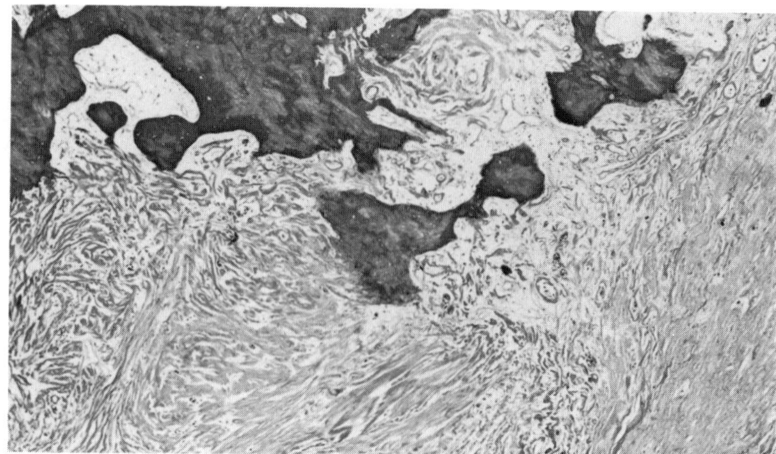

Figure 8–5. Metaplastic bone formation in sclerosing mediastinitis (H&E, ×100).

Tuberculosis, however, is generally not associated with the dense, fibrotic reaction that is typical for histoplasmosis.

The broad differential diagnosis of mediastinal granuloma and fibrosis includes histoplasmosis, tuberculosis, coccidioidomycosis, actinomycosis, sarcoidosis, blastomycosis, syphilis, silicosis, and various malignancies (carcinoma, sarcoma, mesothelioma, lymphoma). An open surgical biopsy with adequate tissue sampling may be necessary to exclude malignancy. In particular, desmoplastic malignant mesothelioma has been reported to simulate sclerosing mediastinitis.[40] (See Chapter 13.) In the absence of malignancy, narrowing the diagnostic possibilities further may be impossible.

Favorable responses to the antifungal drug, ketoconazol, have been reported, even in patients with extensive disease.[37, 38] Interestingly, retroperitoneal fibrosis may also respond to this medication.[37] Surgical intervention may be necessary in selected patients.

SUMMARY

Granulomatous inflammation is an important cause of mediastinal lymphadenopathy. Infectious etiologies include tuberculosis and endemic fungi such as histoplasma. Sarcoidosis commonly involves mediastinal lymph nodes. Silicosis produces sclerohyaline nodules. Infections that spread from adjacent regions may cause acute mediastinitis. Sclerosing mediastinitis is characterized by dense fibrous tissue surrounding and infiltrating mediastinal structures. The fibrosis may result from *Histoplasma* infection, although organisms are difficult to demonstrate.

REFERENCES

1. Goodwin RA, Nickell JA, Des Prez RM. Mediastinal fibrosis complicating healed primary histoplasmosis and tuberculosis. Medicine 1972; 51:227–246.
2. Case records of the Massachusetts General Hospital (Case 3–1993). N Engl J Med 1993; 328:195–202.
3. Im J-G, Song KS, Kang HS, Park JH, Yeon KM, Han MC, Kim C-W. Mediastinal tuberculous lymphadenitis: CT manifestations. Radiology 1987; 164:115–119.
4. Liu C-I, Fields WR, Shaw C-I. Tuberculous mediastinal lymphadenopathy in adults. Radiology 1978; 126:369–371.
5. Bloomberg TJ, Dow CJ. Contemporary mediastinal tuberculosis. Thorax 1980; 35:392–396.
6. Case records of the Massachusetts General Hospital (Case 48–1989). N Engl J Med 1989; 321:1528–1537.
7. Silver CP, Steel SJ. Mediastinal lymphatic gland tuberculosis in Asian and coloured immigrants. Lancet 1961; 1:1254–1256.
8. Ioachim HL. Granulomatous lesions in lymph nodes. *In* Ioachim HL, ed. Pathology of Granulomas. New York: Raven Press, 1983:151–187.
9. Loyd JE, Tillman BF, Atkinson JB, Des Prez RM. Mediastinal fibrosis complicating histoplasmosis. Medicine 1988; 67:295–311.
10. Dovenbarger WV, Tsubura E, Schwarz J, Baum GL. Mediastinal cystic granuloma due to histoplasma capsulatum: a report of three patients treated surgically. J Thorac Cardiovasc Surg 1961; 42:193–199.
11. Rabinowitz JG, Prater W, Silver J, Phillips JC, Wieder S. Mediastinal histoplasmosis. Mt Sinai J Med 1990; 47:356–363.
12. Kirchner SG, Hernanz-Shulman M, Stein SM, Wright PF, Heller RM. Imaging of pediatric mediastinal histoplasmosis. Radiograph 1991; 11:365–381.
13. Clinical records of the Massachusetts General Hospital (Case 15–1991). N Engl J Med 1991; 324:1049–1056.
14. Chambers TF, Stansfeld AG. Histiocytosis and histiocytic neoplasms. *In* Stanfeld AG, ed. Lymph Node Biopsy Interpretation. Edinburgh: Churchill Livingstone, 1985:355–361.
15. Crystal RG. Sarcoidosis. *In* Harrison's Textbook of Medicine. New York: McGraw-Hill, 11th edition, 1987:1445–1450.
16. Bein ME, Putman CE, McLoud TC, Mink JH. A reevaluation of intrathoracic lymphadenopathy in sarcoidosis. AJR 1976; 131:409–415.

17. Soskel NT, Fox R. Sarcoidosis . . . or something like it. South Med J 1990; 83:1190–1202.
18. Reid JD, Andersen ME. Calcium oxalate in sarcoid granulomas: with particular reference to the small ovoid body and a note on the finding of dolomite. Am J Clin Pathol 1988; 90:545–558.
19. Katzenstein A-LA, Askin FB. Systemic diseases involving the lung. *In* Surgical Pathology of Non-Neoplastic Lung Disease. Philadelphia: WB Saunders, 1990:214–251.
20. Ro JY, Luna MA, Mackay B, Ramos O. Yellow-brown (Hamazaki-Wesenberg) bodies mimicking fungal yeasts. Arch Pathol Lab Med 1987; 111:555–559.
21. Moscovic EA. Sarcoidosis and mycobacterial L-forms: a critical reappraisal of pleomorphic chromogenic bodies (Hamazaki corpuscles) in lymph nodes. Pathol Annu 1978; 13:69–164.
22. Stansfeld AG. Inflammatory and reactive disorders. *In* Stansfeld AG, ed. Lymph Node Biopsy Interpretation. Edinburgh: Churchill Livingstone, 1985:85–141.
23. Slavin RE, Swedo JL, Brandes D, Gonzalez-Vitale JC, Osornio-Vargas A. Extrapulmonary silicosis: a clinical, morphologic, and ultrastructural study. Hum Pathol 1985; 16:393–412.
24. Case records of the Massachusetts General Hospital (Case 46–1991). N Engl J Med 1991; 325:1429–1436.
25. Gross BH, Schneider HJ, Proto AV. Eggshell calcification of lymph nodes: an update. AJR 1980; 135:1265–1268.
26. Rosai J. Respiratory tract. *In* Ackerman's Surgical Pathology. St. Louis: CV Mosby, 1989:264–343.
27. Henry K, Farrer-Brown G. Color Atlas of Thymus and Lymph Node Histopathology. Chicago: Year Book, 1982:9–44.
28. Payne WS, Larson RH. Acute mediastinitis. Surg Clin North Am 1969; 49:999–1009.
29. Grossi EA, Culliford AT, Kreiger KH, Kloth D, Press R, Baumann FG, Spencer FC. A survey of 77 major infectious complications of median sternotomy: a review of 7949 consecutive operative procedures. Ann Thorac Surg 1985; 40:214–222.
30. Malnekoff BJ. Acute mediastinal abscess. Am J Dis Child 1930; 39:591–594.
31. Morgan DE, Nath H, Sanders C, Hasson JH. Mediastinal actinomycosis. AJR 1990; 155:735–737.
32. Sobrinho-Simoes MA, Vaz Saleiro J, Wagenvoort CA. Mediastinal and hilar fibrosis. Histopathology 1981; 5:53–60.
33. Drut R. Sclerosing mediastinitis, granulomatous glomerulonephritis, and systemic vasculitis in a child. Pediatr Pathol 1990; 10:439–445.
34. Mitchell IM, Saunders NR, Maher O, Lennox SC, Walker DR. Surgical treatment of idiopathic mediastinal fibrosis: report of five cases. Thorax 1986; 41:210–214.
35. Eggleston JC. Sclerosing mediastinitis. Prog Surg Pathol 1980; 2:1–17.
36. Light AM. Idiopathic fibrosis of mediastinum: a discussion of three cases and review of the literature. J Clin Pathol 1978; 31:78–88.
37. Urschel HC Jr, Razzuk MA, Netto GJ, Disiere J, Chung SY. Sclerosing mediastinitis: improved management with histoplasmosis titer and ketoconazole. Ann Thorac Surg 1990; 50:215–221.
38. Mathisen DJ, Grillo HC. Clinical manifestation of mediastinal fibrosis and histoplasmosis. Ann Thorac Surg 1992; 54:1053–1058.
39. Schowengerdt CG, Suyemoto R, Main FB. Granulomatous and fibrous mediastinitis: a review and analysis of 180 cases. J Thorac Cardiovasc Surg 1969; 57:365–379.
40. Crotty TB, Colby TV, Gay PC, Pisani RJ. Desmoplastic malignant mesothelioma masquerading as sclerosing mediastinitis: a diagnostic dilemma. Hum Pathol 1992; 23:79–82.

Chapter

9

GERM CELL TUMORS

GEORGEAN G. DEBLOIS

PATHOGENESIS
CYTOGENETICS
ASSOCIATION WITH HEMATOLOGIC MALIGNANCY
ASSOCIATION WITH SARCOMAS
IMMUNOHISTOCHEMISTRY
- Cytokeratin
- Epithelial Membrane Antigen
- Alpha-Fetoprotein
- Human Chorionic Gonadotropin
- Placental Alkaline Phosphatase

TERATOMAS
- General
- Clinical Presentation
- Radiographic and Laboratory Features
- Gross and Microscopic Features
- Therapy and Clinical Outcome
- Differential Diagnosis

SEMINOMAS
- Clinical Presentation
- Radiographic and Laboratory Features
- Gross and Microscopic Features
- Differential Diagnosis
- Therapy and Clinical Outcome

NONSEMINOMATOUS MALIGNANT GERM CELL TUMORS
- General
- Clinical Presentation
- Radiographic and Laboratory Features
- Gross Features
- Microscopic Features
  - *Embryonal Carcinoma*
  - *Endodermal Sinus Tumor*
  - *Choriocarcinoma*
- Differential Diagnosis
- Therapy and Clinical Outcome

SUMMARY

Primary mediastinal germ cell tumors have evoked an interest well out of proportion to their incidence. Some reports have questioned the existence of primary extragonadal germ cell tumors and attempted to show that they were, in fact, metastases from an occult or "burned out" testicular primary tumor.[1,2] However, a considerable body of evidence proves otherwise. Daugaard et al. failed to find any carcinoma-in-situ in testicular biopsies obtained from patients with exclusively mediastinal germ cell tumors.[2] In several autopsy series of patients with presumed extragonadal germ cell tumors, meticulous microscopic examination of the testes could not detect either occult tumors or focal scars.[3–7] Furthermore, testicular primary tumors typically metastasize along the retroperitoneum. They rarely masquerade as isolated mediastinal metastases.[4,8,9] Additionally, a number of patients who received only local treatment (i.e., surgical resection or radiotherapy) have been cured, without ever manifesting a testicular primary tumor.[10–14]

More recently, ploidy studies have demonstrated a difference in the DNA content of primary mediastinal germ cell tumors and adult testicular germ cell tumors.[15,16] A significant percentage of mediastinal germ cell tumors, like infantile testicular germ cell tumors, appear diploid. The aneuploid tumors hover in the peritetraploid range. This holds true for both seminomatous and nonseminomatous mediastinal germ cell tumors. In contrast, diploid tumors rarely occur in the adult testicle. Furthermore, in the adult gonad, seminomas are usually hypertriploid, whereas nonseminomatous tumors are typically hypotriploid.[16] Still, the presumptive diagnosis of any extragonadal germ cell tumor should be made only after careful assessment of the gonads. In males, this can be accomplished by a combination of testicular palpation and ultrasonography. In females, ultrasonography of the pelvis can be used to exclude an ovarian primary.

Germ cell tumors account for 1 to 15% of mediastinal tumors in adults and for approximately 25% of mediastinal tumors in children.[13, 17–19] They typically arise in the anterior mediastinum. Although mediastinal germ cell tumors frequently involve the thymus gland, they are histogenetically unrelated to true thymomas.

When considered in the context of all germ cell tumors, those originating in the mediastinum account for only 1 to 6%.[13, 14, 20] However, the mediastinum is the most common extragonadal primary site in most adult series.[21] In children, mediastinal germ cell tumors develop at all ages. Benign and malignant tumors are distributed equally in both sexes.[22] Although men and women exhibit an equal incidence of benign mediastinal germ cell tumors,[14] malignant mediastinal germ cell tumors overwhelmingly are a disease of young men, in whom the peak incidence occurs in the third decade.

Mediastinal germ cell tumors are histologically identical to their gonadal counterparts. Nevertheless, mediastinal germ cell tumors exhibit distinctive clinical features: an association with hematologic malignancies,[23–29] an increased incidence in Klinefelter's syndrome,[30–33] a significant number of pure endodermal sinus tumors,[34–36] and a comparatively poor prognosis.[14, 35, 37–40]

The diagnostic problems surrounding mediastinal germ cell tumors also differ from those of gonadal tumors. When faced with a mediastinal germ cell tumor, the pathologist must often deal with only a small amount of tissue obtained by biopsy. Problems inherent with this type of limited material include crush artifact, necrosis, and sampling error. Furthermore, mediastinal germ cell tumors entail a more extensive differential diagnosis that involves such disparate entities as thymoma, lymphoma, carcinoma, and metastatic melanoma. Treatment of these neoplasms differs considerably, making correct diagnosis imperative. Classification of mediastinal germ cell tumors into teratomas, seminomas (germinomas), and nonseminomatous germ cell tumors (endodermal sinus tumor, embryonal carcinoma, and choriocarcinoma) has clinical, therapeutic, and prognostic implications.

PATHOGENESIS

The origin of mediastinal germ cell tumors remains speculative. Because many mediastinal germ cell tumors arise within the thymus, some earlier researchers suggested that these neoplasms developed from somatic cells misplaced in the thymus during embryogenesis.[41] This hypothesis, however, failed to explain the pathogenesis of extragonadal germ cell tumors in sites other than the mediastinum. One of the most popular hypotheses asserts that mediastinal germ cell tumors and other midline extragonadal germ cell tumors originate from errant primordial germ cells during their midline migration from the yolk sac to the embryonic gonadal ridge.[42] Friedman initially proposed that these tumors originate from "germinal" cells somehow deposited in the thymus during embryogenesis.[43] More recently, he suggested that germ cells distribute widely to the thymus, brain, liver, and bone marrow during embryogenesis. Friedman believed that these germ cells may convey genetic hematologic or immunologic information, or regulate development at somatic sites.[44]

CYTOGENETICS

Chromosomal analysis has revealed an isochromosome of the short arm of chromosome 12 [i(12p)] in more than 90% of germ cell tumors.[45] This appears to be a highly specific marker for germ cell neoplasia that has only rarely been reported in other solid tumors.[46, 47] Another abnormality of chromosome 12, the deletion of part of the long arm [del(12q)], has also been recently identified as a nonrandom occurrence in nonseminomatous germ cell tumors.[45, 46] Although these abnormalities were first described in testicular germ cell tumors, they have since been confirmed in mediastinal germ cell tumors.[46–49] This information is relevant to discussions of pathogenesis, diagnosis, and prognosis of mediastinal germ cell tumors.

Dal Cin et al. suggested that the presence of this characteristic chromosome marker reflects the occurrence of a specific chromosome rearrangement in a primitive germ cell (gonocyte).[48] This genetic aberration persists as the cell proceeds along the pathway of malignant transformation, regardless of whether or not it is in the gonad.

Motzer et al. utilized genetic analysis to elucidate the origins of a series of midline tumors of uncertain histogenesis.[47] Abnormalities of chromosome 12, including multiple copies of 12p, were used as presumptive markers of germ cell origin. Three of four patients with a detectable alteration in chromosome 12 responded completely to cisplatin-based chemotherapy, a treatment regimen successfully pioneered for testicular germ cell tumors. The one patient with this marker who failed to respond to this therapy exhibited multiple copies of 12p, suggesting that this cytogenetic finding heralds a poor prognosis.

Cytogenetic analysis has also confirmed the association of primary mediastinal germ cell tumors and Klinefelter's syndrome, although the pathogenesis remains unclear.[31, 33] Results of two different prospective cytogenetic studies exhibit strikingly similar findings: 21 to 22% of young men with primary mediastinal germ cell tumors demonstrate karyotypic or phenotypic evidence of Klinefelter's syndrome; the incidence of Klinefelter's syndrome in the general population is 0.016%. Furthermore, in patients with Klinefelter's syndrome, primary mediastinal germ cell tumors develop a decade earlier—at a mean age of 16 to 17 years, versus 27 to 29 years for males without Klinefelter's syndrome.[30, 32] Interestingly, Klinefelter's syndrome has been reported exclusively in patients with nonseminomatous tumors, even though seminomas are the most common malignant mediastinal germ cell tumors.[18] Choriocarcinoma reportedly occurs at a higher relative frequency in those with Klinefelter's syndrome.[30]

ASSOCIATION WITH HEMATOLOGIC MALIGNANCY

In 1985, deMent and Nichols independently recognized an association between mediastinal germ cell tumors and hematologic malignancies.[24, 28] Since then, a number of reports have appeared in the literature that associate mediastinal germ cell tumors with such hematologic disorders as acute megakaryocytic leukemia,[27–29, 50] refractory thrombocytopenia,[50] hemophagocytic syndrome,[51] malignant histiocytosis,[26, 52] and, most recently, systemic mastocytosis.[53, 54] Acute nonlymphocytic leukemia is most frequently described. Relatively rare entities, such as erythroleukemia and megakaryoblastic leukemia, appear to be disproportionately represented. Patients with this syndrome have a dismal prognosis and respond poorly to the chemotherapy prescribed for nonseminomatous germ cell tumors. In one series, the median survival following diagnosis was less than 2 months.[25]

An expanding body of literature supports the idea of a true biologic link between mediastinal germ cell tumors and hematologic malignancies. In a number of cases, the hematologic abnormality presents simultaneously with, or even precedes, the germ cell tumor.[23, 24, 28, 29, 50, 51, 55] The remaining cases typically occur within 4 years of treatment; 70% develop within the first 12 months.[55] This contrasts sharply with most treatment-related leukemias that develop after a protracted interval of 25 to 60 months.[29] Moreover, reviews of cisplatin-based chemotherapy suggest that it is not leukemogenic.[29] Cytogenetic studies in several patients have revealed i(12p) in both their leukemic cells and their mediastinal germ cell tumors. This suggests that these two rare malignancies arose from a single progenitor cell.[29, 46, 56] However, not all cases show this association.[6]

Hematologic abnormalities have been described exclusively in patients with nonseminomatous germ cell tumors, especially those with histologic or serologic evidence of endodermal sinus tumor.[29, 55] Ladanyi et al. suggest that in some cases the hematologic malignancy is a non–germ cell malignant component of mediastinal germ cell tumor analogous to the soft tissue sarcomas that develop in germ cell tumors.[25] Nichols et al. point out that germ cells and hematopoietic stem cells share several embryologic characteristics: yolk sac origin, migration during embryogenesis, and the retained capability of differentiation in adulthood.[28] Thus, it is possible that the leukemic stem cell originates within the endodermal sinus tumor, or that the wayward migration of both types of cells results in an abnormal microenvironment that enhances malignant differentiation.[28] Alternatively, the hematologic neoplasia may result from the multipotential differentiation of malignant germ cells.[23, 24, 28, 29] Orazi et al. recently demonstrated morphologic and immunohistochemical evidence of hematologic differentiation within the endodermal sinus component of four of six patients with mediastinal germ cell tumors and leukemia.[56]

No theory, however, adequately explains the striking association of hematologic abnormalities with mediastinal germ cell tumors as opposed to gonadal germ cell tumors. In some way, the mediastinum must provide a unique milieu for the growth and differentiation of abnormal hematopoietic cells. Because mediastinal germ cell tumors often are within or adjacent to the thymus, Ladanyi et al. speculate that growth factors released by thymic epithelial cells induce the proliferation and/or hematopoietic differentiation of primitive germ cells.[26]

ASSOCIATION WITH SARCOMAS

Non–germ cell malignancies have been described as an uncommon phenomenon in both gonadal and extragonadal nonseminomatous germ cell tumors[57–59] (Fig. 9–1). Sarcomas, especially rhabdomyosarcomas and angiosarcomas, have been the most frequently encountered tumors. These neoplasms appear with a relatively greater frequency in mediastinal nonseminomatous germ cell tumors than in their gonadal counterparts. This may reflect the fact that mediastinal germ cell tumors are considerably larger than gonadal germ cell tumors at the time of diagnosis and thus more likely to enable the emergence of new cell lines.[58]

Sarcomas may originate from the totipotential germ cell (embryonal cell) component of the primary tumor[59] or from foci of an immature teratoma.[58] Ulbright et al. reported a series of cytokeratin-positive spindle cell tumors resected from patients with endodermal sinus tumor. These spindle cell lesions may represent overgrowth of the mesenchymal component of endodermal sinus tumor that has been selected out by chemotherapy.[60]

Although the sarcoma often appears as a minor feature of the primary tumor, identification has significant prognostic implications. The sarcomatous component is frequently resistant to the cisplatin-based chemotherapy administered for germ cell tumors and may proliferate locally or metastasize.[57–59, 61]

IMMUNOHISTOCHEMISTRY

Immunohistochemistry is important in differentiating germ cell neoplasms from other malignancies. Immunohistochemistry also helps to identify the particular type of germ cell tumor. The comprehensive report by Niehans et al. confirms that gonadal and extragonadal germ cell tumors display similar patterns of reactivity.[62]

The basic panel of antibodies useful in the diagnosis of mediastinal germ cell tumors includes the following: cytokeratin, epithelial membrane antigen, alpha-fetoprotein (AFP), beta–human chorionic gonadotropin (B-HCG), and placental alkaline phosphatase (PLAP)[63] (Table 9–1).

Cytokeratin

Nonseminomatous germ cell tumors express significantly more cytokeratin than seminomatous germ cell tumors do. Endodermal sinus tumors, choriocarcinomas, and most embryonal carcinomas display diffuse cytoplasmic staining. Occasionally, seminomas can stain either focally or diffusely with cytokeratin. Most of these seminomas will contain either scattered trophoblast cells or elements of nonseminomatous germ cell tumor elsewhere in the tumor. This finding prompted Niehans et

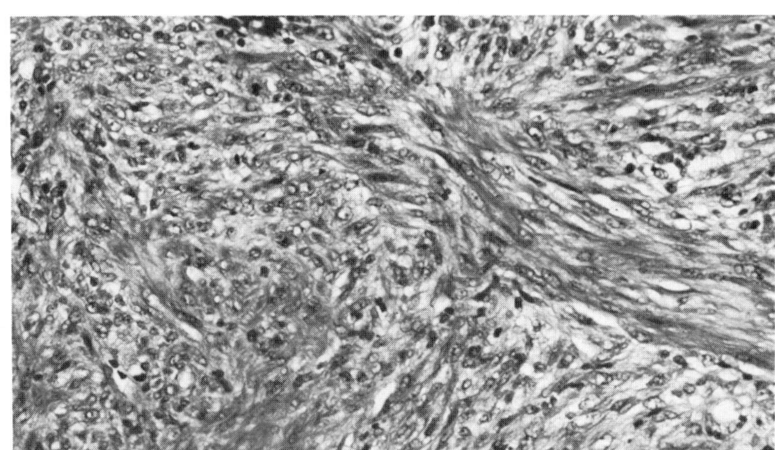

Figure 9–1. Leiomyosarcoma that arose as a nodule in an otherwise typical cystic thymic seminoma. This appears to be a unique case, since, to the best of our knowledge, such non–germ cell malignancies have only been reported in nonseminomatous germ cell tumors (H&E, ×400).

Table 9–1. Mediastinal Germ Cell Tumors: Immunohistochemical Panel

Tumor	AFP	HCG	PLAP	EMA	CK
Seminoma	−	−*	+++	−	−/+
Endodermal sinus tumor	++	−*	++	−	+
Embryonal carcinoma	+	−*	++	−	+
Choriocarcinoma	−	+++	+	−	+
Immature teratoma	+†	−	+	+	+

*Positive in isolated syncytiotrophoblasts.
†Positive in immature neural, hepatic, and intestinal elements.
Abbreviations: AFP, alpha-fetoprotein; HCG, human chorionic gonadotropin; PLAP, placental alkaline phosphatase; EMA, epithelial membrane antigen; CK, cytokeratin.

al. to suggest that cytokeratin production in seminomas is an early manifestation of embryonal, endodermal sinus, or trophoblastic differentiation that occurs before morphologic change at the light-microscopic level.[62]

Epithelial Membrane Antigen

With the exception of syncytiotrophoblast cells and intermediate trophoblast cells, germ cell tumors do not react with this antibody.[62]

Alpha-Fetoprotein

Most endodermal sinus tumors contain scattered clusters of cells that react strongly with antibody to AFP. The hyaline globules may also react. Niehans et al. found that approximately one third of embryonal carcinomas exhibit staining. Primitive hepatic, intestinal, and neural elements within immature teratomas will also react with AFP antibody. Seminomas and choriocarcinomas do not react to this antibody.[62]

Human Chorionic Gonadotropin

Antibodies to HCG identify syncytiotrophoblast cells and intermediate trophoblast cells in various germ cell tumors. The occasional presence of these cells in germ cell tumors other than true choriocarcinomas appears to be of no diagnostic significance but may explain the modest elevation of serum B-HCG seen in such tumors as seminoma and embryonal carcinoma.[62]

Placental Alkaline Phosphatase

PLAP appears to be a sensitive but nonspecific marker for germ cell neoplasia. Seminomas generally exhibit diffuse, membrane-based staining. The majority of embryonal carcinomas, as well as a high percentage of endodermal sinus tumors, choriocarcinomas, and immature teratomas, also react with antibody to PLAP, albeit more variably.[62]

TERATOMAS

General

Primary mediastinal teratomas account for approximately 8 to 20% of mediastinal neoplasms and up to 80% of mediastinal germ cell tumors.[14, 17, 18, 64] In adults, 27% of teratomas arise in the mediastinum. In children, mediastinal teratomas are less common, accounting for approximately 5% of teratomas.[65]

Like their gonadal counterparts, mediastinal teratomas are composed of tissues representing one or more of the embryonic germ cell layers (ectoderm, mesoderm, endoderm) foreign to their anatomic location. Those composed exclusively of mature ectoderm are often termed ''dermoids.'' All tissues contained within a mature teratoma must be fully mature. The presence of any immature neuroectodermal or mesenchymal elements, or blastemas, characterizes the teratoma as immature. Teratocarcinomas are fully malignant tumors in which a seminoma, embryonal carcinoma, endodermal sinus tumor, or choriocarcinoma coexists with a mature or immature teratoma.[66] Unfortunately, the terms teratocarcinoma and malignant teratoma have not always been uniformly applied in the literature. Some authors have used them synonymously with such malignant germ cell tumors as seminoma, embryonal carcinoma, endodermal sinus tumor, and choriocarcinoma.

Clinical Presentation

Most mediastinal teratomas occur in children and young adults.[41, 67, 68] They have been detected in utero as a cause of hydrops fetalis.[69] Rarely, they cause progressive respiratory distress in infants.[70] Mature teratomas can be asymptomatic in 50% of patients, especially children and young adults. Older individuals more typically present with signs and symptoms related to intrathoracic compression such as chest pain, cough, dyspnea, or rarely, superior vena cava syndrome. Constitutional symptoms such as fever, weight loss, and endocrine dysfunction have been reported.[68, 71, 72] These tumors can erode the tracheobronchial tree, resulting in a productive cough of hair or sebaceous material,[72] or in lipoid pneumonia.

Immature teratomas account for approximately 1% of mediastinal teratomas.[73] These tumors occur most often in children and adolescents, with a number reported in infants under 1 year of age.[73] Most patients have symptoms such as chest pain, dyspnea, cough, fatigue, weight loss, and fever.[18, 68, 73]

Teratocarcinomas (malignant teratomas) occur more frequently in young males.[3, 5, 6, 66] These tumors account for approximately 2% of primary mediastinal masses.[17, 19] Overall, 15 to 20% of mediastinal teratomas are classified as malignant.[68] Most patients are symptomatic. Indeed, these tumors can rapidly enlarge, precipitating a critical clinical situation.[41, 68]

Radiographic and Laboratory Features

Most teratomas arise in the anterior-superior mediastinum.[41, 64] Only a few cases have been reported to originate in the posterior mediastinum.[6, 72, 74] The chest radiograph typically reveals a large, rounded, or lobulated mass (Fig. 9–2). The presence of calcification in 20 to 43% of these tumors suggests the diagnosis of benign teratoma. Organized bone or teeth may occasionally be identified.

Computed tomography and magnetic resonance imaging may disclose a cystic component, and they demonstrate different densities corresponding to such tissues as fat.[72, 75] Masses that prove to be solid or that contain areas suspicious for hemorrhage and necrosis generally correspond to histologically malignant teratomas.[22, 65]

Benign teratomas, by definition, lack AFP and B-HCG. Elevated serum AFP or B-HCG indicates a malignant component to the teratoma such as embryonal carcinoma, endodermal sinus tumor, or choriocarcinoma.

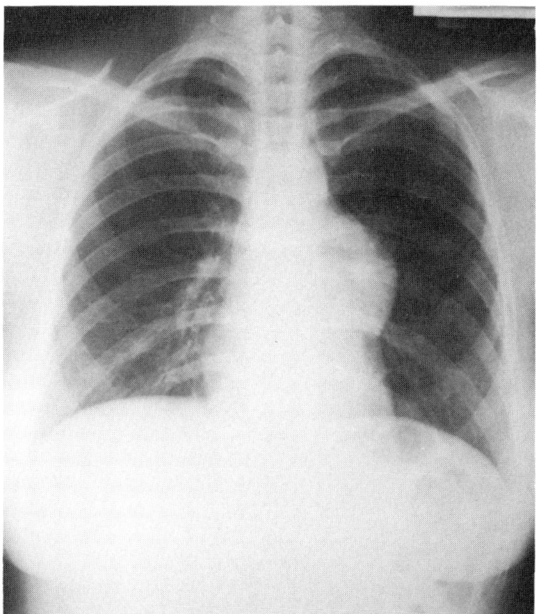

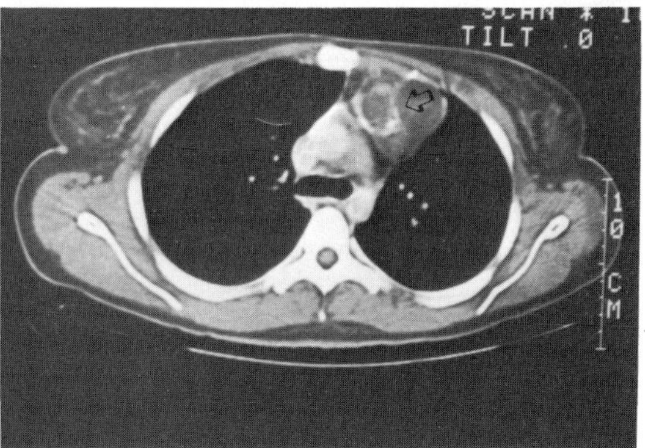

Figure 9–2. Radiographic and computed tomographic appearance of a teratoma. *Top,* Large, rounded mediastinal mass. *Bottom,* Rim of calcification (*arrow*) suggests a diagnosis of teratoma.

Gross and Microscopic Features

The gross appearance correlates well with the microscopic appearance. Most benign teratomas are cystic, representing the "dermoid cyst" of the mediastinum. These form large, rounded masses, often with intramural calcification. Residual thymus may adhere to the wall.[6, 41] Sectioning reveals either a uniloculated or multiloculated cyst containing such ectodermal derivatives as hair and white, yellow, or brown sebaceous or keratinous material (Fig. 9–3). Rupture of these cysts provokes

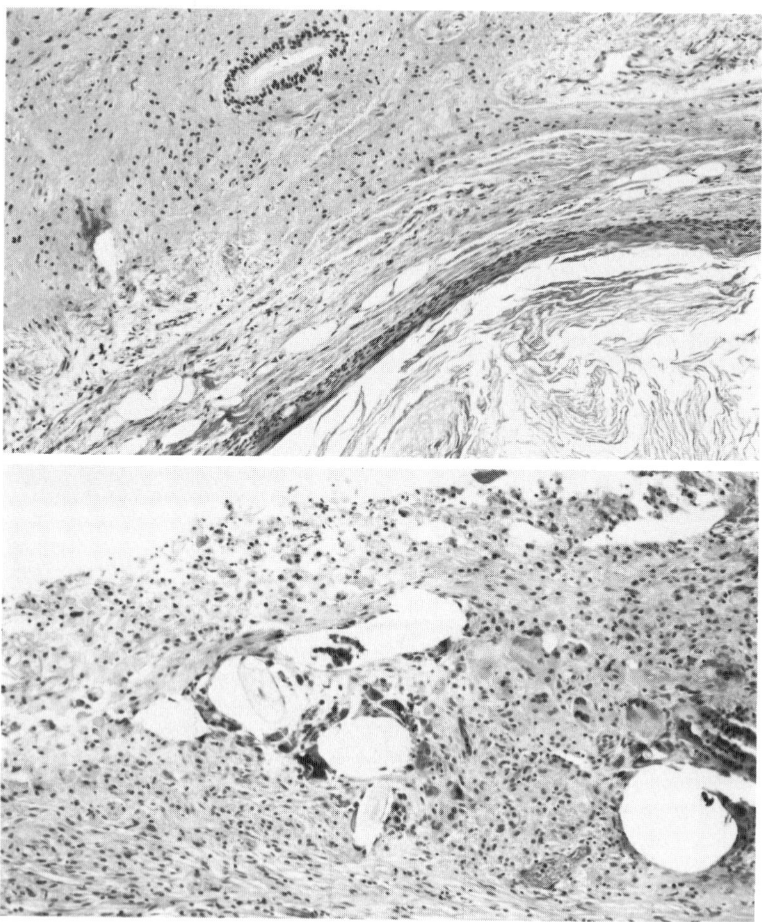

Figure 9–3. Mature cystic teratomas of the mediastinum are often lined by keratin-producing squamous epithelium (H&E, *top,* ×100). These tumors can rupture, provoking an intense granulomatous reaction to fragments of hair and sebaceous material (H&E, *bottom,* ×100).

an intense inflammatory reaction that may be mistaken for tumor extension into the adjacent mediastinal structures or pleural space.[76] Cysts filled with mucin, as well as areas of cartilage and bone, may be recognized. Mature teratomas may also contain solid areas resembling brain. As an answer to the pathologist's perpetual question "How many sections do I need to submit?" Dehner suggests that the absolute number of blocks is not as critical as judicious sampling of the tumor.[22] Enough blocks should be taken to adequately characterize the different components of the teratoma. As with many tumors, areas of hemorrhage and necrosis raise the suspicion of malignancy and should be carefully sampled. Gross penetration into the wall of the cyst or invasion of contiguous structures also portends malignancy.[5, 6, 22, 41]

Almost all mature cystic teratomas contain ectodermal derivatives such as skin and nerve tissue.[6, 41] The larger cysts tend to be lined by keratinizing squamous epithelium. Well-developed dermal appendages are common. Smaller cysts are often lined by foregut derivatives such as respiratory or intestinal epithelium. Pancreatic tissue, rarely identified in gonadal teratomas, has been frequently described as a component of mediastinal teratomas[41, 77] (Fig. 9–4). Mature pancreatic tissue may play an important clinical role. Active proteolytic enzymes can induce tissue necrosis and hemorrhage.[78, 79] Functioning pancreatic tissue can also result in hypoglycemia or elevated serum amylase.[71, 77] Connective tissue, bone, cartilage, and muscle are the most frequently encountered mesodermal derivatives.

Immature teratomas form large, predominantly solid lobulated masses that frequently invade adjacent structures. Sectioning reveals small cysts, often filled with red or brown fluid, surrounded by yellow adipose tissue, bone, cartilage, and/or gray neural tissue. Areas of hemorrhage and necrosis contribute to the variegated gross appearance. Well-developed ectodermal elements such as hair and keratin are usually absent.

Neural elements, including mature glial tis-

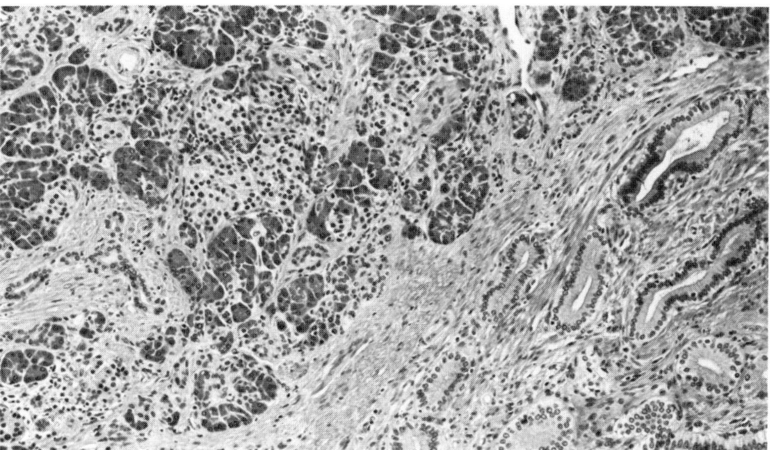

Figure 9–4. Mature pancreatic tissue, here with distinct islet cells and acini, appears more frequently in mediastinal teratomas than in gonadal teratomas (H&E, ×100).

sue as well as immature neuroepithelium, often predominate microscopically (Fig. 9–5). Mature and immature tissues representing the three germinal layers contribute to the diverse microscopic appearance.

Teratocarcinomas are aggressive neoplasms that grow rapidly. Elevated levels of serum AFP or B-HCG may be detected. Symptoms relate to the degree of intrathoracic compression or invasion of mediastinal structures. These tumors often prove too extensive for radical resection.[5, 6, 10, 38] The histologic features depend on the various tissues involved. Embryonal carcinoma is frequently identified as the malignant component (Fig. 9–6). Malignant transformation of a mature teratoma, identified by the presence of squamous cell carcinoma, adenocarcinoma, or undifferentiated carcinoma, has also been reported.[6, 41]

Therapy and Clinical Outcome

Mature teratomas do not metastasize. Complete excision results in cure.[80] Occasionally they induce life-threatening complications by virtue of a mass effect on vital structures.

In immature teratomas, patient age, not histology, appears to be the most significant prognostic factor.[80] This contrasts with ovarian and, to a lesser degree, sacrococcygeal teratomas, in which immature histology denotes malignancy.[65, 81] In the mediastinum, immature teratomas arising in patients younger than 15 years behave as mass lesions. Total resection enables long-term survival.[73] In individuals over 15 years of age, immature teratomas act as highly malignant neoplasms[5, 41] that can metastasize widely. Treatment involves aggressive chemotherapy and radiotherapy,[66] usually with poor results.

Teratocarcinomas also prove to be highly malignant neoplasms.[5, 6, 41] Large size and invasion of vital mediastinal structures usually preclude surgical resection. Hematogenous dissemination is common. These tumors require intensive therapy similar to that administered for nonseminomatous germ cell tumors. Cisplatin regimens may increase survival.[82]

Differential Diagnosis

If a mature teratoma has been completely resected, the diagnosis is readily made after gross and microscopic examination. Difficulties may arise on biopsy if a cyst has ruptured, provoking an intense mediastinitis, which can obscure the underlying neoplasm.[76]

Only a small amount of diagnostic material may be available from immature and malignant teratomas. In adults, other high-grade neoplasms such as carcinoma, sarcoma, and melanoma are often considered in the differential diagnosis. Immunohistochemistry, utilizing a panel of antibodies, can often resolve the diagnosis. Electron microscopy may provide additional diagnostic information.

SEMINOMAS

Seminomas are the most common primary malignant mediastinal germ cell tumor.[14] They almost always arise in the anterior mediastinum and are often intimately associated with the thymus.[91, 93] Seminomas typically afflict

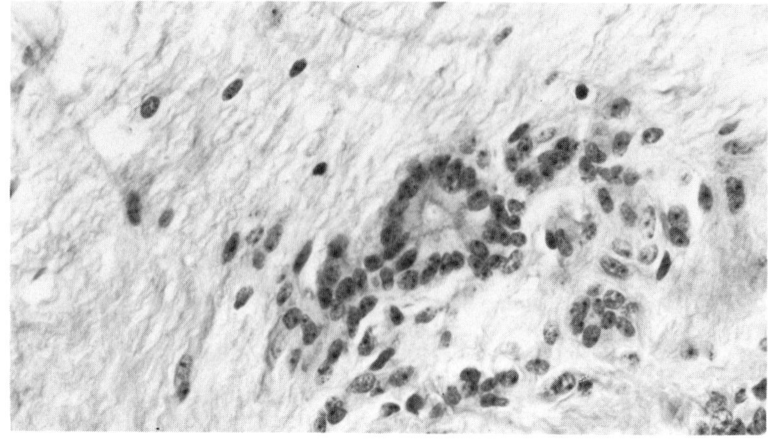

Figure 9–5. A neuroepithelial rosette identifies this teratoma as immature. The surrounding glial tissue appears mature (H&E, ×400).

young men in the third decade of life.[3, 83–86] Reports of this tumor in females are generally limited to individual cases.[87, 88]

Clinical Presentation

Approximately 5 to 25% of patients are asymptomatic at the time of diagnosis. The remaining patients usually present with bulky intrathoracic disease, and up to 26% of these patients suffer from superior vena cava syndrome.[7, 55, 83–85] Symptoms include chest pain, cough, dyspnea, dysphagia, fever, and weight loss.[55, 83, 84]

Radiographic and Laboratory Features

Seminomas typically appear radiographically as large, bulky, well-defined, lobulated anterior mediastinal masses.[75] Computed tomography demonstrates a coarsely lobulated mass that often displays homogeneous attenuation equal to that of soft tissue.[75]

Patients with primary mediastinal seminoma may exhibit low-level elevation of B-HCG (usually less than 100 mIU/ml).[10, 14, 64, 89] Pure seminomas do not produce AFP. The presence of this marker indicates a nonseminomatous component (i.e., endodermal sinus tumor or embryonal carcinoma).[89] Serum lactic dehydrogenase is elevated in approximately 80% of patients with advanced disease. This is a nonspecific marker related to tumor burden and rate of tumor growth.[64, 90]

Gross and Microscopic Features

Mediastinal seminomas typically appear grossly as well-circumscribed, solid, yellow-tan masses. Occasionally, central hemorrhage and necrosis occur. Microscopically, the classic me-

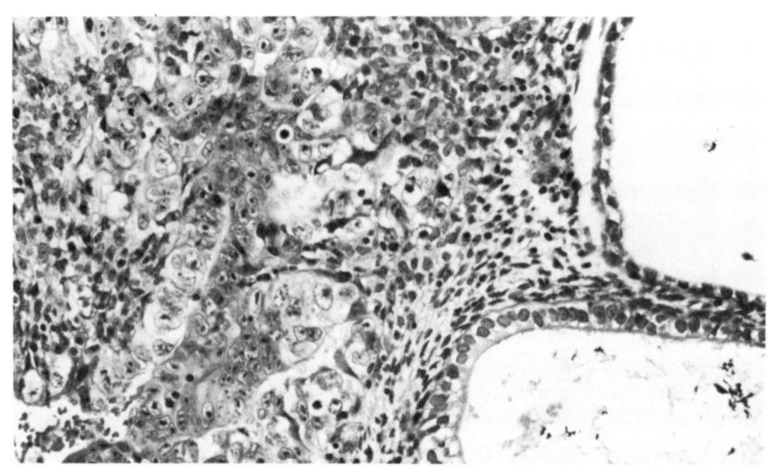

Figure 9–6. Glandular elements *(right)* adjacent to a focus of embryonal carcinoma characterize this tumor as a teratocarcinoma (H&E, ×400).

diastinal seminoma is composed of sheets of uniform round or polygonal cells in a loose fibrovascular stroma. Mitoses are easily identified. Distinct cell membranes enclose abundant clear or faintly eosinophilic cytoplasm. Round, vesicular nuclei with crisply outlined nuclear rims and a single prominent nucleolus stand out on sections stained with hematoxylin and eosin. Lymphocytes, often aggregated along the fibrous septa, are invariably present. Epithelioid histiocytes are regularly associated with the seminoma cells.

A variant of mediastinal seminoma manifests as a thymic cyst.[86, 91] Unlike classic mediastinal seminoma, which is histologically indistinguishable from its gonadal counterpart, this "unusual thymic seminoma" as described by Burns and McCaughey undergoes pronounced secondary changes that easily obscure the diagnosis (Fig. 9–7). Microscopically, low-power examination reveals cystic spaces lined by striking reactive follicular hyperplasia. Prominent aggregates of epithelioid histiocytes and Langhans' giant cells overshadow the neoplastic germ cells that are typically strewn individually and in small clusters among thymic cells. A periodic acid–Schiff stain before and after diastase digestion highlights the glycogen content of the neoplastic cells. The abundant granulomas usually prompt the pathologist to order "special stains" for fungal and acid-fast organisms. These stains are invariably negative.

A clue to the diagnosis of seminoma may be provided by a prominent "tigroid" background evident on cytologic preparations (i.e., needle aspiration or touch-imprint) (Fig. 9–8). Although not specific for seminoma, this tigroid background in conjunction with a dual cell population of lymphocytes and large, uniform malignant cells with prominent nucleoli strongly suggests the diagnosis.

Immunohistochemistry plays a key role in the diagnosis of seminoma.[62, 91, 92] Seminomas display both membrane and cytoplasmic reactivity to PLAP (Fig. 9–9). They may also react with antibodies to neuron specific enolase, but show no reaction with chromogranin. Cytokeratin, which reacts strongly with thymic epithelial cells, will not react with most seminomas. The pathologist must take care not to interpret entrapped thymic epithelial cells as the neoplastic germ cells. Some investigators have suggested that weak or focal cytokeratin positivity within a seminoma represents early development of a nonseminomatous germ cell component.[62] Bailey et al. report an anti-seminoma monoclonal antibody that exhibits both sensitive and specific staining of the cell membrane of seminoma cells.[92]

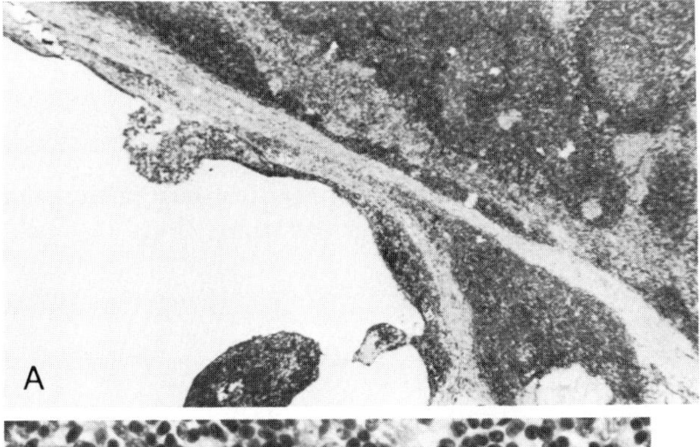

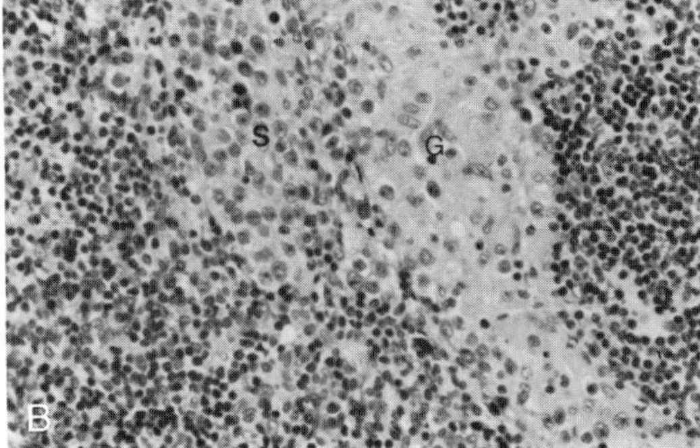

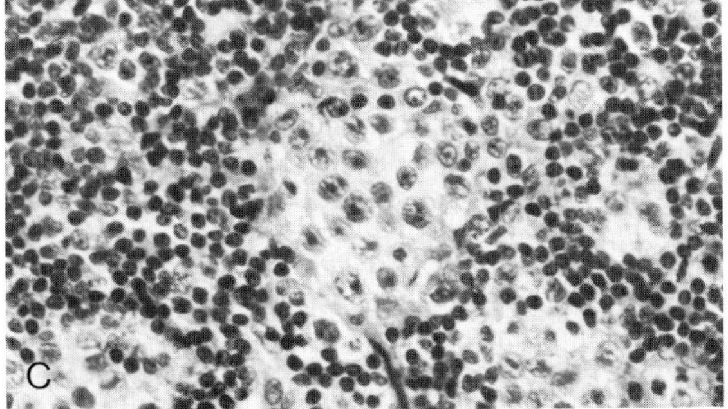

Figure 9–7. Cystic thymic seminoma. *A,* At low power, the cyst wall exhibits marked follicular hyperplasia (H&E, ×100). *B,* A prominent granulomatous component (*G*) often obscures the seminoma cells (*S*) (H&E, ×200). *C,* At high power, typical seminoma cells can be identified scattered among the lymphocytes (H&E, ×400).

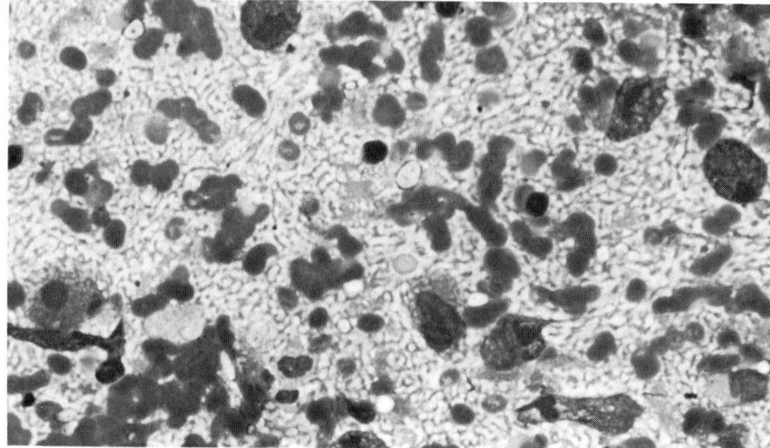

Figure 9–8. Large, single neoplastic cells admixed with lymphocytes in a "tigroid" background suggest a diagnosis of seminoma (Diff-Quik, ×400).

Ultrastructurally, seminoma cells appear as large, round, regular cells containing round nuclei (Fig. 9–10). A prominent, complex, filamentous nucleonema represents a distinctive feature. Cytoplasmic glycogen is present, but organelles tend to be sparse. Rare desmosomes enable cell attachment. Tonofilaments are absent.[93]

Differential Diagnosis

The principal differential diagnoses are (1) thymic cyst, (2) thymoma, (3) nodular sclerosing Hodgkin's disease, and (4) large-cell lymphoma.

1. *Thymic cyst:* The presence of marked follicular hyperplasia and extensive granulomas in a thymic cyst should prompt a diligent search for a seminomatous component.
2. *Thymoma:* In general, the presence of glycogen-rich cells with a prominent nucleolus, associated granulomas, and fibrous septa infiltrated by lymphocytes and plasma cells suggests the diagnosis of seminoma. Strong cytoplasmic reactivity to cytokeratin and ultrastructural evidence of tonofilaments and well-formed desmosomes are characteristic of thymoma.
3. *Nodular sclerosing Hodgkin's disease* may provoke a marked granulomatous reaction in the thymus. Reed-Sternberg cells must be identified. They may be confirmed immunhohistochemically with antibodies to CD15 (Leu M1) and CD30 (Ki-1).
4. *Large-cell lymphoma* will usually react with CD45 (leukocyte common antigen) but not with PLAP and neuron specific enolase. Ultrastructurally, lymphomas lack complex nucleoli and desmosomes.

Therapy and Clinical Outcome

In general, classic mediastinal seminomas have a poorer prognosis than their testicular

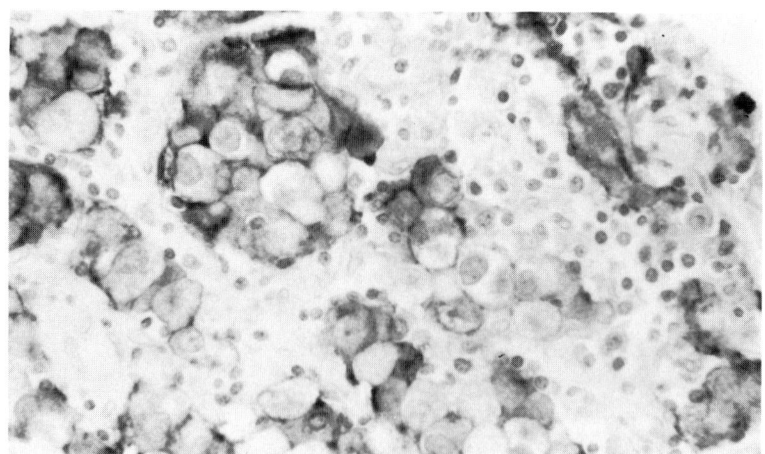

Figure 9–9. Seminoma cells display both membrane and cytoplasmic reactivity for placental alkaline phosphatase. The surrounding lymphocytes are nonreactive to this antibody (immunoperoxidase stain, ×400).

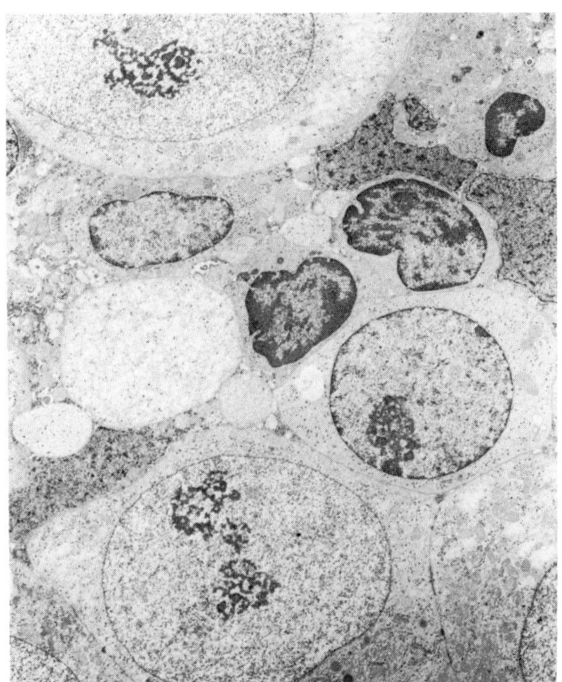

Figure 9–10. Ultrastructurally simple cells with a large, smoothly contoured nucleus and complex nucleonema, in a background of lymphocytes, are the typical electron micrographic appearance of a seminoma (×3000).

counterparts.[13, 55, 64, 80, 86, 93] This may reflect the large tumor burden at the time of diagnosis. Lemairie et al. found that complete resection followed by radiotherapy and/or chemotherapy resulted in long-term disease-free survival.[55] However, seminomas frequently present as bulky, nonresectable tumors, often involving the great vessels. Radiotherapy has been a mainstay of therapy, yielding 60 to 80% long-term survival rates.[9, 10, 12, 13, 55, 84–86, 94, 95] Failure usually occurs at distant sites, predominantly bone and lung.[7, 13, 84–86, 96] More recently, cisplatin-based chemotherapy has been used as primary therapy for mediastinal seminoma[97, 98] with good results. Clinical factors associated with a poor prognosis include age greater than 35 years, superior vena cava syndrome, lymphadenopathy, fever, and hilar involvement at the time of diagnosis.

NONSEMINOMATOUS MALIGNANT GERM CELL TUMORS

General

The malignant nonseminomatous germ cell tumors include endodermal sinus tumor (yolk sac tumor), embryonal carcinoma, choriocarcinoma, teratocarcinoma, and "mixed germ cell tumors." Like seminomas, these tumors typically arise in the anterior mediastinum and display a striking predilection for young males. The mean age of occurrence is in the third decade of life.[39, 61, 99] Unlike mediastinal seminomas, these neoplasms have a clearly documented association with non–germ cell malignancies[23, 24, 28, 29, 57–59] and Klinefelter's syndrome.[31, 33]

Choriocarcinoma is the least common primary mediastinal germ cell tumor. It is also the most difficult to prove, because minute foci of testicular choriocarcinoma, either active or regressed, can result in widely metastatic disease.[100–102] From a practical standpoint, however, both primary testicular and mediastinal choriocarcinoma share a common treatment regimen and outcome.

Clinical Presentation

The majority of these patients have such symptoms as chest pain, dyspnea, cough, weight loss, and superior vena cava syndrome. Distant metastases may be discovered during the initial evaluation. Gynecomastia or complaints of breast tenderness reflect high serum levels of B-HCG and suggest the presence of choriocarcinoma.

Radiographic and Laboratory Features

These tumors manifest as large smooth or lobulated anterior mediastinal masses (Fig. 9–11). There may be evidence of pleural or pericardial effusion.[75] Computed tomography typically reveals large areas of attenuation corresponding to foci of hemorrhage or necrosis.[75]

The serum tumor markers AFP and B-HCG are elevated in over 80% of patients with mediastinal nonseminomatous germ cell tumors.[14, 50, 61, 89, 99, 103] Elevated serum AFP can be seen with either endodermal sinus tumor or embryonal carcinoma. High-level (> 100 IU/ml) serum elevation of B-HCG is invariably present in choriocarcinoma. Indeed, if a young man with a mediastinal mass has significantly elevated levels of serum AFP or B-HCG, some authors recommend that a presumptive diagnosis of germ cell tumor be made and that treatment be initiated without biopsy.[14, 89] These patients also often exhibit increased lev-

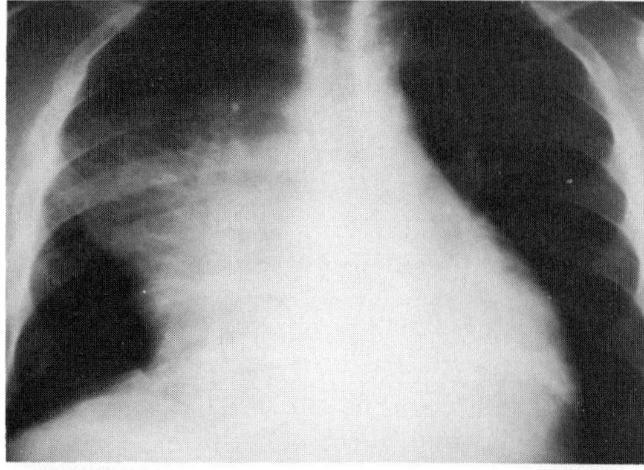

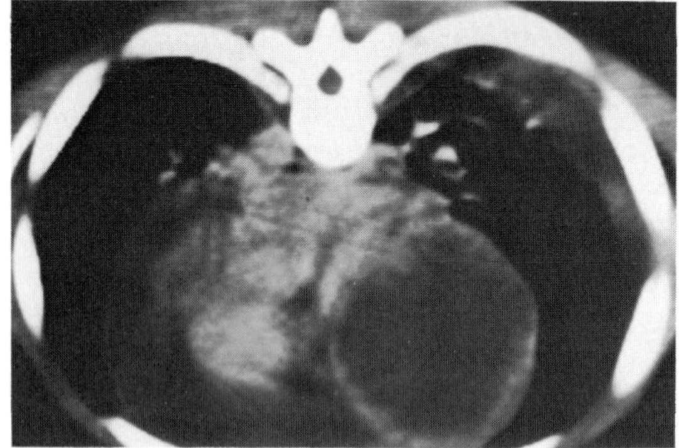

Figure 9–11. Nonseminomatous germ cell tumors often appear as a large mediastinal mass on chest radiograph (*top*). Computed tomography reveals areas of attenuation that correspond to foci of hemorrhage or necrosis (*bottom*).

els of serum lactate dehydrogenase, a nonspecific marker that reflects large tumor size and rapid growth.

Gross Features

Embryonal carcinoma and endodermal sinus tumor appear as bulky, predominantly solid, tan masses, often adherent to adjacent intrathoracic structures. The cut surface displays variegated areas of cyst formation, hemorrhage, and necrosis. Choriocarcinomas are highly vascular tumors that present as solid, hemorrhagic, friable masses. They frequently invade adjacent structures, including the lung.

Microscopic Features

Embryonal Carcinoma

Embryonal carcinoma consists of primitive polygonal cells arranged in solid sheets or in tubular or papillary patterns (Fig. 9–12). Large, often overlapping nuclei with a high nuclear-to-cytoplasmic ratio, indistinct cell borders, and prominent nucleoli are characteristic. These tumors contain numerous, frequently atypical mitotic figures. Rarely, structures recapitulating an early embryo, the "embryoid body," can be seen.

The majority of embryonal carcinomas react with antibodies to PLAP, cytokeratin, and neuron specific enolase. In contrast to the diffuse PLAP staining of seminomas, the staining in embryonal carcinoma may be patchy. Staining tends to be most marked along the cell membrane. Scattered clusters of AFP-positive cells can be identified in approximately one third of these tumors. Areas of syncytiotrophoblasts or intermediate trophoblasts within embryonal carcinoma can be confirmed by their reactivity for B-HCG.[62]

Embryonal carcinoma lacks diagnostic ultrastructural features. The cells appear primitive, with few organelles and rudimentary microvilli.

Endodermal Sinus Tumor

Endodermal sinus tumor displays a variety of patterns. The tumor can be recognized by an intermingling of delicate, microcystic alveolar-glandular and papillary structures in a mesenchymal background (Fig. 9–13). Less commonly, the tumor exhibits a solid pattern. Perivascular Schiller-Duval bodies are pathognomonic (Fig. 9–14). Round, hyaline, intracellular and extracellular, periodic acid–Schiff positive, diastase-resistant globules are a diagnostic feature. These globules may consist of AFP or other plasma proteins.

Endodermal sinus tumor is the germ cell tumor most likely to express AFP. Scattered, strongly positive clusters of AFP-positive cells may be seen in approximately 75% of these tumors.[62] Endodermal sinus tumors also typically exhibit strong, membrane-based staining for cytokeratin and PLAP. Focal neuron specific enolase reactivity may also be detected.

Ultrastructurally, endodermal sinus tumor displays short microvilli, abundant cytoplasmic glycogen, and prominent intracellular and extracellular basement membrane–like material[104, 105] (Fig. 9–15).

Choriocarcinoma

In choriocarcinoma, admixed cytotrophoblast and syncytiotrophoblast give the tumor a

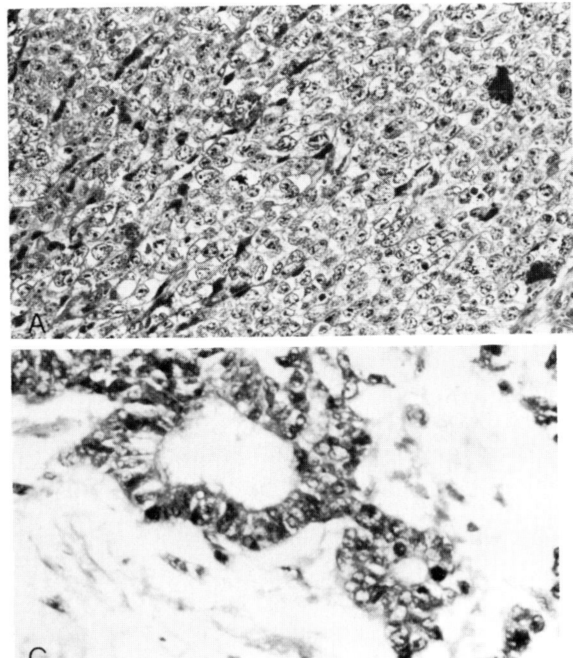

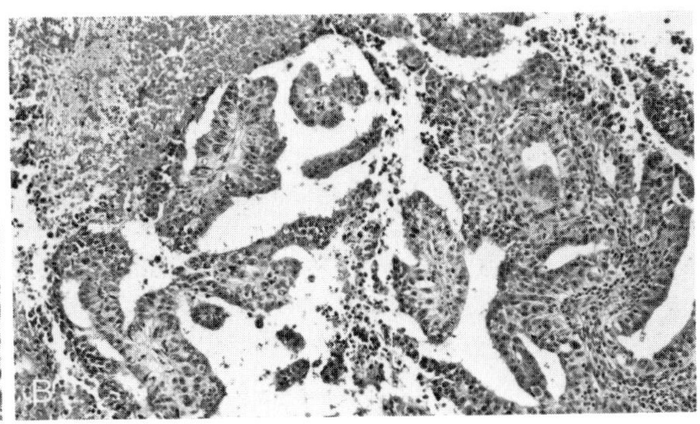

Figure 9–12. Embryonal carcinoma can display a variety of histologic patterns. The solid variant (*A*) is often misdiagnosed as undifferentiated carcinoma (H&E, ×100). The papillary pattern (*B*) can mimic adenocarcinoma (H&E, ×400). The tubular pattern (*C*) consists of primitive polygonal cells. Note the overlapping nuclei (H&E, ×400).

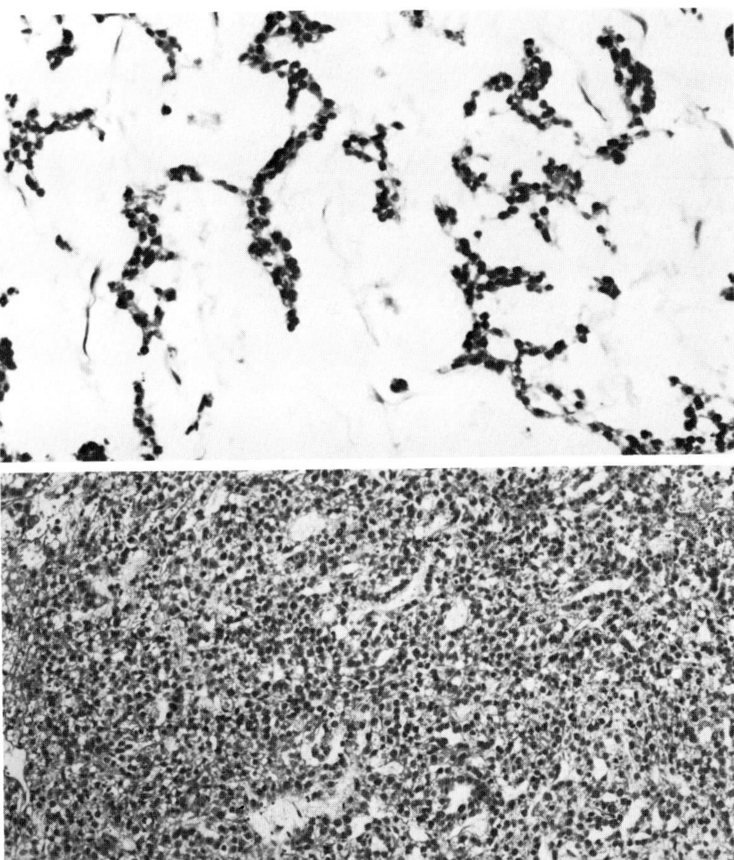

Figure 9–13. One variant of endodermal sinus tumor can be recognized as a delicate microcystic network in a mesenchymal stroma (*top*) (H&E, ×100). Less commonly, small cells with clear cytoplasm and relatively uniform nuclei form a solid aggregate (*bottom*) (H&E, ×100).

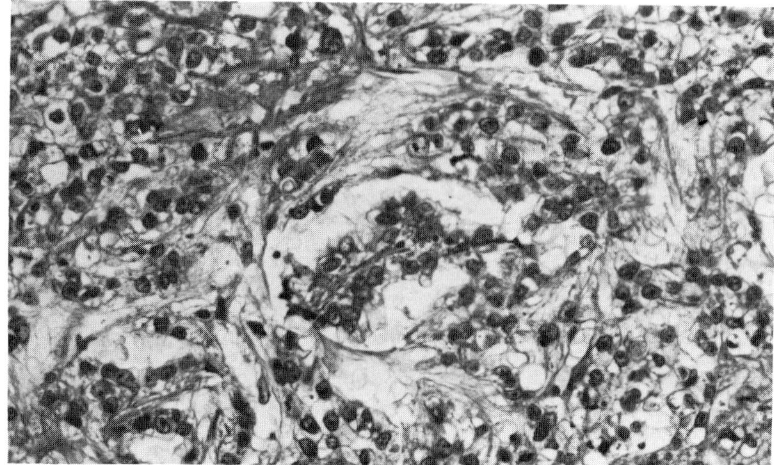

Figure 9–14. Solid variant of endodermal sinus tumor. The central structure suggests a Schiller-Duval body (H&E, ×400).

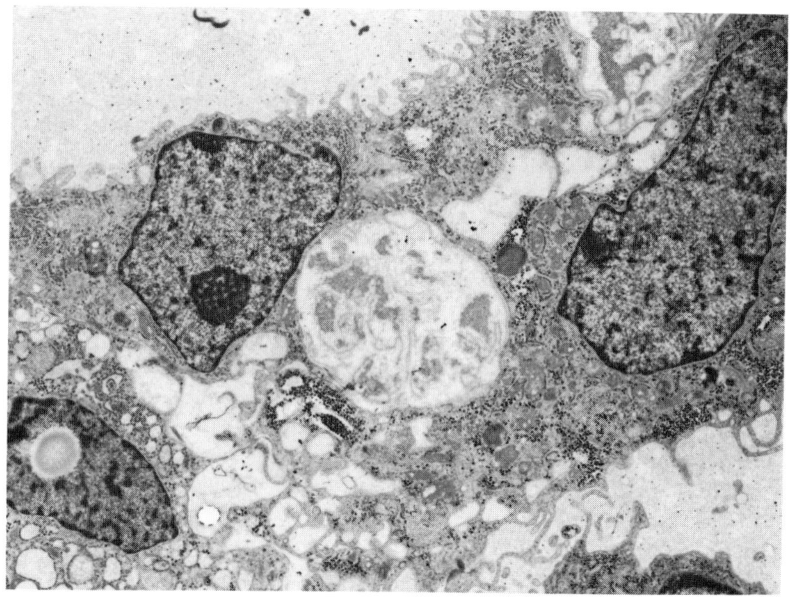

Figure 9–15. Short microvilli and intracellular or extracellular basement membrane–like material can be found ultrastructurally in endodermal sinus tumor (×3000).

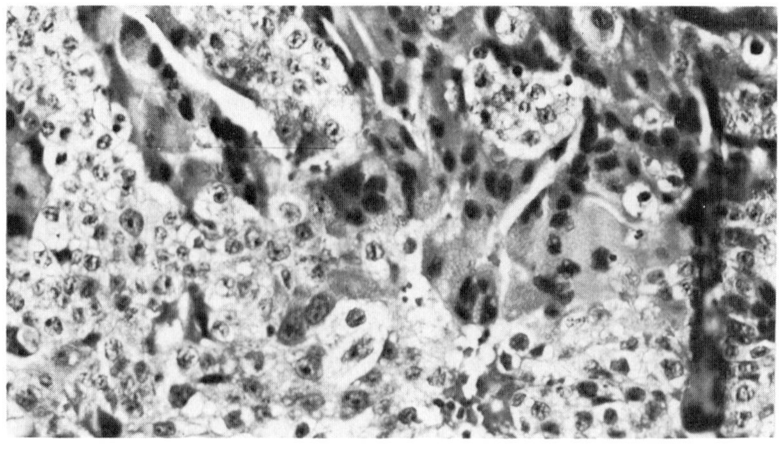

Figure 9–16. The juxtaposition of cytotrophoblast and syncytiotrophoblast identifies this neoplasm as choriocarcinoma (H&E, ×400).

biphasic appearance (Fig. 9–16). The identification of both cell types is critical to the diagnosis of this neoplasm, because isolated syncytiotrophoblastic elements can be found in other germ cell tumors.

All choriocarcinomas exhibit striking syncytiotrophoblastic reactivity to B-HCG[62, 100, 101, 106] (Fig. 9–16). These tumors also display strong cytoplasmic staining with cytokeratin. In addition, approximately 50% of choriocarcinomas will contain foci that stain for neuron specific enolase and PLAP.[62]

The cytotrophoblast ultrastructurally resembles embryonal carcinoma. These are primitive cells that lack well-developed golgi or rough endoplasmic reticulum. One or more nuclei in a common cytoplasm identifies syncytiotrophoblast. Other diagnostic features include numerous microvilli and cisternal stacking of rough endoplasmic reticulum.

Differential Diagnosis

The principal differential diagnoses are (1) undifferentiated carcinoma, (2) malignant lymphoma, and (3) metastatic melanoma.

1. *Undifferentiated carcinoma:* Endodermal sinus tumor and embryonal carcinoma are commonly misdiagnosed as undifferentiated carcinoma or poorly differentiated adenocarcinoma. Richardson et al. coined the term unrecognized extragonadal germ cell cancer syndrome to describe a group of patients initially diagnosed with poorly differentiated or undifferentiated carcinoma.[107] They responded dramatically to the chemotherapy and radiation therapy used for germ cell tumors. In general, carcinomas occur in older individuals and have a more monotonous microscopic pattern. The presence of serum and/or tumor markers for AFP and B-HCG, in conjunction with tumor reactivity for PLAP, suggests a presumptive diagnosis of germ cell tumor. Ultrastructurally, unlike germ cell tumors, most carcinomas feature desmosomes, numerous cytoplasmic organelles, and tonofilaments. They lack the basement membrane–like material found in endodermal sinus tumors.

2. *Large-cell malignant lymphoma* may be differentiated from germ cell tumors by immunohistochemistry. In contrast to germ cell tumors, lymphomas react with CD45 and do not react with cytokeratin, PLAP, AFP, and B-HCG.[62, 63]

3. *Malignant melanoma* can be identified by immunoreactivity to S-100 and HMB-45. Germ cell tumors lack these antigens. Ultrastructurally, even in amelanotic variants, premelanosomes can usually be identified.

Therapy and Clinical Outcome

Before the advent of cisplatin-based chemotherapy, the diagnosis of malignant nonseminomatous germ cell tumor carried an abysmal prognosis.[3, 5, 6, 10, 20, 41] Because most of these tumors are unresectable at the time of presentation, current reports recommend cisplatin-based chemotherapy as the cornerstone of aggressive, multimodality therapy.[10, 21, 36, 38, 55, 61, 80, 90, 97, 99, 108] Normalization of serum tumor markers following chemotherapy is a favorable prognostic indicator. Persistent elevation of markers indicates residual disease. These patients may benefit from adjunctive surgery to resect residual primary tumor.[14, 35, 38, 55, 61, 64, 97, 99] Adjunct radiotherapy may also contribute to increased survival.[12, 34, 61, 94]

Despite therapeutic advances, patients with mediastinal nonseminomatous germ cell tumors still do more poorly than their testicular-affected counterparts.[9, 34, 35, 38, 39] Approximately 50% of these individuals ultimately die of advanced local disease, metastatic disease, or treatment-resistant sarcomas and hematologic malignancies.[38, 61] Choriocarcinoma disseminates especially rapidly along hematogenous routes to the lung, liver, kidney, and brain.[102] High-dose chemotherapy followed by autologous bone marrow rescue has not proven successful in these patients,[109] and treatment protocols continue to evolve.

SUMMARY

The mediastinum is the most common site for extragonadal germ cell tumors. Patients are usually children or young adults. Histologically, mediastinal germ cell tumors are indistinguishable from their gonadal counterparts. They have a similar chromosomal abnormality, although mediastinal seminomas are more often diploid than testicular seminomas. Malignant mediastinal germ cell tumors, particularly the nonseminomatous types, have been associated with sarcomas and with hematologic malignancies (usually acute nonlymphocytic leukemia). Patients with malignant mediastinal nonseminomatous germ cell tumors have an increased incidence of Klinefelter's syndrome.

The histologic differential diagnosis of mediastinal germ cell tumors includes thymoma, undifferentiated carcinoma, Hodgkin's disease, large cell lymphoma, and malignant melanoma. A cystic seminoma may resemble a thymic cyst. Immunohistochemistry is usually helpful in conclusively establishing the diagnosis. With surgery, chemotherapy, and radiation therapy as therapeutic modalities, approximately 50% of patients with mediastinal nonseminomatous germ cell tumors have long-term survival. Those with mediastinal seminoma have a somewhat better prognosis.

REFERENCES

1. Meares EM Jr, Briggs EM. Occult seminoma of the testis masquerading as primary extragonadal germinal neoplasms. Cancer 1972; 30:300–306.
2. Daugaard G, Von der Masse H, Olsen J, Rorth M, Skakkebaek NE. Carcinoma-in-situ testis in patients with assumed extragonadal germ-cell tumors. Lancet 1987; 2:528–530.
3. Cox JD. Primary malignant germinal tumors of the mediastinum. A study of 24 cases. Cancer 1975; 36:1162–1168.
4. Luna MA, Valenzuela-Tamariz J. Germ-cell tumors of the mediastinum, postmortem findings. Am J Clin Pathol 1976; 65:450–454.
5. Oberman HA, Libcke JH. Malignant germinal neoplasms of the mediastinum. Cancer 1964; 17:498–507.
6. Pachter MR, Lattes R. Germinal tumors of the mediastinum: A clinicopathologic study of adult teratomas, teratocarcinomas, choriocarcinomas and seminomas. Dis Chest 1964; 45:301–310.
7. Recondo J, Libshitz HI. Mediastinal extragonadal germ cell tumors. Urology 1978; 11:369–375.
8. Bredael JJ, Vugrin D, Whitmore WF. Autopsy findings in 154 patients with germ cell tumors of the testis. Cancer 1982; 50:548–551.
9. Kiffer JD, Sandeman TF. Primary malignant mediastinal germ cell tumors: a study of eleven cases and a review of the literature. Int J Rad Oncol Biol Phys 1989; 17:835–841.
10. Economou J, Trump D, Holmes E, Eggleston J. Management of primary germ cell tumors of the mediastinum. J Thorac Cardiovasc Surg 1982; 83:643–649.
11. Hainsworth JD, Greco FA. Extragonadal germ cell tumors and unrecognized germ cell tumors. Semin Oncol 1992; 19:119–127.
12. Kersh CR, Eisert DR, Constable WC, Hahn S, Jenrette J, Fitzgerald R, Grayson J. Primary malignant mediastinal germ-cell tumors and the contribution of radiotherapy: A southeastern multi-institutional study. Am J Clin Oncol 1987; 10:302–306.
13. Knapp RH, Hurt RD, Payne WS, Farrow GM, Lewis BD, Hahn RG, Muhm JR, Earle JD. Malignant germ cell tumors of the mediastinum. J Thorac Cardiovasc Surg 1985; 89:82–89.
14. Nichols CR. Mediastinal germ cell tumors. Semin Thorac Cardiovasc Surg 1992; 4:45–50.
15. El-Naggar AK, Ro JY, McLemore D, Ayala AG, Batsakis JG. DNA ploidy in testicular germ cell neoplasms. Histogenetic and clinical implications. Am J Surg Pathol 1992; 16:611–618.
16. Oosterhuis JW, Rammeloo RHV, Cornelisse C, DeJong B, Dam A, Sleijfer D. Ploidy of malignant mediastinal germ-cell tumors. Hum Pathol 1990; 21:729–732.
17. Davis RD, Oldham HN, Sabiston CD Jr. Primary cysts and neoplasms of the mediastinum: recent changes in clinical presentation, methods of diagnosis, management and results. Ann Thorac Surg 1987; 44:229–237.
18. Mullen B, Richardson JD. Primary anterior mediastinal tumors in children and adults. Ann Thorac Surg 1986; 42:338–345.
19. Wychulis AR, Payne WS, Clagett OT, Woolner LB. Surgical treatment of mediastinal tumors: a forty year experience. J Thorac Cardiovasc Surg 1971; 62:379–392.
20. Aliotta PJ, Castillo J, Englander LS, Nseyo U, Huben RP. Primary mediastinal germ cell tumors. Histologic patterns of treatment failures at autopsy. Cancer 1988; 62:982–984.
21. Kuhn M, Weissbach L. Localization, incidence, diagnosis and treatment of extratesticular germ cell tumors. Urol Int 1985; 40:166–172.
22. Dehner L. Gonadal and extragonadal germ cell neoplasms in childhood. Hum Pathol 1983; 14:493–511.
23. DeMent SH. Association between mediastinal germ cell tumors and hematologic malignancies. An update. Hum Pathol 1990; 21:699–703.
24. DeMent SH, Eggleston JC, Spivak JL. Association between mediastinal germ cell tumors and hematologic malignancies. Report of two cases and review of the literature. Am J Surg Pathol 1985; 9:23–30.
25. Ladanyi M, Sanmaniego F, Reuter VE, Motzer RJ, Jhanwar SC, Bosl GJ, Chaganti RSK. Cytogenetic and immunohistochemical evidence for the germ cell origin of a subset of acute leukemias associated with mediastinal germ cell tumors. J Natl Cancer Inst 1990; 82:221–227.
26. Ladanyi M, Roy I. Mediastinal germ cell tumors and histiocytosis. Hum Pathol 1988; 19:586–590.
27. Mihal V, Dusek J, Jarosova M, Zidovah P, Indrak K, Scudla V, Bradova E, Gregurkova J, Spidlova A. Mediastinal teratoma and acute megakaryoblastic leukemia. Neoplasma 1989; 36:739–747.
28. Nichols CR, Hoffman R, Einhorn LH, Williams S, Wheeler L, Garnick M. Hematologic malignancies associated with primary mediastinal germ-cell tumors. Ann Int Med 1985; 102:603–609.
29. Nichols CR, Roth BJ, Heerema NA, Griep J, Tricot G. Hematologic neoplasia associated with primary mediastinal germ-cell tumors. N Engl J Med 1990; 322:1425–1429.
30. Dexeus FH, Logothetis CJ, Chong C, Sella A, Ogden S. Genetic abnormalities in men with cell tumors. J Urol 1988; 140:80–84.
31. Lachman MF, Kim K, Koo B-C. Mediastinal teratoma associated with Klinefelter's syndrome. Arch Pathol Lab Med 1986; 110:1067–1071.
32. Nichols CR, Heerema NA, Palmer C, Loehrer P, Williams S, Einhorn L. Klinefelter's syndrome associated with mediastinal germ cell neoplasms. J Clin Oncol 1987; 5:1290–1294.
33. Hasle H, Jacobsen B, Asschenfeldt P, Andersen K. Mediastinal germ cell tumor associated with Klinefelter syndrome. A report of case and review of the literature. Eur J Pediatr 1992; 151:735–739.
34. Kuzur ME, Cobleigh MA, Greco A, Einhorn LH, Oldham RK. Endodermal sinus tumor of the mediastinum. Cancer 1982; 50:766–774.
35. Saxman S, Nichols CR, Williams SD, Loehrer P, Einhorn L. Mediastinal yolk sac tumor. The Indiana Uni-

versity Experience, 1976–1988. J Thorac Cardiovasc Surg 1991; 102:913–916.
36. Sham JST, Fu KH, Chiu CSW, Lau WH, Choi PHK, Khin MA, Tung SY, Mok CK, Choy D. Experience with the management of primary endodermal sinus tumor of the mediastinum. Cancer 1989; 64:756–761.
37. Hawkins EP, Finegold MJ, Hawkins HK, Krischer J, Starling K, Weinberg A. Nongerminomatous malignant germ cell tumors in children. A review of 89 cases from the pediatric oncology group 1971–1984. Cancer 1986; 58:2579–2584.
38. Nichols CR, Saxman S, Williams SD, Loehrer P, Miller M, Wright C, Einhorn L. Primary mediastinal nonseminomatous germ cell tumors. A modern single institution experience. Cancer 1990; 65:1641–1646.
39. Toner GC, Geller NL, Lin SY, Bosl GJ. Extragonadal and poor risk nonseminomatous germ cell tumors. Cancer 1991; 67:2049–2057.
40. Wright CD, Kesler KA, Nichols CR, Mahomed Y, Einhorn LH, Miller ME, Brown JW. Primary mediastinal nonseminomatous germ cell tumors. Results of a multimodality approach. J Thorac Cardiovasc Surg 1990; 99:210–217.
41. Schlumberger HG. Teratoma of the anterior mediastinum in the group of military age—a study of sixteen cases, and a review of theories of genesis. Arch Pathol 1946; 41:398–444.
42. Gonzalez-Crussi F. The human yolk sac and yolk sac (endodermal sinus) tumors. A review. Perspect Pediatr Pathol 1979; 5:179–215.
43. Friedman NB. The comparative morphogenesis of extragenital and gonadal teratoid tumors. Cancer 1951; 4:265–276.
44. Friedman NB. The function of the primordial germ cell in extragonadal tissues. Int J Androl 1987; 10:43–49.
45. Samaniego F, Rodriguez E, Houldsworth J, Murty V, Ladangi M, Lele K, Chen Q, Dmitrovsky E, Geller N, Reuter V, Jhanwar S, Bosl G, Chaganti R. Cytogenetic and molecular analysis of human male germ cell tumors: chromosome 12 abnormalities and gene amplification. Genes Chromosome Cancer 1990; 1:289–300.
46. Bosl GJ, Dmitrovsky E, Reuter VE, Samaniego F, Rodriguez E, Geller N, Chaganti R. Isochromosome of chromosome 12: clinically useful marker for male germ cell tumors. J Natl Cancer Inst 1989; 81:1874–1878.
47. Motzer RJ, Rodriguez E, Reuter VE, Samaniego F, Dmitrovsky E, Bajorin D, Pfister D, Parsa N, Chaganti R, Bosl G. Genetic analysis as an aid in diagnosis for patients with midline carcinomas of uncertain histogenesis. J Natl Cancer Inst 1991; 83:341–346.
48. Dal Cin P, Drochmans A, Moerman P, Van Den Berghe H. Isochromosome 12P in mediastinal germ cell tumor. Cancer Genet Cytogenet 1989; 42:243–251.
49. Oosterhuis JW, Castedo SMMJ, DeJong B. Cytogenetics, ploidy and differentiation of human testicular, ovarian and extragonadal germ cell tumors. Cancer Surv 1990; 9:321–332.
50. Nichols CR, Hoffman R, Glant M, Goheen M. Malignant disorders of megakaryocytes associated with primary mediastinal germ cell tumors. *In* Levine RF, Williams N, Levin J, Evett Bl, eds. Megakaryocyte Development and Function. New York: Alan R. Liss, 1986:347–353.
51. Myers T, Kessimian N, Schwartz S. Mediastinal germ cell tumor associated with hemophagocytic syndrome. Ann Intern Med 1988; 15:504–505.
52. Ashby MA, Williams CJ, Buchanan RB, Bleehen NM, Arno J. Mediastinal germ cell tumours associated with malignant histiocytosis and high rubella titres. Hematol Oncol 1986; 4:183–194.
53. Chariot P, Monnet I, LeLong F, Chelq C, Droz J-P, deCremoux H. Systemic mast cell disease associated with primary mediastinal germ cell tumor. Am J Med 1991; 90:381–385.
54. Chariot P, Monnet I, Gaulard P, Abd-Alsamad I, Ruffie P, deCremoux H. Systemic mastocytosis following mediastinal germ cell tumor: an association confirmed. Hum Pathol 1993; 24:111–112.
55. Lemarie E, Assouline PS, Diot P, Reynard J, Levasseur P, Droz J, Ruffié P. Primary mediastinal germ cell tumors. Results of a French retrospective study. Chest 1992; 102:1477–1483.
56. Orazi A, Neiman RS, Ulbright TM, Heerema N, John K, Nichols C. Hematopoietic precursor cells within the yolk sac tumor component are the source of secondary hematopoietic malignancies in patients with mediastinal germ cell tumors. Cancer 1993; 71:3873–3881.
57. Caballero C, Gomez S, Matias-Guiu X, Prat J. Rhabdomyosarcomas developing in association with mediastinal germ cell tumors. Virchows Arch [A] Pathol Anat 1992; 420:539–543.
58. Manivel C, Wick MR, Abenoza P, Rosai J. The occurrence of sarcomatous components in primary mediastinal germ cell tumors. Am J Surg Pathol 1986; 10:711–717.
59. Ulbright TM, Loehrer PJ, Roth L, Einhorn L, Williams S, Clark S. The development of non–germ cell malignancies within germ cell tumors. Cancer 1984; 54:1824–1833.
60. Ulbright TM, Michael H, Loehrer PJ, Donohue JP. Spindle cell tumors resected from male patients with germ cell tumors. A clinicopathologic study of 14 cases. Cancer 1990; 65:148–156.
61. Wright CD, Kesler KA, Nichols CR, Mahomed Y, Einhorn LH, Miller ME, Brown JW. Primary mediastinal nonseminomatous germ cell tumors: results of a multimodality approach. J Thorac Cardiovasc Surg 1990; 99:210–217.
62. Niehans GA, Manivel C, Copland G, Scheithauer B, Wick M. Immunohistochemistry of germ cell and trophoblastic neoplasms. Cancer 1988; 62:1113–1123.
63. Wick MR, Simpson RW, Niehans GA, Scheithauer BW. Anterior mediastinal tumors: a clinicopathologic study of 100 cases, with emphasis on immunohistochemical analysis. Progr Surg Pathol 1990; 11:79–119.
64. Nichols CR. Mediastinal germ cell tumors. Clinical features and biologic correlates. Chest 1991; 99:472–479.
65. Gonzalez-Crussi F, Winkler RF, Mirkin DL. Sacrococcygeal teratomas in infants and children: relationship of histology and prognosis in 40 cases. Arch Pathol Lab Med 1978; 102:420–425.
66. Bergh NP, Gatzinsky P, Larsson S, Lundin P, Ridell B. Tumors of the thymus and thymic region: III. Clinicopathologic studies on teratomas and tumors of germ cell type. Ann Thorac Surg 1978; 25:107–111.
67. Lack EE, Weinstein HJ, Welch KJ. Mediastinal germ cell tumors in childhood. A clinical and pathologic study of 21 cases. J Thorac Cardiovasc Surg 1985; 89:826–835.
68. Saabye J, Elbirk A, Andersen K. Teratomas of the mediastinum. Scand J Thorac Cardiovasc Surg 1987; 21:271–272.
69. Weinraub Z, Gembruch U, Fodisch HJ, Hansmann M. Intrauterine mediastinal teratoma associated with

non-immune hydrops fetalis. Prenat Diagn 1989; 9:369–372.
70. Kenny JB, Carty HML. Infants presenting with respiratory distress due to anterior mediastinal teratomas: a report of three cases and a review of the literature. Br J Radiol 1988; 61:241–244.
71. Honicky RE, dePapp EW. Mediastinal teratoma with endocrine function. Am J Dis Child 1973; 126:650–653.
72. Lewis BD, Hurt RD, Payne WS, Farrow GM, Knapp RH, Muhm JR. Benign teratomas of the mediastinum. J Thorac Cardiovasc Surg 1983; 86:727–731.
73. Carter D, Bibro MC, Touloukian RJ. Benign clinical behavior of immature mediastinal teratoma in infancy. Report of two cases and review of the literature. Cancer 1982; 49:398–402.
74. Karl SR, Dunn J. Posterior mediastinal teratomas. J Pediatr Surg 1985; 20:508–510.
75. Rosado-de-Christenson ML, Templeton PA, Moran CA. Mediastinal germ cell tumors. Radiologic and pathologic correlation. Radiographics 1992; 12:1013–1030.
76. Cobb CJ, Wynn J, Cobb SR, Duane GB. Cytologic findings in an effusion caused by rupture of a benign cystic teratoma of the mediastinum into a serous cavity. Acta Cytol 1985; 29:1015–1020.
77. Suda K, Mizuguchi K, Hebisawa A, Wakabayashi T, Saito S. Pancreatic tissue in teratoma. Arch Pathol Lab Med 1984; 108:835–837.
78. Bordi C, DeVita O, Pollice L. Full pancreatic endocrine differentiation in a mediastinal teratoma. Hum Pathol 1985; 16:961–964.
79. Dunn PJS. Pancreatic tissue in benign mediastinal teratoma. J Clin Pathol 1984; 37:1105–1109.
80. Dulmet EM, Macchiariani P, Suk B, Verley JM. Germ cell tumors of the mediastinum: a thirty year experience. Cancer 1993; 72:1894–1901.
81. Norris HJ, Zirkin HJ, Benson WL. Immature teratomas of the ovary: clinicopathologic study of 58 cases. Cancer 1976; 37:2359–2372.
82. Wirtanen GW, Stephenson JA, Wiley AL. Primary anterior mediastinal malignant teratoma. A case report with long-term survival. Cancer 1989; 63:1823–1825.
83. Bush SE, Martinez A, Bagshaw MA. Primary mediastinal seminoma. Cancer 1981; 48:1877–1882.
84. Hurt RD, Bruckman JE, Farrow GM, Bernatz PE, Hahn RG, Earle JD. Primary anterior mediastinal seminoma. Cancer 1982; 49:1658–1663.
85. Lee YM, Jackson SM. Primary seminoma of the mediastinum. Cancer Control Agency of the British Columbia Experience. Cancer 1985; 55:450–452.
86. Schantz A, Sewall W, Castleman B. Mediastinal germinoma. A study of 21 cases with excellent prognosis. Cancer 1972; 30:1189–1194.
87. Brown K, Collins JD, Batra P, Steckel RJ, Kagan AR. Mediastinal germ cell tumor in a young woman. Med Pediatr Oncol 1989; 17:164–167.
88. Moriconi WJ, Taylor S, Huntrakoon M, MacArthur R, Bixler TJ. Primary mediastinal germinomas in females: a case report and review of the literature. J Surg Oncol 1985; 29:176–180.
89. Rapellino M, Cellerino A, Ardissone F, Libertucci D, Coni F, Aimo G, Pecchio F. Alpha-fetoprotein and mediastinal germ cell tumors. J Nucl Med Allied Sci 1989; 33(Suppl):46–52.
90. McLeod DG, Taylor HG, Skoog SJ, Knight RD, Dawson N, Waxman J. Extragonadal germ cell tumors. Clinicopathologic findings and treatment experience in 12 patients. Cancer 1988; 61:1187–1191.
91. Burns BF, McCaughey WTE. Unusual thymic seminomas. Arch Pathol Lab Med 1986; 110:539–541.
92. Bailey D, Bauman R, Marks A. Use of anti-seminoma monoclonal antibody to confirm the diagnosis of mediastinal seminoma. APMIS 1988; 96:206–210.
93. Levine GD. Primary thymic seminoma—a neoplasm ultrastructurally similar to testicular seminoma and distinct from epithelial thymoma. Cancer 1973; 31:729–741.
94. Kersh CR, Constable WC, Hahn S, Spaulding C, Eisert D, Jenrette J, Marks R, Grayson J. Primary malignant extragonadal germ cell tumors. An analysis of the effects of radiotherapy. Cancer 1990; 65:2681–2685.
95. Uematsu M, Kondo M, Dokiya T, Tamai S, Ando Y, Hashimoto S. The role of radiotherapy in the treatment of primary mediastinal seminoma. Radiother Oncol 1992; 24:226–230.
96. Martini N, Golbey RB, Hajdu SI, Whitmore WF, Beattie EJ. Primary mediastinal germ cell tumors. Cancer 1974; 33:763–769.
97. Giaccone G. Multimodality treatment of malignant germ cell tumors of the mediastinum. Eur J Cancer 1991; 27:273–277.
98. Jain K, Bols G, Bains M, Whitmore WF, Golbey RB. The treatment of extragonadal seminoma. J Clin Oncol 1984; 2:820–827.
99. Kay PH, Wells FC, Goldstraw P. A multidisciplinary approach to primary nonseminomatous germ cell tumors of the mediastinum. Ann Thorac Surg 1987; 44:578–582.
100. Knapp RH, Fritz SR, Reiman HM. Primary embryonal carcinoma and choriocarcinoma of the mediastinum. A case report. Arch Pathol Lab Med 1982; 106:507–509.
101. Sangalli G, Livraghi T, Giordano F, Tavani E, Schiaffino E. Primary mediastinal embryonal carcinoma and choriocarcinoma. A case report. Acta Cytol 1986; 30:543–546.
102. Sickles EA, Belliveau RE, Wiernik PH. Primary mediastinal choriocarcinoma in the male. Cancer 1974; 33:1196–1203.
103. Truong LD, Harris L, Mattioli C, Hawkins E, Lee A, Wheeler T, Lane M. Endodermal sinus tumor of the mediastinum. A report of seven cases and review of the literature. Cancer 1986; 58:730–739.
104. Gonzalez-Crussi F, Roth LM. The human yolk sac and yolk sac carcinoma. An ultrastructural study. Hum Pathol 1976; 7:676–691.
105. Mukai K, Adams W. Yolk sac tumor of the anterior mediastinum. Am J Surg Pathol 1979; 3:77–83.
106. Kathuria S, Jablokow VR. Primary choriocarcinoma of mediastinum with immunohistochemical study and review of the literature. J Surg Oncol 1987; 34:39–42.
107. Richardson RL, Schoumacher RA, Fer M, Hande K, Forbes J, Oldham R, Greco FA. The unrecognized extragonadal germ cell cancer syndrome. Ann Intern Med 1981; 94:181–186.
108. Berruti A, Borasio P, Paze E, Mossetti C, Gorzegno G, Dogliotti L. Mediastinal non-seminomatous germ cell tumors: effectiveness of platinum, etoposide, bleomycin combination chemotherapy plus adjunctive surgery [letter]. Eur J Cancer 1992; 28A:1773.
109. Broun ER, Nichols CR, Kneebone P, Williams SD, Loehrer PJ, Einhorn LH, Tricot G. Long-term outcome of patients with relapsed and refractory germ cell tumors treated with high dose chemotherapy and autologous bone marrow rescue. Ann Intern Med 1992; 117:124–128.

Chapter

10

NEUROENDOCRINE TUMORS: CARCINOID AND PARAGANGLIOMA

THYMIC CARCINOID
- Clinical Features
- Pathology
- Therapy and Prognosis
- Cell Origin

PARAGANGLIOMA
- Aortic Body Paraganglioma
- Paravertebral Paraganglioma
- Histochemistry
- Immunoperoxidase Stains and Other Adjunctive Studies
- Differential Diagnosis
- Paraganglioma in Animals

SUMMARY

THYMIC CARCINOID

Thymic carcinoids histologically resemble thymomas but should be distinguished from them because of more aggressive behavior. In 1972, Rosai and Higa clearly separated out a group of mediastinal tumors that histologically and ultrastructurally resembled carcinoids.[1] Previously, such tumors, including those associated with Cushing's syndrome, had been included within the thymoma category.[2] Subsequently, the association of Cushing's syndrome with thymic carcinoid, rather than thymoma, was established.[3]

Thymic carcinoids are less common than thymomas. In a personal series of mediastinal tumors, this author encountered 3 thymic carcinoids and 126 thymomas (unpublished data).[4] This is similar to the experience at the University of Hamburg, where 3 carcinoids and 122 thymomas were identified.[5,6]

Clinical Features

Among 70 thymic carcinoids in the literature, male patients outnumbered females by 3:1.[5] The patients have ranged from 9 to 87 years of age with a median of 43 years.[5,7] In contrast to bronchial carcinoid tumors, most thymic carcinoids are malignant[5] (Table 10–1). Half are invasive at the time of diagnosis. In six series, 21 of 39 thymic carcinoid tumors metastasized, most commonly to regional lymph nodes, skin, and bone.[1,3,5,8–12] Bone metastases may be osteoblastic.

Thymic carcinoids can present with symptoms related to the location of the tumor (e.g., chest pain, cough), or the tumor may be an incidental finding on routine chest radiograph. Less than one third of patients with thymic carcinoid have endocrine symptoms.[5,13] The endocrine symptoms usually relate to production of ectopic adrenocorticotropic hormone (ACTH) with resulting Cushing's syndrome.

Ectopic ACTH production is most common with oat cell carcinoma but is also associated with bronchial and thymic carcinoids.[14–17] Localizing the source of ACTH in a patient with Cushing's syndrome can be difficult.[13,18,19] Computed tomography (CT) scans are valuable for this purpose. Selective venous sampling can be done to look for higher ACTH levels from different sites, such as the petrosal veins

Table 10–1. Thymic Carcinoid Tumors: Summary of Six Published Series

Reference	No. of Cases	No. with Cushing's Syndrome	Age/Male-to-Female Ratio	Invasive	Recurrent	Metastatic
Wick et al.[8]	15	5	15–67/4:1	8/15*		11/15
Rosai and Higa,[1] Rosai et al.[9]	11	0 (3 with MEN)	21–66/ (all male)	4/11	6/11	3/11
Economopoulas et al.[10]	7	0	27–70/6:1	5/7	4/7	3/7
Herbst et al.[11]	5	0			3/5	
Sayler et al.[3]	3	0	35–87/1:2	3/3	2/3	2/3
Muller-Hermelink et al.[12]	3	1	19–42/ (all male)			2/3
Total	44	6	15–87/33:6	20/36 (56%)	15/26 (58%)	21/39 (54%)

MEN, multiple endocrine neoplasia.
*Total number of cases for which information is provided.

(to exclude a pituitary source). However, thymic vein sampling may not be reliable.[13] Ectopic ACTH is usually not suppressed by dexamethasone. Further complicating the diagnosis, the tumor may secrete the hormone intermittently and obscure the diagnostic tests.

Less commonly, the patient with thymic carcinoid has symptoms relating to a multiple endocrine neoplasia (MEN) syndrome.[9] MEN type I (Wermer's syndrome), in particular, has been associated with thymus and foregut-derived carcinoids (bronchus, stomach, duodenum). This syndrome includes parathyroid, pancreatic, and pituitary tumors.[20] Occasional patients, including some with thymic carcinoid, have MEN that overlaps between type I and type II.[21] Type II MEN, or Sipple's syndrome, includes medullary carcinoma of the thyroid, pheochromocytoma, parathyroid enlargement. MEN type IIb or III also includes mucosal neuromas. All types of MEN are autosomal dominant with variable penetrance.

Those patients with thymic carcinoid in association with MEN are usually male (12 of 13 cases in a review of the literature were male).[8, 9, 20, 22–25] In contrast, Cushing's syndrome affects males and females about equally. Thymic carcinoids may be more aggressive if associated with MEN. In one literature review of thymic carcinoids associated with MEN, 14 of 17 were "malignant" (locally invasive or metastatic).[9, 20, 26]

Pathology

Carcinoids of the thymus are usually large (average diameter 11 cm)[27] (Fig. 10–1). Half of the cases are grossly encapsulated. Microscopically, most cases resemble carcinoid tumors of other sites. Growth patterns have been described as "ribbons, festoons, . . . and balls of cells" by Rosai and colleagues.[27] Organoid nests of tumor cells separated by fibrous trabeculae are characteristic. The cells are uniform in size with round to oval nuclei, inconspicuous nucleoli, and pale acidophilic cytoplasm. Mitoses are variable. Lymphocytes are sparse or absent. A morphologic variant composed of spindled cells in solid nests has been described[28] (Fig. 10–2). A thymic carcinoid containing melanin pigment has been reported,[29] as has a thymic tumor resembling medullary carcinoma of the thyroid with amyloid stroma.[27]

Some authors have advocated using a grading system for thymic carcinoids analogous to that used for lung neuroendocrine tumors.[27] Grade I corresponds to the typical bronchial carcinoid ("well differentiated"). Grade II corresponds to atypical carcinoid ("moderately differentiated"). Most thymic carcinoids would be in this category on the basis of necrosis and invasion (Fig. 10–3). Grade III would be oat cell carcinoma ("poorly differentiated"), which does occur as a primary mediastinal neoplasm.[30] Other investigators use the term neuroendocrine carcinoma for malignant thymic carcinoid.[31] Practically, whatever terminology is used must be explained to the clinician.

The histologic differential diagnosis of a thymic carcinoid includes thymic epithelial tumors (thymoma and thymic carcinoma), lymphoma, and germ cell tumor. Immunohistochemistry and electron microscopy would aid in this distinction (see Chapters 5, 6, and 9). Rarely, other neuroendocrine or endocrine tumors may need to be considered. Paraganglioma, or aortic body tumor, is located in the

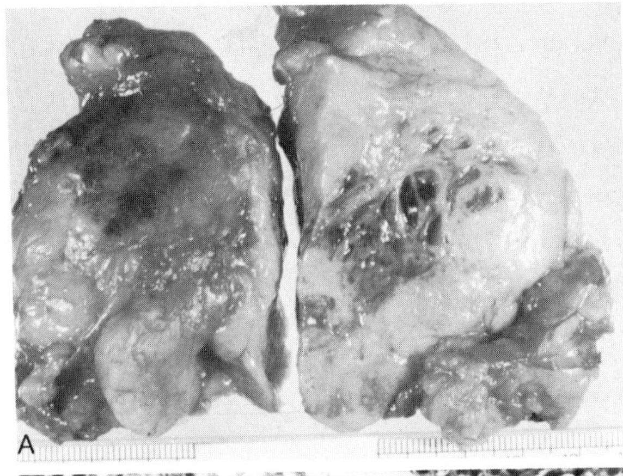

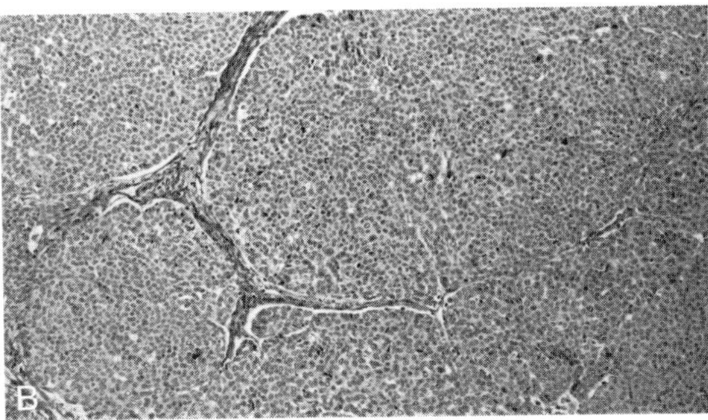

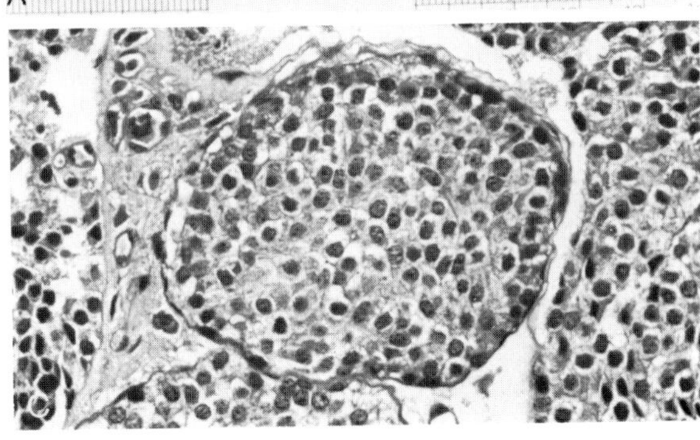

Figure 10–1. *A*, Gross photograph of a thymic carcinoid excised from a 26-year-old female with Cushing's syndrome. The tumor was grossly excised; it did not appear encapsulated. *B* and *C*, Microscopically, the tumor is composed of sheets and nests of monotonous cells with bland nuclei and clear-eosinophilic cytoplasm. The Cushing's syndrome resolved following surgery and radiation therapy. However, it recurred 6 years later. Surgical re-exploration failed to identify the recurrent tumor. Twelve years after initial diagnosis, the patient was alive with persistent Cushing's syndrome (H&E, *B*, ×100; *C*, ×400).

anterior superior mediastinum and is characterized histologically by "zellballen" formation and nuclear pleomorphism (see later). Parathyroid and thyroid neoplasms may also occur in the anterior mediastinum.[32, 33] Another possibility is a tumor metastastic from another site. For example, small-cell carcinoma usually metastasizes to the mediastinum from the lungs but rarely occurs as a primary thymic neoplasm. Prostate carcinoma may present with a metastasis to the mediastinum and may resemble a thymic carcinoid (see Chapter 7).

Histochemical stains often demonstrate cytoplasmic argyrophil granules in scattered tumor cells. Argentaffin stains are generally negative.[27]

Immunohistochemical studies reveal chromogranin (which is in the neuroendocrine granules[34]) and neuron specific enolase (NSE).[26] Herbst et al. reported only two of five thymic carcinoids positive for chromogranin (using a

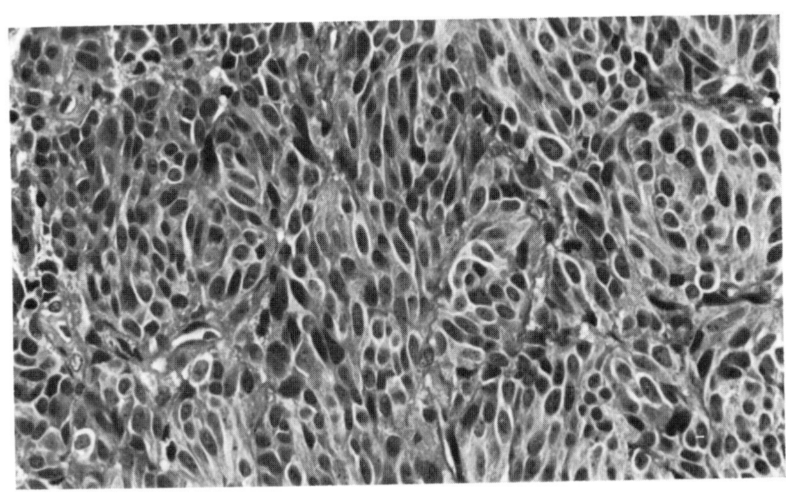

Figure 10–2. Thymic carcinoid with a focal spindled cell pattern (H&E, ×400).

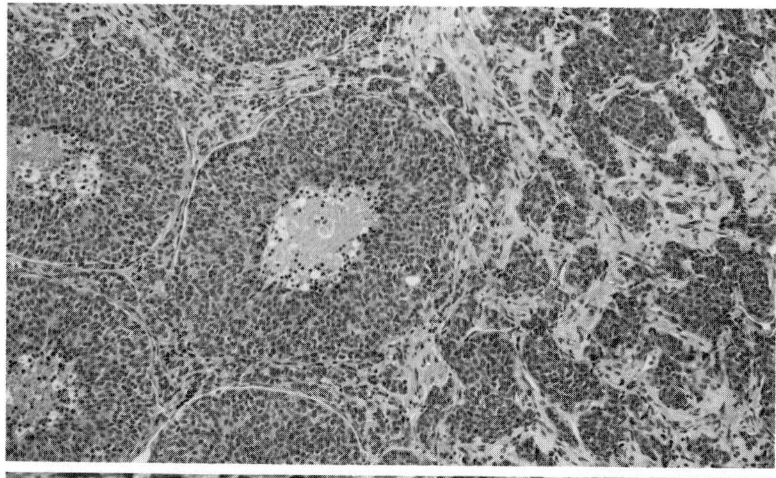

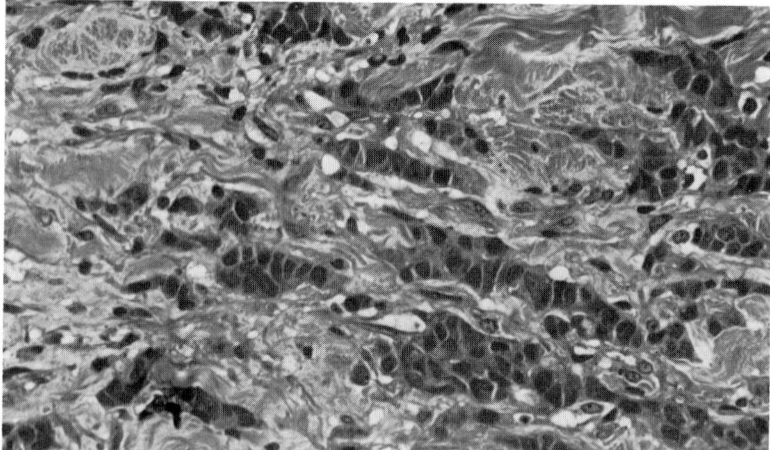

Figure 10–3. Thymic carcinoid with areas of necrosis (*top*) and with tumor cells infiltrating fibrous tissue (*bottom*) (H&E, *top*, ×100; *bottom*, ×400).

polyclonal antibody) and three of five positive for NSE.[11] However, using a monoclonal antibody (such as LK2H10), others have shown excellent correlation between the presence of neurosecretory granules and chromogranin positivity in other tumors. Seven of seven lung carcinoids were chromogranin-positive in one report.[35] Four of four lung carcinoids and two of two thymic carcinoids were chromogranin-positive in this author's experience. Also, Wick et al. reported 11 of 11 thymic carcinoids positive for NSE.[36] Thymomas may be NSE-positive, but the staining is usually focal and weak. Chromogranin is absent in thymoma.[4] Therefore, the presence of chromogranin would distinguish carcinoid from thymoma. Carcinoids are also generally positive for cytokeratin and Leu 7, but this finding would not distinguish them from thymoma.

A variety of other peptides have been identified in thymic carcinoids. As expected, those cases associated with Cushing's syndrome have ACTH. Occasionally, the tumor will contain immunoreactive ACTH in the absence of clinical Cushing's syndrome.[5, 8] The tumors react variably for calcitonin, cholecystokinin, gastrin, somatostatin, and beta-endorphin.[11, 37–39]

Ultrastructurally, dense core granules in the cytoplasm are characteristic (Fig. 10–4). The size of the granules has varied from 600 to 5000 angstroms.[2, 28, 32] Desmosomes have been described in some cases, but the broad tonofilaments and the basal lamina characteristic of thymoma are absent.[32] In a difficult case, electron microscopy may be needed for a definitive diagnosis.

Flow cytometry for DNA analysis[40] has not been of much value for carcinoids of other sites.[41–44] A single case report demonstrated a thymic carcinoid with haploid DNA content (DNA index 0.5).[5] No reported series of thymic carcinoids has studied DNA content.

New techniques using in-situ hybridization for genes or messenger ribonucleic acid

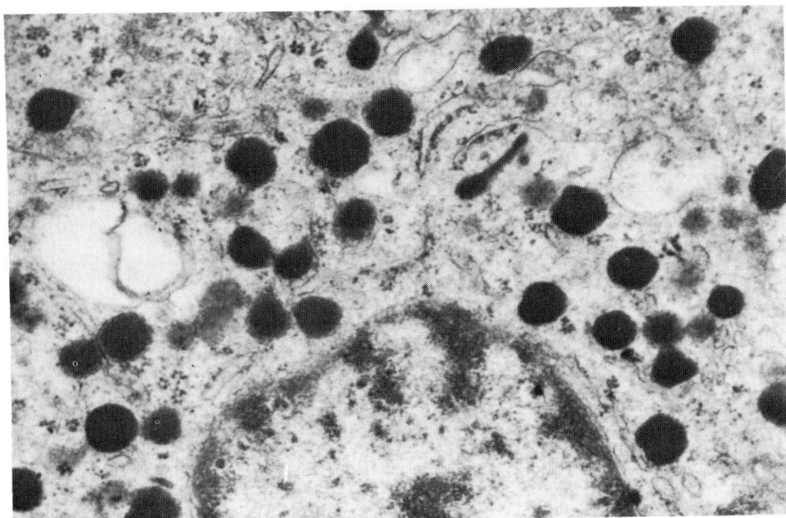

Figure 10–4. Electron micrograph of a thymic carcinoid demonstrating numerous neurosecretory granules (×5000).

(mRNA) are beginning to be applied to carcinoids.[45] The field of oncogenetics is largely unexplored in relation to these tumors.

Therapy and Prognosis

Complete excision is the treatment of choice.[10, 27] The role of radiation therapy in invasive thymic carcinoids is not established. However, these tumors do not appear to be radiosensitive.[46] Similarly, effective chemotherapy has not been found, although drugs such as streptozotocin have been used palliatively for neuroendocrine tumors. In tumors producing Cushing's syndrome, symptomatic relief may be obtained using new agents such as somatostatin analogues.[47] Interferon therapy has been used with variable response in patients with malignant carcinoids of other sites.[48] Reports of the prognosis have varied. Long-term follow-up is necessary, because metastases commonly occur many years after the initial diagnosis. Among eight patients followed for at least five years in the series by Wick and colleagues, only one was free of tumor.[8] The mean survival after the appearance of metastases was three years.

Cell of Origin

The thymus is thought to be the most likely origin for carcinoids of the mediastinum.[1, 32] The location in the anterior mediastinum adjacent to the pericardium, the finding of thymic tissue around the tumor, and the presence of argyrophil cells in the normal thymus all suggest an origin in the thymus. Other less likely origins include ectopic parathyroid, paraganglioma, and metastatic bronchial carcinoid.

Rosai and Higa found plentiful argentaffin cells in the medulla of chicken thymus.[1] In normal human thymus, argyrophilic cells were identified. More recently, calcitonin- and NSE-positive cells have been reported in the thymic medulla.[49]

The concept of a neural crest origin for all neuroendocrine cells and tumors has been challenged. Quail-chick hybrid experiments demonstrated the endodermal origin of amine precursor uptake and decarboxylation (APUD) cells of the digestive tracts.[50] Nevertheless, the neuroendocrine cells do share a common capacity to synthesize related peptides.

The relation of enterochromaffin cells (Kultschitsky's cells) to thymic epithelial cells and lymphocytes is not clear. A relation between neuroendocrine cells and the immune system ("neuroimmuno-modulation") has been postulated.[51]

PARAGANGLIOMA

Paragangliomas derive from the specialized neural crest cells known as paraganglia that are associated with autonomic ganglia.[52–54] Among 400 primary mediastinal tumors and cysts in the series by Davis and colleagues, one paraganglioma was identified.[55] The paraganglia include the adrenal medulla and the extra-adrenal system. The latter is associated with either the sympathetic or the parasympathetic system. In the mediastinum, paraganglia are located in the vicinity of the pulmonary artery and aortic arch or posteriorly along the sympathetic chain. Paraganglia are also located along the pulmonary trunks, ascending aorta, and subclavian artery. Paraganglia in the aorticopulmonary area ("aortic bodies") have a chemoreceptor function. The function of paraganglia in the other mediastinal locations is less well defined.

Historically, paragangliomas were classified by their chromaffin reactions.[53] Catecholamine-secreting tumors were considered chromaffin-positive, whereas nonfunctional tumors were chromaffin-negative. However, the chromaffin reaction is not reliable and does not always correlate with functional activity. Presently, paragangliomas are classified by their anatomic location. Functional activity is assessed clinically.

Mediastinal paragangliomas are more frequent in the anterior compartment than in the posterior compartment.[52, 56, 57] Those in the anterior mediastinum are termed aortic body tumors, whereas those in the posterior location are aorticosympathetic, or paravertebral, paragangliomas. Although the tumors are histologically indistinguishable, clinical differences between aortic body and paravertebral paragangliomas have been described (Table 10–2).

Patients may have multiple paragangliomas. About 10% of patients with aortic body tumors have paragangliomas at other sites such as the carotid body or retroperitoneum. Seven of thirty-one patients (23%) with paravertebral paragangliomas had multiple tumors (including pheochromocytomas, extra-adrenal abdominal paragangliomas, and carotid body paragangliomas).[58] Absolute distinction of second primary paragangliomas from metastases is not possible. If the second tumor is in a site where paragangliomas commonly occur, then it is assumed to be another primary tumor. Functioning extra-adrenal paragangliomas, including those of the anterior and posterior mediastinum, may occur as part of a syndrome with gastric epithelioid leiomyosarcoma and pulmonary chondroma ("Carney's triad").[57, 59]

Table 10–2. Mediastinal Paragangliomas: Clinical Features

Feature and References	Aortic Body	Paravertebral
Average age, years[56, 58]	46	29
Male-to-female ratio[56, 58]	17:24	20:11
Clinically functional[58]	Rare	48%
Completely excised[56, 58, 60]	39–52%	58–93%
Multiple tumors[58]	10%	23%
Metastases (bone, lung, and lymph node are most common sites)[56, 58, 60]	11–18%	7–8%

Aortic Body Paraganglioma

Approximately half of aortic body tumors occur in asymptomatic individuals.[56, 60] When present, the symptoms (cough, hoarseness, dysphagia, chest pain) relate to the location of the tumor. Most patients are over 40 years of age (range 5 to 79 years with an average of 46 years). A slight female predominance has been noted.[56, 60]

Grossly, the tumor appears as a lobulated mass in the superior mediastinum closely related to the aortic arch and base of the heart. Sizes have ranged from two to twelve cm in greatest dimension. The close relationship with major vessels often precludes complete resection.

Microscopically, the tumor consists of cells arranged in nests ("zellballen") with a vascular stroma[53, 54] (Fig. 10–5). The elaborate vascular network surrounds the nests of cells. The cells have central nuclei and abundant granular cytoplasm. Most cases have two cell populations: round cells with clear cytoplasm are admixed with larger cells with eosinophilic cytoplasm. Occasional nuclei are large and hyperchromatic. Multinucleated cells may be present. Mitotic figures are rare or absent. In some tumors, a spindle cell morphology has been noted.[61] Trabecular or pseudoglandular patterns may resemble a carcinoid.

Although approximately 10% of patients develop metastases, no histologic features have clearly distinguished benign from malignant behavior. Even without metastases, the course of aortic body tumors may be aggressive. Of 41 patients reviewed by Olson and Salyer, eight had died of tumor (four with metastases), and eight others had unresectable disease.[56]

Paravertebral Paraganglioma

Gallivan and colleagues reviewed the literature on intrathoracic paravertebral paraganglioma in 1980.[58] Posterior mediastinal paragangliomas tend to occur in younger

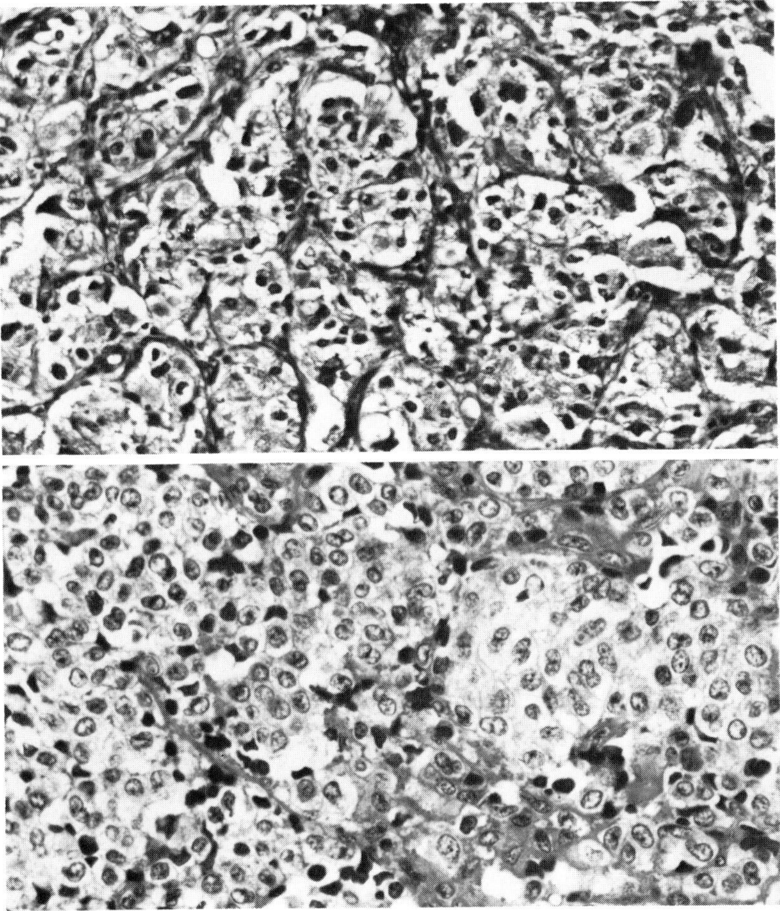

Figure 10–5. *Top,* Aortic body paraganglioma demonstrating prominent nesting ("zellballen") pattern (H&E, ×200). *Bottom,* Compared with a carcinoid, the cells have more nuclear pleomorphism and more prominent nucleoli. Cytoplasm is clear or eosinophilic (H&E, ×400).

individuals (average 29 years of age) and have a male predominance. They are located in the costovertebral sulcus, most frequently in the midthoracic region. They have also been referred to as chemodectomas and pheochromocytomas. About half of patients have symptoms or signs related to catecholamine secretion by the tumor, including headache, sweating, tachycardia, palpitations, chest pain, dyspnea, nausea, and hypertension.[52, 58] Histologically, paravertebral paragangliomas are indistinguishable from those in the anterior mediastinum.

In the Gallivan et al. review, the tumor was completely resected in 25 of the 31 patients. Five tumors were locally invasive, and two patients developed metastatic disease.[58] In a review of the literature on posterior mediastinal paraganglioma in 1990, Odze and Begin concluded that local invasion and metastases are the most significant determinants of aggressive behavior.[62] All seven patients with documented metastases had evidence of local invasion. In contrast, only five of 41 patients without metastases had locally invasive tumors.

Histochemistry

Histochemical stains can be useful in the diagnosis of mediastinal paraganglioma.[52, 53] The reticulin stain highlights the nested pattern of growth. The modified Grimelius stain demonstrates the argyrophilic neurosecretory granules. The tumors do not react with the periodic acid–Schiff reagent.

Immunoperoxidase Stains and Other Adjunctive Studies

In an immunoperoxidase study of mediastinal paragangliomas by Moran and colleagues, chromogranin was strongly positive and cytokeratin was absent in all 10 cases studied.[61] Paragangliomas usually stain for neuron specific enolase (NSE), a relatively nonspecific neuroendocrine marker.[54] These tumors also usually have synaptophysin, a more specific marker of neuroendocrine differentiation. Immunoreactivity for vimentin, ACTH, glucagon, somatostatin, and calcitonin has been described.[63]

S100-positive sustentacular cells were present in 9 of the 10 cases in the Moran et al. study.[61] Sustentacular cells also react for glial fibrillary acid protein.[54] Those paragangliomas that are more clinically aggressive tend to have fewer sustentacular cells.[64] However, too few mediastinal paragangliomas have been studied to assess the significance of sustentacular cells as a prognostic factor.

Similarly, the data on DNA flow cytometry are limited.[57, 65, 66] In a study by Herrera and colleagues, seven mediastinal paraglangliomas were diploid, two were aneuploid, and one was teraploid. All three nondiploid tumors were clinically aggressive. Among the seven diploid tumors, three were malignant.

Ultrastructurally, these tumors have numerous neurosecretory granules.[53, 54, 56, 58] The diameter of the granules varies from 400 to 4000 angstroms. The cells may have intercellular junctions but lack tonofilaments.

Differential Diagnosis

Thymic carcinoid must be considered in the differential diagnosis of paragangliomas in the anterior mediastinum. Both tumors may have similar histologic features and have chromogranin. The tumor cells in a carcinoid appear more uniform in size. The cells tend to be polarized, with the nuclei located nearer the vessels. The diagnosis of paraganglioma is favored by a predominant nesting pattern, nuclear pleomorphism, and the absence of festoons or rosettes.[1, 52] Cytokeratin is found in carcinoid but generally is absent in paraganglioma. Also, the S100-positive sustentacular cells of most (but not all) paragangliomas are absent in carcinoid.[26] Hemangiopericytomas can have spindled cells in concentric arrangements that mimic a paraganglioma. Medullary carcinoma of the thyroid is another consideration. In the posterior mediastinum, paragangliomas should be differentiated from metastatic lesions, including melanoma, renal cell carcinoma, and alveolar soft part sarcoma. The chromogranin positivity typical of paraganglioma along with the other immunoperoxidase stains should help in this differentiation.

Paraganglioma in Animals

The canine aortic body (''heart base'') tumor is a paraganglioma that is predominantly found in Boxer dogs and Boston terriers.[52, 67] Although usually benign, the tumor may invade the atria, pericardium, and adjacent vessels. It appears histologically similar to the paraganglioma in humans.

SUMMARY

Neuroendocrine tumors of the mediastinum include thymic carcinoid and paraganglioma. Thymic carcinoids appear histologically similar to carcinoids of other sites. A few patients with these tumors present with endocrine symptoms, usually Cushing's syndrome. Some are associated with the multiple endocrine neoplasia (MEN) syndrome. Most thymic carcinoids are locally invasive and frequently produce metastases. Immunohistochemistry may help in distinguishing this tumor from thymic epithelial cell tumors. In particular, immunoperoxidase staining demonstrates chromogranin in carcinoid, but not in thymoma.

Mediastinal paragangliomas occur anteriorly in the area of the aortic body or posteriorly along the sympathetic chain. Histologically, these tumors have the characteristic ''zellballen'' pattern of nested cells in a vascular stroma. Immunohistochemistry demonstrates chromogranin within the tumor cells. Approximately 10% of patients with mediastinal paragangliomas develop metastatic disease.

REFERENCES

1. Rosai J, Higa E. Mediastinal endocrine neoplasm, of probable thymic origin, related to carcinoid tumor. Clinicopathologic study of 8 cases. Cancer 1972; 29:1061–1074.
2. Kay S, Willson MA. Ultrastructural studies of an ACTH-secreting thymic tumor. Cancer 1970; 26:445–452.
3. Salyer WR, Salyer DC, Eggleston JE. Carcinoid tumors of the thymus. Cancer 1976; 37:958–873.
4. Kornstein MJ, Curran WJ Jr, Turrisi AT III, Brooks JJ. Cortical versus medullary thymomas: a useful morphologic distinction? Hum Pathol 1988; 19:1335–1339.
5. Viebahn R, Hiddemann W, Klinke F, Bassewitz DB. Thymus carcinoid. Pathol Res Pract 1985; 180:445–448.
6. Otto HF. Letters to the case: thymus carcinoid. Pathol Res Pract 1985; 180:445–448.
7. Kogan J. Carcinoid tumor of the thymus. Postgrad Med J 1984; 75:291–296.
8. Wick MR, Carney JA, Bernatz PE, Brown LR. Primary

mediastinal carcinoid tumors. Am J Surg Pathol 1982; 6:195–205.
9. Rosai J, Higa E, Davie J. Mediastinal endocrine neoplasia in patients with multiple endocrine adenomatosis. A previously unrecognized association. Cancer 1972; 29:1075–1083.
10. Economopoulos GC, Lewis JW Jr, Lee MW, Silverman NA. Carcinoid tumors of the thymus. Ann Thorac Surg 1990; 50:58–61.
11. Herbst WM, Kummer W, Hofmann W, Otto H, Heym C. Carcinoid tumors of the thymus. An immunohistochemical study. Cancer 1987; 60:2465–2470.
12. Muller-Hermelink HK, Marino M, Palestro G. Pathology of thymic epithelial tumors. *In* Muller-Hermelink HK, ed. Current Topics in Pathology: The Human Thymus. Berlin: Springer-Verlag, 1986:208–268.
13. Doppman JL, Pass HI, Nieman LK, Miller DL, Chang R, Cutler GB Jr, Chrousos GP, Jaffe GS, Norton JA. Corticotropin-secreting carcinoid tumors of the thymus: diagnostic unreliability of thymic venous sampling. Radiology 1992; 184:71–74.
14. Felson B, Castleman B, Levinsohn EM, Markarian B. Radiologic-Pathologic Correlation Conference: SUNY Upstate Medical Center. Cushing syndrome associated with mediastinal mass. AJR 1982; 138:815–819.
15. Venkatesh S, Samaan NA. Carcinoid tumors of the thymus. West J Med 1990; 152:72–74.
16. Pass HI. Management of the ectopic ACTH syndrome due to thoracic carcinoids. Ann Thorac Surg 1990; 50:52–57.
17. Gartner LA, Voorhess ML. Adrenocorticotropic hormone-producing thymic carcinoid in a teenager. Cancer 1993; 71:106–111.
18. Thorner MO, Martin WH, Ragan GE, MacLeod RM, Feldman PS, Bruni C, Williamson BR, Orth DN. A case of ectopic ACTH syndrome: diagnostic difficulties caused by intermittent hormone secretion. Acta Endocrinol (Copenh) 1982; 99:364–370.
19. Pass HI, Doppman JL, Nieman L, Stovroff M, Vetto J, Norton JA, Travis W, Chrousos GP, Oldfield EH, Cutler GB Jr. Management of the ectopic ACTH syndrome due to thoracic carcinoids. Ann Thorac Surg 1990; 50:52–57.
20. Duh QY, Hybarger CP, Geist R, Gamsu G, Goodman PC, Gooding GA, Clark OH. Carcinoids associated with multiple endocrine neoplasia syndromes. Am J Surg 1987; 154:142–148.
21. Marchevsky AM, Dikman SH. Mediastinal carcinoid with an incomplete Sipple's syndrome. Cancer 1979; 43:2497–2501.
22. Birnberg FA, Webb WR, Selch MT, Gamsu G, Goodman PC. Thymic carcinoid tumors with hyperparathyroidism. AJR 1982; 139:1001–1004.
23. Vener JD, Zuckerbraun L, Goodman D. Carcinoid tumor of the thymus associated with a parathyroid adenoma. Arch Otolaryngol 1982; 108:324–326.
24. Lokich JJ, Li F. Carcinoid of the thymus with hereditary hyperparathyroidism. Ann Intern Med 1978; 89:364–365.
25. Manes JL, Taylor HB. Thymic carcinoid in familial multiple endocrine adenomatosis. Arch Pathol 1973; 95:252–255.
26. Wick MR, Rosai J. Neuroendocrine neoplasms of the thymus. Pathol Res Pract 1988; 183:188–199.
27. Rosai J, Levine G, Weber WR, Higa E. Carcinoid tumors and oat cell carcinomas of the thymus. Pathol Annu 1976; 11:201–226.
28. Levine GD, Rosai J. A spindle cell varient of thymic carcinoid tumor. A clinical, histologic, and fine structural study with emphasis on its distinction from spindle cell thymoma. Arch Pathol Lab Med 1976; 100:293–300.
29. Ho FC, Ho JC. Pigmented carcinoid tumour of the thymus. Histopathology 1977; 1:363–369.
30. Wick MR, Scheithauer BW. Oat-cell carcinoma of the thymus. Cancer 1982; 49:1652–1657.
31. Lagrange W, Dahm HH, Karstens J, Feichtinger J, Mittermayer C. Melanocytic neuroendocrine carcinoma of the thymus. Cancer 1987; 59:484–488.
32. Rosai J, Levine GD. Tumors of the Thymus. Washington, DC: Armed Forces Institute of Pathology, 1976:34–98.
33. Murphy MN, Glennon PG, Diocee MS, Wick MR, Cavers DJ. Nonsecretory parathyroid carcinoma of the mediastinum: light microcopic, immunocytochemical and ultrastructural features of a case, and review of the literature. Cancer 1986; 58:2468–2476.
34. Angeletti RH. Chromogranins and neuroendocrine secretion [editorial]. Lab Invest 1986; 55:387–390.
35. Said JW, Vimadalal S, Nash G, Shintaku IP, Heusser BA, Sassoon AF, Lloyd RV. Immunoreactive neuron-specific enolase, bombesin, and chromogranin as markers for neuroendocrine lung tumors. Hum Pathol 1985; 16:236–240.
36. Wick MR, Scheithauer BW, Kovacs K. Neuron-specific enolase in neuroendocrine tumors of the thymus, bronchus, and skin. Am J Clin Pathol 1983; 79:703–707.
37. Pullan PT, Clement-Jones V, Corder R, Lowry PJ, Rees GM, Rees LH, Besser GM, Macedo MM, Galvao-Teles A. Ectopic production of methionine enkephalin and beta-endorphin. Br Med J 1980; 280:758–759.
38. Wick MR, Scheithauer BW. Thymic carcinoid. A histologic, immunohistochemical, and ultrastructural study of 12 cases. Cancer 1984; 53:475–484.
39. DeLellis RA, Wolfe HJ. Calcitonin in spindle cell thymic carcinoid tumors [letter]. Arch Pathol Lab Med 1976; 100:340.
40. Coon JS, Landay AL, Weinstein RS. Advances in flow cytometry for diagnostic pathology. Lab Invest 1987; 57:453–479.
41. Tsushima K, Nagorney DM, Weiland LH, Lieber MM. The relationship of flow cytometric DNA analysis and clinicopathology in small-intestinal carcinoids. Surgery 1989; 105:366–373.
42. Thunnissen FB, Van Eijk J, Baak JP, Schipper NW, Uyterlinde AM, Breederveld RS, Meijer S. Bronchopulmonary carcinoids and regional lymph node metastases. A quantitative pathologic investigation. Am J Pathol 1988; 132:119–122.
43. Kujari H, Joensuu H, Klemi P, Asola R, Nordman E. A flow cytometric analysis of 23 carcinoid tumors. Cancer 1988; 61:2517–2520.
44. Wilander E, Bjelkenkrantz K, Risberg B. Nuclear DNA recordings in gastric carcinoids. A cytofluorometric study on single tumour cells. Pathol Res Pract 1987; 182:331–335.
45. Tomita N, Horii A, Doi S, Yokouchi H, Shiosaki K, Higashiyama M, Matsuura N, Ogawa M, Mori T, Matsubara K. A novel type of human alpha-amylase produced in lung carcinoid tumor. Gene 1989; 76:11–18.
46. Lowenthal RM, Gumpel JM, Kreel L, McLaughlin JE, Skeggs DB. Carcinoid tumour of the thymus with systemic manifestations: a radiological and pathological study. Thorax 1974; 29:553–558.
47. Hearn PR, Reynolds CL, Johansen K, Woodhouse NJ. Lung carcinoid with Cushing's syndrome: control of serum ACTH and cortisol levels using SMS 201–995 (sandostatin). Clin Endocrinol (Oxf) 1988; 28:181–185.

48. Dorval T, Pouillart P. Interferons in the treatment of solid tumors. A general review. Bull Cancer (Paris) 1988; 75:885–888.
49. Muller-Hermelink HK, Marino M, Palestro G. Pathology of thymic epithelial tumors. *In* Muller-Hermelink HK, ed. The Human Thymus: Histophysiology and Pathology. Berlin: Springer-Verlag, 1986:207–268.
50. Sidhu GS. The endodermal origin of digestive and respiratory tract APUD cells. Am J Pathol 1979; 96:5–20.
51. Angeletti RH, Hickey WF. A neuroendocrine marker in tissues of the immune system. Science 1985; 230:89–90.
52. Glenner GG, Grimley PM. Atlas of Tumor Pathology, Second Series, Fascicle 9, Tumors of the Extra-Adrenal Paraganglion System (including Chemoreceptors). Washington, DC: Armed Forces Institute of Pathology, 1974.
53. Enzinger FM, Weiss SW. Paraganglioma. *In* Soft Tissue Tumors. St. Louis: CV Mosby, 1988:836–860.
54. Kliewer KE, Cochran AJ. A review of the histology, ultrastructure, immunohistology, and molecular biology of extra-adrenal paragangliomas. Arch Pathol Lab Med 1989; 113:1209–1218.
55. Davis RD Jr, Oldham HN Jr, Sabiston DC Jr. Primary cysts and neoplasms of the mediastinum: recent changes in clinical presentation, methods of diagnosis, management, and results. Ann Thorac Surg 1987; 44:229–237.
56. Olson JL, Salyer WR. Mediastinal paragangliomas (aortic body tumor): a report of four cases and a review of the literature. Cancer 1978; 41:2405–2412.
57. Herrera MF, van Heerden JA, Puga FJ, Hogan MJ, Carney JA. Mediastinal paraganglioma: a surgical experience. Ann Thorac Surg 1993; 56:1096–1100.
58. Gallivan MVE, Chun B, Rowden G, Lack EE. Intrathoracic paravertebral malignant paraganglioma. Arch Pathol Lab Med 1980; 104:46–51.
59. Carney JA. The triad of gastric epithelioid leiomyosarcoma, functioning extra-adrenal paraganglioma, and pulmonary chondroma. Cancer 1979; 43:374–382.
60. Lack EE, Stillinger RA, Colvin DB, Groves RM, Burnette DB. Aortico-pulmonary paraganglioma: report of a case with ultrastructural study and review of the literature. Cancer 1979; 43:269–278.
61. Moran CA, Suster S, Fishback N, Koss MN. Mediastinal paragangliomas: a clinicopathologic and immunohistochemical study of 16 cases. Cancer 1993; 72:2358–2364.
62. Odze R, Begin LR. Malignant paraganglioma of the posterior mediastinum: a case report and review of the literature. Cancer 1990; 65:564–569.
63. Assaf HM, Al-Momen AA, Martin JG. Aorticopulmonary paraganglioma: a case report with immunohistochemical studies and literature review. Arch Pathol Lab Med 1992; 116:1085–1087.
64. Kliewer KE, Wen D-R, Cancilla PA, Cochran AJ. Paragangliomas: assessment of prognosis by histologic, immunohistochemical, and ultrastructural techniques. Hum Pathol 1989; 20:29–39.
65. Granger JK, Houn HY. Head and neck paragangliomas: a clinicopathologic study with DNA flow cytometric analysis. South Med J 1990; 83:1407–1412.
66. Nativ O, Grant CS, Sheps SG, O'Fallon JR, Farrow GM, van Heerden JA, Lieber MM. The clinical significance of nuclear DNA ploidy pattern in 184 patients with pheochromocytoma. Cancer 1992; 69:2683–2687.
67. Moore AS. Chemotherapy for intrathoracic cancer in dogs and cats. Probl Vet Med 1992; 4:351–364.

Chapter

11

TUMORS OF NEURAL ORIGIN

PERIPHERAL NERVE SHEATH TUMORS
TUMORS OF THE SYMPATHETIC GANGLIA
PERIPHERAL PRIMITIVE NEUROECTODERMAL TUMOR OF THORACOPULMONARY REGION ("ASKIN TUMOR")
SUMMARY

Neurogenic lesions account for about 20% of mediastinal tumors.[1, 2] They are usually located in the posterior mediastinum, particularly in the paravertebral area. Rarely, anterior and middle mediastinal locations have been described. Neural lesions include peripheral nerve sheath tumors (neurofibroma, schwannoma, malignant schwannoma), ganglioneuroma, ganglioneuroblastoma, and neuroblastoma. Peripheral primitive neuroectodermal tumors can also be considered in this category.

PERIPHERAL NERVE SHEATH TUMORS

The benign nerve sheath tumors include neurofibroma and neurilemoma. The latter is also termed schwannoma. These lesions usually affect young and middle-aged adults. They are typically found on routine chest radiographs in asymptomatic individuals. Most mediastinal tumors are paravertebral. Some extend into the intraspinal canal as "dumbbell" tumors.[3] Multiple peripheral nerve sheath tumors (usually neurofibromas) are associated with von Recklinghausen's disease, or neurofibromatosis. Ten percent of tumors in patients with von Recklinghausen's disease show evidence of malignancy.[1]

Neurofibromas consist of interlacing bundles of spindled cells with wavy nuclei[4–6] (Fig. 11–1). The cells are within a collagenous and mucoid stroma. "Wire-like" collagen fibrils are admixed with the Schwann cells. The neurofibroma generally lacks the encapsulation of a neurilemoma and lacks the separation into Antoni A and B areas. Neurofibromas may create a fusiform expansion within a major nerve. The nerve may be identified entering and exiting the tumor. The plexiform neurofibroma occurs in von Recklinghausen's disease. This tumor consists of a diffuse expansion of the nerve branches. The nerve fibers become replaced by Shwann cells and thick collagen. S100 may be present in neurofibromas, although less frequently than it is in neurilemomas.

Benign schwannoma is an encapsulated tumor with two components.[4, 5] One component (Antoni A) is an orderly, cellular area composed of compact spindled cells with twisted nuclei, indistinct cytoplasmic borders, and occasional intranuclear vacuoles. Nuclear palisading may be identified (Fig. 11–2). Verocay bodies are formed by two rows of cells with palisaded nuclei. The other element (Antoni B) is loose and myxoid. The spindled cells are arranged haphazardly. Thick-walled vessels are often present (Fig. 11–3). Degenerative changes include cystic areas, calicification, hemorrhage, and hyalinization. Tumors with extensive degenerative features have been termed ancient schwannomas. The nuclei in the ancient schwannoma may be large, hyperchromatic, and multilobed but do not have

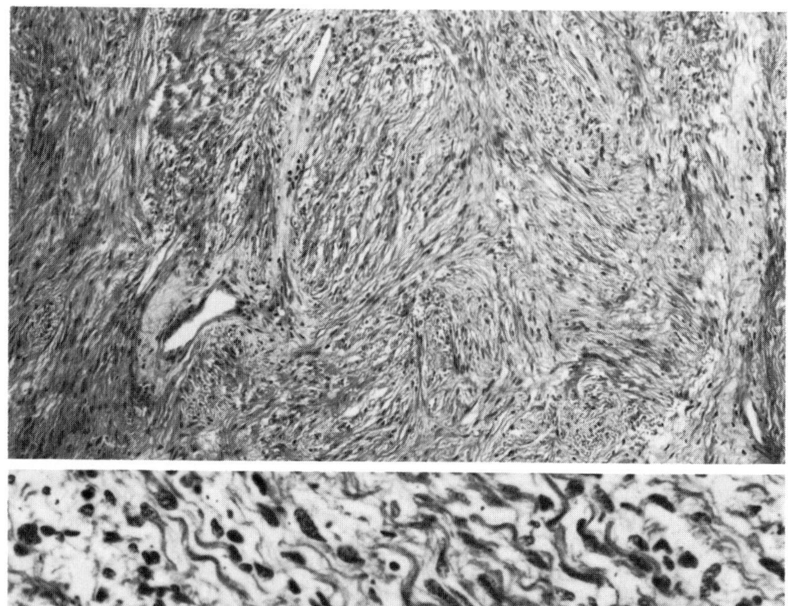

Figure 11–1. *Top,* Neurofibroma is characterized by interlacing bundles of spindled cells in a collagenous stroma (H&E, ×100). *Bottom,* "Wavy" nuclei (Bodian stain, H&E, ×400).

mitotic figures. Most neurilemomas are strongly positive for S100. Electron microscopy demonstrates the features of Schwann cells (i.e., long cytoplasmic processes with continuous basal lamina).

Most mediastinal peripheral nerve sheath tumors are classified as neurilemonas.[1] However, many have features of both neurilemoma and neurofibroma.[5] For example, in a series of 48 neurogenic tumors of the thoracic cavity, Ackerman and Taylor described seven neurofibromas involving the posterior mediastinum.[5] Although all were encapsulated, they had the "tangled" microscopic appearance characteristic of a neurofibroma.

Cellular schwannomas have a predominance of the fascicular spindle cell element.[7–9] A fibrosarcoma-like, "herring-bone" growth pattern has been described. The spindle cells are slender and "wavy." These lesions do not have nuclear palisading or Verocay bodies. They have low mitotic activity (0 to 4 mitoses per 20 high-power fields) and may have moderate pleomorphism. The latter is considered a degenerative phenomenon. Necrosis is not present. By immunohistochemistry, nearly all cellular schwannomas show staining for S-100 and vimentin. Variable staining for glial fibrillary acidic protein is also described. Ultrastructurally, the tumors have long, interdigitating cytoplasmic projections outlined by external lamina.

Cellular schwannomas have a predilection for the paravertebral area of the mediastinum and retroperitoneum. The tumor affects patients in a broad age range (15 to 79 years), with a median of 55 years. Some investigators report a female predominance.[7] Few patients have neurofibromatosis.[7, 9] Clinicopathologic studies have demonstrated the tumor to be benign. These lesions do not metastasize and rarely recur.[8] However, many cases have limited follow-up, and some authors have suggested that cellular schwannomas be regarded as atypical or borderline tumors of uncertain malignant potential.[10]

Melanotic schwannomas contain melanin pigment within melanosomes.[6, 11, 12] These le-

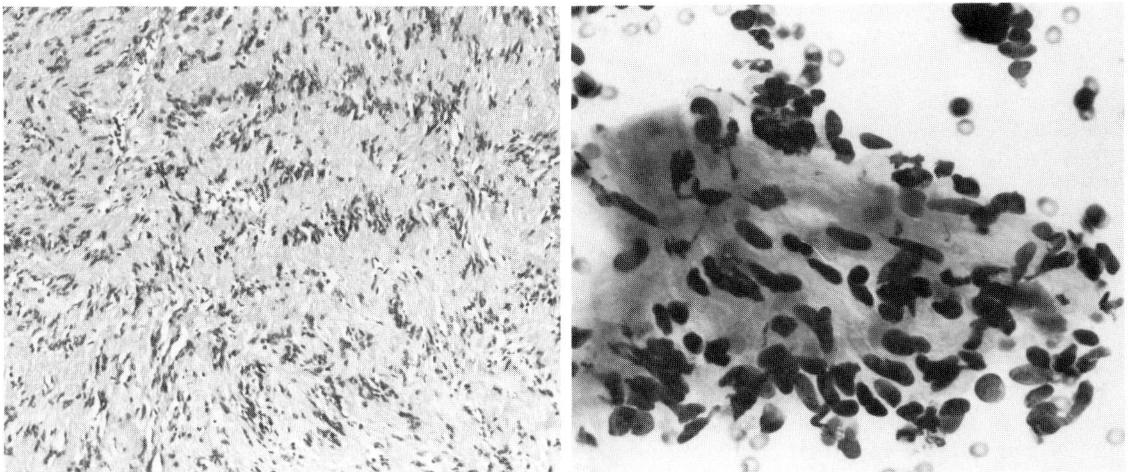

Figure 11–2. Neurilemoma has orderly cellular areas (*left*) with prominent nuclear palisading (H&E, ×100). *Right,* a cluster of cells with elongated nuclei demonstrates the cytologic appearance of a schwannoma (Diff-Quik ×400).

sions may express the melanoma-associated marker, HMB-45. Psammomatous calicification has been described within melanotic schwannomas.[12] These tumors may affect the intramediastinal spinal roots. Carney has described a familial disorder characterized by psammomatous melanotic schwannoma, myxomas, spotty pigmentation, and endocrine overactivity.[12]

Malignant schwannoma is the malignant counterpart of benign schwannoma and neurofibroma.[13] It is uncommon in the mediastinum.[1, 2] Other terms for this entity include neurogenic sarcoma and neurofibrosarcoma. The typical microscopic appearance has long fascicles of spindled cells. Nuclei are twisted or "comma-shaped." These tumors may be difficult to distinguish from other sarcomas. S-100 is present in 50 to 90% of malignant schwannomas. The distinction between a benign and malignant nerve sheath tumor may be difficult to determine.[10] According to Enzinger and Weiss, the major criterion for malignancy in a neurofibroma is the presence of mitotic activity.[13] However, mitotic activity is not useful in separating a benign schwannoma from a malignant one. Benign schwannomas rarely undergo malignant degeneration. Identification of its characteristic features (i.e., Antoni A and B patterns, perivascular hyalinization, and encapsulation) is necessary for proper diagnosis.

Occasionally, malignant schwannomas have evidence of divergent differentiation. Such tumors contain foci of other sarcomatous elements, including rhabdomyosarcoma, osteosarcoma, chondrosarcoma, and angiosarcoma.[14] A neoplasm consisting of rhabdomyo-

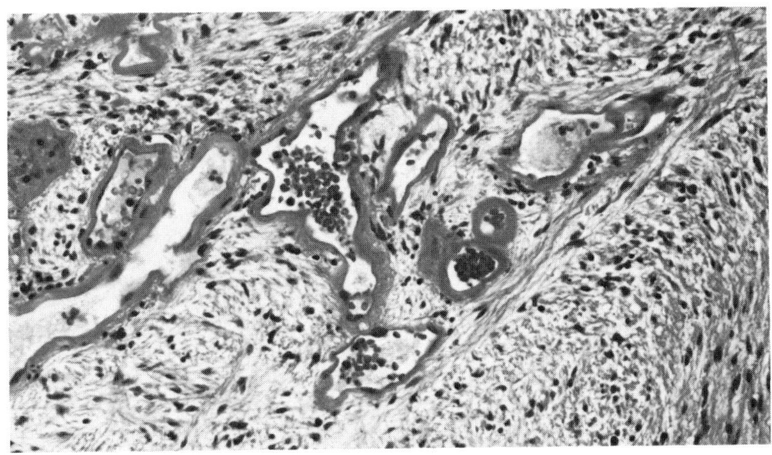

Figure 11–3. Thick-walled vessels are often prominent in a schwannoma, as illustrated in this photograph (H&E, ×200).

sarcoma within a malignant shwannoma has been termed Triton tumor. Epithelial differentiation, including malignant glandular and squamous elements, has also been described.[13, 15] Rarely, malignant schwannomas with divergent differentiation have occurred in the mediastinum, usually in patients with von Recklinghausen's disease.[14–16]

TUMORS OF THE SYMPATHETIC GANGLIA

Neuroblastomas, ganglioneuroblastomas, and ganglioneuromas arise from the sympathetic ganglia and adrenal medulla. Neuroblastomas usually occur in children less than 2 years of age.[17, 18] It is the most common solid, extracranial malignancy in pediatric patients and accounts for approximately 10% of pediatric malignancies. Catecholamines and metabolities are elevated in the urine in over 90% of patients.

Most neuroblastomas are intra-abdominal (adrenal medulla and extra-adrenal retroperitoneum). Their location generally follows that of the sympathetic ganglia, adrenal medulla, and organ of Zuckerkandl. Fourteen percent occur in the thorax, usually in the paraspinal area.[19] They may extend into the spinal column through an intervertebral foramen in an "hourglass" configuration. The tumors may involve the ribs, but invasion of the lungs is uncommon.[20] Neuroblastoma is the most common tumor of the posterior mediastinum in pediatric patients.[21] In adults, however, the tumor is uncommon. Rare cases of adult neuroblastoma have occurred in the posterior mediastinum.[22]

Grossly, the tumors appear well-circumscribed with a smooth or nodular surface. Some have a thickened capsule. The cut section is friable and hemorrhagic. Cystic areas represent necrosis. Calcification is common.

Microscopically, neuroblastoma is a small, round, blue cell tumor[17, 18, 20, 23] (Fig. 11–4). The tumor cells are arranged in sheets or nests. The latter are separated by fibrovascular septa. The cells are uniform in size with round, hyperchromatic nuclei. An eosinophilic, finely fibrillar background is an important clue to the diagnosis of neuroblastoma. Another clue is the presence of Homer-Wright rosettes, which are neuroblasts arranged around a central fibrillary area. Maturing neuroblasts resemble ganglion cells. These are larger cells with a vesicular nucleus, a prominent central nucleolus, and more abundant cytoplasm. Maturing tumors also have a Schwannian spindle cell element.[24] Most neuroblastomas are glycogen-negative using the periodic acid–Schiff reaction.

The classification scheme of Shimada and colleagues based on histologic evidence of differentiation, the mitotic/karyorrhectic index, and age has been useful for prognostication.[24, 25] The favorable prognosis group has a long-term survival rate of over 90%, whereas the unfavorable prognostic group has a 36% survival rate.[23] The thoracic neuroblastomas tend to have a better prognosis than those of other sites.[18, 21, 26]

Ganglioneuroblastoma and ganglioneuroma are designations for tumors with evidence of maturation. Ganglioneuromas are composed only of mature ganglion cells, Schwann cells with neurites, and fibrous tissue. These tumors do not metastasize. Ganglioneuroblastomas represent an intermediate stage of differentiation. They contain both neuroblasts and ganglion cells, but their exact definition varies among authors[23, 25, 27] (Fig. 11–5). Nodular (composite) ganglioneuroblastomas have grossly evident nodules of a neuroblastoma within a ganglioneuroma. The diffuse ("imperfect") ganglioneuroblastoma has a more homogeneous mixture of neuroblasts at different stages of differentiation. The latter has also been termed differentiating neuroblastoma.

Adam and Hochholzer of the Armed Forces Institute of Pathology identified 252 patients with tumors of the sympathetic ganglia arising in the posterior mediastinum.[27] Of the 252 cases, there were 65 neuroblastomas (26%), 107 ganglioneuromas (42%), and 80 ganglioneuroblastomas (32%). The patients with ganglioneuroblastomas were similar in age to patients with neuroblastomas. Most of the ganglioneuroblastomas were grossly encapsulated. Weights varied from 20 to 420 g (mean 126 g). The nodular ganglioneuroblastomas are pale and firm but contain soft hemorragic foci corresponding to the neuroblastomatous areas.

The prognosis of ganglioneuroblastoma is better than that of neuroblastoma, with a 5-year overall survival rate of up to 88%. The stage of disease at diagnosis is a major prognostic factor. The nodular subtype behaves more aggressively. Six of the eight nodular tumors metastasized, versus only 3 of 70 diffuse types.[27] The significance of the nodular versus diffuse categorization emphasizes the importance of careful gross inspection of the tumor and thorough sampling.

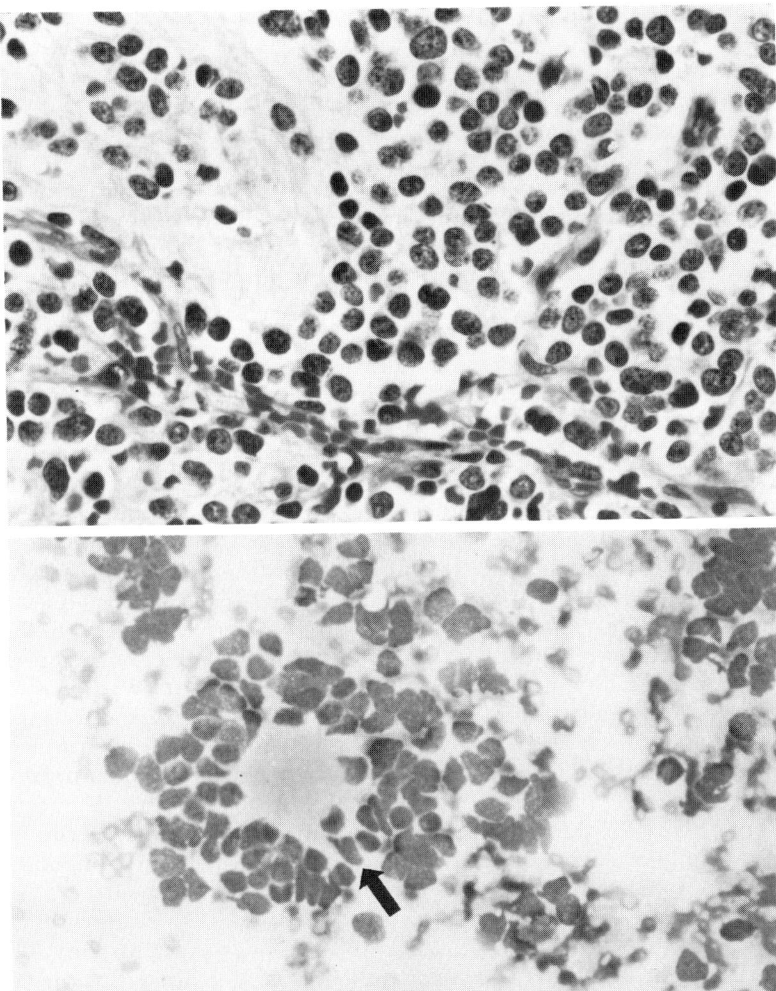

Figure 11–4. *Top,* The histologic appearance of a neuroblastoma. This is a tumor of small, round cells. The fibrillar background is a clue to the diagnosis. (H&E, ×400) *Bottom,* The cytologic appearance of a neuroblastoma in a fine-needle aspirate. Fibrillar material is present within a rosette-like structure (*arrow*). (Diff-Quik, ×400)

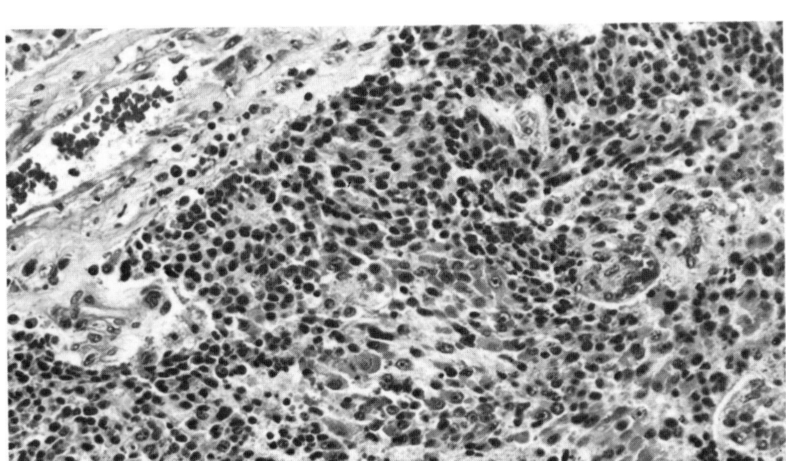

Figure 11–5. A diffuse ganglioneuroblastoma, or differentiating neuroblastoma. Ganglion cells (larger cells with prominent nucleoli) are interspersed among the neuroblasts (H&E, ×200).

Ganglioneuromas are less common than other benign neural tumors.[23] Most are diagnosed in patients older than 10 years. The posterior mediastinum is the most common location. Most are asymptomatic. An association with chronic diarrhea has been related to the presence of vasoactive intestinal peptide within the tumor. Grossly, the tumors appear circumscribed with a fibrous capsule (Fig. 11–6). They have a whorled pattern on cut section similar to that of a leiomyoma. Histologically, ganglion cells are scattered on a background of Schwann cells. The ganglion cells have abundant cytoplasm and one to three nuclei. Pigment related to oxidation of catecholamine products may be present within the ganglion cells. The tumors do not metastasize.

Immunoperoxidase studies demonstrate neuron specific enolase on neuroectodermal tumors regardless of the extent of differentiation.[28] However, neuron specific enolase is nonspecific, because it also stains many other types of tumors. Neurofilaments can be demonstrated in ganglioneuroblastomas and ganglioneuromas more frequently than in neuroblastomas. Similarly, other markers, including chromogranin and synaptophysin, label the more differentiated-appearing cells. S100 stains Schwann cells in ganglioneuroblastomas and ganglioneuromas. Ultrastructurally, neuroblastomas are characterized by neuritic processes containing dense core neurosecretory granules.

The neuroblastoma has been one of the better studied tumors from the molecular biology standpoint.[28] Amplification of the N-myc oncogene has been identified in about 40% of neuroblastomas and has been associated with rapid tumor progression regardless of the stage of the tumor. However, neuroblastomas of the mediastinum and other extra-adrenal sites have not been associated with N-myc amplification.[28, 29] With regard to DNA flow cytometry, hyperdiploid neuroblastomas respond better to chemotherapy than diploid tumors do.[30] Interestingly, aneuploidy is common in ganglioneuromas.[31]

PERIPHERAL PRIMITIVE NEUROECTODERMAL TUMOR OF THORACOPULMONARY REGION ("ASKIN TUMOR")

Askin and colleagues described a small round cell tumor originating in the soft tissues of the chest wall or peripheral lung.[32] The patients ranged from 4 months to 20 years of age, with a median of 14 years. Seventy-five percent were female. Most tumors involved the pleura. Five cases (out of 20) involved the mediastinum: two paravertebral, one in mediastinal lymph nodes, and two pericardial.

Grossly, the tumors ranged from 2 to 14 cm in greatest dimension. Most were circumscribed but not well encapsulated. Microscopically, the tumors have three patterns: compact sheets of cells, nests of cells with interspersed fibrovascular stroma, and serpiginous bands of cells with necrosis. Pseudorosettes have central collagen rather than neurofibrillary substance. Tumor cells are 10 to 14 μm in diameter with coarse but evenly dispersed nuclear chromatin and scant cytoplasm (Fig. 11–7). Ultrastructurally, the tumor cells have infrequent neurosecretory granules. The tumors are distinguished from neuroblastomas by the absence of elevated catecholamine levels, the absence of neurofibillary matrix, and the scarcity of neurosecretory granules. In Askin et al.'s study, they most closely resembled Ewing's sarcoma. However, their lack of primary bone disease and the female preponderance were distinguishing features. Their tendency to recur locally is another feature that distinguishes this tumor from other small round cell tumors of childhood. Median survival was only 8 months.[32]

Subsequent immunoperoxidase studies have shown the Askin tumors to react to neuron specific enolase and to variably react to S100.[28] As with primitive neuroectodermal tumors (PNETs), cytogenetic studies have demonstrated the 11:22 chromosomal translocation. This translocation is also found in Ewing's sarcoma and other PNETs but not in neuroblastomas.[28, 33] This finding suggests a common histogenesis for Askin tumor, Ewing's sarcoma, and PNET.[34]

The small round cell tumor described by Askin and colleagues is now considered a peripheral neuroepithelioma, or PNET.[28, 34] The differential diagnosis, based on histopathology, includes the small round cell tumors of childhood. Unlike neuroblastomas, these tumors do not have the more mature elements (i.e., ganglion cells and neurophil). They also do not have amplification of the N-myc oncogene. The tumor resembles and is evidently closely related to Ewing's sarcoma. Other small round cell tumors can be excluded by immunohistochemistry and electron microscopy. Most PNETs stain for neuron specific enolase and vimentin. They react variably for CD57

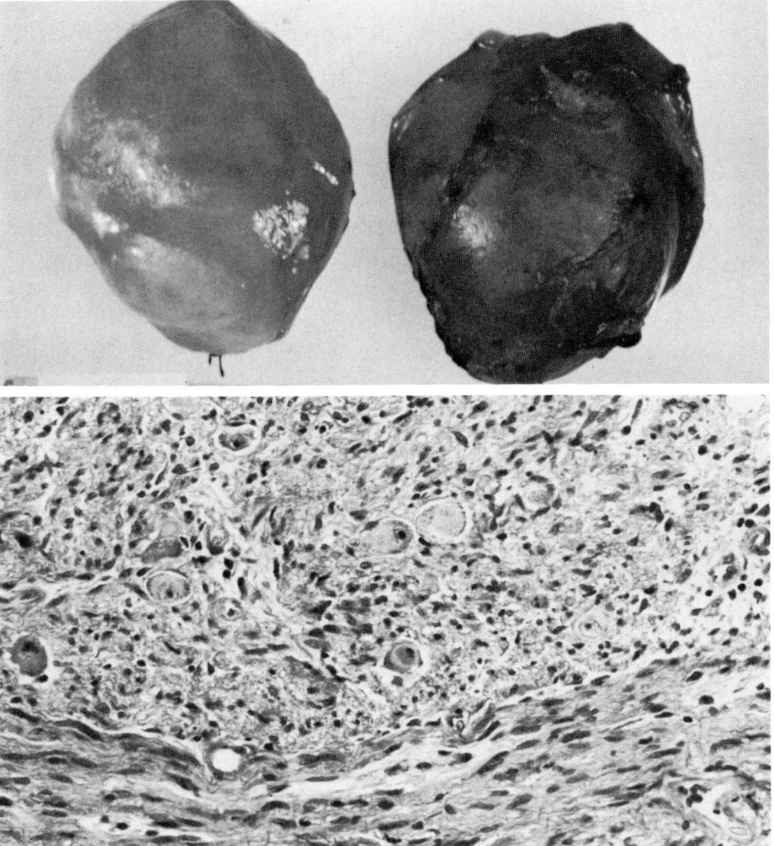

Figure 11–6. *Top,* The ganglioneuroma is a circumscribed tumor with a thin fibrous capsule, as illustrated in this gross photograph. (The tumor is bisected.) This tumor measured 5 cm in greatest diameter. *Bottom,* Microscopically, the lesion is composed of ganglion cells and Schwann cells (H&E, ×200).

(Leu 7).[35] A recently described antibody to the MIC2 gene product, HBA-71, is a relatively specific marker for PNETs and Ewing's sarcoma.[34, 36, 37] However, reactivity with lymphoblastic lymphoma has also been reported.[38]

Another uncommon type of PNET is the melanotic neuroectodermal tumor of infancy.[28, 39] This usually benign, pigmented lesion typically occurs in the maxilla but has been described in other locations, including the posterior mediastinum.[40, 41] Microscopically, the tumor has epithelial-like cells in cords or strands, along with small, dark cells.[39] Melanin pigment is present in many of the epithelial-like cells and in some of the small cells.

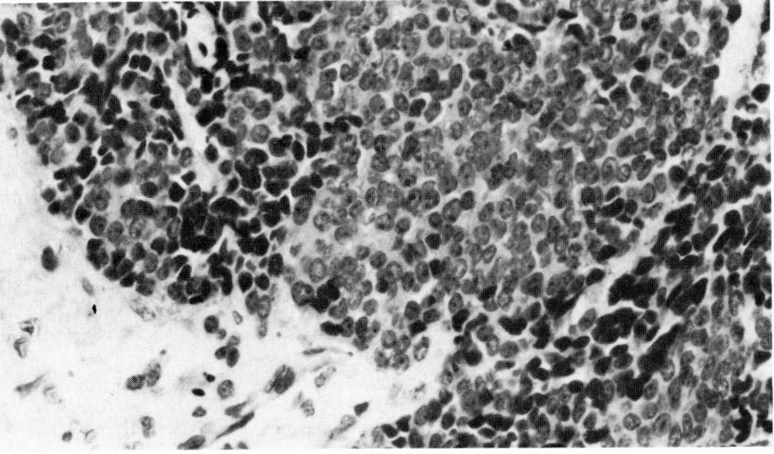

Figure 11–7. Peripheral primitive neuroectodermal tumor of thoracopulmonary region ("Askin tumor"). The tumor consists of small round cells with dispersed nuclear chromatin and scant cytoplasm. (H&E, ×400)

SUMMARY

Neurogenic tumors comprise the majority of neoplasms arising in the posterior mediastinum and are usually in the paravertebral region. The benign tumors of the peripheral nerve sheath are neurofibroma and neurilemoma. Unlike neurofibroma, neurilemoma is encapsulated, is infrequently associated with von Recklinghausen's neurofibromatosis, and has two components: orderly cellular areas (Antoni A) and loose myxoid regions (Antoni B). The malignant peripheral nerve sheath tumor is malignant schwannoma. Mediastinal neuroblastoma, ganglioneuroblastoma, and ganglioneuroma arise from the sympathetic ganglia. Neuroblastoma is the most common posterior mediastinal tumor in children and is one of the "small, round, blue cell tumors." Ganglioneuroblastoma and ganglioneuroma have mature elements. Ganglioneuroma contains only mature ganglion cells, Schwann cells, and fibrous tissue. These tumors do not metastasize. Ganglioneuroblastoma contains both mature ganglion cells and immature neuroblasts. Its prognosis is intermediate between neuroblastoma and ganglioneuroma.

Another small round cell tumor is the primitive neuroectodermal tumor (PNET), or peripheral neuroepithelioma. These tumors may originate in the thoracopulmonary region of children and adolescents. They commonly involve the mediastinum. Like Ewing's sarcoma, these tumors have an 11:22 chromosomal translocation. They must be distinguished from the other small cell neoplasms.

REFERENCES

1. Shields TW, Reynolds M. Neurogenic tumors of the thorax. Surg Clin North Am 1988; 68:645–668.
2. Ingels GW, Campbell DC Jr, Giampetro AM, Kozub RE, Bentlage CH. Malignant schwannomas of the mediastinum: report of two cases and review of the literature. Cancer 1971; 27:1190–1201.
3. Ricci C, Rendina E, Venuta F, Pescarmona EO, Gagliardi F. Diagnostic imaging and surgical treatment of dumbbell tumors of the mediastinum. Ann Thorac Surg 1990; 50:586–589.
4. Enzinger FM, Weiss SW. Benign tumors of peripheral nerves. *In* Soft Tissue Tumors. St. Louis: CV Mosby, 1988:719–780.
5. Ackerman LV, Taylor FH. Neurogenous tumors within the thorax: a clinicopathological evaluation of forty-eight cases. Cancer 1951; 4:669–691.
6. Swanson PE. Soft tissue neoplasms of the mediastinum. Semin Diagn Pathol 1991; 8:14–34.
7. Lodding P, Kindblom L-G, Angervall L, Stenman G. Cellular schwannoma: a clinicopathologic study of 29 cases. Virchows Arch [A] 1990; 416:237–248.
8. Fletcher CDM, Davies SE, McKee PH. Cellular schwannoma: a distinct pseudosarcomatous entity. Histopathology 1987; 11:21–35.
9. Woodruff JM, Godwin TA, Erlandson RA, Susin M, Martini N. Cellular schwannoma: a variety of schwannoma sometimes mistaken for malignant tumor. Am J Surg Pathol 1981; 5:733–744.
10. Hajdu SI. Peripheral nerve sheath tumors: histogenesis, classification, and prognosis. Cancer 1993; 72:3549–3552.
11. Paris F, Cabanes J, Munoz C, Tamarit L. Melanotic spinothoracic schwannoma. Thorax 1979; 34:243–246.
12. Carney JA. Psammomatous melanotic schwannoma: a distinctive, heritable tumor with special associations, including cardiac myxoma and the Cushing syndrome. Am J Surg Pathol 1990; 14:206–222.
13. Enzinger FM, Weiss SW. Malignant tumors of peripheral nerves. *In* Soft Tissue Tumors. St. Louis: CV Mosby, 1988:781–835.
14. Ducatman BS, Scheithauer BW. Malignant peripheral nerve sheath tumors with divergent differentiation. Cancer 1984; 54:1049–1057.
15. Woodruff JM, Christensen WN. Glandular peripheral nerve sheath tumors. Cancer 1993; 72:3618–3628.
16. Krumerman MS, Stingle W. Synchronous malignant glandular schwannomas in congenital neurofibromatosis. Cancer 1978; 41:2444–2451.
17. Burke BA. Pituitary, pineal, adrenal, thyroid, and parathyroid glands. *In* Stocker JT, Dehner LP, eds. Pediatric Pathology. Philadelphia: JB Lippincott, 1992: 941–1001.
18. Triche TJ, Askin FB, Kissane JM. Neuroblastoma, Ewing's sarcoma, and the differential diagnosis of small-, round-, blue-cell tumors. *In* Finegold M, ed. Pathology of Neoplasia in Children and Adolescents. Philadelphia: WB Saunders, 1986:145–195.
19. Carachi R, Campbell PE, Kent M. Thoracic neural crest tumors: a clinical review. Cancer 1983; 51:949–954.
20. Page DL, DeLellis RA, Hough AJ Jr. Adrenal medullary tumors. *In* Atlas of Tumor Pathology Fascicle 23: Tumors of the Adrenal. Washington, DC: Armed Forces Institute of Pathology, 1986:183–260.
21. Saenz NC, Schnitzer JJ, Eraklis AE, Hendren WH, Grier HE, Macklis RM, Shamberger RC. Posterior mediastinal masses. J Pediatr Surg 1993; 28:172–176.
22. Hoover EL, Hsu H-K, Dressler C, Fani K, Webb H, Ketosugbo A, Kharma B. Neuroblastoma: a rare primary intrathoracic neurogenic tumor in adults. Tex Heart Inst J 1988; 15:107–112.
23. Enzinger FM, Weiss SW. Tumors of the sympathetic nervous system. *In* Soft Tissue Tumors. St. Louis: CV Mosby, 1988:816–836.
24. Chatten J, Shimada H, Sather HN, Wong KY, Siegel SE, Hammond GD. Prognostic value of histopathology in advanced neuroblastoma: a report from The Children's Cancer Study Group. Hum Pathol 1988; 19:1187–1188.
25. Joshi VV, Cantor AB, Altshuler G, Larkin EW, Neill JSA, Shuster JJ, Holbrook CT, Hayes FA, Castleberry RP. Recommendations for modification of terminology of neuroblastic tumors and prognostic significance of Shimada classification. Cancer 1992; 69:2183–2196.
26. Punt J, Pritchard J, Pincott JR, Till K. Neuroblastoma: a review of 21 cases presenting with spinal cord compression. Cancer 1980; 45:3095–3101.
27. Adam A, Hochholzer L. Ganglioneuroblastoma of the posterior mediastinum: a clinicopathologic review of 80 cases. Cancer 1981; 47:373–381.
28. Tsokos M. Peripheral primitive neuroectodermal tu-

mors: diagnosis, classification, and prognosis. *In* Garvin AJ, O'Leary TJ, Bernstein J, Rosenberg HS, eds. Pediatric Molecular Pathology: Quantitation and Applications. Basel: Karger, 1992:27–98.

29. Tsuda T, Obara M, Hirano H, Gotoh S, Kubomura S, Higashi K, Kuroiwa A, Nakagawara A, Nagahara N, Shimizu K. Analysis of N-myc amplification in relation to disease stage and histologic types in human neuroblastomas. Cancer 1987; 60:820–826.
30. Gansler T, Chatten J, Varello M, Bunin GR, Atkinson B. Flow cytometric DNA analysis of neuroblastoma: correlation with histology and clinical outcome. Cancer 1986; 58:2453–2458.
31. Taylor SR, Blatt J, Costantino JP, Roederer M, Murphy RF. Flow cytometric DNA analysis of neuroblastoma and ganglioneuroma: a 10 year retrospective study. Cancer 1988; 62:749–754.
32. Askin FA, Rosai J, Sibley RK, Dehner LP, McAlister WH. Malignant small cell tumor of the thoracopulmonary region in childhood: a distinctive clinicopathologic entity of uncertain histogenesis. Cancer 1979; 43:2438–2451.
33. Schneider NR. Cytogenetic evaluation of childhood neoplasms. Arch Pathol Lab Med 1993; 117:1220–1224.
34. Dehner LP. Primitive neuroectodermal tumor and Ewing's sarcoma. Am J Surg Pathol 1993; 17:1–13.
35. Marina NM, Etcubanas E, Parham DM, Bowman LC, Green A. Peripheral primitive neuroectodermal tumor (peripheral neuroepithelioma) in children: a review of the St. Jude experience and controversies in diagnosis and management. Cancer 1989; 64:1952–1960.
36. Ambros IM, Ambros PF, Strehl S, Kovar H, Gadner H, Salzer-Kuntschik M. MIC2 is a specific marker for Ewing's sarcoma and peripheral primitive neuroectodermal tumors: evidence for a common histogenesis of Ewing's sarcoma and peripheral primitive neuroectodermal tumors from MIC2 expression and specific chromosome aberration. Cancer 1991; 67:1886–1893.
37. Seemayer TA, Vekemans M, de Chadarevian J-P. Histological and cytogenetic findings in a malignant tumor of the chest wall and lung (Askin tumor). Virchows Arch [A] 1985; 408:289–296.
38. Riopel MA, Dickman PS, Link M, Perlman EJ. MIC2 analysis in pediatric lymphomas [abstract]. Mod Pathol 1993; 6:128A.
39. Cutler LS, Chaudhry AP, Topazian R. Melanotic neuroectodermal tumor of infancy: an ultrastructural study, literature review, and reevaluation. Cancer 1982; 48:257–270.
40. Misugi K, Okajma H, Newton WA Jr, Kmetz DR, DeLorimier AA. Mediastinal origin of a melanotic progonoma or retinal anlage tumor: ultrastructural evidence for neural crest origin. Cancer 1965; 18:477–484.
41. D'Abrera VSE, Burfitt-Williams W. Melanotic neuroectodermal neoplasm of the posterior mediastinum. J Pathol 1973; 111:165–172.

Chapter

12

MEDIASTINAL CYSTS

BRONCHOGENIC CYSTS
ENTERIC CYSTS
PERICARDIAL/MESOTHELIAL CYSTS
LYMPHATIC CYSTS
PARATHYROID CYSTS
MENINGOCELES
NEOPLASMS
INFECTION
PANCREATIC PSEUDOCYSTS
SUMMARY

Nonthymic cysts account for approximately 20% of primary mediastinal masses.[1–6] Bronchogenic and pericardial cysts are most frequent.[4] The bronchogenic and enteric types derive from malformations of the foregut and can be classified together as foregut cysts.[7] Bronchogenic and pericardial cysts are usually located in the middle mediastinum, where they are the most common mass lesion.[1, 2, 8] Enteric cysts are usually in the posterior mediastinum. Thymic cysts are discussed in Chapter 4. Table 12–1 summarizes the various types of mediastinal cysts.

Fine-needle aspiration has been used in the diagnosis and management of mediastinal cysts.[9, 10] Although one may not be able to establish the origin of the cyst with this technique, the absence of malignant cells supports the diagnosis of a benign cyst. Aspiration of the fluid reduces the size of the cyst and relieves any symptoms. Conservative management rather than a surgical procedure is then an option. However, reports of malignancies arising within benign mediastinal cysts (see later) raise concern. Thoracoscopic resections of mediastinal cysts have been successful.[11–13] Some mediastinal cysts have spontaneously resolved.[14]

BRONCHOGENIC CYSTS

Bronchogenic cysts develop from abnormal budding of the tracheobronchial tree.[15] When the abnormality occurs early in gestation, the cysts are located near the tracheobronchial tree. These cysts infrequently communicate with the trachea or bronchi. Cysts that arise later in gestation are located within the lung parenchyma, where they may communicate with the bronchi. Bronchogenic cysts may cause airway obstruction and life-threatening emergencies.[16, 17] They usually affect infants, children, or young adults but may also be found in older individuals.[8, 15] In adults, most bronchogenic cysts are asymptomatic unless they become infected or exert pressure on adjacent structures.

Bronchogenic cysts are usually attached or adherent to the tracheal bifucation or main bronchi.[4, 18] Some are adjacent to or actually within the esophageal wall. Rarely, they are within the pericardium or adjacent to a congenital pericardial defect. The cysts are usually single and unilocular but may be multiple or septated.[19] They are generally spherical and have a thin, smooth, fibrous wall.[8, 15, 20] They contain milky, mucoid, or gelatinous material. Calcium oxalate crystals within the cyst may produce the appearance of a solid mass on radiographs.[21]

Histologically, ciliated columnar epithelium lines the cyst, but squamous metaplasia is often identified and may be extensive. Chronic inflammation is usually present. Hyaline cartilage, smooth muscle, mucous glands, and

Table 12–1. Mediastinal Cysts*

Type	Histologic Features	Comments
Thymic	Thymic tissue present within cyst wall; cyst lined by flattened, cuboidal, columnar, transitional, or squamous epithelium; may be ciliated; may show pseudoepitheliomatous hyperplasia; cholesterol clefts/granulomas and inflammation are common within cyst wall	Usually in anterior/superior mediastinum; may be unilocular or multilocular; rarely, reported to be associated with squamous cell carcinoma
Bronchogenic	Ciliated columnar epithelium; frequent squamous metaplasia; cartilage; bronchial glands; smooth muscle and fibrous tissue	Usually middle or posterior mediastinum (paratracheal, subcarinal, or hilar); may be attached to or within esophageal wall; unilocular, thin walled, spherical; one case report of a leiomyosarcoma arising in a bronchogenic cyst
Esophageal	Ciliated columnar and/or squamous epithelium; double layer of smooth muscle; may have striated muscle; esophageal glands	Usually superior/posterior mediastinum; unilocular; rare reports of adenocarcinoma arising in esophageal cyst
Gastroenteric	Epithelium may be gastric (chief/parietal cells) or intestinal; muscularis mucosae; two or three layers of smooth muscle; nerve fibers/ganglia; duodenal glands; pancreatic/salivary gland tissue	Posterior mediastinum; most recognized in infancy; male predominance; most unilocular; associated with vertebral anomalies; often symptomatic; acid secretion in gastric type may cause ulcer/rupture; report of adenocarcinoma within cyst
Enterogenous cyst with pancreatic tissue	Lined by columnar epithelium; foci of pancreatic tissue in cyst wall; no other elements	Two reported cases
Pericardial	Fibrous wall with mesothelial lining	Most common location is cardiophrenic angle; usually discovered in asymptomatic adults
Mesothelial	Same as pericardial	Not associated with pericardium or cardiophrenic angle; higher in mediastinum
Thoracic duct	Cyst lined by flat endothelial cells; wall composed of fibrous tissue and smooth muscle	Variable location; origin from thoracic duct can be demonstrated at surgery; chylothorax may develop postoperatively
Parathyroid	Cyst lined by cuboidal epithelium; parathyroid tissue in cyst wall; may also have thymic tissue	Superior mediastinum; most patients are 30–50 years old; minority have hyperparathyroidism
Tumors	Thymoma, teratoma, seminoma, lymphoma (including Hodgkin's disease), metastases	
Cystic lymphangioma (cystic hygroma)	Endothelial-lined spaces; fibrous wall with some smooth muscle; lymphoid aggregates	Usually in superior mediastinum; multilocular
Pancreatic pseudocyst	Inflamed pancreatic tissue	Penetrates into posterior mediastinum from abdomen through esophageal/aortic hiatus
Infections	Hydatid cysts, histoplasmosis, tuberculosis	

*See text for references.

nerve trunks may be found (Fig. 12–1). In some cases, acute inflammation or mucosal ulceration is identified. Calcification may be present. Occasional cases extend below the diaphragm in an "hourglass" configuration.[22, 23] Infection is a common complication in bronchogenic cysts and may lead to the development of a lung abscess.[7] One case report describes a malignant tumor, a leiomyosarcoma, arising within a bronchogenic cyst.[24]

ENTERIC CYSTS

Mediastinal enteric cysts (also called enteric duplication cysts) are either esophageal or gas-

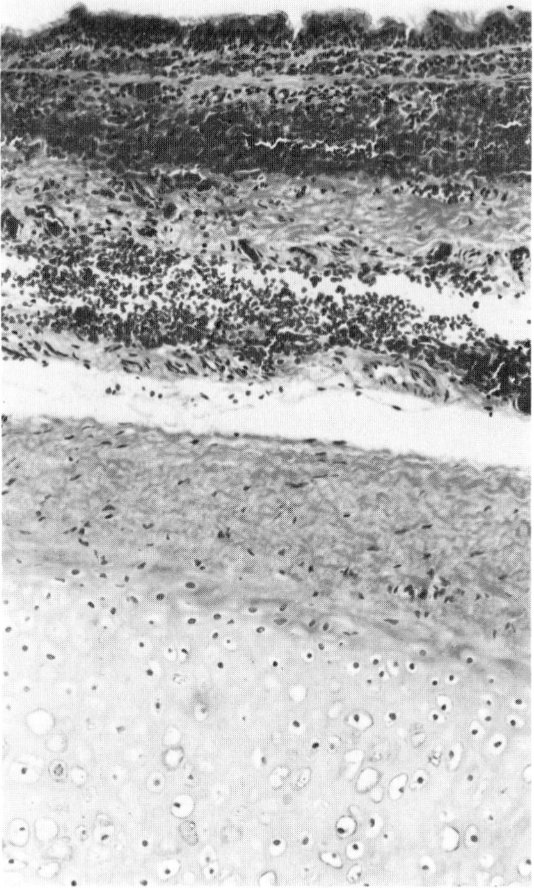

Figure 12–1. Bronchogenic cyst has ciliated columnar epithelium *(top)* and hyaline cartilage *(bottom)*. Chronic inflammation is also evident (H&E, ×100).

troenteric.[4, 25, 26] Most enteric cysts are diagnosed in infants or in children less than 15 years of age. A male predominance has been noted for the gastroenteric type.[4, 20, 25] Patients frequently have respiratory symptoms. Other presenting symptoms include dysphagia, cough, and vomiting. Cysts lined by gastric epithelium may ulcerate, and deaths have resulted from perforation into adjacent structures.[27]

Esophageal cysts may arise from abnormal budding of the foregut.[20] Another theory is that esophageal cysts result from persistence of vacuoles in the foregut wall. Normally, these vacuoles fuse longitudinally to form the esophageal lumen. Lack of proper fusion could result in cyst formation. Esophageal cysts are located within or adjacent to the esophageal wall. If extensive, the cyst, or esophageal duplication, may extend into the abdomen.[23] Occasionally these cysts communicate with the esophagus and may resemble a diverticulum.[28] They are usually lined by ciliated or nonciliated columnar epithelium. Squamous epithelium is also common. Esophageal-type glands may be identified. A double layer of smooth muscle is characteristic. Some esophageal cysts also have striated muscle.

Gastroenteric cysts are frequently associated with vertebral abnormalities, including hemivertebrae and spina bifida.[4, 20, 29] Lower cervical and upper thoracic vertebrae are usually affected. To explain this association, investigators have postulated that the developing foregut adheres focally to the notochord.[6] With further development, a "traction diverticulum" forms that results in a gastroenteric cyst and an associated vertebral anomaly. Another theory is that the gut anlage herniates into a gap formed by a "split" notochord.[30] Alternatively, a persistent neuroenteric canal has been postulated.[31]

Patients may develop two cystic lesions: one posterior mediastinal and the other intraspinal.[17] However, the cyst may be present in one location and not the other. The term "neuroenteric cyst" has been used for these lesions. The gastroenteric cyst in the posterior mediastinum is frequently attached to the vertebra by a fibrous band.[4] The cyst may extend intraspinally through a spinal defect. Completely intraspinal cysts are commonly associated with gastroenteric cysts.[32] Cord compression can develop.[29] Occasional cases are associated with intra-abdominal enteric duplications.[4]

Gastroenteric cysts are located in the posterior mediastinum close to the esophagus, typically in a retrocardiac position.[4, 20, 25] Grossly, they have a variably thick muscular wall with a smooth mucosal lining. They may be unilocular or septated. Microscopically, a thick muscle wall with two or three layers is characteristic. Gastroenteric cysts have gastric- or intestinal-type epithelium. The gastric epithelium may include chief and parietal cells. Acid secretion by gastric epithelium may erode and perforate the cyst wall.[27, 30] Preoperative technetium pertechnetate nuclear medicine scans can arouse suspicion of gastric mucosa in the cyst.[17] Muscularis mucosae and the nerve fibers and ganglia of the myenteric plexus are usually identifiable in gastroenteric cysts.[4] Duodenal glands may be present.[20] Pancreatic and salivary gland tissues have been described.[25] Microscopic descriptions of the intraspinal cyst have noted squamous, columnar, or gastric epithelium.[33, 34]

Rarely, carcinoma arises within a mediastinal cyst. Olsen and colleagues described an adenocarcinoma arising within an esophageal cyst in a 61-year-old patient.[35] The cyst had been followed for 39 years because the patient was asymptomatic. When sudden growth occurred, the cyst was excised. It measured 14 cm in greatest dimension and was contiguous with the esophageal wall. Histopathologic examination revealed foci of adenocarcinoma infiltrating the cyst wall. The cyst wall had a double layer of smooth muscle and was lined mostly by cuboidal and ciliated columnar epithelium. Focal dysplasia was identified. Another report describes a squamous cell carcinoma within an esophageal cyst.[28]

Chuang and colleagues reported an adenocarcinoma within a gastroenteric cyst.[36] It was discovered on a chest radiograph from a 41-year-old asymptomatic man. The cyst was located in the superior mediastinum behind the trachea and measured 6 cm in diameter. The surgeon noted a pedicle running from the cyst to the fourth dorsal vertebra. Microscopically, the cyst was lined by intestinal epithelium consisting of columnar cells and many goblet cells. Muscularis mucosa and double layers of smooth muscle along with myenteric nerve plexuses were present. Epithelial dysplasia was identified. In one half of the specimen, a moderately differentiated adenocarcinoma infiltrated the entire thickness of the cyst wall. The patient had no evidence of metastatic disease at follow-up 4 years after diagnosis.

Distinction between bronchogenic and esophageal cysts can be difficult.[20] A bronchogenic cyst may become attached to the esophageal wall and lose connection with the respiratory tree. The bronchogenic cyst may become entirely incorporated within the wall of the esophagus. Ciliated columnar epithelium can be present in either type of cyst. The presence of cartilage is the most unequivocal feature of bronchogenic origin. In equivocal cases, the term foregut cyst is appropriate.[26]

The term foregut cyst can also be applied to "combination" lesions whose structures represent different origins. For example, tracheoesophageal cysts have features of both bronchogenic and esophageal origin.[4] The lining has both squamous and columnar epithelium. Cartilage, esophageal-type glands, and two layers of smooth muscle may be present. Dehner used the term bronchopulmonary foregut malformation for a cyst that had both bronchial cartilage and gastric mucosa.[26]

Mediastinal cysts with pancreatic tissue have been described in two case reports.[37, 38] They occurred in females 15 and 57 years old. The wall of the cysts contained ducts, acini, and islets of Langerhans typical of the pancreas. No other elements were present.

PERICARDIAL/MESOTHELIAL CYSTS

Pericardial cysts usually arise in the cardiophrenic angle.[4, 8, 20, 39] They are more likely to be located at the right cardiophrenic angle than the left. Some are in the upper mediastinum and are connected to the pericardium.[40] Pericardial cysts are thought to arise during the embryologic development of the pleuropericardial membranes. Some are attached to the pericardium by a pedicle. They are usually noticed in adults but have been described in children. Most patients are asymptomatic. Computed tomography demonstrates a thin cyst wall with fluid contents of water density. Grossly, the cysts resemble peritoneal hernia sacs and consist of fibrovascular tissue with a smooth lining. The cysts contain clear fluid. Microscopically, the cyst is composed of fibrous tissue lined by mesothelial cells. Although usually arranged in a single layer, the mesothelial cells may become hyperplastic. Surgical excision is curative. Mesothelial (pleural) cysts are histologically similar but are located higher up in the anterior mediastinum without a connection to the pericardium.[41, 42]

LYMPHATIC CYSTS

Cystic lymphangioma, or cystic hygroma, is a cystic lesion of lymphatic vessels. This lesion is discussed in Chapter 14.

Thoracic duct cysts are described in case reports that have been reviewed by Tsuchiya and colleagues.[43] The eight reported patients were 20 to 49 years of age and included five females and three males. The cysts were in various mediastinal locations: below the azygos vein in the posterior mediastinum, above the aortic arch, at the right hilus, in the epiphrenic area, and behind the heart. Origin from the thoracic duct could be demonstrated at surgery. In one case, the diagnosis was supported by lymphangiography. Grossly, the cysts measured up to 15 cm in greatest dimension. The microscopic appearance is characterized by fibrous connective tissue with endothelial cells lining the internal surface. Occasionally, patients develop a chylothorax postoperatively.[43, 44]

Similar to thoracic duct cysts are mediastinal lymphoceles, or lymphocysts.[45] These are cystic lesions usually resulting from trauma to the thoracic duct. Most reported cases have followed cardiothoracic surgery and trauma. Diagnosis can be established by injection of contrast material into lymphatic vessels of the foot followed by a computed tomography scan. This demonstrates a cystic cavity communicating with the thoracic duct.

Hurlburt has described lymphocysts within hilar lymph nodes in patients without any history of surgery or trauma.[46] He reported two patients with hilar masses on chest radiographs. At surgery, cystic lesions 4 cm in diameter were excised. They contained up to 20 ml of clear fluid. Microscopically, the wall of the cysts contained lymphoid tissue with reactive germinal centers and anthracotic pigment. No thymic tissue was identified.

PARATHYROID CYSTS

Parathyroid cysts are rare in the mediastinum and usually present as asymptomatic mass lesions.[8, 47–50] Histologically, they are similar to thymic cysts but have parathyroid tissue within the cyst wall (Fig. 12–2). Thymic tissue may also be present. Given the similar developmental origin of the thymus and parathyroid, the presence of both parathyroid and thymic tissue within a cyst is not surprising. If neither element predominates, then the term third pharyngeal pouch cyst may be used.[8]

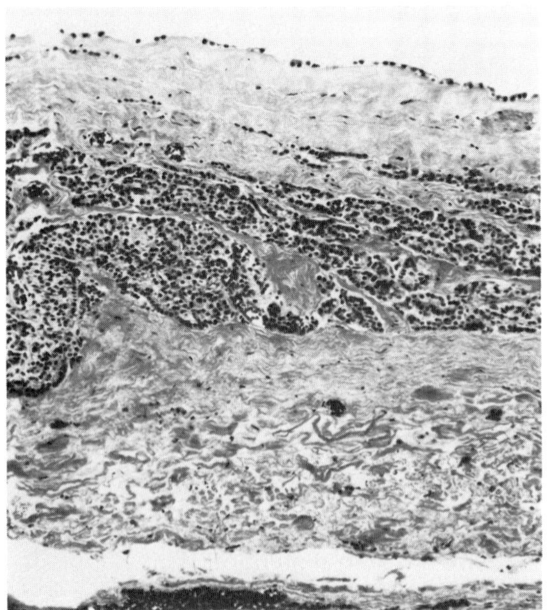

Figure 12–2. Parathyroid cyst. Parathyroid tissue is present in cyst wall *(center)*. The cyst is lined by cuboidal epithelium *(top)*. (H&E, ×100).

MENINGOCELES

Meningoceles should be considered in the differential diagnosis of a posterior mediastinal cyst.[4, 6] The cyst communicates with the subarachnoid space. Most intrathoracic meningoceles are associated with neurofibromatosis. Meningoceles are smooth-walled and unilocular. They contain clear fluid. The wall has an inner arachnoid layer composed of arachnoid lining cells and connective tissue. The outer layer is fibrous dura containing small nerves or ganglia.

NEOPLASMS

As discussed in other chapters, a variety of neoplasms may appear cystic. In particular, thymomas, teratomas, lymphomas (including Hodgkin's disease), and seminomas must be considered in the differential diagnosis of mediastinal cysts. Metastases to mediastinal lymph nodes may also appear cystic.

INFECTION

Hydatid cysts, caused by tapeworms of the genus *Echinococcus,* may occur as primary mediastinal lesions.[47, 51] They may be located in any compartment of the mediastinum. Hydatid cysts are usually multivesicular and filled with colorless fluid. The cyst wall has a laminated, acellular membrane lined by a germinal layer. Scolices and hooklets can be identified in the cyst or in aspirates of the cyst fluid. Extensive caseous necrosis of enlarged lymph nodes from tuberculosis or histoplasmosis may result in mediastinal cystic structures.[52, 53] The cystic lesions may reach 10 cm or more in diameter. Residual lymph node may be identified at the periphery.

PANCREATIC PSEUDOCYSTS

Pancreatic pseudocysts rarely present as a mediastinal mass.[13, 54] Patients have ranged in age from 10 months to 73 years. In most cases, clinical history or laboratory evaluation suggests the diagnosis of pancreatitis. Alcoholism is a common factor in adults, whereas trauma is more often the cause in children. In most cases, the pseudocyst extends from the pancreas to the posterior mediastinum through the esophageal hiatus. Less commonly, the mass may penetrate through the aortic hilus, foramen of Morgagni, or a diaphragmatic erosion. Presentation as an anterior and middle mediastinal mass has been reported.

SUMMARY

The mediastinum is the site of various types of cysts. Thymic cysts were discussed in Chapter 4. Foregut cysts may be bronchogenic or enteric. Enteric cysts may be either esophageal or gastroenteric. Distinction among the various cysts is based on location and histologic appearance. Both bronchogenic and esophageal cysts have ciliated columnar or squamous epithelium. Gastroenteric cysts have epithelium of the gastric or intestinal type. The presence of cartilage is a clue to bronchogenic origin. The term foregut cyst may be used in equivocal cases or in lesions with evidence of multiple origins. Pericardial and mesothelial cysts consist of fibrous tissue with a mesothelial lining. The former usually arise at the cardiophrenic angle; the latter are more superior in the mediastinum. Cysts of lymphatic vessels include cystic lymphangioma (discussed in Chapter 14) and thoracic duct cysts. Parathyroid cysts contain parathyroid tissue within the cyst wall. Meningoceles, neoplasms, infections, and pancreatic pseudocysts are other possible cystic lesions in the mediastinum.

REFERENCES

1. Davis RD, Oldham HN Jr, Sabiston DC Jr. Primary cysts and neoplasms of the mediastinum: recent changes in clinical presentation, methods of diagnosis, management, and results. Ann Thorac Surg 1987; 44:229–237.
2. Cohen AJ, Thompson L, Edwards FH, Bellamy RF. Primary cysts and tumors of the mediastinum. Ann Thorac Surg 1991; 51:378–386.
3. Boyd DP, Midell AI. Mediastinal cysts and tumors: an analysis of 96 cases. Surg Clin North Am 1968; 48:493–505.
4. Abell MA. Mediastinal cysts. Arch Pathol 1956; 61:360–379.
5. Marchevsky AM, Kaneko M. Mediastinal cysts. *In* Surgical Pathology of the Mediastinum. New York: Raven Press, 1984:217–234.
6. Flinner RL, Hammond EH. Cysts. *In* Pathology of the Mediastinum. Chicago: ASCP Press, 1989:116–126.
7. Sirivella S, Ford WB, Zikria EA, Miller WH, Samadani SR, Sullivan ME. Foregut cysts of the mediastinum: results in 20 consecutive surgically treated cases. J Thorac Cardiovasc Surg 1985; 90:776–782.
8. Wick MR. Mediastinal cysts and intrathoracic thyroid tumors. Semin Diagn Pathol 1990; 7:285–294.
9. Nath PH, Sanders C, Holley HC, McElvein RB. Percutaneous fine needle aspiration in the diagnosis and management of mediastinal cysts in adults. South Med J 1988; 81:1225–1228.
10. Walker WJ. Fine needle mediastinal cyst aspiration—a new therapeutic approach. Br J Radiol 1985; 58:679–681.
11. Lewis RJ, Caccavale RJ, Sissler GE. Imaged thoracoscopic surgery: a new thoracic technique for resection of mediastinal cysts. Ann Thorac Surg 1992; 53:318–320.
12. Naunheim KS, Andrus CH. Thoracoscopic drainage and resection of giant mediastinal cyst. Ann Thorac Surg 1993; 55:156–158.
13. Hazelrigg SR, Landreneau RJ, Mack MJ, Acuff TE. Thoracoscopic resection of mediastinal cysts. Ann Thorac Surg 1993; 56:659–660.
14. Martin KW, Siegel MJ, Chesna E. Spontaneous resolution of mediastinal cysts. AJR 1988; 150:1131–1132.
15. St Georges R, DesLauriers J, Duranceau A, Vaillancourt R, Deschamps C, Beauchamp G, Page A, Brisson J. Clinical spectrum of bronchogenic cysts of the mediastinum and lung in the adult. Ann Thorac Surg 1991; 52:6–13.
16. Eraklis AJ, Griscom NT, McGovern JB. Bronchogenic cysts of the mediastinum in infancy. N Engl J Med 1969; 281:1150–1155.
17. Haddon MJ, Bowen A'D. Bronchopulmonary and neurenteric forms of foregut anomalies: imaging for diagnosis and management. Radiol Clin North Am 1991; 29:241–254.
18. Maier HC. Bronchiogenic cysts of the mediastinum. Ann Surg 1948; 127:476–501.
19. Ramenofsky ML, Leape LL, McCauley RGK. Bronchogenic cyst. J Pediatr Surg 1979; 14:219–224.
20. Salyer DC, Salyer WR, Eggleston JC. Benign developmental cysts of the mediastinum. Arch Pathol Lab Med 1977; 101:136–139.
21. Yernault J-C, Kuhn G, Dumortier P, Rocmans P, Ketelbant P, de Vuyst P. "Solid" mediastinal bronchogenic cyst: mineralogic analysis. AJR 1986; 146:73–74.
22. Amendola MA, Shirazi KK, Brooks J, Agha FP, Dutz W. Transdiaphragmatic bronchopulmonary foregut anomaly: "dumbbell" bronchogenic cyst. AJR 1982; 138:1165–1167.
23. Snyder ME, Luck SR, Hernandez R, Sherman JO, Raffensberger JG. Diagnostic dilemmas of mediastinal cysts. J Pediatr Surg 1985; 20:810–815.
24. Bernheim J, Griffel B, Versano S, Bruderman I. Mediastinal leiomyosarcoma in the wall of a bronchial cyst [letter]. Arch Pathol Lab Med 1980; 104:221.
25. Spock A, Schneider S, Baylin GJ. Mediastinal gastric cysts: a case report and review of English literature. Am Rev Respir Dis 1966; 94:97–103.
26. Dehner LP. Mediastinum, lungs, and cardiovascular system. *In* Pediatric Surgical Pathology. Baltimore: Williams & Wilkins, 1987:229–333.
27. Chitale AR. Gastric cyst of the mediastinum: a distinct clinicopathological entity. J Pediatr 1969; 75:104–110.
28. Tapia RH, White VA. Squamous cell carcinoma arising in duplication cyst of the esophagus. Am J Gastroenterol 1985; 80:325–329.
29. Piramoon AM, Abbassioun K. Mediastinal enterogenic cyst with spinal cord compression. J Pediatr Surg 1974; 9:543–545.

30. Kirwan WO, Walbaum PR, McCormack RJM. Cystic intrathoracic derivatives of the foregut and their complications. Thorax 1973; 28:424–428.
31. Holcomb GW Jr, Matson DD. Thoracic neuroenteric cyst. Surgery 1954; 35:115–121.
32. Superina RA, Ein SH, Humphreys RP. Cystic duplications of the esophagus and neurenteric cysts. J Pediatr Surg 1984; 19:527–530.
33. Tekkok IH, Palaoglu S, Erbengi A, Onol B. Intramedullary epidermoid cyst of the cervical spinal cord associated with an extraspinal neuroenteric cyst: case report. Neurosurgery 1992; 31:121–125.
34. Kantrowitz LR, Pais MJ, Burnett K, Choi B, Pritz MB. Intraspinal neuroenteric cyst containing gastric mucosa: CT and MRI findings. Pediatr Radiol 1986; 16:324–327.
35. Olsen JB, Clemmensen O, Andersen K. Adenocarcinoma arising in a foregut cyst of the mediastinum. Ann Thorac Surg 1991; 51:497–499.
36. Chuang MT, Barba FA, Kaneko M, Teirstein AS. Adenocarcinoma arising in an intrathoracic duplication cyst of foregut origin: a case report with review of the literature. Cancer 1981; 47:1887–1890.
37. Shillitoe AJ, Wilson JE. Enterogenous cyst of thorax with pancreatic tissue as a constituent. J Thorac Surg 1957; 34:810–814.
38. Carr MJT, Deiraniya AK, Judd PA. Mediastinal cyst containing mural pancreatic tissue. Thorax 1977; 32:512–516.
39. Lillie WI, McDonald JR, Clagett OT. Pericardial celomic cysts and pericardial diverticula. J Thorac Surg 1950; 20:494–504.
40. Stoller JK, Shaw C, Mathay RA. Enlarging, atypically located pericardial cyst: recent experience and literature review. Chest 1986; 89:402–406.
41. Ovrum E, Birkeland S. Mediastinal tumours and cysts. Scand J Thorac Cardiovasc Surg 1979; 13:161–168.
42. Klein DL. Pleural cyst of the mediastinum. Br J Radiol 1978; 51:548–549.
43. Tsuchiya R, Sugiura Y, Ogata T, Suemasu K. Thoracic duct cyst of the mediastinum. J Thorac Cardiovasc Surg 1980; 79:856–859.
44. Mori M, Kidogawa H, Isoshima K. Thoracic duct cyst in the mediastinum. Thorax 1992; 47:325–326.
45. Sullivan KL, Wechsler RJ. CT diagnosis of mediastinal lymphocele. J Comput Assist Tomogr 1985; 9:1110–1111.
46. Hurlburt WB. Spontaneous intrathoracic lymphocyst. Am Rev Respir Dis 1972; 105:283–286.
47. von Sinner WN, Linjawi T, Al Watban J. Mediastinal hydatid disease: report of three cases. J Can Assoc Radiol 1990; 41:79–82.
48. Rosenberg J, Orlando R, Ludwig M, Pyrtek LJ. Parathyroid cysts. Am J Surg 1982; 143:473–480.
49. Petri N, Holten I. Parathyroid cyst: report of case in the mediastinum. J Laryngol Otol 1990; 104:56–57.
50. Thacker WC, Wells VH, Hall ER Jr. Parathyroid cyst of the mediastinum. Ann Surg 1971; 174:969–975.
51. Sparks AK, Connor DH, Neafie RC. Echinococcosis. *In* Binford CH, Connor DH, eds. Pathology of Tropical and Extraordinary Diseases, volume 2. Washington, DC: Armed Forces Institute of Pathology, 1976:530–533.
52. Rasmussen LD, Madsen KM. [Tuberculous cysts of the mediastinum]. Radiologe [QRL] 1990; 30:299–300.
53. Schwarz J, Schaen MD, Picardi JL. Complications of the arrested primary histoplasmic complex. JAMA 1976; 236:1157–1161.
54. Kirchner SG, Heller RM, Smith CW. Pancreatic pseudocyst of the mediastinum. Radiology 1977; 123:37–42.

Chapter

13

PLEURAL TUMORS

SOLITARY FIBROUS TUMOR
Clinical Features
Pathology
Clinical Course
Differential Diagnosis
DIFFUSE PLEURAL MESOTHELIOMA
SUMMARY

SOLITARY FIBROUS TUMOR

Solitary (or localized) fibrous tumor of the pleura is a neoplasm thought to originate from submesothelial connective issue.[1-3] In a series of 230 cases from the Armed Forces Institute of Pathology (AFIP), 19 (8%) were located within the mediastinum.[1]

Clinical Features

In the AFIP series, patients ranged from 9 to 86 years of age (median 57) with an even distribution of males and females. Approximately half of the patients were asymptomatic. When present, symptoms included chest pain, dyspnea, cough, and hemoptysis. Twelve patients had hypoglycemia, and eight had clubbing of fingers. A pleural effusion was present in 36 cases. Superior vena cava syndrome has been reported.[4]

In general, the solitary fibrous tumors have similar features whether they are in the mediastinum or in other intrathoracic sites. A series by Witkin and Rosai reported 14 mediastinal solitary fibrous tumors.[5] Patients ranged from 27 to 70 years of age (median 54). Most tumors were in the anterosuperior compartment. Two cases were in the middle mediastinum, and one was posterior. One case in this series was attached to a pedicle from the thymus. Another case appeared to be arising from the thymus.

Pathology

Grossly, these lesions appear well-circumscribed[1, 5, 6] (Fig. 13–1). Tumors have ranged from 12 to 3800 g. Many are encapsulated by a thin membrane. The tumors frequently are attached to the pleura by a single pedicle. The cut surface appears lobulated. Focal cystic changes may be present, particularly near the pleural attachment.

Microscopically, the tumors are composed predominantly of fibroblasts and collagen in varying proportions[1, 2, 5] (Fig. 13–2). A disordered, random ("patternless") pattern is characteristic. The tumor cells are ovoid or spindled with round-to-oval nuclei having diffuse chromatin and inconspicuous nucleoli. Cytoplasm is usually poorly defined but may be vacuolated or foamy. Multinucleated tumor

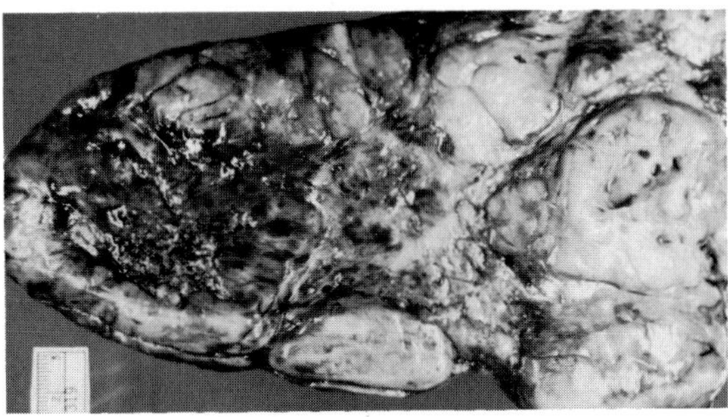

Figure 13–1. This solitary fibrous tumor of the pleura occupied half of the left thoracic cavity in a 76-year-old patient. Grossly, the circumscribed, lobulated appearance on cross-section is evident.

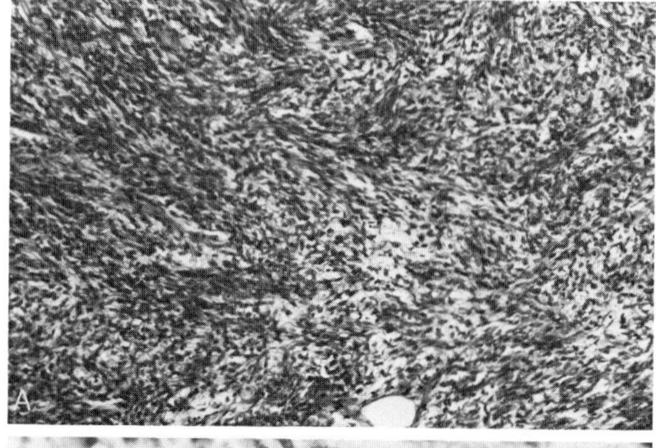

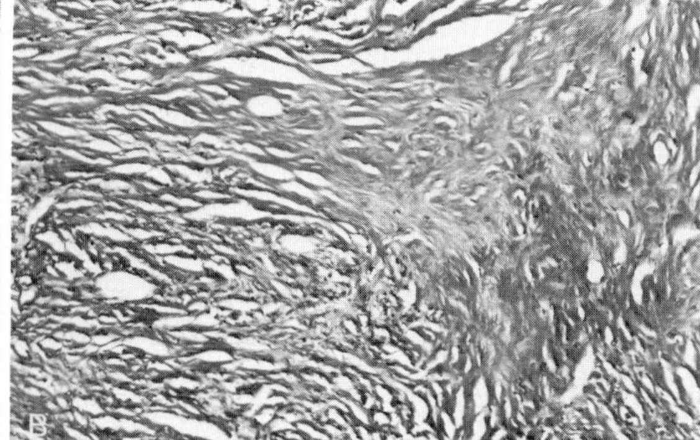

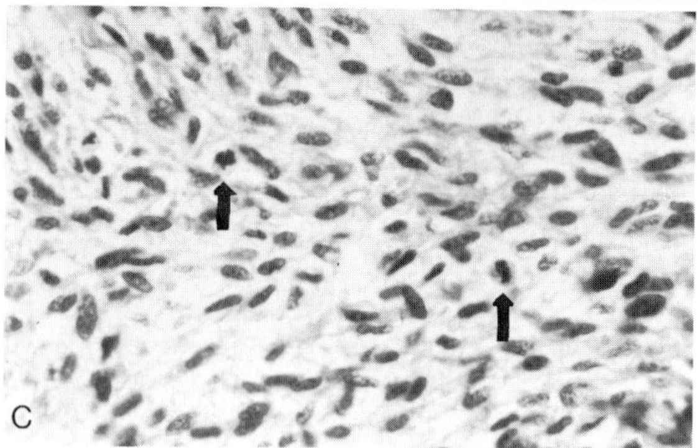

Figure 13–2. Solitary fibrous tumor of the pleura. *A*, Disordered proliferation of spindled cells is characteristic (H&E, ×200). *B*, The tumor also has areas of dense fibrous tissue (H&E, ×100). *C*, Mitotic activity (*arrows*) correlates with a more aggressive clinical course (H&E, ×400).

giant cells may be present. Cellularity varies within the same tumor. Accellular areas contain hyalinized collagen. Hypercellular and hypocellular areas may alternate. Hypocellular areas may be edematous and myxoid. Hypercellular areas may appear sarcomatous with mitotic figures and necrosis. Cytology smears demonstrate a predominance of small, bland, oval, naked nuclei.[7]

Many tumors have hemangiopericytoma-like areas with branching capillaries and thick-walled larger vessels. Vascular areas within the tumor stalk may resemble an arteriovenous malformation.[6] Less commonly, portions of the tumor may appear storiform. A "herringbone pattern" may be present. Some tumors have foci where the cells are arranged in fascicles as with a leiomyoma or palisade as with a neurofibroma. An inflammatory cell infiltrate may be present.

Certain microscopic features are more common in clinically aggressive tumors. Tumor size, cellularity, mitotic figures, and pleomorphism are greater in the aggressive tumors. England and colleagues considered the solitary fibrous tumor malignant if one or more of the following features were present: (1) high cellularity with crowded, overlapping nuclei, (2) more than four mitotic figures per 10 high-power fields or abnormal mitotic figures, (3) pleomorphism of nuclei.[1] By these criteria, 82 of 223 tumors (37%) were considered malignant. In the series of mediastinal solitary fibrous tumors, more than one mitotic figure per 10 high-power fields was considered helpful in identifying the clinically aggressive neoplasms.[5] The pathologist should thoroughly sample the tumor to search for areas that have these features.

Histochemical stains may be useful.[8] Reticulin stain shows thin fibers surrounding individual cells or nests of cells. Trichome stain confirms the presence of dense collagen. Tumor cells react negatively with the periodic acid–Schiff test. The tumor cells may react positively with the colloidal iron test; the positivity persists after treatment with hyaluronidase. In contrast, the hyaluronidase treatment blocks the colloidal iron positivity of mesothelial cells.

By immunoperoxidase studies, the solitary fibrous tumors usually express vimentin and CD34.[1, 5, 8a] Some express the muscle markers desmin or actin. They consistently fail to express epithelial markers (cytokeratin and epithelial membrane antigen), carcinoembryonic antigen, and S-100.

By electron microscopy, the tumor cells appear to be primitive mesenchymal cells or fibroblasts.[1, 5, 6] The cells have rough endoplasmic reticulum and a paucity of other cytoplasmic organelles. They have indistinct cell borders. Collagen is abundant. The tumor cells may have intercellular junctions. Tonofilaments are absent.

Clinical Course

Among 90 patients in the AFIP study with tumors considered benign by histologic criteria, 88 were free of disease and without recurrence at a median follow-up period of 57 months. The other two patients each had a single recurrence that was excised. Among patients whose tumors were classified as malignant, 32 of 71 were free of disease at a median follow-up time of 31 months. The remaining 39 patients experienced a more aggressive course with recurrences and/or metastases. Sixteen patients had metastastic disease. Sites of metastases include liver, central nervous system, spleen, peritoneum, adrenal glands, gastrointestinal tract, kidney, lymph nodes, and bone. Six patients had metastases to mediastinal lymph nodes. The malignant tumors were usually greater than 10 cm in diameter, hemorrhagic, and necrotic.

The single best predictor of a benign course was complete excision. Thus, histologically malignant tumors that were pedunculated and easily excised usually behaved benignly. Not all solitary fibrous tumors are predictable. Some tumors that appear histologically benign may behave aggressively. Some clinically benign tumors have aggressive pathologic features. Tumors that invade adjacent structures (e.g., chest wall, diaphragm, lung) and cannot be completely resected are likely to recur and may metastasize. Overall, approximately 15% of all solitary fibrous tumors prove fatal. Most deaths occur within 5 years of diagnosis. However, recurrences as long as 16 years after the original excision have been reported.[6]

Mediastinal solitary fibrous tumors tend to have a more aggressive course.[1, 5] Perhaps this reflects a greater difficulty in achieving a complete resection. In the Witkin and Rosai series, 64% of mediastinal fibrous tumors had an aggressive course characterized by intrathoracic recurrences.[5] No patient in this series developed extrathoracic metastases.

Differential Diagnosis

The differential diagnosis of mediastinal solitary fibrous tumors includes thymoma, mesothelioma, neurofibroma, leiomyoma, sarcoma, and other spindle cell neoplasms. Immunohistochemistry is useful in that thymoma and mesothelioma express cytokeratin, whereas the solitary fibrous tumor does not. Electron microscopy demonstrates the fibroblast-like cells of the solitary fibrous tumor in contrast to epithelial differentiation in thymoma and mesothelial cell features in mesothelioma.

There has been confusion in the literature between solitary fibrous tumor and mesothelioma.[6, 8] The former has been termed localized mesothelioma. This designation is inappropriate. The tumor cells are not mesothelial according to immunohistochemical and ultrastructural evidence. Diffuse mesothelioma could be confused with solitary fibrous tumor, particularly on the basis of a small biopsy. As noted above, immunohistochemistry and electron microscopy are helpful. These two tumors must be clearly distinguished. In contrast to diffuse mesotheliomas, solitary fibrous tumors are not associated with asbestos exposure. Importantly, most patients with solitary fibrous tumors have a good prognosis, whereas most diffuse mesotheliomas behave aggressively.

As noted above, solitary fibrous tumors may have areas resembling peripheral nerve sheath tumors, leiomyomas, and sarcomas. Thorough histologic sampling of the tumor is necessary to identify its characteristic features. Immunohistochemistry and electron microscopy are often required. Another spindle cell tumor in the mediastinum was recently described by Witkin and colleagues.[9] They reported four cases of a mediastinal tumor resembling a synovial sarcoma. All cases contained a mixture of cytokeratin-positive epithelial cells and vimentin-positive spindle cells.

DIFFUSE PLEURAL MESOTHELIOMA

Diffuse pleural malignant mesotheliomas typically spread to the mediastinum in advanced stages.[10, 11] Within the mediastinum, the tumor may involve the pleura, pericardium, and/or mediastinal lymph nodes. Mesotheliomas may also arise in the pericardium and spread to the adjacent pleura and mediastinum.[12–15] All diffuse pleural mesotheliomas are considered malignant. "Benign" mesothelioma is better characterized as mesothelial hyperplasia.[10] Cases of localized mesothelioma are thought to represent the solitary fibrous tumor (see earlier).

Rarely, malignant mesothelioma predomi-

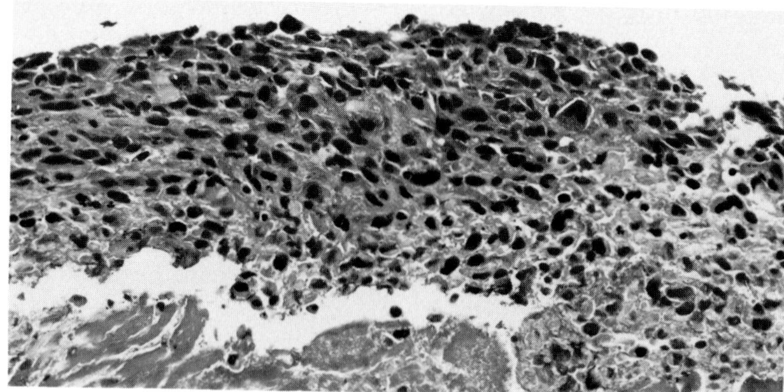

Figure 13–3. Sarcomatous mesothelioma is characterized by pleomorphic, malignant-appearing cells (H&E, ×200).

nantly involves the mediastinum.[13, 16] Such a case was reported by Crotty and colleagues.[16] They describe a desmoplastic diffuse mesothelioma that closely resembled sclerosing mediastinitis on biopsies. At autopsy, the mediastinum was encased by sclerotic tissue. Focal areas of the tumor had a high-grade sarcomatous appearance. Strong cytokeratin immunoreactivity in both the initial biopsies and autopsy material supported the diagnosis of mesothelioma. This case was complicated by an additional finding of histoplasmosis within mediastinal lymph nodes. Thus, sclerosing mediastinitis may have contributed to the extensive fibrosis.

Sussman and Rosai reported six patients with malignant mesothelioma who presented with metastases to lymph nodes.[17] A mediastinal lymph node was the initial biopsy site in one of the six. Most of the patients had widespread tumor at the time of diagnosis. The patient with mediastinal disease had lymphadenopathy resulting from metastastic malignant mesothelioma of the peritoneum. Brooks and colleagues reported mesothelial cell inclusions within mediastinal lymph nodes.[18] Thorough clinical and radiographic evaluation of the patient is necessary in such a situation to rule out metastatic malignant mesothelioma.

Microscopically, a wide range of patterns have been described for mesothelioma[10] (Figs. 13–3 and 13–4). In the common form, mesothelioma cells are round to polygonal with a fairly uniform, bland appearance. Nucleoli may be prominent or inconspicuous. The tumor cells may be cohesive. They may also be arranged individually or form alveolar and tubulopapillary patterns. Both epithelial and sarcomatous patterns may be present. Within lymph nodes, the tumor cells fill the sinuses and must be distinguished from sinus histiocytosis.[17]

Additional studies are useful. Pretreatment with hyaluronidase and diastase reverses positive reactions with the alcian blue and colloidal iron reaction tests.[10] Immunoperoxidase stains for cytokeratin are positive. Unlike carcinomas, mesotheliomas usually do not express carcinoembryonic antigen and CD15 (Leu M1). Ultrastructurally, the tumor cells have long microvilli and complex desmo-

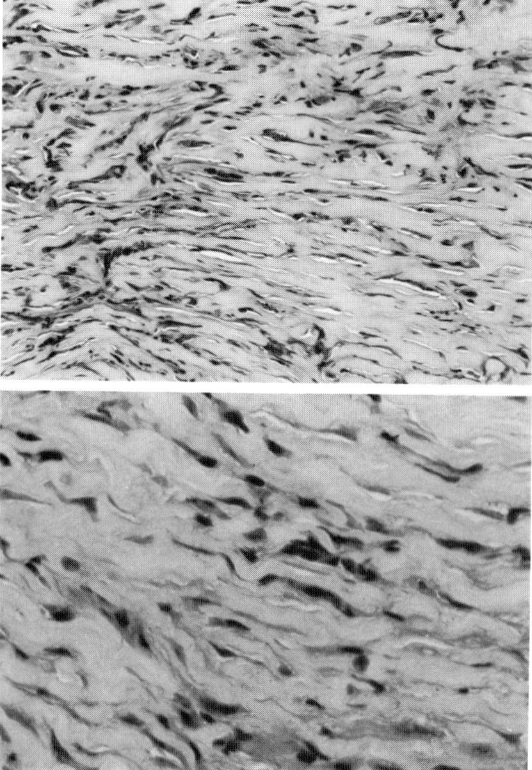

Figure 13–4. Desmoplastic mesothelioma has malignant cells within a dense fibrous stroma. (*Top,* H&E, ×100; *Bottom,* H&E, ×400.)

somes. Intermediate filaments are concentrated in the perinuclear area.

The differential diagnosis must include metastases from other sites. In certain cases, sarcomas and lymphomas may need to be considered. Thymomas can present with diffuse pleural involvement similar to malignant mesothelioma.[19, 20] Some mesotheliomas resemble spindle cell tumors, such as leiomyomas and nerve sheath tumors. Solitary fibrous tumors appear similar microscopically. As discussed above, sclerosing mediastinitis may be a consideration in cases with extensive fibrosis. Sinus histiocytes in lymph nodes must be distinguished from metastatic mesothelioma. Immunoperoxidase and ultrastructural studies may be necessary.

Benign multicystic mesothelioma is a rare, multifocal lesion of mesothelial cells that typically occurs in the peritoneal cavity of young adult females. One report describes a case that involved the pleura.[21] The patient, a 37-year-old woman, had multicystic pleural-based masses in the lateral thorax and paravertebral area. Histologically, they consisted of cystic spaces lined by flattened or cuboidal cells. They are distinguished from cystic lymphangioma in that they lack smooth muscle, have a well-developed basement membrane, and express cytokeratin. Unlike lymphangioma, multicystic mesothelioma rarely recurs.

SUMMARY

Tumors of the pleura may involve the mediastinum and, on occasion, must be considered in the differential diagnosis of a mediastinal lesion. A solitary fibrous tumor of the pleura consists of fibroblasts and collagen in a disordered pattern. On the basis of cellularity, mitoses, and pleomorphism, most of those tumors that are likely to recur and metastasize can be identified. Immunohistochemistry can help to distinguish a solitary fibrous tumor from mesothelioma, thymoma, and various spindle cell neoplasms. Malignant mesothelioma may involve the mediastinum in advanced stages or, rarely, produce predominant mediastinal disease. Mesotheliomas have a wide range of histologic patterns, including a desmoplastic form that must be distinguished from sclerosing mediastinitis. Immunohistochemistry and electron microscopy may be needed for diagnosis.

REFERENCES

1. England DM, Lochholzer L, McCarthy MJ. Localized benign and malignant fibrous tumors of the pleura: a clinicopathologic review of 223 cases. Am J Surg Pathol 1989; 13:640–658.
2. Steinetz C, Clarke R, Jacobs GH, Abdul-Karim FW, Petrelli M, Tomashefski JF Jr. Localized fibrous tumors of the pleura: correlation of histopathological, immunohistochemical and ultrastructural features. Pathol Res Pract 1990; 186:344–357.
3. El-Naggar AK, Ro JY, Ayala AG, Ward R, Ordonez NG. Localized fibrous tumor of the serosal cavities: immunohistochemical, electron-microscopic, and flow-cytometric DNA study. Am J Clin Pathol 1989; 92:561–565.
4. Balassiano M, Reichert N, Rosenman Y, Hertcheg E, Lieberman Y, Yellin A. Localized fibrous mesothelioma of the mediastinum devoid of pleural connections. Postgrad Med J 1989; 65:788–790.
5. Witkin GB, Rosai J. Solitary fibrous tumor of the mediastinum: a report of 14 cases. Am J Surg Pathol 1989; 13:547–557.
6. Briselli M, Mark EJ, Dickersin R. Solitary fibrous tumors of the pleura: eight new cases and review of 360 cases in the literature. Cancer 1981; 47:2678–2689.
7. Dusenbery D, Grimes MM, Frable WJ. Fine-needle aspiration cytology of localized fibrous tumor of pleura. Diagn Cytopathol 1992; 8:444–450.
8. Scharifker D, Kaneko M. Localized fibrous "mesothelioma" of pleura (subpleural fibroma): a clinicopathologic study of 18 cases. Cancer 1979; 43:627–635.

8a. Renshaw AA, Pinkus GS, Corson JM. CD34 and AE1/AE3: Diagnostic discriminants in the distinction of solitary fibrous tumor of the pleura from sarcomatoid mesothelioma. Appl Immunohistochem 1994; 2:94–102.

9. Witkin GB, Miettinen M, Rosai J. A biphasic tumor of the mediastinum with features of synovial sarcoma: a report of four cases. Am J Surg Pathol 1989; 13:490–499.
10. Mackay B, Lukeman JM, Ordonez NG. Tumors of the pleura and chest wall. *In* Tumors of the Lung. Philadelphia: WB Saunders, 1991:323–364.
11. Kawashima A, Libshitz HI. Malignant pleural mesothelioma: CT manifestations in 50 cases. AJR 1990; 155:965–969.
12. McMallister HA Jr, Fenoglio JJ Jr. Tumors of the Cardiovascular System. Washington, DC: Armed Forces Institute of Pathology, 1977:73–81.
13. Tagliamonti JA, Yannopoulos K, Kryle LS. Malignant epithelial mesothelioma of the anterior mediastinum. N Y State J Med 1984; 84:127–129.
14. Chun P, Leeburg W, Coggin J, Zajtchuck R. Primary pericardial malignant epithelioid mesothelioma causing acute myocardial infarction. Chest 1980; 77:559–561.
15. Aggarwal P, Wali JP, Agarwal J. Pericardial mesothelioma presenting as a mediastinal mass. Singapore Med J 1991; 32:185–186.
16. Crotty TB, Colby TV, Gay PC, Pisani RJ. Desmoplastic malignant mesothelioma masquerading as sclerosing mediastinitis: a diagnostic dilemma. Hum Pathol 1992; 23:79–82.
17. Sussman J, Rosai J. Lymph node metastasis as the initial manifestation of malignant mesothelioma: report of six cases. Am J Surg Pathol 1990; 14:819–828.
18. Brooks JSJ, LiVolsi VA, Pietra GG. Mesothelial cell inclusions in mediastinal lymph nodes mimicking metastatic carcinoma. Am J Clin Pathol 1990; 93:741–748.

19. Moran CA, Travis WD, Rosado-de-Christenson M, Koss MN, Rosai J. Thymomas presenting as pleural tumors: report of eight cases. Am J Surg Pathol 1992; 16:138–144.
20. Honma K, Shimada K. Metastasizing ectopic thymoma arising in the right thoracic cavity and mimicking diffuse pleural mesothelioma—an autopsy study of a case with review of literature. Wien Klin Wochen 1986; 98:14–20.
21. Ball NJ, Urbanski SJ, Green FHY, Kieser T. Pleural multicystic mesothelial proliferation: the so-called multicystic mesothelioma. Am J Surg Pathol 1990; 14:375–378.

Chapter

14

MISCELLANEOUS LESIONS

THYMOLIPOMA
LIPOMA
VASCULAR LESIONS
LYMPHANGIOMA
LYMPHANGIOMYOMA
HEMANGIOPERICYTOMA
BENIGN MUSCLE TUMORS
BENIGN TUMORS OF BONE AND CARTILAGE
OTHER BENIGN LESIONS
SARCOMA
ENDOCRINE LESIONS
MENINGIOMA
EPENDYMOMA
CHORDOMA
SUMMARY

THYMOLIPOMA

Thymolipoma is a rare benign tumor of the anterior mediastinum characterized by adipose tissue with interspersed strands of thymus. Thymolipoma has been the subject of numerous case reports.[1–17] Among 72 thymic tumors collected by Otto and colleagues, five (7%) were thymolipomas.[17] The tumor may occur at any age, including children as young as 4 years.[18] In a literature review of 91 cases, the mean age was in the third decade of life.[19] Patients may be asymptomatic or have symptoms related to the tumor mass (usually dyspnea, chest pain, or cough).

Like thymomas, thymolipomas have been reported in patients with other disorders, including myasthenia gravis.[4, 17, 20] The 10 reported thymolipoma patients with myasthenia gravis are somewhat older than those without myasthenia (ranging from 31 to 62 years with a mean age of 53 years).[20] The symptoms of myasthenia gravis usually improve after thymectomy. Thymolipomas have also been described in patients with aplastic anemia, hypogammaglobulinemia, Graves' disease, Hodgkin's disease, and chronic lymphocytic leukemia.[2, 12, 13, 17, 21]

The tumor has a characteristic appearance on computed tomography. High- and low-density areas are interspersed within the mass. Linear soft tissue densities are identifiable within the adipose tissue.[14, 15, 19] A similar pattern has been described with massive thymic hyperplasia. On chest radiographs, the tumor may be mistaken for cardiomegaly.[11, 22]

Grossly, the tumor is a lobulated mass with a thin fibrous capsule. Thymolipomas commonly weigh several kilograms.[19, 23, 24] A well-illustrated report from 1955 by Dunn and Frkovich documents a thymolipoma weighing 6 kg[6] (Fig. 14–1). It was diagnosed at autopsy in a 47-year-old patient admitted to the hospital with shortness of breath.

Microscopically, most of the tumor is mature adipose tissue. Intervening strands of normal-appearing thymus have cortex and medulla in varying proportions. Hassall's corpuscles can be identified. Myoid cells have been described.[25] Germinal centers have not been identified, even in those cases associated with myasthenia gravis. On fine-needle aspiration biopsies, the presence of adipose tissue and thymic cells, together with the appropriate clinical and radiographic findings, suggests the diagnosis.[26]

The pathogenesis of thymolipoma has been debated.[20, 24] According to one theory, the tu-

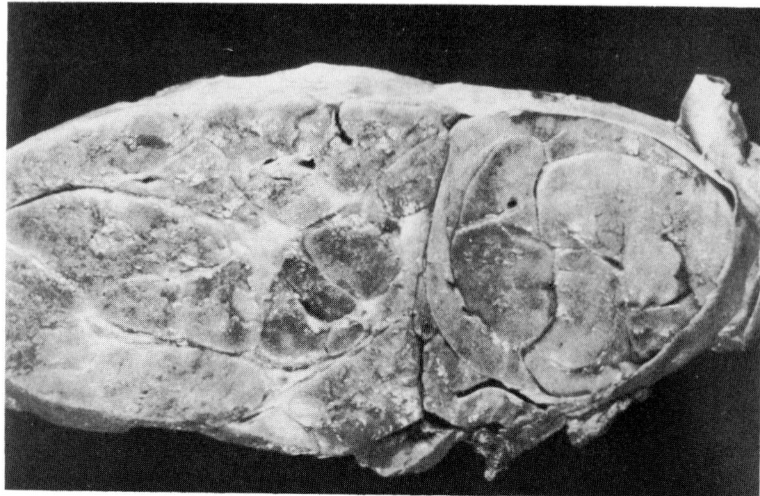

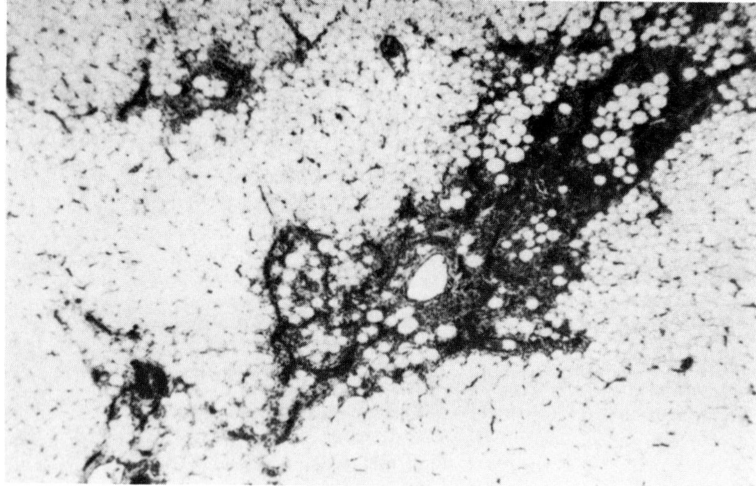

Figure 14–1. *Top,* Gross photograph of cross-sectioned thymolipoma demonstrates the encapsulated, lobulated appearance. This 6-kg tumor (34 cm in greatest dimension) was removed at autopsy from the anterior mediastinum of a 47-year-old male. *Bottom,* Microscopically, the tumor consists of fat with strands of thymic tissue interspersed (H&E, ×28). (From Dunn BH, Frkovich G. Lipomas of the thymus gland with an illustrative case report. Am J Pathol 1956; 32:41–50.)

mor is a hamartoma. In support of this concept, Jagadha and Ramaswamy describe a thymolipoma with "hamartomatous elements": epithelial nests, cords, and trabeculae, with ductular structures.[3] Squamous and oncocytic metaplasia was prominent. Others speculate that the thymolipoma is a thymoma with fatty involution. Some suggest that the tumor is a lipoma or hyperplasia of adipose tissue occurring within the thymus. Another theory is that thymolipomas represent fatty replacement of an enlarged thymus. None of the theories is entirely satisfactory.

True thymic hyperplasia, an enlargement of the normal thymus, should be considered in the differential diagnosis of thymolipoma. (See Chapter 4.) In contrast to thymolipoma, true thymic hyperplasia consists mostly of thymic lymphoid tissue, although some fat may be present.

LIPOMA

Lipomas (i.e., tumors of adipose tissue without thymic elements) may occur in the mediastinum. In a classic series of articles on mediastinal mesenchymal tumors in 1956, Pachter and Lattes found lipomas to be among the most common tumors of mesenchymal origin in this location.[27–29] Of 22 mesenchymal neoplasms of the mediastinum, 4 were classified as lipomas.[27] Most mediastinal lipomas are in the anterior compartment. Both adults and children may be affected.[30] Patients have ranged in age from 4 to 61 years.

Grossly, the tumors can be quite large, measuring up to 30 cm in diameter and weighing several kilograms.[27] A thin fibrous capsule is present. Microscopically, the tumors are composed of mature adult adipose tissue with occasional lymphocytes. Pleomorphism and mitotic figures are absent. No thymic tissue is identified.

"Hourglass" lipomas are both intra- and extra-thoracic with extensions from the mediastinum into the neck or outside the thoracic cage.[30] One case report describes a lipoma that presented as a mass in the upper mediastinum and extended into the spinal canal.[31] A mediastinal lipoma with a prominent vascular component (angiolipoma) has been described adjacent to the esophagus.[32] Mediastinal angiomyolipoma and myelolipoma have also been reported.[33-36] The former is a tumor composed of vessels, smooth muscle, and fat. The latter has mature hematopoietic elements and fat. Mediastinal lipomatosis refers to a diffuse increase in fatty tissue.[37] It may produce mediastinal widening on radiographic studies.[38]

Lim described another fatty tumor of the mediastinum, a chondrolipoma.[39] The tumor was excised from the superior-posterior mediastinum of a 32-year-old male. The mass appeared lobulated and on cross-section had a central cartilaginous area. Histologic examination revealed lobulated, benign cartilage surrounded by mature adipose tissue.

A single case of a mediastinal hibernoma has been reported.[40, 41] Hibernoma is a benign tumor usually affecting adults. It is composed of granular or multiloculated fat cells similar to fetal brown fat. Golden brown, coarsely granular pigment with staining characteristics of lipofuscin is common. Its name derives from a morphologic similarity to cells of the so-called "hibernating gland" of animals. The tumor is most often located in the scapular or interscapular regions. Of 91 reported tumors, 7 were intra-thoracic (5 subpleural, 1 intramyocardial, 1 in the anterior-superior mediastinum). The one reported mediastinal tumor was attached to the thymus in a 16-year-old patient. Surgical excision is curative.

Lipoblastoma is a benign fatty tumor occurring in infants and children usually less than 3 years of age.[41-43] The upper and lower extremities are most commonly affected. Tabrisky and colleagues reported an 11-month-old infant with a lipoblastoma attached to the posterior superior mediastinum and filling the right hemithorax.[43] Another case occurred in the anterior mediastinum.[43] Some authors differentiate the lipoblastoma, a circumscribed tumor, from a diffuse form, lipoblastomatosis.[42, 44] Either lesion is composed of adipocytes arranged in lobules. The adipocytes range from lipoblasts to mature lipocytes. The lipoblasts include stellate, spindled mesenchymal cells. The mature cells are more centrally located within the tumor. The stroma may be myxoid. The vascular pattern of myxoid liposarcoma is not present. Nuclear atypia and mitotic activity are absent. The diffuse form may be difficult to excise completely and may recur.

VASCULAR LESIONS

Hemangiomas are uncommon in this location, accounting for less than 1% of mediastinal masses.[45, 46] Cohen and colleagues reviewed 15 patients with mediastinal hemangiomas,[47] four of whom were less than 2 years of age. The remainder were adults. In other series, about half of the mediastinal hemangiomas occur in those under the age of 20 years.[45, 48] These lesions have been associated with multiple hemangiomas and with Osler-Weber-Rendu disease.[48, 49] In the Cohen series, seven patients were asymptomatic; the others had chest pain, dyspnea, hemoptysis, persistent respiratory infections, or back pain. Eight tumors were in the anterior mediastinum; seven were posterior. Two of the anterior mediastinal lesions were in the thymus. Tumors ranged from 3 to 16 cm in diameter. Histologically, the hemangiomas were of the cavernous, capillary, venous, or mixed types. Five patients underwent total excision. The remaining cases could not be completely removed, because the tumors invaded adjacent structures. Subtotal excision was not associated with massive hemorrhage. Follow-up information was obtained for 14 patients. One patient with a subtotal excision underwent re-excision and was stable for 10 years. One patient thought to have a complete excision had a recurrence noted radiographically that remained unchanged for 6 years. One patient had only a biopsy but developed no subsequent evidence of tumor growth. Radiation therapy was not effective. Citing these data, Cohen et al. believe that radical resection is not indicated. If necessary, local recurrences can be excised.

Most mediastinal hemangiomas are of the cavernous type.[28, 45] These lesions are composed of large, dilated blood vessels lined by flattened endothelium.[50] The vessels may be arranged haphazardly or in a lobular configuration. Capillary hemangiomas are characterized by plump endothelial cells with small, inconspicuous lumina. As the capillary hemangioma ages, the endothelial cells become more flattened. Venous hemangiomas have thick-walled vessels. The smooth muscle in the vessel often merges into the surrounding soft tissue.

Epithelioid hemangioendothelioma (hemangioendothelioma, histiocytoid hemangioma) is a vascular tumor that is more aggressive than a hemangioma. Rare cases have been reported in the mediastinum.[51–55] This tumor consists of nests or short cords of rounded or slightly spindled endothelial cells. The endothelial cells look epithelioid. Strands of cells are within a hyaline matrix. Some areas have solid nests of tumor cells. Transition to vascular channels may be found. Foci of osteoclast-like giant cells and metaplastic bone may be identified. In contrast to angiosarcoma, epithelioid hemangioendothelioma lacks nuclear pleomorphism, mitoses, and necrosis.[37]

LYMPHANGIOMA

Lymphangiomas of the mediastinum are usually of the cystic type. Cystic lymphangioma (also called cystic hygroma) is thought to be a developmental malformation of lymphatic vessels.[56–58] Most are found in the cervical and axillary regions of children less than 2 years of age. Two or three percent of the cervical lesions extend into the mediastinum. Rarely, cystic lymphangiomas may be confined to the mediastinum, usually in the anterior-superior region. Posterior and inferior mediastinal locations have been reported.

In contrast to the cervical and axillary lesions, those in the mediastinum often are diagnosed in adults. Cystic lymphangiomas are commonly associated with respiratory distress in infants but are usually asymptomatic in adults. These are slow-growing lesions. Rapid growth may result from hemorrhage or infection in the cyst. Malignant transformation rarely occurs.[37] Cystic lymphangiomas are multilocular and consist of dilated endothelial-lined spaces containing clear fluid. Smooth muscle and fibrous tissue compose the cyst wall. Lymphocytic aggregates are commonly present (Fig. 14–2). Complete excision is the treatment of choice. When complete resection is not possible, recurrences may develop.

Lymphangiomatosis is a generalized disorder characterized by proliferating lymphatic vessels in bone, viscera, and soft tissues, including the mediastinum.[59–61] Patients are usually children. Respiratory symptoms are often associated with chylothorax. A mediastinal mass may be present and consists of anastomosing, thin-walled lymphatics and occasional germinal centers. Immunoperoxidase studies demonstrate expression of endothelial cell markers, factor VIII–related antigen, and CD31.[59] Ulex Europaeus lectin binding and immunoreactivity for another endothelial cell antigen, CD34, is variable. Prognosis is related to the extent of disease. Pleural and lung involvement is associated with an unfavorable outcome.[59]

LYMPHANGIOMYOMA

Lymphangiomyoma (or lymphangioleiomyoma) is an uncommon lesion involving lymphatic vessels of the mediastinum, lung, retroperitoneum, and lymph nodes.[62, 63] The lesion is often multifocal. It affects adult females (average age about 40 years). Patients usually present with dyspnea associated with a chylothorax. Honeycombing of the lung may also contribute to the respiratory symptoms. Most cases involve the mediastinum, usually the thoracic duct and/or mediastinal lymph nodes.[63, 64] The lesions may be discrete, circumscribed, red-to-gray, spongy masses. They may also manifest as diffuse proliferations of smooth muscle along the lymphatics.[64] The latter type has been referred to as the diffuse form of lymphangiomyoma, or lymphangiomyomatosis.

Histologically, lymphangiomyomas have prominent smooth muscle around anastomosing lymphatic channels.[29, 64] The smooth muscle is present as "cords" enclosing the lymphatic spaces. The channels are lined by endothelium and contain proteinaceous fluid, some lymphocytes, and occasional red blood cells. Aggregates of lymphocytes may be adjacent to the muscle. Cellular pleomorphism and mitoses are absent. These lesions do not metastasize or invade adjacent structures. Patients with pulmonary involvement usually develop progressive respiratory insufficiency. Long survival has been reported after surgery in patients with localized lesions.

Regarding the differential diagnosis, partial replacement of a lymph node may resemble a metastatic sarcoma. Helpful features in a lymphangiomyoma include the constant orientation of smooth muscle cells around endothelial spaces, lack of cellular pleomorphism, and absence of mitoses.

HEMANGIOPERICYTOMA

Hemangiopericytoma is a tumor of pericytic origin.[65] Most are located in the lower extrem-

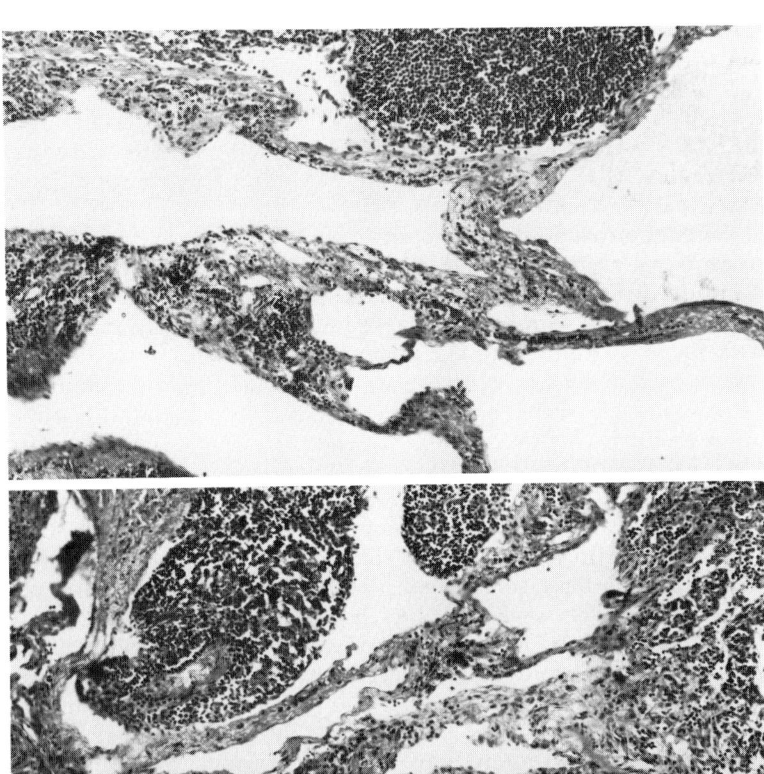

Figure 14–2. Cystic lymphangioma. Dilated, endothelial-lined spaces with lymphocytic aggregates are evident. (*Top* and *Bottom*, H&E, ×200.)

ities and retroperitoneum. Mediastinal hemangiopericytomas are uncommon.[37] In the series by Pachter and Lattes, seven hemangiopericytomas among 43 mediastinal vascular lesions (including 32 hemangiomas) were described.[28] Several types of tumors may look like hemangiopericytoma. In the absence of electron microscopy and/or immunoperoxidase studies, a reliable diagnosis may not be possible.[65]

Histologically, the tumor is well circumscribed and has prominent, anastomosing vascular channels of varying sizes. Typically, the branching vessels have a "staghorn" appearance. The tumor cells have round-to-oval nuclei with indistinct cytoplasm. More than four mitoses per 10 high-power fields is helpful in predicting recurrence and metastases. Malignant hemangiopericytomas are more cellular and more likely to have cellular pleomorphism, necrosis, and hemorrhage. Infiltration into adjacent structures is another indicator of aggressive behavior.[37] The microscopic appearance may resemble various tumors, including a thymoma, solitary fibrous tumor, hemangioma, leiomyoma, schwannoma, mesothelioma, liposarcoma, and fibrosarcoma.[65] Immunohistochemistry with endothelial cell markers highlights the distinction between endothelial cells and surrounding pericytes. Reactivity of the tumor cells for actin, vimentin, and S100 has been described.

BENIGN MUSCLE TUMORS

Mediastinal leiomyomas usually arise from the walls of the esophagus, trachea, or great vessels.[37, 66, 67] Thirteen cases were collected from a literature review by Uno and colleagues.[67] The tumors have a whorled, trabeculated appearance on cut surface and microscopically consist of interlacing bundles of fusiform cells. Cellular atypia or mitotic figures are absent. A rhabdomyoma has been reported in the anterosuperior mediastinum of an 80-year-old patient.[68] The lesion was unattached to the heart. Although no thymus could be identified, the authors speculated that the tumor originated from thymic myoid cells.

BENIGN TUMORS OF BONE AND CARTILAGE

Osteochondromas and chondromas may arise from the chest wall or vertebrae and secondarily extend into the mediastinum.[69] Fibrous dysplasia of the paravertebral aspect of the ribs may extend into the posterior mediastinum.

OTHER BENIGN LESIONS

Several examples of mediastinal myxomas have been reported in the mediastinum.[69, 70] These lesions have stellate cells within a mucoid matrix. They should be distinguished from liposarcoma. Feigin and colleagues reported a pleomorphic adenoma presenting as a well-circumscribed mass in the mediastinum.[71] The lesion was beneath the aortic arch. It was adherent to, but separate from, the trachea. Immunoperoxidase and ultrastructural studies supported the diagnosis. Extramedullary hematopoiesis may produce a mediastinal mass, such as in a patient with a hemoglobinopathy.[72]

SARCOMA

Liposarcomas are among the most common mediastinal sarcomas. Well-documented cases have occurred in both children and adults.[73–82] All histologic types of liposarcoma have been described. In children, most mediastinal liposarcomas are myxoid. The differential diagnosis in these pediatric cases includes lipoblastoma. Lipoblastomas occur in young children and have fibrous septa that divide the tumor into small lobules. They have a uniform growth pattern and do not have the mucoid lakes frequently seen in myxoid liposarcoma.[73] Havlicek and Rosai reported a liposarcoma-like malignant neoplasm arising in the thymic stroma.[83] These authors suggest that the tumor is the malignant counterpart of a thymolipoma.

Rare reports of other types of primary mediastinal sarcomas have been published. In the recent literature, these include malignant fibrous histiocytoma,[84, 85] fibrosarcoma,[86] rhabdomyosarcoma,[86a, 86b] leiomyosarcoma,[87–89] angiosarcoma,[90] extraskeletal osteogenic sarcoma,[91–94] extraskeletal mesenchymal chondrosarcoma,[95] and myxoid chondrosarcoma.[96] Two case reports describe infants with a mediastinal rhabdoid tumor.[97, 98] Witkin et al. reported mediastinal synovial sarcoma.[99]

In children, mediastinal rhabdomyosarcoma and extraosseous Ewing's sarcoma have been reported.[100] In pediatric patients, these mediastinal sarcomas are associated with advanced disease. The tumors tended to occur in older children and often had an undifferentiated histologic type.

Rarely, sarcomas have been associated with mediastinal nonseminomatous germ cell tumors in young adult male patients.[101–103] (See Chapter 9.) In particular, rhabdomyosarcoma and angiosarcoma have been most commonly reported. Recurrences and metastases may consist only of the sarcomatous element. The finding of a mediastinal sarcoma in a young adult male should prompt a search for evidence of a nonseminomatous germ cell component. Serologic studies (especially for alpha-fetoprotein) and thorough sampling of the tumor may be helpful.

Sarcomas may have differentiation along different cell lines. For example, Heinemann and Lehman described an anterior mediastinal tumor diagnosed as a liposarcoma.[104] Subsequently, the patient developed metastases with differentiation to a chondrosarcoma and osteosarcoma. Different metastatic sites had different appearances. The term malignant mesenchymoma has been used to define a sarcoma showing two or more differentiated tissue types (excluding fibrous tissue)—for example, rhabdomyosarcoma and liposarcoma within the same tumor.[105]

Another tumor with divergent differentiation is the pleuropulmonary blastoma in childhood.[106] This rare, aggressive tumor involves the lung and/or mediastinum and occurs in early childhood. Microscopically, the lesion consists of a diffuse proliferation of undifferentiated cells. In addition, foci of chondroblastic differentiation are commonly present. Some tumors also have a storiform pattern, alveolar pattern, or lipoblastic differentiation. The tumors frequently express desmin and actin. S-100 is positive in chondroblastic areas. Histiocytic markers, including CD68, also are expressed within the tumor. Cytokeratin is expressed only in entrapped epithelial or mesothelial cells. Ultrastructurally, the tumor contains a variety of cell types: primitive fibroblasts, myofibroblasts, and rhabdomyoblasts along with histiocytoid and fibrohistiocytoid elements.

ENDOCRINE LESIONS

Lesions of the thyroid and parathyroid may involve the mediastinum. In large series, intrathoracic goiters account for 5 to 25% of mediastinal masses.[107–109] Intrathoracic goiters are defined as enlarged thyroid glands that have a greater mass inferior to the thoracic inlet.[110] Most are extensions of thyroid tissue from the neck. Seventy-five percent are located in the anterior mediastinum.[111] Those in the posterior mediastinum may be more difficult to excise.[110, 112, 113] Rarely, a goiter may arise from ectopic thyroid tissue within the mediastinum. These "aberrant" goiters do not have any connection to the cervical thyroid gland and do not have a cervical blood supply.

Completely intrathoracic goiters account for less than 1% of all surgically removed goiters.[110] Histologic examination usually demonstrates features similar to those of other nodular goiters.[110] They are multinodular and composed of thyroid follicles of varying sizes. Old hemorrhage, calcification, cyst formation, fibrosis, and focal thyroiditis may be present.[114] Follicular adenomas and Hashimoto's thyroiditis may be identified within the mediastinum.[114] Rarely, malignancies of the thyroid occur in this location. Papillary carcinoma, follicular carcinoma, Hürthle cell carcinoma, and lymphoma have all been described as arising within mediastinal goiters.[114, 115]

In large series of parathyroid adenomas, 10 to 20% are in the mediastinum.[108, 116, 117] Usually they are discovered after neck exploration fails to identify an adenoma in a patient with hyperparathyroidism.[107, 118–121] Within the mediastinum, most parathyroid adenomas are located in the anterosuperior compartment. Approximately two thirds are in or near the thymus. Most presumably originate in the lower parathyroid glands, because these are the glands that develop in close association with the thymus. About 20% arise from supernumerary (fifth) parathyroid glands.[121, 122]

Histologically, a parathyroid adenoma has a fibrous capsule and is composed of polyhedral cells with round, bland nuclei.[123, 124] Mitoses are rare or absent. The lesion may have a nodular or acinar pattern. Occasionally, a mediastinal parathyroid adenoma will have a prominent component of adipose tissue. This lesion has been described as "lipoadenoma."[125] Parathyroid cysts also occur in the mediastinum. (See Chapter 12.)

Rare cases of mediastinal parathyroid carcinoma have been reported.[126, 127] Murphy and colleagues reported a 51-year-old male with parathyroid carcinoma that presented as a mass in the anterosuperior mediastinum.[127] At surgery, the tumor was adherent to the esophagus and trachea. A biopsy was obtained. Histologically, the tumor had fibrous septa creating prominent lobules. The tumor resembled the parathyroid with chief cells, oxyphil cells, and water-clear cells. Slight nuclear pleomorphism and inconspicuous nucleoli were present. Numerous mitoses, capsular penetration, and vascular invasion were identified. Immunoperoxidase stains for parathormone and chromogranin were positive. Ultrastructurally, the tumor had regular cuboidal cells with interdigitating membranes, intercellular junctions, and dense core granules.

In distinction from adenomas, parathyroid carcinomas have a trabecular pattern with thick fibrous septa.[123, 124, 127] They tend to be unencapsulated, to be invasive, and to have mitoses. Vascular invasion may or may not be present. Cellular atypia and pleomorphism are not useful criteria, because they are as likely to be present in an adenoma as in a carcinoma.

The differential diagnosis of a parathyroid tumor in the mediastinum includes carcinoid, thymic carcinoma or metastatic carcinoma, seminoma, paraganglioma, and thyroid tumors. Hypercalcemia is usually present in patients with parathyroid tumors. Immunohistochemistry may be helpful in difficult cases.[127]

Meijer and Hoitsma reported a malignant oncocytoma of the superior mediastinum.[1] Microscopic examination demonstrated a tumor composed of polygonal cells with eosinophilic, granular cytoplasm. Ultrastructurally, the cytoplasm was packed with mitochondria. The tumor was locally invasive and could not be completely resected. The patient died 2 years later of an unrelated cause. Although no normal adjacent tissue could be identified, the authors speculated that the tumor may have originated from thyroid or parathyroid tissue in the mediastinum.

MENINGIOMA

Wilson and colleagues reported a mediastinal meningioma arising near the apex of the pleural space.[128] The mass was thought to be arising from the stellate ganglion. Microscopically the tumor cells formed nests and clusters with cellular whorls. Psammoma bodies were present. Electron microscopy supported the diagnosis of a meningioma. In a study of 22 meningiomas by Schnitt and Vogel, all expressed epithelial membrane antigen.[129] Nine were at least focally expressive of S-100, and two had focal reactivity for cytokeratin (using the AE1/AE3 antibody cocktail). In contrast, all eight schwannomas failed to express epithelial membrane antigen and cytokeratin.

EPENDYMOMA

Doglioni and colleagues reported a 51-year-old patient with an ependymoma of the posterior mediastinum.[130] The tumor was not attached to the spine. Microscopically, the tumor had papillary and solid areas. The tumor cells were columnar with apically located nuclei and elongated fibrillary cytoplasmic process. Rare psammoma bodies were identified. Elongated tubules and ependymal rosettes were present in solid areas. The tumor expressed glial fibrillary acid protein and did not stain for cytokeratin.

CHORDOMA

Chordomas are tumors originating from the primitive notochord. Most are spheno-occipital or sacral. They have occurred as primary posterior mediastinal masses, usually adjacent to or extending from the spine.[37, 131–133] Histologically, these tumors have the characteristic, vacuolated "physaliferous" cells.

SUMMARY

Virtually any type of mesenchymal tumor can be located in the mediastinum. One tumor unique to the mediastinum is the thymolipoma, a lesion composed of mature adipose tissue with interspersed strands of thymus. Lipoma, hemangioma, hemangiopericytoma, and other benign mesenchymal tumors occur in the mediastinum as elsewhere. Mediastinal lymphangiomas are usually of the cystic type. Lymphangiomyoma occurs in adult females and is characterized by prominent smooth muscle around anastomosing lymphatic channels. All types of sarcomas have occurred in the mediastinum. In young adult men, the sarcomas may be associated with mediastinal germ cell tumors.

Any lesions of the thyroid and parathyroid may occur in the mediastinum. With regard to the thyroid, intrathoracic goiters, adenomas, and carcinomas have all been described. Ten to 20% of parathyroid adenomas and unusual cases of parathyroid carcinomas are mediastinal. Other unusual mediastinal tumors include meningioma, ependymoma, and chordoma.

REFERENCES

1. Boetsch CH, Swoyer GB, Adams A, Walker JH. Lipothymoma: report of two cases. Dis Chest 1966; 50:539–543.
2. Barnes RDS, O'Gorman P. Two cases of aplastic anaemia associated with tumours of the thymus. J Clin Pathol 1962; 15:264–268.
3. Jagadha V, Ramaswamy G. An unusual case of thymolipoma with hamartomatous changes [letter]. Arch Pathol Lab Med 1984; 108:611–612.
4. Reintgen D, Fetter BF, Roses A, McCarty KS Jr. Thymolipoma in association with myasthenia gravis. Arch Pathol Lab Med 1978; 102:463–466.
5. Yeh H-C, Gordon A, Kirschner PA, Cohen BA. Computed tomography and sonography of thymolipoma. AJR 1983; 140:1131–1133.
6. Dunn BH, Frkovich G. Lipomas of the thymus gland with an illustrative case report. Am J Pathol 1956; 32:41–50.
7. Peake JB, Ziegler MG. Thymolipoma: report of three cases. Am Surg 1977; 43:477–479.
8. Mok CK, Ho FCS, Nandi P, Ong GB. Lipothymoma. Med J Aust 1980; 1:272–274.
9. Hall GFM. A case of thymolipoma with observations on possible relations to intrathoracic lipomata. Br J Surg 1948; 36:321–324.
10. Korhonen LK, Laustela E. Thymolipoma: report of a case. Scand J Thorac Cardiovasc Surg 1968; 2:147–150.
11. Almog Ch, Weissberg D, Herczeg E, Pajewski M. Thymolipoma simulating cardiomegaly: a clinicopathological rarity. Thorax 1977; 32:116–120.
12. Lebrun E, Ajchenbaum F, Troussard X, Galateau F, Leporrier M, Lacombe C, Casadavall N, Varet B, Vernant JP, Dumont J, Binet JL, Piette M, Dreyfus B. Leucemie lymphoide chronique, erythroblastopenie, thymolipome. Nouv Rev Fr Hematol 1985; 27:29–37.
13. Pillai R, Yeoh N, Addis B, Peckham M, Goldstraw P. Thymolipoma in association with Hodgkin's disease. J Thorac Cardiovasc Surg 1985; 90:306–308.
14. Faerber EN, Balsara RK, Schidlow DV, Marmon LM, Zaeri N. Thymolipoma: computed tomographic appearances. Pediatr Radiol 1990; 20:196–197.
15. Shirkhoda A, Chasen MH, Eftekhari F, Goldman AM, Decaro LF. MR imaging of mediastinal thymolipoma. J Comput Assist Tomogr 1987; 11:364–365.
16. Chew FS, Weissleder R. Mediastinal thymolipoma. AJR 1991; 157:468.
17. Otto HF, Loning Th, Lachenmayer L, Janzen RWC, Gurtler KF, Fischer K. Thymolipoma in association with myasthenia gravis. Cancer 1982; 50:1623–1628.

18. Dyon JF, Paramelle B, Perdrix A, Pasquier B, Sarrazin R. [A case of thymolipoma in a child]. J Chir (Paris) 1979; 116:123–128.
19. Nishimura O, Naito Y, Noguchi Y, Matsuoka S, Takenaka K. Thymolipoma: a report of three cases. Jpn J Surg 1990; 20:234–237.
20. Le Marc'hadour F, Pinel N, Paszuier B, Dieny A, Stoebner P, Couderc P. Thymolipoma in association with myasthenia gravis. Am J Surg Pathol 1991; 15:802–809.
21. Benton C, Gerard P. Thymolipoma in a patient with Graves' disease. J Thorac Cardiovasc Surg 5193; 51:428–433.
22. Winarso P, Isherwood I, Photiou S, Donnelly RJ. Thymolipoma simulating cardiomegaly: use of computed tomography in diagnosis. Thorax 1982; 37:941–942.
23. Rubin M, Mishkin S. The relationship between mediastinal lipomas and the thymus. J Thorac Surg 1954; 27:494–502.
24. Rosai J, Levine GD. Tumors of the thymus. Washington, DC: Armed Forces Institute of Pathology, 1976:34–98.
25. Iseki M, Tsuda N, Kishikawa M, Shimada O, Hayashi T, Kawahara K, Tomita M. Thymolipoma with striated myoid cells: histological, immunohistochemical, and ultrastructural study. Am J Surg Pathol 1990; 14:395–398.
26. Heimann A, Sneige N, Shirkhoda A, Decaro LF. Fine needle aspiration cytology of thymolipoma: a case report. Acta Cytol 1987; 31:335–339.
27. Pachter MR, Lattes R. Mesenchymal tumors of the mediastinum: I. Tumors of fibrous tissue, adipose tissue, smooth muscle and striated muscle. Cancer 1963; 16:74–94.
28. Pachter MR, Lattes R. Mesenchymal tumors of the mediastinum: II. Tumors of blood vessel origin. Cancer 1963; 16:95–107.
29. Pachter MR, Lattes R. Mesenchymal tumors of the mediastinum: III. Tumors of lymph vascular origin. Cancer 1963; 16:108–117.
30. Handorf CR. Intrathoracic lipomas in children. South Med J 1982; 75:1403–1405.
31. Quinn SF, Monson M, Paling M. Spinal lipoma presenting as a mediastinal mass: diagnosis by CT. J Comput Assist Tomogr 1983; 7:1087–1089.
32. Kline ME, Patel BU, Agosti SJ. Noninfiltrating angiolipoma of the mediastinum. Radiology 1990; 175:737–738.
33. Bertrand G, Bidabe MC, George P, Dubin P, Touzard C. [Angiomyolipoma of the central mediastinum]. Ann Chir 1984; 38:679–681.
34. Fukuzawa J, Shimizu T, Sakai E, Ido A, Fujita Y, Tsuji T, Ohki Y, Kimura T, Fujita M, Onodera S. [Case report of angiomyolipoma of the posterior upper mediastinum]. Nippon Kyobu Shikkan Gakkai Zasshi 1992; 30:464–467.
35. Kim K, Koo BC, Davis JT, Franco-Saenz R. Primary myelolipoma of mediastinum. J Comput Assist Tomogr 1984; 8:119–123.
36. Suzuki T, Mushiaki T, Hori G, Tonozuka H, Suzuki H, Noguchi H, Sagawa F, Mitsuya T. [A case of primary myelolipoma of the posterior mediastinum]. Nippon Kyobu Shikkan Gakkai Zasshi 1988; 26:1318–1322.
37. Swanson PE. Soft tissue neoplasms of the mediastinum. Semin Diagn Pathol 1991; 8:14–34.
38. Homer MJ, Wechsler RJ, Carter BL. Mediastinal lipomatosis: CT confirmation of a normal variant. Radiology 1978; 128:657–661.
39. Lim YC. Mediastinal chondrolipoma. Am J Surg Pathol 1980; 4:407–409.
40. Ahn C, Harvey JC. Mediastinal hibernoma, a rare tumor. Ann Thorac Surg 1990; 50:828–830.
41. Enzinger FM, Weiss SW. Benign lipomatous tumors. *In* Soft Tissue Tumors. St. Louis: CV Mosby, 1988:301–346.
42. Coffin CM, Dehner LP. The soft tissues. *In* Stocker JT, Dehner LP, eds. Pediatric Pathology. Philadelphia: JB Lippincott, 1992:1091–1132.
43. Tabrisky J, Rowe JH, Christie SG, Weinstein ED, Asch M. Benign mediastinal lipoblastomatosis. J Pediatr Surg 1974; 9:399–401.
44. Dudgeon DL, Haller JA. Pediatric lipoblastomatosis: two unusual cases. Surgery 1984; 95:371–373.
45. Gindhart TD, Tucker WY, Choy SH. Cavernous hemangioma of the superior mediastinum: report of a case with electron microscopy and computerized tomography. Am J Surg Pathol 1979; 3:353–361.
46. Kelley MJ, Mannes EJ, Ravin CE. Mediastinal masses of vascular origin. A review. J Thorac Cardiovasc Surg 1978; 76:559–572.
47. Cohen AJ, Sbaschnig RJ, Hochholzer L, Lough FC, Albus RA. Mediastinal hemangiomas. Ann Thorac Surg 1987; 43:656–659.
48. Kings GLM. Multifocal haemangiomatous malformation: a case report. Thorax 1975; 30:485–488.
49. Kissel P, Andre JM, Regent D. Hemangiome tumoral du mediastin au cours d'une malade de Rendu-Osler. Evolution pendant 17 ans. Semin Hop Paris 1976; 52:2159–2160.
50. Enzinger FM, Weiss SW. Benign tumors and tumorlike lesions of blood vessels. *In* Soft Tissue Tumors. St. Louis: CV Mosby, 1988:489–532.
51. Lamovec J, Sobel HJ, Zidar A, Jerman J. Epithelioid hemangioendothelioma of the anterior mediastinum with osteoclast-like giant cells: light microscopic, immunohistochemical, and electron microscopic study. Am J Clin Pathol 1990; 93:813–817.
52. Weiss SW, Enzinger FM. Epithelioid hemangioendothelioma: a vascular tumor often mistaken for a carcinoma. Cancer 1982; 50:970–981.
53. Moreno A, Canadas MA, Minguella J, Torras J. Histiocytoid hemangioma of the innominate vein. Pathol Res Pract 1988; 183:785–788.
54. Yousem SA, Hochholzer L. Unusual thoracic manifestations of epithelioid hemangioendothelioma. Arch Pathol Lab Med 1987; 111:459–463.
55. Weidner N. Atypical tumor of the mediastinum: epithelioid hemangioendothelioma containing metaplastic bone and osteoclastlike giant cells. Ultrastruct Pathol 1991; 15:481–488.
56. Curley SA, Ablin DS, Kosloske AN. Giant cystic hygroma of the posterior mediastinum. J Pediatr Surg 1989; 24:398–400.
57. Shenoy SS, Barua NR, Patel AR, Culver GJ, Jennings EC. Mediastinal lymphangioma. J Surg Oncol 1978; 10:523–528.
58. Shin MS, Berland LL, Ho K-J. Mediastinal cystic hygromas: CT characteristics and pathogenetic consideration. J Comput Assist Tomogr 1985; 9:297–301.
59. Ramani P, Shah A. Lymphangiomatosis: histologic and immunohistochemical analysis of four cases. Am J Surg Pathol 1993; 17:329–335.
60. Gilsanz V, Yeh HC, Baron MG. Multiple lymphangiomas of the neck, axilla, mediastinum, and bones in an adult. Radiology 1976; 120:161–162.
61. Watts MA, Gibbons JA, Aaron BL. Mediastinal and osseous lymphangiomatosis: case report and review. Ann Thorac Surg 1982; 34:324–328.
62. Enzinger FM, Weiss SW. Tumors of lymph vessels. *In* Soft Tissue Tumors. St. Louis: CV Mosby, 1988:614–637.

63. Wolff M. Lymphangiomyoma: clinicopathologic study and ultrastructural confirmation of its histogenesis. Cancer 1973; 31:988–1007.
64. Cornog JL Jr. Lymphangiomyoma, a benign lesion of chyliferous lymphatics synonymous with lymphangiopericytoma. Cancer 1966; 19:1909–1930.
65. Enzinger FM, Weiss SW. Hemangiopericytoma. *In* Soft Tissue Tumors. St. Louis: CV Mosby, 1988:596–613.
66. Shaffer K, Pugatch RD, Sugarbaker DJ. Primary mediastinal leiomyoma. Ann Thorac Surg 1990; 50:301–302.
67. Uno A, Sakurai M, Onuma K, Yamane Y, Kurita K, Hayashi I, Ikeda M, Hagiwara N, Tominaga K, Hakozaki H. A case of giant mediastinal leiomyoma with long-term survival. Tohoku J Exp Med 1988; 156:1–6.
68. Miller R, Kurtz SM, Powers MJ. Mediastinal rhabdomyoma. Cancer 1978; 42:1983–1988.
69. Schlumberger HG. Tumors of mesenchymal derivatives. *In* Tumors of the Mediastinum. Washington, DC: Armed Forces Institute of Pathology, 1951:34–45.
70. Jaituni S, Arkee MSK, Caterine JM. Mediastinal myxoma. A case report. J Iowa Med Soc 1974; 64:107–110.
71. Feigin GA, Robinson B, Marchevsky A. Mixed tumor of the mediastinum. Arch Pathol Lab Med 1986; 110:80–81.
72. Verani R, Olson J, Moake JL. Intrathoracic extramedullary hematopoiesis. Report of a case in patient with sickle-cell disease-beta-thalassemia. Am J Clin Pathol 1980; 73:133–137.
73. Castleberry RP, Kelly DR, Wilson ER, Cain WS, Salter MR. Childhood liposarcoma. Report of a case and review of the literature. Cancer 1984; 54:579–584.
74. Plukker JT, Joosten HJ, Rensing JB, Van Haelst UJ. Primary liposarcoma of the mediastinum in a child. J Surg Oncol 1988; 37:257–263.
75. Razzuk MA, Urschel HC Jr, Race GJ, Kingsley WB, Paulson DL. Liposarcoma of the mediastinum. Case report and review of the literature. J Thorac Cardiovasc Surg 1971; 61:819–826.
76. Schweitzer DL, Aguam AS. Primary liposarcoma of the mediastinum. Report of a case and review of the literature. J Thorac Cardiovasc Surg 1977; 74:83–97.
77. Okumori M, Mabuchi M, Nakagawa M. Malignant thymoma associated with liposarcoma of the mediastinum—a case report. Jpn J Surg 1983; 13:512–518.
78. Shibata K, Koga Y, Onitsuka T, Wake N, Ishii K, Sekiya R, Sumiyoshi A. Primary liposarcoma of the mediastinum—a case report and review of the literature. Jpn J Surg 1986; 16:277–283.
79. Ferretti G, Pittet L, Pison C, Ranchoup Y, Le Marc'hadour F, Sarrazin R, Coulomb M. [Primary liposarcoma of the mediastinum: contribution of MRI to the diagnosis. Apropos of a case]. Rev Mal Respir 1992; 9:467–469.
80. Prohm P, Winter J, Ulatowski L. Liposarcoma of the mediastinum. Case report and review of the literature. Thorac Cardiovasc Surg 1981; 29:119–121.
81. Standerfer RJ, Armistead SH, Paneth M. Liposarcoma of the mediastinum: report of two cases and review of the literature. Thorax 1981; 36:693–694.
82. Sharma BS, McGuigan JA, Bharucha H, Bailey IC. Aggressive myxoid liposarcoma of mediastinum. Ulster Med J 1992; 61:193–197.
83. Havlicek F, Rosai J. A sarcoma of thymic stroma with features of liposarcoma. Am J Clin Pathol 1984; 82:217–224.
84. Morshuis WJ, Cox AL, Lacquet LK, Mravunac M, Barentsz JO. Primary malignant fibrous histiocytoma of the mediastinum. Thorax 1990; 45:154–155.
85. Muneta S, Kohno N, Matsuoka H, Hiwada K, Ueda N. Prolonged partial remission of malignant fibrous histiocytoma in posterior mediastinum by immunotherapy. Chest 1992; 101:1163–1165.
86. Pescarmona E, Remotti D, Marzullo A, Faraggiano T, Muda AO, Baroni CD. Fibrosarcoma of the thymic region: a case report. Tumori 1991; 77:363–366.
86a. Suster S, Moran CA, Koss MN. Rhabdomyosarcomas of the anterior mediastinum: Report of 4 cases unassociated with germ cell, teratomatous, or thymic carcinomatous components. Am J Surg Pathol 1994; 24:349–356.
86b. Begin LR, Schurch W, Lacoste J, Hiscott J, Melnychuk DA. Glycogen-rich clear cell rhabdomyosarcoma of the mediastinum. Am J Surg Pathol 1994; 18:302–308.
87. Eng J, Murday AJ. Leiomyosarcoma of the pulmonary artery. Ann Thorac Surg 1992; 53:905–906.
88. Bernheim J, Griffel B, Versano S, Bruderman I. Mediastinal leiomyosarcoma in the wall of a bronchial cyst [letter]. Arch Pathol Lab Med 1980; 104:221.
89. Steen BC, Florez Martin S, Fernandez Fau L, Garcia Tirado J, Jareno Esteban J, Ancochea Bermudez J. [Mediastinal leiomyosarcoma]. An Med Interna 1993; 10:83–85.
90. Gibbs AR, Johnson NF, Giddings JC, Powell DEB, Jasani B. Primary angiosarcoma of the mediastinum: light and electron microscopic demonstration of factor VIII–related antigen in neoplastic cells. Hum Pathol 1984; 15:687–691.
91. Greenwood SM, Meschter SC. Extraskeletal osteogenic sarcoma of the mediastinum. Arch Pathol Lab Med 1989; 113:430–433.
92. Ikeda T, Ishihara T, Yoshimatsu H, Kikuchi K, Murakami M, Kobayashi K, Inoue H, Kasahara M. Primary osteogenic sarcoma of the mediastinum. Thorax 1974; 29:582–588.
93. Yoshitake T, Takahama T, Suzuki T, Itoyama S, Oka T. [Osteosarcoma developing after radiation and chemotherapy for primary mediastinal seminoma]. Nippon Kyobu Geka Gakkai Zasshi 1991; 39:424–429.
94. Tarr RW, Kerner T, McCook B, Page DL, Nance EP, Kaye JJ. Primary extraosseus osteogenic sarcoma of the mediastinum: clinical, pathologic, and radiologic correlation. South Med J 1988; 81:1317–1319.
95. Chetty R. Extraskeletal mesenchymal chondrosarcoma of the mediastinum. Histopathology 1990; 17:261–278.
96. Pescarmona E, Rendina EA, Venuta F, Pisacane A, Baroni CD. Myxoid chondrosarcoma of the mediastinum. Appl Pathol 1989; 7:318–321.
97. Maschek H, Werner M, Busche G, Weinel P. Kongenitaler rhabdoidtumor in mediastinum und leber. Pathologe 1992; 13:172–178.
98. Lynch HT, Shurin SB, Dahms BB, Izant RJ, Lynch J, Danes BS. Paravertebral malignant rhabdoid tumor in infancy: in vitro studies of a familial tumor. Cancer 1983; 52:290–296.
99. Witkin GB, Miettinen M, Rosai J. A biphasic tumor of the mediastinum with features of synovial sarcoma: a report of four cases. Am J Surg Pathol 1989; 13:490–499.
100. Crist WM, Raney RB, Newton W, Lawrence W Jr, Tefft M, Foulkes MA. Intrathoracic soft tissue sarcomas in children. Cancer 1982; 50:598–694.
101. Ritchey ML, Bagnall JW, McDonald EC, Sago AL. Development of nongerm cell malignancies in nonseminomatous germ cell tumors. J Urol 1985; 134:146–149.

102. Manivel C, Wick MR, Abenoza P, Rosai J. The occurrence of sarcomatous components in primary mediastinal germ cell tumors. Am J Surg Pathol 1986; 10:711–717.
103. Cabellero C, Gomez S, Matias-Guiu X, Prat J. Rhabdomyosarcomas developing in association with mediastinal germ cell tumors. Virchows Arch [A] 1992; 420:539–543.
104. Heinemann MW, Lehman WL. Mediastinal mesenchymoma masquerading as liposarcoma. Cancer 1951; 4:692–696.
105. Enzinger FM, Weiss SW. Malignant tumors of uncertain histogenesis. *In* Soft Tissue Tumors. St. Louis: CV Mosby, 1988:929–965.
106. Hachitanda Y, Aoyama C, Sato JK, Shimada H. Pleuropulmonary blastoma in childhood: a tumor with divergent differentiation. Am J Surg Pathol 1993; 17:382–391.
107. Wychulis AR, Payne WS, Clagett OT, Woolner LB. Surgical treatment of mediastinal tumors: a 40 year experience. J Thorac Cardiovasc Surg 1971; 62:379–392.
108. Blegvad S, Lippert H, Simper LB, Dybdahl H. Mediastinal tumours. A report of 129 cases. Scand J Thorac Cardiovasc Surg 1990; 24:39–42.
109. Silverman NA, Sabiston DC Jr. Mediastinal masses. Surg Clin North Am 1980; 60:757–777.
110. Katlic MR, Wang C-A, Grillo HC. Substernal goiter. Ann Thorac Surg 1985; 39:391–399.
111. Mullen B, Richardson JD. Primary anterior mediastinal tumors in children and adults. Ann Thorac Surg 1986; 42:338–345.
112. Landreneau RJ, Nawarawong W, Boley TM, Johnson JA, Curtis JJ. Intrathoracic goiter: approaching the posterior mediastinal mass. Ann Thorac Surg 1991; 52:134–136.
113. De Andrade MA. A review of 128 cases of posterior mediastinal goiter. World J Surg 1977; 1:789–797.
114. Katlic MR, Grillo HC, Wang C-A. Substernal goiter: analysis of 80 patients from Massachusetts General Hospital. Am J Surg 1985; 149:283–287.
115. LiVolsi VA. Thyroid lesions in unusual places. *In* Surgical Pathology of the Thyroid. Philadelphia: WB Saunders, 1990:351–363.
116. Conn JM, Goncalves MA, Mansour KA, McGarity WC. The mediastinal parathyroid. Am Surg 1991; 57:62–67.
117. Nathaniels EK, Nathaniels AM, Wang CA. Mediastinal parathyroid tumors: a clinical and pathological study of 84 cases. Ann Surg 1970; 171:165–170.
118. Oldham HN Jr, Sabiston DC Jr. Primary tumors and cysts of the mediastinum. Monogr Surg Sci 1967; 4:243–279.
119. Doherty GM, Doppman JL, Miller DL, Gee MS, Marx SJ, Spiegel AM, Aurbach GD, Pass HI, Brennan MF, Norton JA. Results of a multidisciplinary strategy for management of mediastinal parathyroid adenoma as a cause of persistent primary hyperparathyroidism. Ann Surg 1992; 215:101–106.
120. Schlinkert RT, Whitaker MD, Argueta R. Resection of select mediastinal parathyroid adenomas through an anterior mediastinotomy. Mayo Clin Proc 1991; 66:1110–1113.
121. Russell CF, Edis AJ, Scholz DA, Sheedy PF, van Heerden JA. Mediastinal parathyroid tumors: experience with 38 tumors requiring mediastinotomy for removal. Ann Surg 1981; 193:805–809.
122. Wang C, Mahaffey JE, Axelrod L, Perlman JA. Hyperfunctioning supernumerary parathyroid glands. Surg Gynecol Obstet 1979; 148:711–714.
123. Wick MR, Rosai J. Neuroendocrine neoplasms of the mediastinum. Semin Diagn Pathol 1991; 8:35–51.
124. Castleman B, Roth SI. Tumors of the Parathyroid Glands. Washington, DC: Armed Forces Institute of Pathology, 1978.
125. Wolff M, Goodman EN. Functioning lipoadenoma of a supernumerary parathyroid. Head Neck Surg 1980; 2:302–307.
126. Putnam JB Jr, Schantz SP, Pugh WC, Hickey RC, Samaan NA, Garza R, Suda RW. Extended en bloc resection of a primary mediastinal parathyroid carcinoma. Ann Thorac Surg 1990; 50:138–140.
127. Murphy MN, Glennon PG, Diocee MS, Wick MR, Cavers DJ. Nonsecretory parathyroid carcinoma of the mediastinum: light microcopic, immunocytochemical and ultrastructural features of a case, and review of the literature. Cancer 1986; 58:2468–2476.
128. Wilson AJ, Ratliff JL, Lagios MD, Aguilar MJ. Mediastinal meningioma. Am J Surg Pathol 1979; 3:557–562.
129. Schnitt SJ, Vogel H. Meningiomas: diagnostic value of immunoperoxidase staining for epithelial membrane antigen. Am J Surg Pathol 1986; 10:640–649.
130. Doglioni C, Bontempini L, Iuzzolino P, Furlan G, Rosai J. Ependyoma of the mediastinum. Arch Pathol Lab Med 1988; 112:194–196.
131. Castellano GC, Johnston HW. Intrathoracic chordoma presenting as a posterior mediastinal tumor. South Med J 1975; 68:109–112.
132. Gregorius FK, Batzdorf U. Removal of thoracic chordoma by staged laminectomy and thoracotomy: case report. Am Surg 1979; 45:535–537.
133. Clemons RL, Blank RH, Hutcheson JB, Ruffolo EH. Chordoma presenting as a posterior mediastinal mass. A choristoma. J Thorac Cardiovasc Surg 1972; 63:922–924.

Appendix Nomenclature for Leukocyte Surface Antigens[1-3]

Cluster of Differentiation	Antibody*	Specificity
1	T6, Leu 6	Cortical thymocyte, Langerhans cell
2	T11, Leu 5	T cells (E-rosette receptor)
3	T3, Leu 4	T cells (antigen-receptor associated)
4	T4, Leu 3	T helper/inducer cells
5	T1, Leu 1	T cells, subset of B cells
6	T12	T cells, subset of B cells
7	Leu 9, 3A1	T cells, NK cells
8	T8, Leu 2	T suppressor/cytotoxic cells, NK cells
9	BA-2	Precursor B, B subset, neutrophils
10	CALLA	Common acute lymphoblastic leukemia antigen
11a	LFA-1 α chain	Leukocytes
11b	Mo1, Leu 15	C3bi receptor of monocytes, granulocytes, NK cells (CR3)
11c	Leu M5	C3bi receptor of monocytes, granulocytes, NK cells, hairy cell leukemia (CR4)
13	MY7, Leu M7	Granulocytes, monocytes
14	MY 4, Leu M3, Mo2	Monocytes
15	Leu M1	Granulocytes, monocytes
16	Leu 11a, b, c	IgG Fc receptor of NK cells, granulocytes
19	Leu 12, B4	B cells
20	Leu 16, B1	B cells
21	B2, CR2	C3d receptor of B cells, follicular dendritic cells
22	Leu 14, B3	B cells
23	Leu 20, B6	Activated B cells, activated monocytes
25	IL-2r	Interleukin-2 receptor of activated T and B cells, monocytes
30	Ki-1, BerH2	Activated lymphocytes
33	Leu M9, MY9	Early myeloid
34	MY10, HPCA-1	Early hematopoietic cell
35	CRI, To5	Complement receptor 3b of B cells, neutrophils, monocytes
38	Leu 17, T10	Immature and activated T cells, NK, plasma cells
41	Plt-1	Platelet glycoprotein IIb/IIIa
42b	AN51	Platelet glycoprotein Ib
43	Leu 22, L60, MT1	T cells, subset of B cells, neutrophils, monocytes, NK cells
45	LCA, T29/33, and 2B11	Pan-leukocyte
45RA	MB1, MT2, 4KB5	B cells, monocytes, subset of T cells, neutrophils
45RB	PD7/26	T-cell subset, B cells, granulocytes, monocytes
45RO	UCHL1	T cells, monocytes/macrophages, subset of B cells
56	Leu 19, NKH-1	NK cells, activated T cells
57	Leu 7, HNK-1	NK cells, subset of T cells
68	KP-1, EMB11	Monocytes/macrophages
69	Leu 23	Activated B and T cells, activated macrophages, NK cells
71	T9	Transferrin receptor on activated B and T cells, macrophages
74	LN2	HLA invariant chain on B cells, monocytes
w75	LN1, OKB4	B cells

*Leu antibodies are marketed by Becton-Dickinson (Mountain View, CA); B1, B2, B3, B4, B6, and MY are from Coulter Corp. (Hialeah, FL); UCHL1 and L26 are from Dako (Carpinteria, CA); L60 (Leu 22), Becton-Dickinson; Ber-H2 (CD30), L26 (CD20), 4KB5 (CD45RA), and UCHL1 (CD45RO), Dako; LN1 (CDw75) and LN2 (CD74), ICN (Lisle, IL) or Biotest (Fairfield, NJ); MT1 from Biotest; LCA from various companies.

Abbreviations: NK, natural killer; LCA, leukocyte common antigen.

Index

Note: Page numbers in *italics* refer to illustrations; numbers followed by t indicate tables.

A2B5 antibody, *18*, 20, 21, 25, 27
Abscess, Dubois', 53
ABVD (doxorubicin, bleomycin, vinblastine, and dacarbazine), for Hodgkin's disease, 139
Accutane (isotretinoin), thymic hypoplasia and, 58–59
Acetylcholine receptor (AchR), myasthenia gravis and, 34–36
  thymoma and, 105
Acid phosphatase, 22t
Acquired immunodeficiency syndrome (AIDS), angiofollicular lymphoid hyperplasia and, 141
  Hodgkin's disease and, 132
  thymic cyst and, *56*, 58
  thymic germinal centers and, 38
  thymoma and, 69
  thymus in, 48–51, 48t, *49*, 50t
  tuberculous mediastinal lymphadenopathy in, 164
ACTH. See *Adrenocorticotropic hormone (ACTH).*
Actin, in hemangiopericytoma, 227
  in pleuropulmonary blastoma, 220
  in solitary fibrous tumor, 218
  in thymic myoid cells, 23
ADA (adenosine deaminase), severe combined immunodeficiency disease and, 45, 47
Addison's disease, thymic germinal centers and, 38
  true thymic hyperplasia and, 43
Adenocarcinoma, poorly differentiated, metastases from, 159–160
Adenosine deaminase (ADA), severe combined immunodeficiency disease and, 45, 47
Adenosquamous carcinoma of thymus, histopathology of, 95, 95t, 96t, *98*
Adenovirus, 52
Adhesion molecules, 19, 125
Adrenal steroids, thymus and, 24t
Adrenalectomy, thymus and, 24t
Adrenocorticotropic hormone (ACTH), in paraganglioma, 198
  in thymic carcinoid, 191–192, 194
  in thymus, 24, 24t, 39
AIDS. See *Acquired immunodeficiency syndrome (AIDS).*
Allergic angiitis, thymus and, 53–54
Alopecia areata, thymoma and, 69t
Alpha-fetoprotein (AFP), in mediastinal germ cell tumors, 176, 176t, 179, 180, 184, 187
Alpha-thymosin, in normal thymus, 18t, 20, 24–25, 24t
  in stress-related thymic involution, 40
  in thymus of acquired immunodeficiency syndrome, 51
Anaplastic carcinoma of thymus, histopathology of, 95t, 96, 99–101, *100*
Anatomy, of mediastinum, 2–3, *2*, *3*
  of thymus, 14–16
Anemia, aplastic, thymic cyst and, 58
    thymoma and, 68, 69t
  autoimmune hemolytic, thymoma and, 69t
  pernicious, thymoma and, 69t
Anencephaly, true thymic hyperplasia and, 43
Angiitis, allergic, thymus and, 53–54
Angiofollicular lymphoid hyperplasia, 42, 139–144
  clinical features of, 139, 140t
  histopathology of, 139–142, 140t, *141*, *142*
  hyaline vascular, 139–141, *141*
  localized, 141–143
  pathogenesis of, 143–144
  plasma cell, 141, *142*
  systemic, 143
Angiolipoma, 225
Angiosarcoma, 228
  malignant schwannoma and, 203
  mediastinal germ cell tumors and, 175
Animals, mediastinal lymphoma in, 130–131
  mouse thymic virus in, 52
  paraganglioma in, 198
  thymic epithelial tumors in, 104
  with graft-vs.-host disease, 52
Ann Arbor staging system, for Hodgkin's disease, 132, 132t
Anoxia, in newborn, thymus and, 53
Anthrasilicotic nodule, in silicosis, 167, *168*
Antigen(s), heat-stable, 17
  leukocyte surface, 234t
  of lymphomas, 116–118, 117t, 118t, 123–125, 124t, 129–130, 135–137, 137t
  of thymic epithelial cells, *18*, 20–21
  of thymic lymphocytes, 17–19, *18*
  of thymomas, 87–88, 87t

Antigen receptor, T-cell, 17–19
 in Hodgkin's disease, 137
 in lymphoblastic lymphomas, 118–120
 in mediastinal lymphoma, 137
 in multicentric angiofollicular lymphoid hyperplasia, 143
 in thymoma, 88
 in thymoma-associated lymphocytosis, 69
Anti-P19. See *P19.*
Aortic body paraganglioma, 196–197
Aplastic anemia, thymic cyst and, 58
 thymoma and, 68, 69t
Apoptosis, 19
Askin tumor (peripheral primitive neuroectodermal tumor, peripheral neuroepithelioma), 206–207, *207*
Aspiration, fine needle. See *Fine needle aspiration biopsy (FNAB).*
Asteroid bodies, in sarcoidosis, 166, *167*
Asteroid cells, 19, *19*
Ataxia-telangiectasia, thymus in, 48
ATPase, 22t
Auditory meatus, external, embryology of, *27*

B lymphocytes, thymic, 19
 in myasthenia gravis, 36
 in thymoma, 88
B72.3, 104
Bands, fibrous. See *Fibrous bands.*
Bare lymphocyte syndrome, 45, 47
 thymus in, 47
Basal lamina, in thymoma, 89
Basaloid carcinoma of thymus, histopathology of, 95t, 96t, 99, *102*
Basedow's disease. See *Graves' disease.*
B-cell lymphoma, of mediastinum, 123
 of mucosa-associated lymphoid tissue (MALT), 127–128, *127*
Bcl–2 gene rearrangement, absence of, in large cell lymphoma, 127
Beckwith-Weidemann syndrome, true thymic hyperplasia and, 43
Beta-endorphin, thymic, 24
Beta-enolase, in thymic myoid cells, 23
Beta-F1 antibody, in lymphoblastic lymphoma, 118–119, 118t
Beta–2 microglobulin, 28
Biopsy, fine needle aspiration. See *Fine needle aspiration biopsy (FNAB).*
Birbeck granules, 22, 38, 145
Blalock, Alfred, 11–12, 12t
Blastoma, pleuropulmonary, 228
Blastomycosis, 166
Bone, benign tumors of, 228
Bone marrow transplantation, for Hodgkin's disease, 139
 for immunodeficiency, 48
 for lymphoblastic lymphoma, 121
 thymus and, 47, 51–52
Bronchogenic cyst, 210–211, 211t, *212*

Calcitonin, in paraganglioma, 198
CALLA (common acute lymphoblastic leukemia antigen). See *CD10.*
Canal, of Kursteiner, 26, *28*
Candidiasis, mucocutaneous, thymoma and, 69t
Carcinoembryonic antigen (CEA), absence of, in mesothelial cells, 162
 in mesothelioma, 220
 in thymic carcinoma, 104
 in thymic epithelial cell tumors, 87t, 88
Carcinoid, thymic, 191–195
 cell of origin of, 195
 clinical features of, 191–192, 192t
 histologic differential diagnosis of, 192–193
 immunohistochemistry of, 193–194
 paraganglioma vs., 198
 pathology of, 192–195, *193–195*
 therapy and prognosis for, 195
 ultrastructure of, 194, *195*
Carcinoma, embryonal, differential diagnosis of, 187
 embryoid body in, 184
 immunohistochemistry of, 176t
 microscopic features of, 184, *185*
 follicular, of thyroid, in mediastinal goiter, 229
 metastatic, 158–162
  from extrathoracic sites, 158–159, 159t, 160
  from lung, 158
  from unknown primary tumor, 159–160
  immunohistochemistry of, 160–161, *161*
  karyotypic analysis for, 161–162
 papillary, of thyroid, in mediastinal goiter, 229
 primary, frequency of, 1t
 squamous cell, metastatic, 158
  of thymus, 95t, 96, *96–97,* 99, *99,* 101
   pseudoepitheliomatous hyperplasia vs., 54
   thymic cyst and, 58, 212t
 thymic, 94–104. See also specific carcinoma.
  clinical features of, 94–95
  defined, 67, 68t
  differential diagnosis of, 101–104
  gross pathology of, 95, *96*
  histologic grading of, 95, 96t, 101
  histopathology of, 95–101, 95t, 96t, *97–102*
  immunopathology of, 103
  prognostic factors for, 96t, 101
  therapy and prognosis for, 96t, 101, 103, 162
  thymoma vs., 71, 103, 104
  undifferentiated, 99
 undifferentiated, differential diagnosis of, 187
Carcinoma showing thymus-like differentiation (CASTLE), 70–71
Carney's triad, 196
Cartilage, benign tumors of, 228
Caseating granuloma, from tuberculosis, 164, *165*
CASTLE (carcinoma showing thymus-like differentiation), 70–71
Castleman's disease. See *Angiofollicular lymphoid hyperplasia.*
Castration, thymic size and, 24t, 43
Catecholamine, thymic size and, 24t
CD (cluster of differentiation) number, 17, 234t
CD1, in histiocytosis X, 146
 in myasthenic thymus, 36
 in normal thymus, *18, 19,* 22, 22t
 in T-cell lymphoblastic lymphoma, 117–119, 117t, 118t
 in thymic carcinoma, 103
 in thymic involution, 40
 in thymoma, 82t, 85, 88
CD2, in Hodgkin's disease, 136
 in normal thymus, *18*

CD2 *(Continued)*
in T-cell lymphoblastic lymphoma, 117–119, 117t, 118t
in thymoma-associated lymphocytosis, 69
in thymus of severe combined immunodeficiency, 46
CD3, in normal thymus, 17, *18,* 24
in T-cell lymphoblastic lymphoma, 117–119, 117t, 118t
in thymoma, 88
in thymoma-associated lymphocytosis, 69
CD4, OKT4 epitope of, in Good's syndrome, 68
in normal thymus, 17, *18, 28–29*
in T-cell lymphoblastic lymphoma, 117t, 118t, 119
in thymus of acquired immunodeficiency syndrome, 51
in thymus of severe combined immunodeficiency, 46
CD5, in mediastinal large-cell lymphoma, 124t
in normal thymus, *18*
in T-cell lymphoblastic lymphoma, 118t, 119
in thymoma-associated lymphocytosis, 69
CD7, in normal thymus, *18*
in T-cell lymphoblastic lymphoma, 117t, 118t, 119
in thymoma-associated lymphocytosis, 69
CD8, in normal thymus, 17, *18,* 28–29
in T-cell lymphoblastic lymphoma, 117t, 118t, 119
in thymus of acquired immunodeficiency syndrome, 51
in thymus of severe combined immunodeficiency, 46
CD10, in mediastinal lymphoma, 124, 124t
in T-cell lymphoblastic lymphoma, 117, 118t
CD11c, in mediastinal large cell lymphoma, 124, 124t
CD11-CD18, immunodeficiency, 48
CD15, in Hodgkin's disease, 136–138, 137t, 182
in large cell anaplastic lymphoma, 130
mesothelioma vs. carcinoma, 220
CD16, in T-cell lymphoblastic lymphoma, 117, 118t
CD19, in mediastinal large cell lymphoma, 123, 124t
in thymus, 19
CD20, in evaluation of poorly differentiated neoplasms, 160
in Hodgkin's disease, 136–138, 137t
in mediastinal large cell lymphoma, 123, 124t
in myasthenic thymus, 36
in thymoma, 88
in thymus, 19, *19*
CD21, in mediastinal large cell lymphoma, 124–125, 124t
in thymus, 19
CD22, in mediastinal large cell lymphoma, 124t
in thymus, 19
CD25, 118t
CD30 (Ki–1), in Hodgkin's disease, 136–137, 137t
in large cell anaplastic lymphoma, 129–130, *129,* 161, 182
in mediastinal large cell lymphoma, 126
CD34, in solitary fibrous tumors, 218
in thymus, 19
CD38, in mediastinal large cell lymphoma, 124t
CD43, in acute leukemia, 147
in Hodgkin's disease, 137t
CD43 *(Continued)*
in large cell anaplastic lymphoma, 130
in large cell lymphoma, 124, 124t
in T-cell lymphoblastic lymphoma, 118t
in Wiskott-Aldrich syndrome, 48
CD44, in thymus, 19
CD45 (leukocyte common antigen), in evaluation of poorly differentiated neoplasms, 160
in Hodgkin's disease, 136–138, 137t
in large cell anaplastic lymphoma, 129
in large cell lymphoma, 123, 124t, 182, 187
CD45RA, in Hodgkin's disease, 137t
CD45RO, in Hodgkin's disease, 137t
in large cell lymphoma, 124, 124t
in T-cell lymphoblastic lymphoma, 118t
CD57 (Leu 7), in carcinoid, 194
in primitive neuroectodermal tumor (PNET), 206
in T-cell lymphoblastic lymphoma, 117, 118t
in thymomas, 87, 87t
in thymus, 18
CD68 (KP–1), in acute myeloid leukemia, 147
in pleuropulmonary blastoma, 228
CD74 (LN2), in Hodgkin's disease, 137, 137t
in thymic interdigitating cells, 22t
CDw45 antigen, 124
CDw75 (LN1), in Hodgkin's disease, 137, 137t
in mediastinal large cell lymphoma, 124, 124t
CEA. See *Carcinoembryonic antigen (CEA).*
Cell adhesion, integrin and, 19
Cell proliferation indices, for lymphoblastic lymphoma, 119
Cell-mediated immune system, thymus and, 10, 29
Cellular atypia, in thymoma, 75, 78
Cellular schwannoma, 202
Chemotherapy, for carcinoid, 195
for germ cell tumors, 183, 187
for Hodgkin's disease, 139
for large cell lymphoma, 127
for lymphoblastic lymphoma, 121
for thymic carcinoma, 101
for thymoma, 94
thymic enlargement and, 42–43
Chloroma, 146–147
Cholesterol granuloma, in thymic cyst, *58*
Chondrolipoma, 225
Chondroma, 228
Chondrosarcoma, 228
malignant schwannoma and, 203
CHOP (cyclophosphamide, doxorubicin, vincristine, and prednisone), for large-cell lymphoma, 127
Chordoma, 230
Choriocarcinoma, antigens expressed by, 176t
microscopic features of, 184–187, *186*
Chorionic gonadotropin, human (HCG), in mediastinal germ cell tumors, 176, 176t
thymic, 24–25
Choristoma of the thymus, 55
Chromaffin reactivity, in paraganglioma, 196
Chromatin, in thymoma, 89
Chromogranin, in neuroectodermal tumors, 206
in paraganglioma, 196
in thymic carcinoid, 87, 193–194
in thymic epithelial cell tumor, 87, 87t
Chromosome 12, in germ cell tumors, 173–174
Chromosome 22, in DiGeorge syndrome, 44–45
Churg-Strauss syndrome, thymus and, 53–54

Cisplatin, for germ cell tumor, 161–162
CK. See *Cytokeratin (CK).*
Clear cell carcinoma of thymus, 95t, 96t, 99–101
Cluster of differentiation (CD) number, 17, 234t
CMV (cytomegalovirus), thymus and, 52–53
C-myc oncogene, in large cell lymphoma, 127
Coccidioidomycosis, 166
Colitis, ulcerative, thymoma and, 69t
Collagen vascular disease, mixed, thymoma and, 69t
Colony stimulating factor, 25
Common acute lymphoblastic leukemia antigen (CALLA, CD10), 124, 124t
 in lymphoblastic lymphoma, 117, 118t
Computed tomography (CT), in detection of mediastinal tumors, 4
Cortical epithelial cells, in thymus, electron microscopy of, 20, *20*
"Cortical" thymoma, 82t, 83–85, *84*
Corticomedullary differentiation, in myasthenia gravis, 37
 in thymus, after bone marrow transplantation, 51
  age-related changes of, 25
  embryology of, 28
  in acquired immunodeficiency syndrome, 48–50, 48t, 49, 50t
  in congenital immunodeficiencies, 45, *46,* 47–48, 50t
  in histiocytosis X, 146
  stress-related changes, 39, 50t
Creatine kinase, in thymic myoid cells, 23
Crohn's disease, thymoma and, 69t
Cryptococcosis, 166
CT. See *Computed tomography (CT).*
Cushing's syndrome, endocrine tumor and, 2
 thymic carcinoid and, 191–192, 194, *195*
Cyclophosphamide, doxorubicin, vincristine, and prednisone (CHOP), for large cell lymphoma, 127
Cyclosporin A, thymic involution with, 52
Cyst, 54–58, *55–58,* 210–215, 211t, *212, 214*
 bronchogenic, 210–211, *212*
 distribution of, 2t
 enteric, 211–213, 211t
 frequency of, 1t
 gastroenteric, 211t, 212–213
 hydatid, 5, 214
 in mediastinal Hodgkin's disease, 134, *134*
 in mediastinal lymphomas, 122
 in thymoma, frequency of, 72t
 lymphatic, 211t, 213–214
 meningocele, 214
 mesothelial, 211t, 213
 neoplasm vs., 211t, 213
 of thoracic duct, 211t, 213
 parathyroid, 211t, 214
 pericardial, 213
 pseudoepithelial hyperplasia in, 54–55, *57*
 thymic, 54–58, *55–58*
  acquired immunodeficiency syndrome and, *56,* 58
  aplastic anemia and, 58
  cholesterol granuloma in, *58*
  differential diagnosis, 58
  germinal centers in, 55, *57*
  gross features, 54–55
  histopathology of, 54–55, *55–57*
  lymphoma and, 58
  mediastinal seminoma vs., 181–182
Cyst *(Continued)*
  multilocular, 55–58, *56, 57*
  myasthenia gravis, 58
  radiographic appearance, 54
  Sjögren's syndrome and, 58
  squamous cell carcinoma and, 58, *96*
  surgical trauma and, 58
  thymic carcinoma and, 58
  thymoma and, 58
  unilocular, 54–55, *55*
Cystic Hassall's corpuscles, 21, 53
Cystic hygroma. See *Cystic lymphangioma.*
Cystic lymphangioma, 211t, 226, *227*
Cystic teratoma, 177–178, *178*
Cystic thymic seminoma, 58, 181, *181*
Cystic thymoma, 58, 71, 78, *82*
Cytogenetics, of germ cell tumors, 173
 of large cell anaplastic lymphoma, 129
 of lymphoblastic lymphoma, 119
Cytokeratin (CK), in carcinoid, 194
 in entrapped thymic epithelium, 123
 in germ cell tumors, 175–176, 176t
 in melanoma, absence of, 161
 in mesothelioma, 220
 in mesothelioma vs. solitary fibrous tumor, 219
 in paraganglioma, 197
 in pleuropulmonary blastoma, 228
 in thymic epithelial cell tumors, 87, 87t
 in thymic epithelial cells, 20, *21,* 22
Cytokine, thymic, 25
Cytologic atypia, in thymoma, *75,* 78
Cytomegalovirus (CMV), thymus and, 52–53
Cytopathology, Diff-Quik stain for, 86
 of Hodgkin's disease, 137–138, *138*
 of large cell lymphoma, 125–126, *126*
 of lymphoblastic lymphoma, 116, *117,* 120
 of neuroblastoma, *205*
 of schwannoma, *203*
 of seminoma, 181, *182*
 of thymic carcinoma, 103–104, *103*
 of thymoma, 86–87, *86*

del(12q), germ cell tumors and, 173
Dendritic cells, interdigitating, 22, *22*
Dermatomyositis, thymoma and, 69t
Dermoid, 176
Desmin, in pleuropulmonary blastoma, 228
 in solitary fibrous tumor, 218
 in thymic myoid cells, 23
Desmoplastic mesothelioma, 220, *220*
Desmosomes, in thymoma, 88–89
DiGeorge, A.M., 43–44
DiGeorge syndrome, 28, 43–45
 thymus in, 50t
Dioxin, thymus and, 58
DNA ploidy, in carcinoid tumor, 194
 in germ cell tumor, 172–173
 in Hodgkin's disease, 137
 in large cell lymphoma, 125
 in lymphoblastic lymphoma, 119
 in neuroblastoma, 206
 in paraganglioma, 198
 in thymic carcinoma, 103–104
 in thymoma, 91
Down's syndrome, thymus and, 54
Doxorubicin, bleomycin, vinblastine, and dacarbazine (ABVD), for Hodgkin's disease, 139

Dubois' abscess, 53
Dysinvolution, of thymus, in AIDS, 48t, 49–50
Dysplasia, of thymus, defined, 43

Ear, embryology, *27*
EBV. See *Epstein-Barr virus (EBV).*
Echinococcosis, hydatid cyst and, 5, 214
Ectopic hamartomatous thymoma, 70
Eggshell radiographic pattern, in silicosis, 167
Electron microscopy, of carcinoid, 194, *195*
  of endodermal sinus tumor, 184, *186*
  of meningioma, 230
  of mesothelioma, 220
  of neuroblastoma, 206
  of paraganglioma, 198
  of pleuropulmonary blastoma, 228
  of primitive neuroectodermal tumor, 206
  of schwannoma, 202
  of seminoma, 182, *182*
  of solitary fibrous tumor, 218
  of thymoma, 88–89, *89*
  of thymus, 20, *20*
Embryoid body, in embryonal carcinoma, 184
Embryology, of thymus, 25–29, *27*
Embryonal carcinoma, antigens expressed by, 176t
  differential diagnosis of, 187
  microscopic features of, 184, *185*
Encephalitis, limbic, thymoma and, 69t
Endocrine interactions, with thymus, 24t
Endocrine lesions, 229
Endocrine tumor, Cushing's syndrome and, 2
  distribution of, 2t
  frequency of, 1t
Endodermal sinus tumor, antigens expressed by, 176t
  differential diagnosis of, 187
  microscopic features of, 184, *185, 186*
Endorphin, thymic, 24
Enteric cyst, 211–213, 211t
Enterochromaffin cells, 25
  thymic carcinoid and, 195
Eosinophils, thymic, 16, 23
Ependymoma, 230
Epidermal growth factor, 105
Epidermal growth factor receptors, 25
Epithelial cells, thymic, 19–21
    cytokeratin in, 20, *21,* 22
    electron microscopy of, 20, *20*
    immunoreactivity of, 18
    subcapsular vs. medullary, 20–21
    tumors of, 67–106. See also *Carcinoma, thymic; Thymoma;* specific tumor.
      definitions of, 67, 68t
      in animals, 104
      Leu-7 (CD57) antigen in, 87t
      pathogenesis of, 104–106
Epithelial membrane antigen (EMA), in CD30-positive large cell anaplastic lymphoma, 129
  in Hodgkin's disease, 137t
  in mediastinal germ cell tumors, 176, 176t
  in meningioma, 228
  in thymic epithelial cell tumors, 87, 87t, 103–104
  mediastinal lymphoma and, 123
Epithelial thymoma, cytopathology of, 86
  histopathology of, 72, *75, 79–81, 84*
  immunohistochemistry of, 88
Epithelial thymoma *(Continued)*
  prognosis, 91, 92t, 93t
  reticular pattern in, *72, 80*
  thymic carcinoma vs., 103
Epithelioid hemangioendothelioma, 226
Epstein-Barr virus (EBV), Hodgkin's disease and, 131, 138–139
  in angiofollicular lymphoid hyperplasia, 144
  in large cell lymphoma (absence of), 127
  thymic epithelial tumors and, 104–106
Erythroleukemia, mediastinal germ cell tumors and, 174
Esophageal cyst, 211–213, 211t
Esterase, 22t
Ewing's sarcoma, primitive neuroectodermal tumor and, 206

Fibronectin, 36, 88
Fibronectin receptor, 18
Fibrosarcoma, 228
Fibrous bands, in large cell lymphoma, 122
  in thymoma, 72, 72t, *78*
Fibrous histiocytoma, malignant, 228
Fibrous tumor, solitary, 217–219, *217, 218*
Fine needle aspiration (FNA), 4, 5
Fine needle aspiration biopsy (FNAB), 4–5
  Diff-Quik stain for, 86
  in Hodgkin's disease, 137–138, *138*
  in large cell lymphoma, 125–126
  in lymphoblastic lymphoma, 116, 120
  in mediastinal cyst, 210
  in mediastinal Hodgkin's disease, 137–138, *138*
  in neuroblastoma, *205*
  in seminoma, 181, *182*
  in thymoma, 86
  in true thymic hyperplasia, 41
FK506, 52
FNA. See *Fine needle aspiration biopsy (FNAB).*
FNAB. See *Fine needle aspiration biopsy (FNAB).*
Follicle stimulating hormone, in thymus, 24
Follicular carcinoma, of thyroid, in mediastinal goiter, 229
Follicular center cell lymphoma, extra-mediastinal, mediastinal large cell lymphoma vs., 124t
Frozen sections, 85, 103, 125

Galen, 9
Ganglia, sympathetic, tumors, 204–206, *205, 207*
Ganglioneuroblastoma, 204, *205*
Ganglioneuroma, 204–206, *207*
Gastroenteric cyst, 211t, 212–213
Gene rearrangement, in Hodgkin's disease, 137
  in mediastinal lymphoma, 125
  in multicentric angiofollicular lymphoid hyperplasia, 143
  in T-cell lymphoblastic lymphoma, 118–120
  in thymoma, 88
  in thymoma-associated lymphocytosis, 69
Gene therapy, for congenital immunodeficiency, 40
Germ cell tumors, mediastinal, 172–188
    chemotherapy for, 161–162
    cytogenetics of, 173–174
    distribution of, 2t

Germ cell tumors *(Continued)*
DNA ploidy in, 172
frequency of, 1t
hematologic malignancy and, 174–175
immunopathology of, 175–176, 182, 187
nonseminomatous malignant, 183–187, *184–186*
pathogenesis of, 173
sarcoma and, 175, *175*
seminoma, 179–183, *181–183*
teratoma, 176–179, *177–180*
Germinal center hyperplasia, of thymus, 19, 34–39, 35
Germinal centers, in thymic cyst, 55, *57*
in thymoma, 78, *83*
thymic, 35, *38*
Giant lymph node hyperplasia. See *Angiofollicular lymphoid hyperplasia.*
Giant lymphoma, benign. See *Angiofollicular lymphoid hyperplasia.*
Gland-like structures, in thymoma, 78, *81*
Glucagon, in paraganglioma, 198
Glucocorticoid receptors, 40
Gonadotropin, human chorionic, in mediastinal germ cell tumor, 176, 176t
Good's syndrome, thymus and, 68, 69t
Graft-vs.-host disease, thymus and, 47, 51–52
Granulocytic sarcoma, 146–147
Granuloma, caseating, from tuberculosis, 53, 164, *165*
cholesterol, in thymic cyst, *58*
with ruptured thymic cyst, 53
Granulomatous lymphadenopathy, 164–168
acute mediastinitis and, 168
histoplasmosis and, 165–166
sarcoidosis and, 166, *167*
sclerosing mediastinitis and, 168–170
silicosis and, 166–168, *168*
tuberculous, 164–165, *165*
Granulomatous thymoma. See *Hodgkin's disease.*
Graves' disease, thymic enlargement and, 43
thymic germinal centers and, 30
thymoma and, 69t
Growth factors, thymic, 25
Growth hormone, 24
GVH (graft-vs.-host disease), thymus and, 47, 51–52

Hairy cell leukemia, 147
Hamartomatous thymoma, ectopic, 70
Hamazaki-Wesenberg bodies, in sarcoidosis, 166, *167*
Harington, H., 43–44
Hashimoto's disease, thymic germinal centers and, 38
Hassall, A.H., 10
Hassall's corpuscle (HC), *35*
after bone marrow transplantation, 51
after cyclosporin A therapy, 52
in acquired immunodeficiency syndrome, 48t, 49–50, 50t
in congenital immunodeficiency, 45–47, 50t
in graft-vs.-host disease, 52
in malnutrition, 53
in stress-related changes, 40
in thymic carcinoma, 103
in thymoma, 72, 72t, 73, 87
in thymus, 10, *17, 18,* 21–22, *21,* 29
HC. See *Hassall's corpuscle (HC).*
H-CAM antigen, 19
HCG. See *Human chorionic gonadotropin (HCG).*
Heat stable antigen (HSA), 17
Hemangioendothelioma, epithelioid, 226
Hemangioma, 225–226
Hemangiopericytoma, 226–227
paraganglioma vs., 198
Hematologic malignancy, mediastinal germ cell tumor and, 174–175
Hematopoiesis, in thymus, 23
Hemolytic anemia, autoimmune, thymoma and, 69t
Hemophagocytic syndrome, mediastinal germ cell tumor and, 174
Herbicides, thymus and, 58
Hibernoma, 225
Hilar lymph nodes, 3, 4t
Histiocytoid hemangioma, 226
Histiocytoma, malignant fibrous, 228
Histiocytosis, malignant, mediastinal germ cell tumor and, 174
Histiocytosis X, 144–146, *145*
Histioeosinophilic granuloma, histiocytosis X vs., 146
in thymus, myasthenia gravis and, 38
Histochemistry, of carcinoid, 193
of paraganglioma, 197
of thymoma, 87
Histoplasma capsulatum, histoplasmosis and, 165–166
Histoplasmosis, 105–106
sclerosing mediastinitis and, 168, 169
HIV–1. See *Human immunodeficiency virus (HIV–1).*
HLA antigens, association with myasthenia gravis, 38
classes, 21, 29
in T-cell lymphoblastic lymphoma, 118t
in thymoma, 88
in thymus, 21, 29
HLA-DR, in thymoma, 88
in thymus, 21, 22t
after bone marrow transplantation, 51
stress-related changes of, 40
HMB–45, in melanoma, 161
in melanotic schwannoma, 203
Hodgkin's disease, 2, 131–139
Ann Arbor staging system for, 132, 132t
clinical features of, 131–132
cytopathology of, 137–138, *138*
epidemiology of, 131
histiocytosis X vs., 145–146
histopathology of, 132–136, *133–136*
in AIDS patients, 132
lymphocyte depleted type, 135–136
lymphocyte predominant type, 134–135, *135*
mixed cellularity type, 135, *136*
molecular pathology of, 137
nodular sclerosing type, 132–134
seminoma vs., 182
pathogenesis of, 138–139
prognosis and therapy for, 139
Rye classification of, 132
thymic cyst and, 58
Homing receptors, 19
Hormones, thymic, 23–25, 24t
Horner's syndrome, 2
"Hourglass" lipoma, 225
HSA (heat stable antigen), 17

Human chorionic gonadotropin (HCG), in mediastinal germ cell tumor, 176, 176t
  thymic, 25
Human immunodeficiency virus (HIV–1), thymus and, 51
Hürthle cell carcinoma, in mediastinal goiter, 229
Hydatid cyst, 5, 214
Hygroma, cystic, 211t, 226, *227*
Hypercalcemia, endocrine tumor and, 2
Hyperplasia, angiofollicular. See *Angiofollicular lymphoid hyperplasia.*
  pseudoepitheliomatous, 57
  thymic, with massive enlargement. See *True thymic hyperplasia (TTH).*
Hypertension, endocrine tumor and, 2
Hyperthyroidism, endocrine tumor and, 2
  true thymic hyperplasia and, 43
Hypogammaglobulinemia, thymoma and, 68, 69t
Hypophysectomy, thymic size and, 24

i(12p), germ cell tumor and, 173
Imaging, of mediastinum, 3–4
Immune response, cell-mediated, thymus and, 29
  T lymphocytes and, 29
  thymus and, 10
Immunodeficiency disorders, primary, thymic dysplasia and, 45–48, *46*
Immunoglobulin, cell surface, in large cell lymphoma, 124–125
  in thymus, 19
Immunoglobulin gene rearrangements, in angiofollicular lymphoid hyperplasia, 143
  in Hodgkin's disease, 137
  in large cell lymphoma, 125
  in lymphoblastic lymphoma, 119
  in thymoma, 88
Immunohistochemistry, for diagnosis of carcinoma of unknown primary site, 160–161
  of angiofollicular lymphoid hyperplasia, 142–143
  of carcinoid, 193–194
  of germ cell tumors, 175–176, 176t, 182, 187
  of granulocytic sarcoma, 147
  of histiocytosis X, 146
  of Hodgkin's disease, 136–137, 137t, 138
    in differential diagnosis of, 134
  of large cell anaplastic lymphoma, 129
  of large cell lymphoma, 123–125, 124t
  of lymphoblastic lymphoma, 116–118, 117t, 118t
  of meningioma, 230
  of mesothelioma, 220
  of metastatic disease, 160–162
  of neuroectodermal tumors, 206–207
  of paraganglioma, 197
  of pleuropulmonary blastoma, 228
  of schwannoma, 202–203
  of solitary fibrous tumor, 218
  of thymoma, 87–88
  of thymus, 18–21, 23
    in acquired immunodeficiency syndrome, 50
    in myasthenia gravis, 36
  of true thymic hyperplasia, 42
Immunopathology. See *Immunohistochemistry.*
Immunoperoxidase. See *Immunohistochemistry.*
Infection, 164–170
  thymus and, 52–53
Inflammation, 164–170
Integrins, 19
Interdigitating dendritic cells, thymic, 22, *22*
Interleukin–1, 23
Interleukin–2, cyclosporin A and, 52
Interleukin–6, 25
  angiofollicular lymphoid hyperplasia and, 143–144
"Inverted" histologic pattern, in thymus, 39–40, *40*
Isotretinoin (Accutane), thymic hypoplasia and, 58–59

Kaposi's sarcoma, thymoma and, 69t
Karyotypic analysis. See also *DNA ploidy;* specific chromosome.
  for diagnosis of metastases, 162
Ketoconazole, for sclerosing mediastinitis, 170
Ki–1 large-cell anaplastic lymphoma, 122, 129–130, *129*
Ki–67 immunoreactivity, in large-cell lymphoma, 125
  in lymphoblastic lymphoma, 119
  in thymoma, 88
  in thymus, stress-related changes of, 40
Klinefelter's syndrome, primary mediastinal germ cell tumor and, 174
Kultschitsky's cells, thymic, 25
  thymic carcinoid and, 195
Kursteiner, canal of, 26, *28*
Kwashiorkor, 53

Laminin, 18, 34, 37
  in thymoma, 88
Langerhans cell(s), 22
Langerhans cell histiocytosis, 144–146, *145*
Large-cell lymphoma, 121–127
  anaplastic, CD30-positive, 129–130, *129*
    CD43 in, 129
    epithelial membrane antigen (EMA) in, 129
  clinical features of, 121, 122t
  cytopathology of, 125–126
  differential diagnosis of, 126
  DNA ploidy and cell proliferation indices for, 125
  germ cell tumor vs., 187
  histopathology of, 121–123, *123*
  immunopathology of, 123–125, 124t
  molecular pathology of, 125
  pathogenesis of, 127
  prognosis and therapy for, 122t, 127
  seminoma vs., 182
  with tropism for germinal centers, 128, *128*
LCA (leukocyte common antigen). See *CD45 (leukocyte common antigen).*
Leiomyoma, 227–228
Leiomyosarcoma, 175, *175*, 211, 228
Leu 7 (CD57), 18, 21
  in carcinoid, 194
  in PNET, 194
  in thymic epithelial tumors, 87t
Leu 8, 19

Leukemia(s), acute myeloid, 147
  hairy cell, 147
  mediastinal germ cell tumor and, 174
  T-cell lymphoblastic lymphoma vs., 117, 117t
Leukemia/lymphoma, T cell, 128–129
Leukocyte common antigen (LCA). See *CD45 (leukocyte common antigen).*
Lewis X antigen, in Hodgkin's disease, 136
Limbic encephalitis, thymoma and, 69t
Lipoblastoma, 225, 228
Lipoma, 224–225
Liposarcoma, 228
LN1 (CDw75), 124
  in Hodgkin's disease, 137t
LN2 (CD74), 137–138
LN3, 87t
Lung, metastases from, 158
Lupus erythematosus, systemic, thymoma and, 69t
Luteinizing hormone, 24
Lymph node hamartoma. See *Angiofollicular lymphoid hyperplasia.*
Lymph nodes, intrathoracic, 4t
  mediastinal, 1, *2*, 3
    classification of, 3, 4t
    hilar, 3, 4t
    mesothelial cells in, *161*, 162
Lymphadenopathy, granulomatous. See *Granulomatous lymphadenopathy.*
  tuberculous mediastinal, AIDS and, 164
Lymphangioleiomyoma, 226
Lymphangioma, cystic, 211t, 226, *227*
Lymphangiomatosis, 226
Lymphangiomyoma, 226
Lymphatic cyst, 211t, 213–214
Lymphoblastic leukemia, T-cell acute, lymphoblastic lymphoma vs., 117, 117t
Lymphoblastic lymphoma, 115–121
  clinical features of, 115–116
  cytochemistry of, 120
  cytogenetics of, 119–120
  cytopathology of, *117*, 120
  differential diagnosis of, 117, 117t, 120
  DNA ploidy and cell proliferation indices for, 119
  histopathology of, 116, *116*, *117*
  immunopathology of, 116–118, 117t, 118t
  molecular pathology of, 118–119
  prognosis and therapy for, 120–121, 121t
  true thymic hyperplasia vs., 41
Lymphocele, mediastinal, 214
Lymphocyst, 214
Lymphocytes, surface antigens of, nomenclature for, 234t
  thymic, 16–19, *20*
    CD1-positive, *19*
    differentiation of, 17–19, *18*
    double-negative, 28
    double-positive, 17
    maturational stages of, *18*
    single-positive, 17
Lymphocytic thymoma, histopathology of, *71*, 72, 72t, *73*, *74*, *76*, *78*, *79*, *81–84*, *86*, *90*
  true thymic hyperplasia vs., 41
Lymphocytosis, associated with thymoma, 68–69
Lymphoepithelioma-like thymic carcinoma, histopathology of, 95–96, 95t, 96t, *98*
Lymphofollicular hyperplasia, of thymus, 34–39, *35–37*
Lymphoglandular bodies, in lymphoma, 86
Lymphoid hyperplasia, angiofollicular. See *Angiofollicular lymphoid hyperplasia.*
Lymphoma, 114–147. See also specific lymphoma.
  distribution of, 2t
  fever and, 2
  frequency of, 1t
  histopathologic classification of, 82t, 83–85
  in mediastinal goiter, 229
  large-cell, germ cell tumor vs., 187
    seminoma vs., 182
  mediastinal, in animals, 130–131
    T-cell, 128–130, *129*
Lymphoma/leukemia, T-cell, adult, 128–129
Lymphoproliferative syndrome, X-linked, thymus in, 47–48
Lymphosarcoma, 115. See also *Lymphoblastic lymphoma.*
Lysosomes, 22t
Lysozyme, 22t

MAC-1 and 2, in thymic mononuclear phagocytes, 22t
MACOP-B (methotrexate with leucovorin, doxorubicin, cyclophosphamide, vincristine, prednisone, and bleomycin), 127
Macrophages, foamy, in thymoma, 78, *81*
  thymic, 22–23, 22t
Magnetic resonance imaging (MRI), in detection of mediastinal tumors, 4
Major histocompatibility complex (MHC) antigens, 21. See also *HLA antigens.*
Major histocompatibility complex deficiency syndrome, thymus in, 45, 47
Malignancy, hematologic, mediastinal germ cell tumor and, 174–175
Malignant fibrous histiocytoma, 228
Malnutrition, thymus and, 53
MALT (mucosa-associated lymphoid tissue), B-cell lymphoma of, 127–128, *127*
Mass(es), biopsy of, 4
  mediastinal, primary, 1, 1t
    distribution of, 2t
Massive thymic hyperplasia. See *True thymic hyperplasia (TTH).*
Mast cells, in thymoma, 87
  thymic, 23
Mastocytosis, systemic, 174
MB2 antigen, 124
M-BACOD (methotrexate, bleomycin, doxorubicin, cyclophosphamide, vincristine, and dexamethasone), 127
Median sternotomy, transcervical approach vs., 6
Mediastinal lymphocele, 214
Mediastinal neoplasms, distribution of, 2t
Mediastinitis, acute, 168
  median sternotomy and, 6
  sclerosing, 168–170, *169*, *170*
Mediastinoscopy, 5–6
  metastases diagnosed by, 159, 159t
  transcervical, 5–6
Mediastinum, access to, 4–6
  anatomy of, 2–3, *2*, *3*
  compartments of, 3, *3*
  definition of, 1
  imaging of, 3–4
  overview of, 1–2, 1t, 2t
  primary masses in, 1, 1t

Mediastinum *(Continued)*
distribution of, 2t
Medullary differentiation, in thymoma, *73*
frequency of, 72t
Medullary epithelium, hyperplasia of, myasthenia gravis and, 36–37, *37*
"Medullary" thymoma, *77*, 82t, 83–85
Megakaryocytic leukemia, mediastinal germ cell tumor and, 174
Melanoma, germ cell tumor vs., 187
immunoreactivity of, 161
Melanotic schwannoma, 202–203
MEN (multiple endocrine neoplasia) syndrome, thymic carcinoid and, 192
Meningioma, 229–230
Meningocele, 214
Mesenchymal tumor, distribution of, 2t
frequency of, 1t
Mesothelial cells, in mediastinal lymph nodes, *161*, 162
Mesothelial cyst, 213
histologic features of, 211t
Mesothelioma, benign multicystic, 221
desmoplastic, *220*
diffuse pleural, 219–221, *220*
sarcomatous, *220*
Metastases, 158–162
from extrathoracic sites, 158–159, 159t, *160*
from lung, 158
from unknown primary sites, 159–160
diagnosis of, immunoperoxidase for, 160–161, *161*
karyotypic analysis for, 161–162
Methotrexate, bleomycin, doxorubicin, cyclophosphamide, vincristine, and dexamethasone (M-BACOD), 127
Methotrexate with leucovorin, doxorubicin, cyclophosphamide, vincristine, prednisone, and bleomycin (MACOP-B), 127
MG. See *Myasthenia gravis (MG).*
MHC (major histocompatibility complex) antigens, 21, 29. See also *HLA antigens.*
MHC (bare lymphocyte) syndrome, 45, 47
MIC2, 207
Microcystic pattern, in epithelial thymoma, 72, *80*
Microcytic thymoma, 78
Minimal change nephropathy, thymoma and, 69t
Mixed collagen vascular disease, thymoma and, 69t
"Mixed" thymoma, *82*, 82t, 83–85
histopathology of, 72, 72t
Molecular pathology, of Hodgkin's disease, 137
of large cell lymphoma, 125
of lymphoblastic lymphoma, 118–119
of neuroblastoma, 206
of thymoma, 88
Monoclonal antibodies, 20–21
Mononuclear phagocytes, thymic, 22–23, 22t
MOPP (nitrogen mustard, vincristine, procarbazine, and prednisone), for Hodgkin's disease, 139
Mors thymica, 10
MR3, 18, 20
MR6, 18, 20
MR10, 18
MR19, 18
MRI (magnetic resonance imaging), in detection of mediastinal tumors, 4
Mucocutaneous candidiasis, thymoma and, 69t
Mucoepidermoid carcinoma of thymus, 95t, 96t, 99
Multiple endocrine neoplasia (MEN) syndrome, thymic carcinoid and, 192
Multiple sclerosis, thymic germinal centers and, 38
Muscle, benign tumor of, 227–228
Myasthenia gravis (MG), germinal center hyperplasia in, 34–39, *35*
histioeosinophilic granuloma and, 38
hyperplasia of medullary epithelium and, 36–37, *37*
involution of thymus in, 37–38, *37*
myoid cells in, 23
thymectomy for, 11–12, 38
thymic cyst and, 58
thymoma and, 34, 68, 68t, 105–106
thymus in, 11, *15*
Myeloid leukemia, 147
Myocarditis, thymoma and, 69t
Myoid cells, thymic, 23, *23*
myasthenia gravis and, 35
Myopathy, thymoma and, 69t
Myxoma, 228

Neoplasms. See *Tumors.*
Nephropathy, minimal change, thymoma and, 69t
Nerve sheath, peripheral, tumors of, 201–204, *202*, *203*
Neural crest, maldevelopment of, DiGeorge syndrome and, 44
thymic embryology and, 27, 28
Neurilemoma (schwannoma), 201–203, *203*
Neuroblastoma, 204, *205*, 206
opsomyoclonus and, 2
Neuroectodermal tumor, peripheral primitive, 206–207, *207*
Neuroendocrine carcinoma, 192. See also *Carcinoid, thymic.*
Neuroendocrine tumor, 191–198. See also *Carcinoid, thymic; Paraganglioma.*
Neuroepithelioma, peripheral (PNET), 206–207, *207*
Neurofibroma, 201, *202*
Neurofibromatosis (von Recklinghausen's disease), multiple peripheral nerve sheath tumor and, 201
Neurofibrosarcoma, 203–204
Neurofilament, in neuroectodermal tumors, 206
Neurogenic tumors, mediastinal, 201–208. See also specific tumor.
distribution of, 2t
frequency of, 1t
Neuron-specific enolase (NSE), in neuroectodermal tumors, 206
in paraganglioma, 197–199
in thymic carcinoid, 193–194
in thymic epithelial tumors, 87t
New Zealand mouse, 38
Nezelof syndrome, thymus and, 46
NHL. See *Non-Hodgkin's lymphoma (NHL).*
Nitrogen mustard, vincristine, procarbazine, and prednisone (MOPP), for Hodgkin's disease, 139
N-myc, in neuroblastoma, 206
Non-Hodgkin's lymphoma (NHL), histiocytosis X vs., 145–146

Non-Hodgkin's lymphoma (NHL) *(Continued)*
lymphocyte-depleted Hodgkin's disease vs., 135–136
thymic cysts and, 58
Nonseminomatous malignant germ cell tumor, 183–187
clinical presentation of, 183
differential diagnosis of, 187
gross features of, 184
microscopic features of, 184–187, *185, 186*
radiographic and laboratory features of, 183–184, *184*
therapy and clinical outcome, 187
NSE. See *Neuron-specific enolase (NSE).*
Nuclear atypia, in thymoma, *75,* 78
Nurse cells, thymic, 22
Nutrition, thymus and, 53

Omenn's syndrome, thymus in, 47
Oncocytoma, malignant, of superior mediastinum, 229
OPD4 antigen, in T-cell lymphoblastic lymphoma, 118t
Opsomyoclonus, neuroblastoma and, 2
"Organoid" thymoma, 78
Organotins, thymus and, 58
Osteochondroma, 228
Osteogenic sarcoma, extraskeletal, 228
Osteosarcoma, malignant schwannoma and, 203
Oxytocin, in thymus, 24

p19, in thymic epithelial cell tumor, 87
in thymus, *18,* 21, 25
Paltauf, 10, 12t
Pancreatic pseudocyst, 214–215
histologic features of, 211t
Papillary carcinoma, in mediastinal goiter, 229
Paraganglioma, 195–198, 196t, *197*
aortic body, 196, *197*
chromaffin reactivity of, 196
clinical features of, 196, 196t
differential diagnosis of, 198
DNA flow cytometry of, 198
electron microscopy of, 198
histochemistry of, 197
immunohistochemistry of, 197
in animals, 198
paravertebral, 196–197
tests for, 197–198
Parathyroid, embryologic, *27*
lesions of, 229
within thymus, 23, *24*
Parathyroid cyst, 214
histologic features of, 211t, *214*
PC–1, in large cell lymphoma, 125
PCNA (proliferating cell nuclear antigen, cyclin), in large cell lymphoma, 125
Peanut agglutinin (PNA), 17
in Hodgkin's disease, 137t
Pemphigus vulgaris, thymoma and, 69t
Pericardial cyst, 213
histologic features of, 211t
Peripheral nerve sheath, tumors of, 201–204, *202, 203*
Peripheral neuroepithelioma (PNET, Askin tumor), 206–207, *207*
Peripheral primitive neuroectodermal tumor of thoracopulmonary region (PNET, Askin tumor), 206–207, *207*
Perivascular spaces, in thymoma, 72, *79*
frequency of, 72t
Pernicious anemia, thymoma and, 69t
Phagocytes, mononuclear, 22–23, 22t
Phagolysosomes, 22t
Pharyngeal cleft, *27*
Pharyngeal pouch, *27*
Pharyngotympanic tube, embryologic, *27*
Phenotypes, of thymomas, 85
Phylogeny, of thymus, 29
Physaliferous cells, in chordoma, 230
Pituitary, anterior, thymectomy and, 24
Pituitary hormones, thymus and, 24
Placental alkaline phosphatase (PLAP), in mediastinal germ cell tumor, 176, 176t
in nonseminomatous malignant germ cell tumor, 184, 187
Plasma cells, thymic, 23
Plasmacytoma, 146
Platter, Felix, 10, 127
Pleural tumor, 217–221
diffuse pleural mesothelioma, 219–221, *220*
Pleural tumors, solitary fibrous, *217,* 217–219, *218*
Pleuropulmonary blastoma, 228
Ploidy. See *DNA ploidy.*
PNA (peanut agglutinin), 17
in Hodgkin's disease, 137t
PNET (peripheral neuroepithelioma, Askin tumor), 206–207, *207*
Pneumomediastinum, diagnostic, 38
POEMS, 143
Polymyositis, thymoma and, 69t
Prevertebral structures, 3
Prolactin, 24
Prostate carcinoma, metastatic to mediastinum, 159–160
Prothymocytes, 16
Pseudocyst, pancreatic, 214–215
histologic features of, 211t
Pseudoepitheliomatous hyperplasia, *57*
Pseudorosettes, in thymoma, 72–78
Pure red cell aplasia, thymoma and, 68, 69t

Radiation, thymus and, 54
Radiation therapy, for carcinoid, 195
for enlarged thymus, 11
for germ cell tumors, 183, 187
for Hodgkin's disease, 137
for large cell lymphoma, 127
for thymic carcinoma, 101
for thymoma, 92–94
Radiography, of chest, for detection of mediastinal tumors, 3–4
Ras oncogene, 105
Rebound true thymic hyperplasia, 42–43
Receptors, homing, 19
Red cell aplasia, pure, thymoma and, 68, 69t
Reed-Sternberg cells, Epstein-Barr virus in, 139
in Hodgkin's disease, 133, *133,* 134, 135, *135,* 136, *136, 138,* 138–139
Reticular pattern, in epithelial thymoma, 72, *80*
Reticuloendotheliosis with eosinophilia, familial, thymus in, 47
Retrosternal structures, 3

RFD1, 22t
RFD4, 18
RFD7, 22t
Rhabdomyoma, 227
"Rhabdomyomatous" thymoma, 78
Rhabdomyosarcoma, 228
  malignant schwannoma and, 203–204
  mediastinal germ cell tumor and, 175
Rheumatoid arthritis, thymic germinal centers and, 38
Rheumatoid heart disease, thymic germinal centers and, 38
Rib, first, *2*
Rosettes, in thymoma, 72–78
Rufus of Ephesus, 9

S100 antigen, in hemangiopericytoma, 220
  in melanoma, 161
  in meningioma, 230
  in neuroectodermal tumors, 206
  in paraganglioma, 198
  in pleuropulmonary blastoma, 228
  in schwannoma, 202
  in thymic epithelial cell tumors, 87
  in thymic interdigitating cells, 22t
Salivary gland tissue, thymic, 23
Sarcoidosis, 166, *167*
  thymoma and, 69t
  true thymic hyperplasia and, 43
Sarcoma, 228–229
  extraskeletal osteogenic, 228
  mediastinal germ cell tumor and, 175, *175*
  neurogenic, 203–204
  Sternberg, 115
Sarcomatoid carcinoma of thymus, histopathology of, 95t, 96–99, 96t, *100*
Sarcomatous mesothelioma, *220*
Schaumann bodies, in sarcoidosis, 166
Schwannoma, benign, 201–202, *203*
  cellular, 202
  malignant, 203–204
  melanotic, 202–203
SCID (severe combined immunodeficiency disease), 45–48, *46*
  thymus in, 50t
Sclerohyaline nodules, in extrapulmonary sites, 166–168, *168*
Sclerosing mediastinitis, 168–170, *169, 170*
Sebaceous glands, thymic, 23
Self-tolerance, 29
Seminoma, 179–183
  antigens expressed by, 176t
  clinical presentation of, 180
  cytopathology of, 86, 181, *182*
  differential diagnosis of, 182
  gross and microscopic features of, 180–182, *181–183*
  mediastinal, 67
  radiographic and laboratory features of, 180
  therapy and clinical outcome, 182–183
Seminoma-like thymoma, 67
SETTLE (spindle epithelial tumor with thymus-like differentiation), 70–71
Severe combined immunodeficiency disease (SCID), 45–48, *46*
  thymus in, 50t
Sex hormones, thymic size and, 24t
Signet-ring-like cells, in thymoma, 78
Silica, in sclerohyaline nodules, visualization of, 167, 168
Silicosis, 166–168, *168*
Simian immunodeficiency virus (SIV), thymus and, 51
Simon, Sir John, 10
Sipple's syndrome, thymic carcinoid and, 192
SIV. See *Simian immunodeficiency virus (SIV).*
Sjögren's syndrome, lymphoma and, *127,* 128
  thymic cyst and, 58
  thymoma and, 69t
SLE (systemic lupus erythematosus), thymoma and, 69t
Small-cell carcinoma of thymus, 95t, 96t, 99
Somatostatin, in paraganglioma, 198
  in thymus, 24
Spinal cord compression, 2
Spindle cell carcinoma of thymus. See *Sarcomatoid carcinoma of thymus.*
Spindle epithelial tumor with thymus-like differentiation (SETTLE), 70–71
Spindled thymoma, histopathology of, 72, 72t, *77*
  staghorn-shaped vessels in, 72, *80*
Spindling squamous cell carcinoma of thymus, 96, 99. See also *Sarcomatoid carcinoma of thymus.*
Squamous cell carcinoma of thymus, cystic, 58
  histopathology of, 95, 95t, 96t, *97*
  poorly differentiated, histopathology of, 95–96, 95t, 96t, *98*
  well differentiated, histopathology of, 95t, 96, 96t, *99*
Squamous differentiation, in thymoma, 78, *84*
  frequency of, 72t
Staghorn-shaped vessels, in spindled thymoma, 72, *80*
Staging, of Hodgkin's disease, 132, 132t
  of thymoma, 89, 90t
"Starry sky" appearance, in lymphoblastic lymphoma, 116, *116*
  in lymphocytic thymoma, 72, *74*
  of thymic cortex, 39, *39*
Status Lymphaticus Investigation Committee, 11
Status thymicolymphaticus, 9, 10–11, 15
Sternberg sarcoma, 115
Sternotomy, median, transcervical approach vs., 6
Steroid therapy, for true thymic hyperplasia, 42
Stress, thymus and, 50t
  true thymic hyperplasia and, 41, 41t
Subcapsular cortex, *18*
Subcapsular epithelial cells, 20
Superior vena cava, *2*
Superior vena cava syndrome, 2
Surface antigens, leukocyte, nomenclature for, 234t
Sympathetic ganglia, tumors of, 204–206, *205, 207*
Sympathetic trunk, *2*
Synaptophysin, in neuroectodermal tumors, 206
  in paraganglioma, 198
Syphilis, congenital, thymus and, 53
Systemic lupus erythematosus (SLE), thymic germinal centers and, 38
  thymoma and, 69t
Systemic mastocytosis, 174

T lymphocytes, development of, 10, 17–19

T lymphocytes *(Continued)*
function of, 29
T-ALL. See *T-cell acute lymphoblastic leukemia (T-ALL).*
T-cell acute lymphoblastic leukemia (T-ALL), lymphoblastic lymphoma vs., 117, 117t
T-cell antigen receptor (TCR), 17–19
T-cell leukemia/lymphoma, adult, 128–129
T-cell lymphoblastic lymphoma (T-LL), 117–118, 117t, 118t
T-cell lymphoma of mediastinum, 128–130, *129*
TCR. See *T-cell antigen receptor (TCR).*
TDT. See *Terminal deoxynucleotidyl transferase (TDT).*
TE–3, *18,* 20
TE–4, *18,* 20, 21, 25
TE–7, 27
Teratocarcinoma, 176, 177
Teratoma, 176–179
antigens expressed by, 176t
clinical presentation of, 177
differential diagnosis of, 179
gross and microscopic features of, 177–179, *178–180*
radiographic and laboratory features of, 177, *177*
therapy and clinical outcome, 179
Terminal deoxynucleotidyl transferase (TDT), *18*
in fine needle aspirates, 41
in T-cell lymphoblastic lymphoma, 118t
thymic, 25
Thoracic duct, cysts of, 213
histologic features of, 211t
Thoracic vertebra, fourth, *12*
Thoracoscopy, 6
Thoracotomy, 6
Thrombocytopenia, refractory, mediastinal germ cell tumors and, 174
Thrombocytosis, essential, thymoma and, 69t
Thy–1 antigen, *18,* 21
Thyme plant, 8, *8*
Thymectomy, anterior pituitary cells and, 24
for myasthenia gravis, 11–12, 38
median sternotomy vs. transcervical approach, 6
Thymic carcinoid. See *Carcinoid, thymic.*
Thymic carcinoma. See *Carcinoma, thymic.*
Thymic cyst. See *Cyst, thymic.*
Thymic dysplasia, primary immunodeficiency disorders and, 45–48, *46*
Thymic epithelial cell tumor, 67–106. See also *Carcinoma, thymic; Thymoma;* specific tumor.
definitions of, 67, 68t
in animals, 104
pathogenesis of, 104–106
Thymic hormones, 24, 24t
Thymic hyperplasia, tri-iodothyronine and, 43
with massive enlargement. See *True thymic hyperplasia (TTH).*
Thymic hypoplasia, isotretinoin (Accutane) and, 58–59
Thymic neoplasms, distribution of, 2t
Thymic seminoma, cystic, *181*
Thymitis, 34
Thymocytes, 16. See also *Lymphocytes.*
Thymolipoma, 223–224, *224*
true thymic hyperplasia vs., 41, 224
Thymoma, 67–94
acquired immunodeficiency syndrome and, 69

Thymoma *(Continued)*
association with other tumors, 69
chemotherapy for, 94
childhood, 91
classification, histologic, 72, 72t, 82t, 83, 91
clinical features of, 67–71
cortical, 82t, 83, *84,* 85
cystic changes in, 71, *71*
cytopathology of, 86, *86,* 87
defined, 67
disorders associated with, 68, 69t
ectopic hamartomatous, 70
electron microscopy of, 88–89, *89*
epithelial, 72, 75, 79–81, 84, 86. See also *Epithelial thymoma.*
frequency of, 1t, 72t
frozen sections of, 85–86
germinal centers in, 72t, 78
granulomatous. See *Hodgkin's disease.*
gross pathology of, *70,* 71, *71*
Hassall's corpuscles in, 72, 72t, 73
histiocytosis X vs., 87
histochemistry of, 87
"histogenetic" classification of, 82t, 83–85
histopathology of, 72–85, 72t
immunohistochemistry of, 87–88, 87t
invasive, 71, *90,* 90t
defined, 68t
lymphocytic, 72, *73, 74*
true thymic hyperplasia vs., 41
lymphocytosis and, 68–69
malignant, type 1, 67, 68t. See also *Thymoma, invasive.*
type 2, 67, 68t. See also *Thymoma, invasive.*
medullary, 82t, 83, 85, 91
medullary differentiation in, 72, 72t, *73*
metastases, sites of, 71
microcytic, 78
mixed cortical and medullary, 82t, 83
mixed lymphocytic and epithelial, 72, 72t, *76*
molecular pathology of, 88
myasthenia gravis and, 34, 105–106
noninvasive, *70, 90,* 90t
defined, 68t
organoid, 78
perivascular spaces, 72, 72t, *79*
phenotypes of, 82t, 85
prognosis and therapy in, 91–94, 92t–93t, *93*
prognostic factors in, 89–91, *90,* 91t–93t
radiation therapy of, 92, 94
recurrence and survival rates for, 92t–93t
rhabdomyomatous, 78
seminoma vs., 182
seminoma-like, 67
spindled, 72, *77*
staghorn-shaped vessels in, 72, *80*
squamous differentiation in, 78, *84*
staging systems for, 90t
"starry sky" pattern in, 72, *74*
surgical pathology report for, 91
therapy of, 92, 94
thymic carcinoma vs., 71
tonofilaments in, 88–89, *89*
traditional classification of, 72, 72t, 91
unusual locations of, 69–70
Thymopoietin, *18,* 20, 24, 24t
Thymosin-alpha–1, 20, 24, 24t
Thymulin, 24, 24t, 51
Thymus, 1, 2
age-related changes of, 25, *26*

Thymus *(Continued)*
anatomy of, 14–16, *15*, 16t
biopsy of, 45
blood supply of, 14
cell markers in, 18
congenital disorders of, 43–48, *46*
ectopic, 26
embryology of, 25–29, *27*
endocrine interactions with, 24t
enlarged. See *True thymic hyperplasia (TTH).*
etymology of "thymus," 8–9, *8*
function of, 9–10, 29
germinal centers in, 19, 34–36, *35*
histology of, 16–23, *17*, *18*
historical overview of, 8–12, 12t
hormones of, 23, 24, 24t
immunodeficiencies and, 45–50, *46*, 50t
innervation of, 15
involution of, acute, 40
in myasthenia gravis, 37–38, *37*
lymphatics of, 4t, 14–15
neuroendocrine features of, 23–25, 24t
non-neoplastic pathology of, 34–59
normal, 14–30
phylogeny of, 29
stress-related changes in, 39–40, *39*, *40*
toxic agents and, 58–59
vasculitis and, 53–54
volume of, 16t
weight of, 15–16, 16t
Thymus serpyllum, 8, *8*
Thyroid, 27
lesions of, 229
Thyroid hormones, thymic size and, 24, 24t, 43
Thyroid stimulating hormone, 24
Thyroidectomy, thymic size and, 24t
Thyroiditis, chronic, thymic enlargement and, 43
Thyrotoxicosis, thymic enlargement and, 43
L-Thyroxine, thymic enlargement and, 43
"Tigroid" background, in seminoma, 86, 181, *182*
T-LL. See *T-cell lymphoblastic lymphoma (T-LL).*
TNM staging system for lung cancer, mediastinal lymph nodes in, 3
Tonofilaments, in thymoma, 88–89, *89*
Toxic agents, thymus and, 58–59
Trachea, *2*
Transcervical mediastinoscopy, 5–6
Transforming growth factor-beta, 25
Trauma, surgical, thymic cysts and, 58
Tri-iodothyronine, thymic hyperplasia and, 43
Triton tumor, 203–204
True thymic hyperplasia (TTH), 40–43, *41*, 41t, 42t
True thymic hyperplasia (TTH) *(Continued)*
thymolipoma vs., 41, 224
Tuberculosis, 164–165, *165*
Tumors, endocrine, distribution of, 2t
frequency of, 1t
germ cell. See *Germ cell tumors.*
mesenchymal, distribution of, 2t
frequency of, 1t
neurogenic. See *Neurogenic tumors.*

Ulcerative colitis, thymoma and, 69t
Ultrasonography, in biopsy of mediastinal masses, 4
Ultrastructure. See *Electron microscopy.*

Vascular lesions, 225–226
Vasculitis, thymus and, 53–54
Vasoactive inhibitory peptide, in ganglioneuroma, 206
Vasopressin, in thymus, 24
Vena cava, superior, *2*
Vertebra, fourth thoracic, *2*
Very late activation antigens (VLA), 19
Vimentin, in hemangiopericytoma, 220
in paraganglioma, 198
in primitive neuroectodermal tumors, 206
in schwannoma, 202
Virus, mouse thymic, 52
Vocal cord paralysis, 2
von Recklinghausen's disease (neurofibromatosis), multiple peripheral nerve sheath tumors and, 201

Weigert, 11, 12t
Wermer's syndrome, thymic carcinoid and, 192
Wiskott-Aldrich syndrome, thymus in, 48

X-linked lymphoproliferative syndrome, thymus in, 47–48

Yellow-brown bodies, in sarcoidosis, 166, *167*

Zellballen, in paraganglioma, 192–193, 196, *197*
Zellweger-Kallmann syndrome, 44

ISBN 0-7216-4337-X